Lecture Notes of the Institute for Computer Sciences, Social Informatics and Telecommunications Engineering 572

The LNICST series publishes ICST's conferences, symposia and workshops.
LNICST reports state-of-the-art results in areas related to the scope of the Institute.
The type of material published includes

- Proceedings (published in time for the respective event)
- Other edited monographs (such as project reports or invited volumes)

LNICST topics span the following areas:

- General Computer Science
- E-Economy
- E-Medicine
- Knowledge Management
- Multimedia
- Operations, Management and Policy
- Social Informatics
- Systems

Dario Salvi · Pieter Van Gorp · Syed Ahmar Shah
Editors

Pervasive Computing Technologies for Healthcare

17th EAI International Conference, PervasiveHealth 2023
Malmö, Sweden, November 27–29, 2023
Proceedings

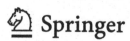 Springer

Editors
Dario Salvi
Malmö University
Malmö, Sweden

Pieter Van Gorp ⓘ
Eindhoven University of Technology
Eindhoven, The Netherlands

Syed Ahmar Shah ⓘ
University of Edinburgh
Edinburgh, UK

ISSN 1867-8211   ISSN 1867-822X (electronic)
Lecture Notes of the Institute for Computer Sciences, Social Informatics
and Telecommunications Engineering
ISBN 978-3-031-59716-9   ISBN 978-3-031-59717-6 (eBook)
https://doi.org/10.1007/978-3-031-59717-6

This Springer imprint is published by the registered company Springer Nature Switzerland AG
The registered company address is: Gewerbestrasse 11, 6330 Cham, Switzerland

If disposing of this product, please recycle the paper.

Preface

We are very happy to introduce the proceedings of the 17th European Alliance for Innovation (EAI) International Conference on Pervasive Computing Technologies for Healthcare (PervasiveHealth 2023), held on 27–29 November 2022 in Malmö, Sweden. This year, we brought together a diverse community of researchers with an interest in pervasive health for healthcare and well-being, including engineers, computer scientists, designers, but also clinicians, ethicists, and experts in law.

The conference was held within the evocative venue of a converted slaughterhouse, surrounded by the mix of history and modernity that the city of Malmö offers. We had the pleasure of being hosted by Carina Nilsson, Chairman of the Malmö City Council, at the historic Town Hall in the heart of the city. At the end of the second day, we were also blessed with a gentle snowfall, enhancing the ambience and making the surroundings more captivating.

We had the privilege to host two excellent keynote lectures: one by Per Carlbring, from the Department of Psychology of Stockholm University, at the start of the conference, and one the day after, by Jakob Eyvind Bardam, from the Department of Computer Science of the Technical University of Denmark. Prof. Carlbring talked about "From Face-to-Face to Cyberspace", covering a futuristic view of mental health treatments, while Prof. Bardram talked about "Digital Phenotyping", covering technologies and methods for the longitudinal collection and analysis of health data in the wild.

The focus of this year's conference was the use of smart technologies such as wearable devices, mobile phones, sensors, the Internet of Things, and medical devices to monitor patients in the hospital, at home, and in the community. Novel interventions made possible by these technologies, such as behavioural interventions and digital therapies, were also considered within scope. These proceedings contain 35 papers, with a mix of long papers, short papers, and poster presentations. The topics span clinical applications (such as those in mental health, remote monitoring, and rehabilitation), technical aspects (such as the processing of big datasets, machine learning, and artificial intelligence), as well as human aspects (such as usability, ethical, and regulatory considerations). All works are of high quality and relevant to the topics of the conference.

The conference also hosted the "Workshop on the Internet of Things in Health Research", the papers of which were selected with the same rigorous review process as the ones in the main conference. The workshop aimed to explore the challenges of solutions based on the Internet of Things for healthcare together with researchers and practitioners from academia and industry. Workshop paper presentations were merged into a session with posters and demo presentations, where two local companies (i.e., Infonomy and Arjo) presented two of their products, respectively the Snubblometer and the Provizio SEM Scanner. The session sparked engaging conversations and allowed participants to interact in a more informal setting.

This year's conference was possible thanks to the hard work of the EAI, the organising committee, and the Technical Programme Committee. We would like to thank particularly the general co-chair and local chair Carl Magnus Olsson (for arranging most of the practical issues, from the venue to social activities), Radka Vasileiadis, Patricia Gabajova, and Martin Hochel from the EAI, for their logistical and organisational support. We are also grateful to the reviewers who provided extensive and constructive feedback to our authors. Last but not least, we would like to express our gratitude to all enthusiastic presenters and other conference participants, for their thought-provoking contributions and engagement at the event.

Dario Salvi
Syed Ahmar Shah
Pieter Van Gorp

Organization

Steering Committee

Imrich Chlamtac   University of Trento, Italy
Liming Chen   Ulster University, UK
Panos Makropoulos   Eindhoven University of Technology,
                         The Netherlands

Organizing Committee

General Chair

Dario Salvi   Malmö University, Sweden

General Co-chair

Carl Magnus Olsson   Malmö University, Sweden

TPC Chairs and Co-chairs

Syed Ahmar Shah   University of Edinburgh, UK
Pieter Van Gorp   Eindhoven University of Technology,
                         The Netherlands
Haridimos Kondylakis   University of Crete, Greece
Andreas Triantafyllidis CERTH-ITI, Greece

Sponsorship and Exhibit Chair

Dario Salvi   Malmö University, Sweden

Local Chair

Carl Magnus Olsson   Malmö University, Sweden

Workshops Chair

Francesco Potortì   ISTI-CNR, Italy

Publicity and Social Media Chair

Manuel Ottaviano   Universidad Politécnica de Madrid, Spain

Publications Chair

Dario Salvi   Malmö University, Sweden

Clinical Chairs

Elizabeth Orchard   Oxford University NHS Trust, UK
Igor Rudan   University of Edinburgh, UK
Gerd Tinkhauser   Universitätsspital Bern, Switzerland
Carmen Carrazco Lopez   Malmö University, Sweden

Posters and Demos Chair

Dario Salvi   Malmö University, Malmö, Sweden

Technical Program Committee

Thanasis Tsanas   University of Edinburgh, UK
Hadas Lewy   Holon Institute of Technology, Israel
Paula Toledo   Universidad Carlos Tercero, Spain
Filippo Palumbo   ISTI-CNR, Italy
Laura Lopez   Universidad Politécnica de Madrid, Spain
Beatriz Merino   Universidad Politécnica de Madrid, Spain
Andreas Ziegl   Telbiomed, Austria
Leila Aflatoony   Georgia Institute of Technology, USA
Kevin Tsang   University of Edinburgh, UK
Steven Kerr   University of Edinburgh, UK
Holly Tibble   University of Edinburgh, UK
Fasih Haider   University of Edinburgh, UK
Saturnino Luz Filho   University of Edinburgh, UK
Priyanka Chaurasia   Ulster University, UK
Kamala Payyapilly   PennState University, USA
    Thiruvenkatanathan

Dieff Vital	University of Illinois Chicago, USA
Johan Holmgren	Malmö University, Sweden
Reza Malekian	Malmö University, Sweden
Dipak Surie	Malmö University, Sweden
Gent Ymeri	Malmö University, Sweden
Dario Salvi	Malmö University, Sweden
Sara Caramaschi	Malmö University, Sweden
Dimitrios Katehakis	FORTH-ICS, Greece
Eiman Kanjo	Nottingham Trent University, UK
José Manuel Molina	Universidad Carlos 3 Madrid, Spain
Konstantinos Votis	Centre for Research and Technology Hellas, Greece
Luigi Borzí	Politecnico di Torino, Italy
Salvatore Tedesco	University College Cork, Ireland
Stefan Wagner	Aarhus University, Denmark
Silvia Imbesi	University of Ferrara, Italy
Anastasios Alexiadis	CERTH-ITI, Greece
Özlem Durmaz İncel	Boğaziçi University, Turkey
Frank Wallhoff	Jade University of Applied Science, Germany
Gianluca Amprimo	CNR-IEIIT, Italy
Alessandra Angelucci	Politecnico di Milano, Italy
Stefano Canali	Politecnico di Milano, Italy

Contents

Pervasive Health for Carers

Pervasive Health in Clinical Practice

Motion and Rehabilitation

Workshop on the Internet of Things in Health Research

Posters and Demos (Non Indexed Annex)

Pervasive Mental Health

Gaze Behaviour in Adolescents with Obsessive-Compulsive Disorder During Exposure Within Cognitive-Behavioural Therapy

Annika Thierfelder[1]([✉])(iD), Björn Severitt[2](iD), Carolin S. Klein[3],
Annika K. Alt[3](iD), Karsten Hollmann[3](iD), Andreas Bulling[4](iD),
and Winfried Ilg[1](iD)

[1] Hertie Institute for Clinical Brain Research, Section for Computational
Sensomotorics, University Hospital Tübingen, Tübingen, Germany
{annika.thierfelder,winfried.ilg}@uni-tuebingen.de
[2] Department of Computer Science, Human-Computer Interaction,
University of Tübingen, Tübingen, Germany
bjoern.severitt@uni-tuebingen.de
[3] Department of Child and Adolescent Psychiatry,
Psychosomatics and Psychotherapy, University Hospital Tübingen,
Tübingen, Germany
{carolin.klein,annika.alt,karsten.hollmann}@med.uni-tuebingen.de
[4] Institute for Visualisation and Interactive Systems, University Stuttgart,
Stuttgart, Germany
andreas.bulling@vis.uni-stuttgart.de

Abstract. Digital health interventions that involve monitoring patient behaviour increasingly benefit from improvements in sensor technology. Eye tracking in particular can provide useful information for psychotherapy but an effective method to extract this information is currently missing. We propose a method to analyse natural gaze behaviour during exposure exercises for obsessive-compulsive disorder (OCD). At the core of our method is a neural network to detect fixations based on gaze patch similarities. Detected fixations are clustered into *exposure-relevant, therapist,* and *other* locations and corresponding eye movement metrics are correlated with subjective stress reported during exposure. We evaluate our method on gaze and stress data recorded during video-based psychotherapy of four adolescents with OCD. We found that fixation duration onto *exposure-relevant* locations consistently increases with the perceived stress level as opposed to fixations onto *other* locations. Fixation behaviour towards the *therapist* varied largely between patients. Taken together, our results not only demonstrate the effectiveness of

This work is funded by the German Federal Ministry of Health (BMG) project SSTeP KiZ (2520DAT700) and the European Research Council (ERC SYNERGY Grant RELEVANCE). The authors thank the International Max Planck Research School for Intelligent Systems (IMPRS-IS) for supporting A. Thierfelder. A. Bulling was funded by the European Research Council (ERC; grant agreement 801708).

D. Salvi et al. (Eds.): PH 2023, LNICST 572, pp. 3–17, 2024.
https://doi.org/10.1007/978-3-031-59717-6_1

our method for analysing natural gaze behaviour during exposure sessions. The fixation analysis shows that patients allocate more attention towards exposure-related objects under higher stress levels, suggesting higher mental load. As such, providing feedback on fixation behaviour holds significant promise to support therapists in monitoring intensity of exposure exercises.

Keywords: mobile eye tracking · obsessive-compulsive disorder · sensor-assisted therapy · exposure exercises · real life gaze behaviour

1   Introduction and Related Work

Digital health interventions are becoming increasingly important to ensure that affected patients have easy access to treatment and to personalize said treatment. Video-based online therapy has proven its effectiveness in treating anxiety [11], including obsessive-compulsive disorder (OCD) [12]. OCD is a psychiatric disorder characterized by a combination of obsessions and compulsions [1]. Obsessions are repeated intrusive thoughts or urges that cause anxiety, whereas compulsions are mental or behavioural repetitions or rituals that the person with OCD feels the urge to do in order to reduce anxiety [33]. In children and adolescents, OCD affects around 0.5–4% of the population [9,10] and if not treated in young age, patients are at high risk to develop chronic symptoms [28].

The state-of-the-art treatment for OCD is cognitive behavioural therapy (CBT) based on exposure and response prevention (E/RP) sessions [1]. In the E/RP sessions, patients confront their obsession whilst refraining from the urge to perform the compulsion and instead enduring the anxiety until it, in the desired case, reduces without the compulsion. Given that obsessions are often linked to specific places or objects, which can be challenging to recreate in clinical environments, moving therapy into patients' homes through video-based CBT allows for a more direct confrontation with the obsession, thereby improving the effectiveness of the treatment [25].

A key limitation of such video-based approaches for CBT is the limited field of view of the web camera. Here, eye tracking devices can add valuable information about what is within sight of the patient, what the patient is focusing on at any point in time, and emerging gaze behaviour throughout therapy.

1.1   Fixations in Mobile Eye Tracking

What constitutes a fixation in mobile eye tracking differs from what is typically considered a fixation in laboratory-based eye tracking research [15,27]. There, fixations are temporal episodes during which the eyes remain stationary. In mobile eye tracking this definition is too narrow given that neither the body nor the head is necessarily still: Gaze may follow a moving object (smooth pursuit) or the head moves while the eyes keep fixating a still object. Thus, a fixation is typically defined as an episode during which gaze stays on a fixed object or location. This difference renders common methods based on eye movement velocity or gaze dispersion unsuitable for mobile eye tracking [15,27]. We therefore adapt the method from [27] that detects fixations based on the similarity of small regions around each gaze location within the visual scene.

1.2 Eye Tracking in Patients with OCD

Eye tracking is being increasingly used to study attention of patients with psychiatric disorders [3], including OCD [4,6,19]. The recording paradigm closest to real-life gaze behaviour is the free-viewing task in which patients are shown a neutral and an OCD-related stimulus at the same time without instructions on where to look. Studies using the free-viewing paradigm have shown evidence for a maintenance bias [4]: Patients with OCD show sustained attention towards OCD-related stimuli resulting in an increased number and duration of fixations on these stimuli [6,19].

An important marker during exposure exercises is the perceived stress triggered by the confrontation with the obsession. In healthy subjects, several studies investigated the effect of stress on gaze behaviour during real-life situations, e.g., flight simulation [30], interview settings [5] or the work day of ICU nurses [2]. These studies have shown that with increased stress the fixation duration drops [5,30] or, similarly, the number of fixations increases [2].

In these studies, stress has usually been induced by a time-pressured increase in mental effort to create anxiety. During exposure sessions, in contrast, stress is induced by confrontation with the obsessive thought without time constraints. Studies in healthy subjects have shown that an increase in mental effort without time pressure leads to longer fixation duration [8,16] and sometimes a concurrent increase in variability of fixation duration [22]. Longer fixations are thought to reflect the narrowed but increased attention allocated to the fixated goal [16] and therefore to be dependent on the task type [8].

Due to the lack of methods to analyse fixation behaviour in patients with OCD during real-life situations, the study of attention in said patients has been constrained to laboratory settings. While the effect of stress and mental effort on fixation behaviour in real-life situations has been well studied for healthy subjects, studies on their influence on real-life gaze behaviour in patients with OCD are still missing.

In this work we propose a method to detect and cluster fixations in mobile eye tracking during real-life therapy sessions, and analyse the effect of the subjective stress levels on fixation behaviour. Based on existing evidence for maintenance bias from laboratory eye tracking studies and the effect of mental effort on fixation behaviour, we hypothesised that attention on exposure-relevant locations increases with rising stress levels, showing in a higher fixation count and longer fixations towards these locations. If the predominant influence on gaze behaviour are stress and anxiety, the number of fixations onto other objects should also increase but fixations should become shorter.

2   Method

2.1   Study Details

Eye tracking data for this work was collected within the SSTeP KiZ study [13]. In this study, different sensor modalities were integrated into video-based CBT for children and adolescents with OCD, allowing patients to receive treatment in their home environments. An overview of the sensor-assisted therapy setup can be seen in Fig. 1. The sensor modalities included eye tracking, heart rate monitoring and hand movements, which have been shown to be promising candidates for measuring stress and compulsive behaviour [29]. The procedure was approved by the local ethics committee (877/2020BO1). In this work, we will focus on the eye tracking recordings of four patients from this study.

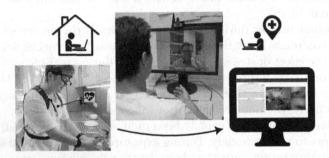

Fig. 1. Patients were equipped with a system to record their therapy sessions in their home environment. The data was streamed to the therapist UI, where the therapist had access to the egocentric video including gaze estimation and physiological measures. All icons are attributed to Flaticon.com

Treatment consisted of 14 session of video-based CBT. There was no exposure exercise within the first four sessions, since these were dedicated to building a therapist-patient relationship and psychoeducation in preparation for E/RP exercises. Afterwards, the amount of sessions including an exposure exercise was dependent on condition and therapy progress of the individual patient.

2.2   Data Collection and Labelling

The software architecture to record, transmit and display sensor data was custom designed for the purpose of the study [21]. Sensor data was recorded and synchronised locally and streamed to a therapist User Interface (UI), where the therapist could access the egocentric video of the patient together with the current gaze estimation and physiological parameters.

The therapist UI additionally served as a platform for data labelling where the therapists tagged time points defining the course of the therapy session, including start and end point of the exposure exercise. Throughout therapy, patients were asked to rate their perceived stress level on a scale from 0 to 10, which was also provided as label through the therapist UI.

Gaze data was recorded using the *Look!* head-mounted eye tracking device [14]. It included a scene camera with a resolution of 640×280 px and two eye cameras with a resolution of 320×240 px each. All videos were recorded at 30 Hz. Gaze estimation was computed using a convolutional neural network designed to be robust against small movements of the eye tracker to reduce the need for frequent recalibration [23]. Patients were asked to calibrate the system regularly, but at least before the first session and towards the middle of therapy.

2.3 Patients

We investigated a sample of four patients that participated in the SSTeP KiZ study. Symptom severity was assessed with the CY-BOCS score (Children's Yale-Brown Obsessive Compulsive Scale) before (t_0) and after treatment (t_1) [24]. A general reference for therapy success is a reduction of the CY-BOCS score by at least 35% [17], however, numerical symptom reduction can differ from personal experience. CY-BOCS values for all patients as well as demographic information and the amount and duration of exposure exercises can be found in Table 1.

Table 1. Overview of the patients included in this work. The table shows the amount of recorded exposure exercises per patient, mean and standard deviation of their durations, and the CY-BOCS score before and after treatment.

Patient			exposure exercises		CY-BOCS		
	age (year)	sex	n	length (min)	t_0	t_1	reduction
P1	17	f	9	38.6 ± 15.6	28	25	10.71%
P2	16	f	10	30.1 ± 11.9	21	13	38.10%
P3	17	m	7	28.9 ± 9.3	28	0	100%
P4	18	f	8	23 ± 6.4	29	12	58.62%

Manifestations of OCD are very heterogeneous across patients, which reflected in the four patients investigated in this work.

P1 showed a manifestation of OCD caused by the thought that certain objects are contaminated, triggering a strong feeling of disgust. To neutralise, these objects as well as both hands were cleaned excessively. Exposure exercises involved physical contact with "contaminated" objects such as doorknobs or contaminating "clean" objects such as one's bed. Subjectively, P1 reported a beneficial impact of the treatment, even though numerical symptom reduction was minor.

P2 showed the a repetition compulsion, repeating actions until they felt "just right", and a counting compulsion, mentally reciting certain number sequences over and over. Exposure for P2 included performing certain actions only once, e.g., closing the lid of a pen, and writing down a number included in the number sequence several times without mentally reciting the entire sequence.

P3 showed a contamination-based manifestation of OCD accompanied by the urge to perform frequent hand-washing. Exposures mainly consisted of touching "disgusting" objects like glue, the bathroom sink or toilet bowl. P3 started therapy with severe symptoms, but showed a surprisingly successful therapeutic effect, managing to reduce symptom severity by 100% to a minimum.

P4 showed a repetition-based manifestation of OCD with the urge to repeat actions with a positive thought until they felt "just right". Exposure sessions consisted mainly of selecting an item once and then performing the action with that item once (e.g., selecting and wearing the clothing item). The exercises were intensified by having to think of a negative event during the one-time execution.

2.4   Fixation Analysis Pipeline

To analyse the fixation behavior in the introduced patients, we adapted a fixation detection method for mobile eye tracking [27], structured the fixations using unsupervised clustering and assigned each cluster to *exposure-relevant*, *therapist* or *other* locations. The complete pipeline can be seen in Fig. 2.

Fixation Detection. First, we reduced noise in the gaze estimation by applying a moving average filter over a window of five frames. We then adapted an approach specifically designed for mobile eye tracking based on the assumption that image patches around the gaze estimation stay similar during a fixation [27].

We cropped an image patch of 50 × 50 px around the gaze estimation for every frame in the video. Each pair of consecutive frames served as input for a convolutional neural network (CNN) pretrained to predict patch similarity on the liberty dataset [7,34], resulting in a vector containing the patch similarity for each pair of frames. Sequences with similarities above the threshold of 1.3 were kept as fixation candidates. To remove outliers and ensure validity of fixations, we discarded candidates shorter than 3 frames (i.e., 100 ms) or longer than 95% of the data which corresponded to a maximal fixation length of 1 s.

The pipeline including the architecture of the CNN is shown in Fig. 2. It consists of two parallel 2-channel streams, one processing both full patches ("periphery") and one processing the central crops in a higher resolution ("fovea") that are integrated by two fully connected layers. Details on the network architecture can be found in the original publication [34].

To adapt the approach to our data, we tuned three hyperparameters: (1) image patch size, (2) similarity threshold and (3) the dataset for pretraining the patch similarity network. For tuning, we created a validation dataset consisting of a total video length of 15 min (i.e., roughly 27.000 frames) taken from three different subjects of the SSTeP KiZ study. All videos were labeled by at least two and at most three annotators to form the ground truth labels "fixation" and "no fixation" for each frame. The parameters were tuned by evaluating the fixations with event detection performance metrics [31].

Fixation Clustering. For each detected fixation, we extracted the centre frame as a representative and replaced its patch by a larger 256 × 256 px image cropped around the gaze estimation to obtain more context information. Since especially

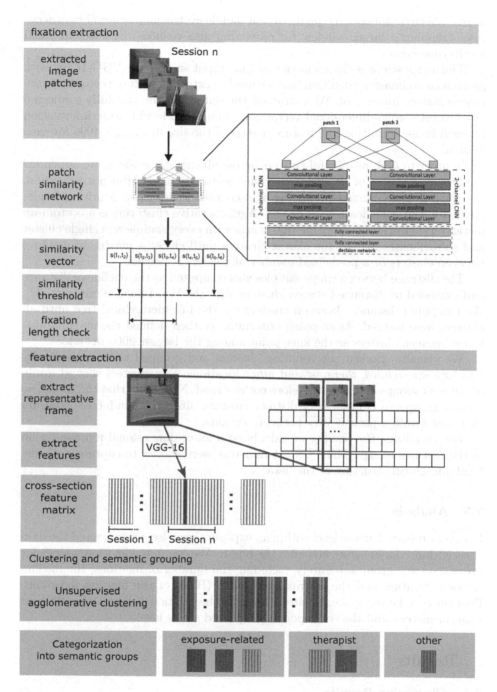

Fig. 2. Visualisation of the fixation processing pipeline, including fixation detection, feature extraction and unsupervised clustering. The network figure is adapted from [34].

in real-life environments the prediction of mobile eyetracking is not always accurate, cropping a larger window for clustering also reduces the effect of small localisation errors.

The image size was chosen as the optimal input size for the VGG-16 network pretrained on image recognition that we used to extract a feature vector for every representative image [26]. We extracted the output of the last fully-connected layer to get a 4096-dimensional vector containing high-level feature information for each image, resulting in a feature matrix of the size $n_{\text{fixations}} \times 4096$ for each session.

In order to find meaningful clusters across all therapy sessions, we appended the feature matrices of all sessions into one feature matrix. After normalization, the features were clustered with the agglomerative clustering algorithm implemented in the scikit-learn toolbox [20]. Agglomerative clustering is a bottom-up hierarchical clustering algorithm that starts with every sample as a single cluster and subsequently merges the closest clusters until either a maximum distance between clusters or a predefined number of clusters is reached.

The distance between single samples was computed as the euclidean distance and extended to distance between clusters with the Ward linkage criterion [32]. We computed distances between clusters for the full hierarchical tree until all clusters were merged. As stopping criterium, we then defined the maximal distance between clusters as the knee point among the largest 2000 distances.

We visually checked the resulting clusters and grouped them semantically into *exposure-related*, *therapist* and *other* locations. Few clusters showed a mix of different groups and were therefore not assigned. Note here, that the *exposure-related* group can contain very distinct clusters, since the conducted exposure exercises within a patient vary between sessions.

For visualising the results, we calculated a lower-dimensional representation of the features using UMAP [18]. Parameters were chosen to capture both the local and global structure of the data.

2.5   Analysis

For every reported stress level within an exposure exercise, we extracted the fixations within 1.5 min before and after the report. We computed fixation metrics for every semantic group separately, including the number of fixations, the median fixation duration and the interquartile range (IQR) of the fixation durations. Pearson correlation was calculated to assess the relation between the different fixation metrics and the corresponding reported stress level.

3   Results

3.1   Clustering Results

The clustering resulted on average in 31.25 clusters per subject of which on average 25 could be assigned to one of the semantic groups (P1: 25 cluster (21 assigned), P2: 25 (17), P3: 47 (40), P4: 28 (22)).

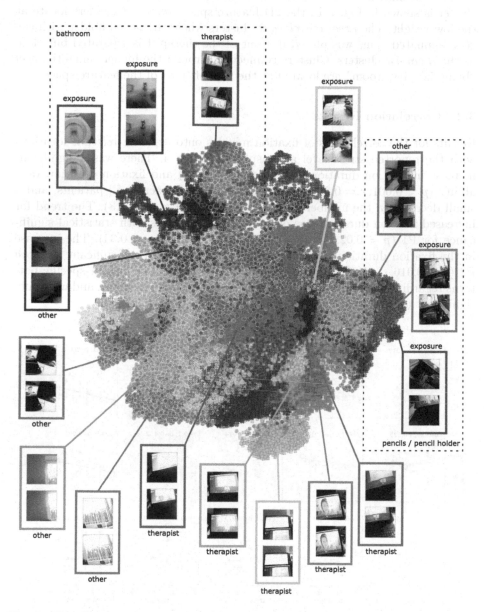

Fig. 3. Visualisation of the clustering results for P3. clusters were projected into a 2D space using UMAP. Clusters are colour-coded, while semantic groups are displayed as different shapes (X-shape: *exposure-relevant*, square: *therapist*, and circle: *other*). For exemplary clusters, the two images closest to the cluster centre are shown for illustration. Semantically meaningful grouped clusters are indicated by dashed lines.

The visualisation of clustering results for P3 along with examples for each cluster is shown in Fig. 3. In the 2D feature space, *therapist* clusters locate at the lower right. The *exposure-relevant* clusters where the pencil holder with the "contaminated" glue was placed in front of the therapist is separated but close to the *therapist* clusters. Clusters connected through the higher semantic level "being in a bathroom" are located at the top left part of the feature space.

3.2 Correlation Results

Results for the correlations of fixation metrics onto *exposure-relevant* locations with the reported stress level are displayed in Fig. 4. There was a significant increase in fixation duration ($p < 0.001, r = 0.41$) and fixation duration variability ($p < 0.001, r = 0.3$) with the perceived stress across all patients, and a small decrease in the number of fixations ($p = 0.01, r = -0.18$). The trend for increased fixation duration was observed in all subjects with statistical significance for P1 ($p = 0.02, r = 0.37$) and P2 ($p = 0.004, r = 0.34$). The increase in the fixation duration IQR did not occur in P1, but was significant for both P2 ($p = 0.016, r = 0.29$) and P3 ($p = 0.01, r = 0.42$). The patient-specific patterns regarding the number of fixations were individually different, and were only significant for P2 ($p = 0.01, r = -0.3$).

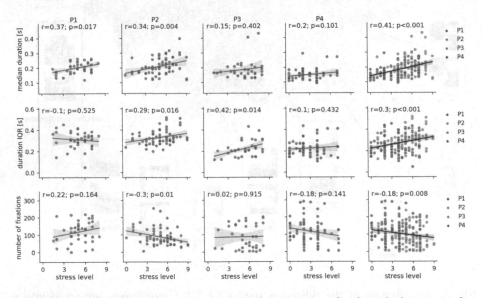

Fig. 4. Correlation of the patients' reported subjective stress levels with the metrics for fixations onto the *exposure-relevant* cluster. The first four columns represent a patient each, while the last column presents the results taken across all patients.

For fixations onto *other* locations, displayed in Fig. 5, we found small correlations of the stress level with fixation duration ($p = 0.04, r = 0.16$) and fixation

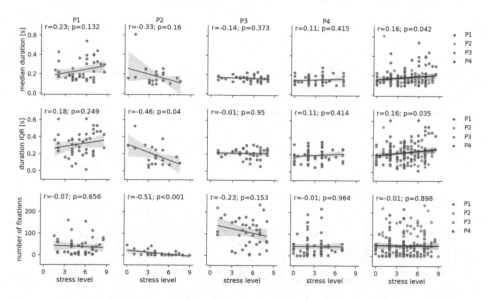

Fig. 5. Correlation of the patients' reported subjective stress levels with the metrics for fixations onto the *other* cluster. The first four columns represent a patient each, while the last column presents the results taken across all patients.

duration variability ($p = 0.04, r = 0.16$), but no correlation with the number of fixations ($p = 0.9$) across all patients. There was no consistent trend of duration increase in single patients and none showed significant results. We observed similar results for duration IQR, which was only significant for P2, where correlation was strongly negative ($p = 0.04, r = -0.46$) as opposed to the positive correlation across all patients. P2 was also the only patient that showed a significant correlation with the number of fixations ($p < 0.001, r = -0.51$).

Correlation results for fixations onto the *therapist* are shown in Fig. 6. For fixation duration and duration variability, there was no correlation with stress levels across all patients ($p > 0.48$) and no common trend across single patients. Correlation was only significant in P2 for fixation duration ($p = 0.01, r = 0.39$) and variability ($p = 0.002, r = 0.48$). The number of fixations across all patients decreased with reported stress level ($p < 0.001, r = -0.25$), which was not consistent across single patients, where the number of fixations decreased with stress for P1 ($p = 0.007, r = -0.35$) but increased for P2 ($p = 0.02, r = 0.34$).

4 Discussion

We proposed a method to analyse the fixation behaviour of children and adolescents with OCD during exposure exercises within video-based CBT. The method was specifically designed for challenges caused by real-life behaviour recorded with mobile eye tracking in home environments. For fixation detection we adapted an approach based on gaze patch similarity that is robust to head

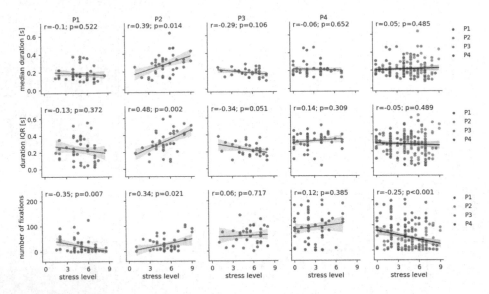

Fig. 6. Correlation of the patients' reported subjective stress levels with the metrics for fixations onto the *therapist* cluster. The first four columns represent a patient each, while the last column presents the results taken across all patients.

movements. We extended the method with unsupervised clustering to automatically identify targets in the real world from the fixated locations. We demonstrated that these clusters have semantic meaning and represent three categories of gaze targets: *exposure-relevant*, *therapist* and *other* locations.

We found that fixation duration onto *exposure-relevant* locations consistently reflected reported stress levels of the patient, i.e., fixation duration correlated positively with higher stress levels. This was accompanied by an increase in fixation variability, suggesting that fixation duration did not change systematically but that only some fixations lasted longer. While similar effects could be observed for *other* locations, these proved smaller and inconsistent across subjects.

Our results reveal that during real-life exposures patients put more attention on exposure-relevant locations if the subjective stress level, and thus the intensity of the exposure, increased. Given that fixation duration has been shown to increase with higher mental load, our results suggest that the patients' mental load and perceived stress level are closely connected.

There was no increase in the amount of fixations, neither onto *exposure-relevant* nor *other* locations, which we would have expected as an effect of the rising stress. In contrast, some patients even showed a decrease in the amount of fixations. Together with the increase in fixation duration, this indicates that reported stress reflects mental effort during exposure rather than anxiety.

Fixation behaviour towards the therapist was highly individual and there was no common effect across patients. This is not surprising given that fixation behaviour towards the therapist can depend on many variables that differ between patients, like the type of conversation during exposure or the patient-therapist relationship.

Our results underline the effectiveness of our method. However, it should be noted that the method assumes that exposure sessions contain a physical exposure to objects or locations. Therefore, this approach is most suitable for manifestations of OCD where obsessive thoughts are connected to a physical counterpart like an action, an object or a specific location.

In general, our findings stress the importance of analysing fixation behaviour during real-life exposure sessions as an extension of controlled eye tracking studies in the laboratory. Especially fixation duration and variability promise to be valuable parameters for therapists to monitor and adapt the patient's stress level and the connected mental load during exposure sessions. Since our analysis is exemplary on four patients, future studies would have to replicate and validate these results with a larger population.

4.1 Conclusion

We proposed a pipeline suitable for analysing gaze behaviour of patients with OCD during exposure sessions in their home environments. Although further research is needed to validate our findings, our work provides a preliminary argument for the usefulness of eyetracking for patients with OCD. Providing feedback about gaze behaviour could therefore support therapists in monitoring stress and mental load of patients, helping them to adapt to the needs of the patient. Next steps will be to use our approach for behavioural feedback to therapists in exposure exercises practised as homework outside of therapy sessions, to ensure correctness and prevent avoidance behaviour. In future research, it will also be interesting to connect the gaze features not only with perceived stress but also with physiological measures of stress such as heart rate.

References

1. Abramowitz, J.S., Taylor, S., McKay, D.: Obsessive-compulsive disorder. Lancet **374**(9688), 491–499 (2009)
2. Ahmadi, N., et al.: Quantifying Workload and Stress in Intensive Care Unit Nurses: Preliminary Evaluation Using Continuous Eye-Tracking. Human Factors (2022)
3. Armstrong, T., Olatunji, B.O.: Eye tracking of attention in the affective disorders: a meta-analytic review and synthesis. Clin. Psychol. Rev. **32**(8), 704–723 (2012)
4. Basel, D., Hallel, H., Dar, R., Lazarov, A.: Attention allocation in OCD: a systematic review and meta-analysis of eye-tracking-based research. J. Affect. Disord. **324**, 539–550 (2023)
5. Behroozi, M., Lui, A., Moore, I., Ford, D., Parnin, C.: Dazed: measuring the cognitive load of solving technical interview problems at the whiteboard. In: Proceedings of the 40th International Conference on Software Engineering: New Ideas and Emerging Results, pp. 93–96. ACM, Gothenburg Sweden (2018). https://doi.org/10.1145/3183399.3183415

6. Bradley, M.C., Hanna, D., Wilson, P., Scott, G., Quinn, P., Dyer, K.F.W.: Obsessive-compulsive symptoms and attentional bias: an eye-tracking methodology. J. Behav. Ther. Exp. Psychiatry **50**, 303–308 (2016)
7. Brown, M., Gang Hua, Winder, S.: Discriminative learning of local image descriptors. IEEE Trans. Pattern Anal. Mach. Intell. **33**(1), 43–57 (2011). https://doi.org/10.1109/TPAMI.2010.54
8. Chen, S., Epps, J., Ruiz, N., Chen, F.: Eye activity as a measure of human mental effort in HCI. In: Proceedings of the 16th International Conference on Intelligent User Interfaces, pp. 315–318. IUI 2011. ACM, New York (2011). https://doi.org/10.1145/1943403.1943454
9. Douglass, H.M., Moffitt, T.E., Dar, R., McGee, R., Silva, P.: Obsessive-compulsive disorder in a Birth Cohort of 18-Year-Olds: prevalence and predictors. J. Am. Acad. Child Adolesc. Psychiatry **34**(11), 1424–1431 (1995)
10. Heyman, I., Fombonne, E., Simmons, H., Ford, T., Meltzer, H., Goodman, R.: Prevalence of obsessive-compulsive disorder in the British nationwide survey of child mental health. British J. Psychiatry J. Mental Sci. **179**, 324–329 (2001)
11. Hollis, C., Falconer, C.J., Martin, J.L., Whittington, C., Stockton, S., Glazebrook, C., Davies, E.B.: Annual research review: digital health interventions for children and young people with mental health problems - a systematic and meta-review. J. Child Psychol. Psychiatry **58**(4), 474–503 (2017)
12. Hollmann, K., et al.: Internet-based cognitive behavioral therapy in children and adolescents with obsessive-compulsive disorder: a randomized controlled trial. Front Psychiatry **13** (2022)
13. Klein, C.S., et al.: Smart sensory technology in tele-psychotherapy of children and Adolescents with Obsessive-Compulsive Disorder (OCD): a feasibility study. preprint, SSRN (2023). https://doi.org/10.2139/ssrn.4395216
14. Kübler, T.: Look! Technical specifications, Blickschulungsbrille (2021)
15. Lappi, O.: Eye movements in the wild: oculomotor control, gaze behavior & frames of reference. Neurosci. Biobehav. Rev. **69**, 49–68 (2016)
16. Marquart, G., Cabrall, C., De Winter, J.: Review of eye-related measures of drivers' mental workload. Procedia Manuf. **3**, 2854–2861 (2015)
17. Mataix-Cols, D., de la Cruz, L.F., Nordsletten, A.E., Lenhard, F., Isomura, K., Simpson, H.B.: Towards an international expert consensus for defining treatment response, remission, recovery and relapse in obsessive-compulsive disorder. World Psychiatry **15**(1), 80–81 (2016)
18. McInnes, L., Healy, J., Melville, J.: UMAP: uniform manifold approximation and projection for dimension reduction. arXiv preprint arXiv:1802.03426 (2018)
19. Mullen, M., Hanna, D., Bradley, M., Rogers, D., Jordan, J.A., Dyer, K.F.W.: Attentional bias in individuals with obsessive-compulsive disorder: a preliminary eye-tracking study. J. Behav. Cogn. Ther. **31**(2), 199–204 (2021)
20. Pedregosa, F., et al.: Scikit-learn: machine learning in Python. J. Mach. Learn. Res. **12**, 2825–2830 (2011)
21. Primbs, J., et al.: The SSTeP-KiZ system-secure real-time communication based on open web standards for multimodal sensor-assisted tele-psychotherapy. Sensors **22**(24), 9589 (2022)
22. Recarte, M.A., Nunes, L.M.: Effects of verbal and spatial-imagery tasks on eye fixations while driving. J. Exp. Psychol. Appl. **6**(1), 31–43 (2000)
23. Santini, T., Niehorster, D.C., Kasneci, E.: Get a grip: slippage-robust and glint-free gaze estimation for real-time pervasive head-mounted eye tracking. In: Proceedings of the 11th ACM Symposium on Eye Tracking Research & Applications, pp. 1–10. ACM (2019). https://doi.org/10.1145/3314111.3319835

24. Scahill, L., Riddle, M.A., McSwiggin-Hardin, M., Ort, S.I., King, R.A., Goodman, W.K., Cicchetti, D., Leckman, J.F.: Children's yale-brown obsessive compulsive scale: reliability and validity. J. Am. Acad. Child Adolesc. Psychiatry **36**(6), 844–852 (1997)
25. Selles, R.R., et al.: Effects of treatment setting on outcomes of flexibly-dosed intensive cognitive behavioral therapy for pediatric ocd: a randomized controlled pilot trial. Front Psychiatry **12** (2021)
26. Simonyan, K., Zisserman, A.: Very Deep Convolutional Networks for Large-Scale Image Recognition. arXiv preprint arXiv:1409.1556 (2015)
27. Steil, J., Huang, M.X., Bulling, A.: Fixation detection for head-mounted eye tracking based on visual similarity of gaze targets. In: Proceedings of the 2018 ACM Symposium on Eye Tracking Research & Applications, pp. 1–9. ACM (2018). https://doi.org/10.1145/3204493.3204538
28. Stewart, S.E., Geller, D.A., Jenike, M., Pauls, D., Shaw, D., Mullin, B., Faraone, S.V.: Long-term outcome of pediatric obsessive-compulsive disorder: a meta-analysis and qualitative review of the literature. Acta Psychiatr. Scand. **110**(1), 4–13 (2004)
29. Thierfelder, A., et al.: Multimodal sensor-based identification of stress and compulsive actions in children with obsessive-compulsive disorder for telemedical treatment. In: 2022 44th Annual International Conference of the IEEE Engineering in Medicine & Biology Society (EMBC), pp. 2976–2982 (2022). https://doi.org/10.1109/EMBC48229.2022.9871899
30. Tichon, J.G., Wallis, G., Riek, S., Mavin, T.: Physiological measurement of anxiety to evaluate performance in simulation training. Cognition, Technol. Work **16**(2), 203–210 (2014)
31. Ward, J.A., Lukowicz, P., Gellersen, H.W.: Performance metrics for activity recognition. ACM Trans. Intell. Syst. Technol. **2**(1), 1–23 (2011). https://doi.org/10.1145/1889681.1889687
32. Ward, J.H.: Hierarchical grouping to optimize an objective function. J. Am. Stat. Assoc. **58**(301), 236–244 (1963)
33. World Health Organization: International classification of diseases for mortality and morbidity statistics (11th revision). https://icd.who.int/browse11/l-m/en. Accessed 9 July 2023
34. Zagoruyko, S., Komodakis, N.: Learning to compare image patches via convolutional neural networks. In: Proceedings of the IEEE Conference on Computer Vision and Pattern Recognition, pp. 4353–4361 (2015)

Individual Behavioral Insights in Schizophrenia: A Network Analysis and Mobile Sensing Approach

Andy Davies[1]([✉]) [iD], Eiko Fried[2] [iD], Omar Costilla-Reyes[3] [iD], and Hane Aung[1] [iD]

[1] School of Computer Sciences, University of East Anglia, Norwich NR9 7TJ, UK
{andy.davies,Min.aung}@uea.ac.uk
[2] Faculty of Social Sciences, Institute of Psychology, Leiden University,
Rapenburg 70, 2311 Leiden, Netherlands
e.i.fried@fsw.leidenuniv.nl
[3] Computer-Aided Programming Research Group,
MIT Computer Science and Artificial Intelligence Laboratory (CSAIL),
Cambridge, MA 02139, USA
costilla@mit.edu

Abstract. Digital phenotyping in mental health often consists of collecting behavioral and experience-based information through sensory and self-reported data from devices such as smartphones. Such rich and comprehensive data could be used to develop insights into the relationships between daily behavior and a range of mental health conditions. However, current analytical approaches have shown limited application due to these datasets being both high dimensional and multimodal in nature. This study demonstrates the first use of a principled method which consolidates the complexities of subjective self-reported data (Ecological Momentary Assessments - EMAs) with concurrent sensor-based data. In this study the CrossCheck dataset is used to analyse data from 50 participants diagnosed with schizophrenia. Network Analysis is applied to EMAs at an individual (n-of-1) level while sensor data is used to identify periods of various behavioral context. Networks generated during periods of certain behavioral contexts, such as variations in the daily number of locations visited, were found to significantly differ from baseline networks and networks generated from randomly sampled periods of time. The framework presented here lays a foundation to reveal behavioural contexts and the concurrent impact of self-reporting at an n-of-1 level. These insights are valuable in the management of serious mental illnesses such as schizophrenia.

Keywords: Schizophrenia · CrossCheck · n-of-1 · Digital Phenotyping · Network Analysis · Mobile Sensing

1 Introduction

Schizophrenia is a complex, Serious Mental health Illness (SMI) that develops in approximately 1% of the global population [41] and represents a significant

D. Salvi et al. (Eds.): PH 2023, LNICST 572, pp. 18–33, 2024.
https://doi.org/10.1007/978-3-031-59717-6_2

personal and economic burden at an individual, familial and societal level [15,44]. Symptoms can include hallucinations (both visual and auditory), disordered and delusional thinking, impaired cognitive ability, disorganized speech and behavior [37], as well as increased social isolation, withdrawal and amotivation [29]. Although characterised as a chronic condition, the disease course is not static, with diagnosed individuals typically fluctuating between periods of partial remission and periods of symptomatic relapse [17,35,46]. Studies have identified symptomatic and behavioral changes that can manifest prior to relapse [3,9,17,20], however, these changes often remain undetected until the occurrence of significant negative consequences [45]. Evidence further suggests that timely clinical intervention poses an effective strategy in the prevention of further deterioration, and the transition into a state of full relapse [33,45].

In this paper, we seek to demonstrate a method which consolidates the complexities of subjective self-reported Ecological Momentary Assessments (EMAs) when accounting for variations in behavioral context. Using the CrossCheck dataset, a first of its kind dataset combining real-world, longitudinal behavioral data, and self-reported EMAs specific to schizophrenia [45]; we aim to demonstrate the effectiveness of using sensor-based data to identify periods of various behavioral context, from which network analysis can be applied to observe and compare differences in network connectivity and the relationships between corresponding EMAs. Specifically, we focus on behaviors that can be categorised according to periods of sociability and social isolation, both noted symptoms associated with schizophrenia symptom severity [20]. Figure 1 provides a high-level overview of this process, from individual-level (n-of-1) data through to behavioral filtering and network analysis. Ultimately, the goal of this framework is to reveal behavioral contexts and their resulting impact on self-reported EMAs at an n-of-1 level, in particular providing insights into symptomatic improvement or disease exacerbation.

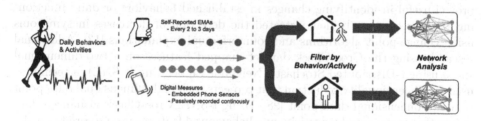

Fig. 1. Overview of the processes involved in this study; networks are generated using EMA responses concurrent with specific sensor-based behavioral contexts.

2 Related Work

Conventional research into human behavior often relies on time and resource intensive data collection through face-to-face engagement in a controlled or clinical environment. However, the pervasiveness of mobile technology [42] in everyday life is affording researchers and clinicians access to vast quantities of moment-by-moment, in-situ, individual-level data captured by personal digital devices; the granular level quantification of which is referred to as digital phenotyping [32,43]. These personal phenotypes [5,36] provide a digital fingerprint from which psychological, cognitive and behavioural characteristics can be measured and assessed [16,22,23,31]; providing valuable insights into symptomatic markers and effective psychiatric treatments [38]. Within mental health research, digital phenotyping has been employed in a number of studies, including student mental health [30], depression [26], prediction of suicidal urges [12], anxiety disorders [24], social anxiety [25], and psychosis spectrum illnesses [8].

With an increasing emphasis on patient-centred healthcare and individualised medicine [11], digital phenotyping lends itself to move away from the population level [18] and instead conduct n-of-1 trials (or single subject trials); these focus on an individual patient as the sole unit of observation throughout a study [27]. Typically, n-of-1 studies have been used within both clinical and research settings to assess pharmaceutical efficacy and treatment viability within individual participants [39]. The focus of these trials enables the identification of observations or characteristics that may not be evident in a collective population-level analysis. However for larger population samples, the insights gained from n-of-1 trials can contribute to larger-scale Randomized Control Trials (RCTs).

The CrossCheck collection emulated a Randomized Control Trial (RCT) design [14] that explored the viability of continuous remote patient monitoring through a multimodal sensing system; the core aim of which sought to accurately predict indicators of symptomatic and psychotic relapse in Schizophrenia Spectrum Disorders (SSD) [45]. CrossCheck's digital phenotyping dataset identified unique digital indicators of psychotic relapse; for some participants changes in self-reported EMAs provided actionable descriptors of symptom exacerbation, whilst in others, passively recorded behavioural and sensory data proved useful in identifying changes in established behaviors or daily functioning [7]. A recent study demonstrated the detection of decreases in symptoms using change-point algorithms and counterfactual explanations [13]. Additional research using the CrossCheck dataset mapped features on a two-dimensional space using t-Distributed Stochastic Neighbor Embedding (t-SNE), a technique used for dimensionality reduction that projects each high-dimensional data point to a two-dimensional data point [28]. Using t-SNE, CrossCheck visualized data points that represented a participant's behavioural features used to predict EMA responses; when plotted, these data points clustered according to each specific study participant. This clearly demonstrated that there are observable differences between study participants and that CrossCheck's sensor data is highly person dependent [45]. At a population level, the initial study found significant associations between recorded behavioral features and changes in mental health indicators; in particular decreased levels of physical activity and sociability was associated with negative mental health, whilst improvements in established sleep patterns and getting up earlier collated with positive mental health

[45]. These findings were further supported through research into behavioral stability using the same dataset, this stability index drew on participant's passively recorded features and behaviours to assess the extent to which a diagnosed participant adheres to a stable routine. This study identified correlations between the stability index of recorded features and symptomatic severity, the results of which demonstrated that greater periods of stability in social activities - such as calls and SMS messages - was associated with reduced symptoms. In contrast, increased stability in periods of inactivity - time spent still - exhibited an association with increased symptom severity [20]. The findings of these studies highlight not only the highly person-centric nature of CrossCheck's multimodal data, but also the close association between daily behaviors and symptom severity; both of which are of particular importance to this study as we seek to analyse the impact recorded behavioral contexts have on self-reported EMAs at an individual level.

In recent years the use of network analysis within psychological research has become an important tool in the estimation and visualization of psychological data, and can be used to identify multivariate patterns and relationships [10, 21]. Within these networks, nodes represent variables such as mood states collected via EMAs, with edges between nodes denoting statistical relationships between said nodes [21]. The process by which these associations and relationships are calculated can vary depending on the initial dataset and selected statistical model [10]. In recent years, network analysis techniques have been applied to a large number of datasets in order to gain deeper insights into a range of mental health problems, including drug and alcohol dependency [40], suicidal behavior in adolescents [19], depression and anxiety [6], and the treatment of psychosis [4]. Network analysis consists of three stages; network structure estimation, network description, and network stability analysis [10]. Network structure estimation refers to the process by which the underlying structure of a network is inferred, involving the selection of relevant nodes and edges as well as selecting an optimal statistical model. Network description is the characterisation of a network which involves understanding network topology and node centrality. Finally, network stability analysis refers to the examination of a network's robustness, consistency and the accuracy of edge weights [10]. Recently, estimating network models on time-series data with numerous repeated observations using EMA data has gained traction, however this presents three distinct challenges. First, most work is estimated at the group level, ignoring potential variation across participants in network structures. Second, networks are stationary, i.e., one network is obtained throughout the time period, assuming network structure does not vary by context. Third, it is unclear how network analysis ought to deal with multimodal (e.g., sensor and EMA) data. Here we tackle all three challenges, by estimating n-of-1 networks according to a selected behavioral (sensor-based) context prior to EMA network generation, as a result enabling more nuanced, context-dependent qualitative networks.

3   Dataset

The CrossCheck [45] dataset originally consisted of 150 participants, each of whom met the criteria for schizophrenia as defined in the DSM-IV [1] and DSM-V [2], whilst also meeting CrossCheck's inclusion criteria [7,45]. Organised into two groups of 75, participants within the CrossCheck study arm were each issued with a smartphone that continuously recorded a range of behavioral, sensory and self-reported EMA data over a 12 month period [7,45,47]. Embedded smartphone sensors passively record daily behaviours and activities continuously, whilst EMAs were self-reported every 2 to 3 days [45]. Of particular relevance to this paper are the following features:

Ecological Momentary Assessment (EMA): EMAs afford a viable way of capturing real-time psychological data within a natural environment. Every 2 to 3 days, CrossCheck administered a 10-item self-reporting assessment designed to measure schizophrenia-related thoughts, feelings, and behaviors [7,45]. Each question (see Table 1) was answered on a scale from 0 ("Not at all") to 3 ("Extremely"). For ease of analysis and understanding, each EMA is grouped according to either its positive or negative association.

Table 1. CrossCheck EMA Questions

Positive EMAs	Negative EMAs
+ Have you been feeling **CALM**?	- Have you been **DEPRESSED**?
+ Have you been **SOCIAL**?	- Have you been feeling **STRESSED**?
+ Have you been **SLEEPING** well?	- Have you been bothered by **VOICES**?
+ Have you been able to **THINK** clearly?	- Have you been **SEEING THINGS** other people can't see?
+ Have you been **HOPEFUL** about the future?	- Have you been worried about people trying to **HARM** you?

Behavioural Sensing: Study smartphones continuously collected a wide range of behavioral features for each participant, however only the following behavioral features are relevant to this paper due to their close association with sociability and social isolation. - *Geo-spatial Activity:* refers to timestamped locational data derived using a combination of device GPS, Wifi and cellular network towers [7,45]. - *Speech Frequency & Duration:* periods of human speech was inferred from ambient sound using the inbuilt device microphone [7]. - *Calls & SMS:* The frequency and duration of incoming and outgoing calls, as well as the number of incoming and outgoing SMS messages is passively logged and recorded by the CrossCheck application [7,45].

4 Method

The following section presents the proposed methodology employed in this study, from prerequisite data pre-processing, through to initial network generation and statistical analyses. Data pre-processing requires basic resampling and thresholding, with network generation simply based on the correlations within the 10 set EMA questions (see Table 1). As such giving low computational requirements and ease of re-implementation.

4.1 Data Pre-processing

From CrossCheck's original study arm, 50 participants have been identified from which further analysis can be conducted, these individuals were selected for the quantity and quality of their recorded data. Participants whose engagement was limited, or who recorded inconsistent and unusable data were omitted from further analysis. Whilst both sensory and device usage data is temporally continuous, self-reported EMA responses are only given every 2 to 3 days [45]. However, each EMA question also pertains to days prior to a given response, as such we can retrospectively replicate each EMA score to also be concurrent with sensor data recorded between EMA responses. Any days that fall outside of the 2 day back fill window are omitted from a participant's dataset.

Selection of sensor features was based on their ability to effectively capture defined behavioral contexts, without the need for further processing to map sensor data to a particular context (e.g. it is a reasonable assumption that no location data outside of the primary residence indicates not leaving the home, and that no calls or detected conversations indicates not verbally socializing). Table 2 lists these selected features and their corresponding categories. These categories are created based on 2 factors; first relating to the veracity of the behavioral context that the data represents as stated above, with the second factor being based on well understood behavioral contexts for this SMI, such as social isolation and sociability. Along side these features random sampling of unfiltered data is also conducted from which an empirical distribution is generated, this serves as a baseline from which comparisons can then be made.

Table 2. Selected behavioral contexts and their corresponding categories.

Behavioral Feature in a 24 h period	Periods of Social Isolation	Periods of Sociability
Baseline	*Random Unfiltered Sample*	*Random Unfiltered Sample*
Locations Visited	*No locations visited*	≥ 1 *locations visited*
Calls Made	*No calls made*	≥ 1 *calls made*
Calls Received	*No calls received*	≥ 1 *calls received*
SMS Messages Sent	*No SMS messages sent*	≥ 1 *messages sent*
SMS Messages Received	*No SMS messages received*	≥ 1 *messages received*
Conversations Detected	*No detected conversations*	≥ 1 *detected conversations*

4.2   Network Structure Estimation and Description

Although participant data is initially chronologically ordered, filtering according to a selected behavioral category, either social isolation or sociability, results in time-series segmentation. This segmentation necessitates the identification of a statistical model that can account for this lack of temporal consistency. Correlation network models applied to cross-sectional data deal well with this lack of consistency, as they are effective at visualizing relationships between variables at a specific point in time [10]. As a result we can use this model to generate networks for each person that represent an aggregated average for a sample taken from each selected behavioral category. This allows us to compare network structures of EMAs when participants are, for instance, spending time socially isolated (e.g. remaining at home) or engaging socially (e.g. visiting locations outside of their home). Structurally, EMAs are represented as network nodes with edges between nodes visualizing the linear relationship between each. The strength and sign of any given relationship is defined by the correlation coefficient. Numerically, correlations between nodes range between -1 and 1; with -1 indicating a perfect negative relationship, 1 a perfect positive relationship, and 0 no relationship at all. Pearson's R Correlation Coefficient is used to calculate the associations between all 10 EMA nodes. For each behavioral context two networks are generated, one for each category within a given behavior (Table 2).

4.3   Permutation Testing

To discern whether variations in each behavioral context and their observed network structures differ in statistically meaningful ways, permutation testing is used. The goal of which is to evaluate the null hypothesis that these variations have no discernible concurrence with a participant's self-reported EMAs.

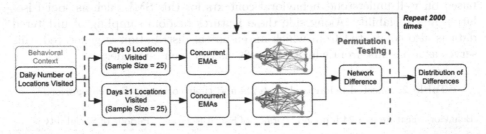

Fig. 2. Permutation testing process for **Daily Number of Locations Visited**, networks are generated using concurrent EMAs from each behavioral category, in turn allowing for the calculation of differences in network connectivity.

Procedurally, permutation testing requires a selected behavior to be filtered according to predefined categories (see Table 2). A network is generated for each category using a 25 day sample, at the end of each permutation the observed difference in network connectivity is calculated by subtracting the sum of the network matrices from each other. In probability theory, Central Limit Theorem (CLT) suggests a sample size of approximately 30, however, to maximise the number of viable participants a reduced sample size of 25 days is used throughout the permutation testing process. Repeated 2000 times, a new observed difference in network connectivity is calculated for each permutation, from which a distribution of these differences is then produced. Figure 2 demonstrates this process using the daily number of locations visited as an example.

The resulting distribution of differences in network connectivity for a given behavior can then be compared with a baseline distribution. This baseline undergoes the same testing process but is generated using randomly sampled data, and serves as an empirical distribution from which comparisons can then be made. To measure statistical significance, paired-sample t-testing is used to compare a given behavioral distribution with the empirical baseline distribution. The resulting t-score and p-value can then be used to confirm or reject the null hypothesis that a selected sensor based behavioural context has no discernible influence over an individual's network connectivity.

5   Results

In this section we present the findings of our analysis; first detailing results for a single participant, and then at a wider level for multiple participants.

5.1   Example of an Individual CrossCheck Participant

Having recorded 330 days of usable data, this individual returned results across 5 of the 6 selected behavioral contexts. Figure 3 visualizes the results produced during permutation testing for each behavior according to networks generated using only positive, and only negative EMAs (see Table 1).

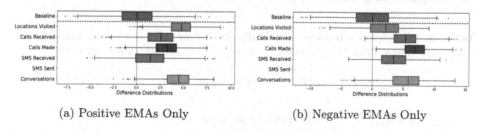

(a) Positive EMAs Only   (b) Negative EMAs Only

Fig. 3. Side-by-side comparison of permutation test results for a single individual across all selected behavioral contexts as well a baseline test - networks generated during testing process used positive EMAs only versus negative EMAs only

In each instance, we observe differences when comparing each behavior to a baseline distribution, for example in Fig. 3a, we observe a baseline mean of 0 compared to a mean of 4.7 in detected conversations. Focusing in on daily number of locations visited, there is not only an observable difference between behavior and baseline, but there is a notable difference when comparing positive and negative EMAs.

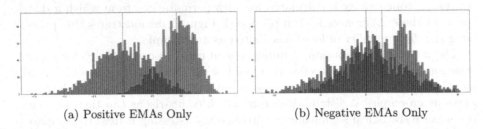

(a) Positive EMAs Only   (b) Negative EMAs Only

Fig. 4. More detailed analysis of participants results for both their baseline distribution (Blue) and **Number of Locations Visited** distribution (Red). Figure 4a clearly shows an observable difference between the baseline distribution and the behavioral context distribution for positive EMAs. (Color figure online)

Figure 4 provides a more detailed visualization of this participant's baseline distribution (in blue) and variations in their daily number of locations visited (in red). Upon visual inspection, there is a clear observable difference in distributions produced using positive EMAs (Fig. 4a) when compared to those produced using negative EMAs (Fig. 4b). This suggests that, for this participant, there is a noticeable impact on their self-reported positive EMAs when factoring in variations in the daily number of locations visited. Table 3 provides a breakdown of these results across all EMA groups, with a consistent p-value < 0.001 indicating these results are statistical significant. Moreover, we see a more sizeable t-score for this participant's positive EMAs (-72.78), further suggesting that variations in this behavioral context impacts this individual's self-reporting habits - particularly for their positive EMAs.

Table 3. Participant's baseline and **Daily Number of Locations Visited** test results, including mean ($\bar{x}$), standard deviation (σ), t-score (t) and p-value (p)

	Baseline		Daily Number of Locations Visited		
	$\bar{x}$	σ	$\bar{x}$	σ	t
All EMAs	-0.44	9.06	17.30	6.22	-55.62 *
Positive EMAs	0.05	2.28	4.61	1.55	-72.72 *
Negative EMAs	-0.05	3.80	1.83	3.07	-13.21 *

* $p < 0.001$

Whilst numerically these results indicate a statistical significance for this particular behavioral context; network generation provides a visualization of the relationship between EMAs. Figure 5 provides a side-by-side comparison between two networks that each visualize one of the two categories for variations in the daily number of locations this individual participant has visited.

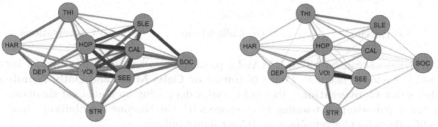

(a) Days with 0 locations visited   (b) Days with 1 or more locations visited

Fig. 5. Cross-Sectional Networks for **Daily Number of Locations Visited**. Nodes: **DEP**ressed, **HAR**m, **SEE**ing Things, **STR**essed, Hearing **VOI**ces, **CAL**m, **HOP**e, **SLE**ep, **SOC**ial, **THI**nking Clearly. Thicker edges denote stronger relationships with blue edges indicating positive correlations and red negative. As expected, one can observe positive relations between positive EMAs (i.e., when this person reports one positive EMA, they are more likely to report others, too); positive relations between negative EMAs; and negative relations between positive and negative EMAs. (Color figure online)

Both networks in Fig. 5 present strong positive relationships between auditory and visual hallucinations, however, on days where this participant remained at home (see Fig. 5a) we see a much more complex network with the presence of stronger edges in greater numbers. A visual analysis of these two networks suggests that, for this particular participant, there is a beneficial link between social engagement (interacting with locations away from home) and improvements in self-reported EMAs. In particular, Fig. 5a illustrates strong negative relationships between each hallucinatory node and feelings of calm and hopeful, this suggests that increased instances of one has a detrimental impact on the other. For example, hallucinations experienced at home could have a more noticeable detrimental impact on this participant's ability to feel calm and hopeful; likewise it could also suggest that feeling calm within this participant's own home reduces the likelihood of them experiencing increased hallucinations.

5.2   By Behavioral Context

In the interest of brevity the following results focus on the analysis of all 10 EMAs for three specific behavioral contexts. The daily number of calls made, daily number of conversations detected and daily number of locations visited.

Daily Number of Calls Made & Detected Conversations: Fig. 6 presents the distributions of 6 participants who each returned results for both the daily number of calls made and number of conversations detected.

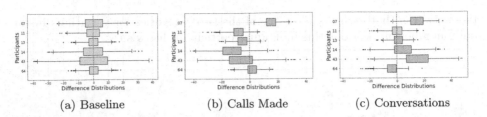

(a) Baseline   (b) Calls Made   (c) Conversations

Fig. 6. Results across for **all 10 EMAs** for participants who returned results for both selected behavioral contexts - **Daily Number of Calls Made** and **Daily Number of Detected Conversations**. Plot color varies depending on statistical significance when using pair-sampled t-testing to compare with the baseline distribution - blue if $p < 0.05$ otherwise plot remains grey. (Color figure online)

As expected, the baseline distributions in Fig. 6a indicate a mean close to 0, demonstrating the consistency of randomized sampling. However following the same process as with the previous individual's results, a comparison between each participant's baseline distribution and behavioral context distribution demonstrates varying degrees of difference - further highlighting the individuality of participant data.

Table 4. Participant results for paired-sample t-testing between their baseline distribution and **both** Number of Calls Received and Calls Made. For each behavior results include; mean ($\bar{x}$), standard deviation (σ), t-score (t), and p-value (p).

ID	Baseline		Daily Number of Calls Made			Daily Number of Conversations		
	$\bar{x}$	σ	$\bar{x}$	σ	t	$\bar{x}$	σ	t
07	−0.18	8.75	15.45	4.97	−49.65 *	14.67	6.57	−46.80 *
11	−0.02	6.81	−8.47	5.43	44.06 *	0.24	5.41	−1.24
13	−0.01	5.33	−4.73	4.90	19.93 *	1.00	4.09	−4.91 *
14	−0.27	10.62	−12.40	9.58	39.43 *	3.88	9.51	−13.01 *
43	−0.42	13.63	−5.45	12.12	12.91 *	14.43	11.44	−37.31 *
64	−0.11	4.88	1.55	4.61	−9.79 *	−4.16	5.00	23.47 *

* $p < 0.001$

Table 4 provides a breakdown of results for each participant visualized in Fig. 6. Whilst in most cases analysis of these two behaviors produces a statistically significant p-value ($p < 0.001$), there is one instance where this is not the case - participant 11 for daily number of detected conversations. A population level analysis, or an unfiltered analysis would have obscured this outlier individual given the variability in distributions across each participant. Moreover participant 07, the same participant analysed previously (see Sect. 5.1), presents significant differences for each of these behavioral contexts; further strengthening the hypothesis that for this participant activities associated with sociability and social engagement have a marked influence on their self-reported EMAs.

Daily Number of Locations Visited: The following results are from 8 participant's who returned distributions for this behavioral context across all 10 EMAs.

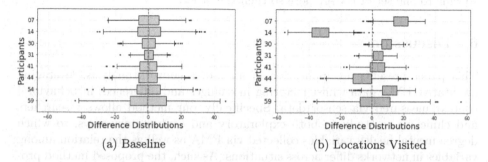

(a) Baseline

(b) Locations Visited

Fig. 7. Results across for **all 10 EMAs** for participants who only returned results for **Daily Number of Locations Visited**. Plot color varies depending on statistical significance when using pair-sampled t-testing to compare with the baseline distribution - blue if $p < 0.05$ otherwise plot remains grey. (Color figure online)

The side-by-side plots in Fig. 7a visualize both the baseline and behavioral context distributions for each valid participant, again, we observe statistical significance ($p < 0.05$) across each individual. Table 5 provides a numerical breakdown of these distributions.

Table 5. Results across for **all 10 EMAs** for participants who returned results for **Daily Number of Locations Visited**. Results include; mean ($\bar{x}$), standard deviation (σ), t-score (t), and p-value (p).

ID	Baseline		Daily Number of Locations Visited		
	$\bar{x}$	σ	$\bar{x}$	σ	t
07	−0.07	8.76	17.42	6.40	−55.33 *
14	0.44	10.28	−32.71	8.16	112.87 *
30	0.09	5.60	8.96	4.15	−56.95 *
31	0.10	4.43	3.80	4.39	−21.34 *
41	−0.03	7.84	3.34	7.14	−6.05 *
44	−0.09	8.21	−6.26	8.56	22.57 *
54	0.09	10.32	10.81	6.80	−35.19 *
59	0.13	16.00	1.54	13.96	−2.25 **

* $p < 0.001$, ** $p < 0.05$

As with previous behavioral contexts, the results presented in Table 5 further demonstrate the unique behavioral patterns of each participant. Whilst in certain participants we observe a reduced difference between distributions, participant 14 returns a significantly larger result ($t = 112.87$), suggesting that visiting locations outside of the home has an influence over how this individual reports their EMAs. Continued analysis of each behavioral context at a positive and negative EMA level would yield insights into whether or not this influence is specific to one set of EMAs more so then the other.

6 Discussion

This paper presents an application of an n-of-1 network analysis, leveraging qualitative EMA data whilst factoring in changes and differences in behavioral context measured via sensor data. Specifically, our method allows researchers and clinicians to study, in both exploratory and confirmatory ways, to which degree mental health variables collected via EMA as well as the relation among variables in networks differ across situations. As such, the proposed method provides an inroad to combining multimodal data sources in clinical research and practice, with the goal to enable the potential development of bespoke treatment/management pathways. As an example, the results produced in Fig. 4 reveal that, for this participant at least, not leaving the home significantly changes the way this person reports on his/her positive EMA questions. This new insight coupled with the structure of generated networks could give qualitative actionable information, enabling timely and adaptive interventions for this person's care going forward [34]. The next step from this approach will be to expand this methodology and to represent this information in a format this is comprehensible and explainable to the larger psychiatry community.

In summary, the task of how to meaningfully analyse multimodal behavioral sensor data with a complex array of concurrent qualitative self reported data is not well understood, particularly for SMI applications. In this analysis we demonstrate an n-of-1 network analysis approach applied solely to self-reported contextual behavioral data. Networks generated from these distinct periods of behavioral context reveal differences in self-reporting habits, differences beyond chance. This is a first stage indicative approach for datasets similar to Cross-Check which is computationally inexpensive, easily deployed and may lead to actionable clinical insights. However further studies are required to better understand how such insights can be utilized in practice, which are clinically effective but that are also compliant of ethical, regulator and legal requirements.

References

1. American Psychiatric Association, A., Association, A.P., et al.: Diagnostic and statistical manual of mental disorders: DSM-IV, vol. 4. American psychiatric association Washington, DC (1994)
2. American Psychiatric Association, D., Association, A.P., et al.: Diagnostic and statistical manual of mental disorders: DSM-5, vol. 5. American psychiatric association Washington, DC (2013)

3. Ascher-Svanum, H., et al.: The cost of relapse and the predictors of relapse in the treatment of schizophrenia. BMC Psychiatry **10**, 1–7 (2010)
4. Bak, M., Drukker, M., Hasmi, L., van Os, J.: An n= 1 clinical network analysis of symptoms and treatment in psychosis. PLoS ONE **11**(9), e0162811 (2016)
5. Barnett, I., Torous, J., Staples, P., Sandoval, L., Keshavan, M., Onnela, J.P.: Relapse prediction in schizophrenia through digital phenotyping: a pilot study. Neuropsychopharmacology **43**(8), 1660–1666 (2018)
6. Beard, C., Millner, A.J., Forgeard, M.J., Fried, E.I., Hsu, K.J., Treadway, M.T., Leonard, C.V., Kertz, S., Björgvinsson, T.: Network analysis of depression and anxiety symptom relationships in a psychiatric sample. Psychol. Med. **46**(16), 3359–3369 (2016)
7. Ben-Zeev, D., et al.: Crosscheck: integrating self-report, behavioral sensing, and smartphone use to identify digital indicators of psychotic relapse. Psychiatr. Rehabil. J. **40**(3), 266 (2017)
8. Benoit, J., Onyeaka, H., Keshavan, M., Torous, J.: Systematic review of digital phenotyping and machine learning in psychosis spectrum illnesses. Harv. Rev. Psychiatry **28**(5), 296–304 (2020)
9. Birchwood, M., Spencer, E., McGovern, D.: Schizophrenia: early warning signs. Adv. Psychiatr. Treat. **6**(2), 93–101 (2000)
10. Borsboom, D., et al.: Network analysis of multivariate data in psychological science. Nature Rev. Methods Primers **1**(1), 58 (2021)
11. Bradbury, J., Avila, C., Grace, S.: Practice-based research in complementary medicine: could n-of-1 trials become the new gold standard? In: Healthcare, vol. 8, p. 15. MDPI (2020)
12. Brown, L.A., et al.: Digital phenotyping to improve prediction of suicidal urges in treatment: study protocol. Aggress. Violent. Beh. **66**, 101733 (2022)
13. Canas, J.S., Gomez, F., Costilla-Reyes, O.: Counterfactual explanations and predictive models to enhance clinical decision-making in schizophrenia using digital phenotyping. arXiv preprint arXiv:2306.03980 (2023)
14. Chalmers, T.C., et al.: A method for assessing the quality of a randomized control trial. Control. Clin. Trials **2**(1), 31–49 (1981)
15. Chong, H.Y., Teoh, S.L., Wu, D.B.C., Kotirum, S., Chiou, C.F., Chaiyakunapruk, N.: Global economic burden of schizophrenia: a systematic review. Neuropsychiatric disease and treatment, pp. 357–373 (2016)
16. Davidson, B.I.: The crossroads of digital phenotyping. Gen. Hosp. Psychiatry **74**, 126–132 (2022)
17. Emsley, R., Chiliza, B., Asmal, L., Harvey, B.H.: The nature of relapse in schizophrenia. BMC Psychiatry **13**, 1–8 (2013)
18. Fisher, A.J., Medaglia, J.D., Jeronimus, B.F.: Lack of group-to-individual generalizability is a threat to human subjects research. Proc. Natl. Acad. Sci. **115**(27), E6106–E6115 (2018)
19. Fonseca-Pedrero, E., Al-Halabí, S., Pérez-Albéniz, A., Debbané, M.: Risk and protective factors in adolescent suicidal behaviour: a network analysis. Int. J. Environ. Res. Public Health **19**(3), 1784 (2022)
20. He-Yueya, J., Buck, B., Campbell, A., Choudhury, T., Kane, J.M., Ben-Zeev, D., Althoff, T.: Assessing the relationship between routine and schizophrenia symptoms with passively sensed measures of behavioral stability. NPJ Schizophr. **6**(1), 35 (2020)
21. Hevey, D.: Network analysis: a brief overview and tutorial. Health Psychol. Behav. Med. **6**(1), 301–328 (2018)

22. Insel, T.R.: Digital phenotyping: technology for a new science of behavior. JAMA **318**(13), 1215–1216 (2017)
23. Insel, T.R.: Digital phenotyping: a global tool for psychiatry. World Psychiatry **17**(3), 276 (2018)
24. Jacobson, N.C., Feng, B.: Digital phenotyping of generalized anxiety disorder: using artificial intelligence to accurately predict symptom severity using wearable sensors in daily life. Transl. Psychiatry **12**(1), 336 (2022)
25. Jacobson, N.C., Summers, B., Wilhelm, S.: Digital biomarkers of social anxiety severity: digital phenotyping using passive smartphone sensors. J. Med. Internet Res. **22**(5), e16875 (2020)
26. Kamath, J., Barriera, R.L., Jain, N., Keisari, E., Wang, B.: Digital phenotyping in depression diagnostics: Integrating psychiatric and engineering perspectives. World J. Psychiatry **12**(3), 393 (2022)
27. Lillie, E.O., Patay, B., Diamant, J., Issell, B., Topol, E.J., Schork, N.J.: The n-of-1 clinical trial: the ultimate strategy for individualizing medicine? Pers. Med. **8**(2), 161–173 (2011)
28. Van der Maaten, L., Hinton, G.: Visualizing data using t-sne. J. Mach. Learn. Res. **9**(11) (2008)
29. McCutcheon, R.A., Marques, T.R., Howes, O.D.: Schizophrenia-an overview. JAMA Psychiatry **77**(2), 201–210 (2020)
30. Melcher, J., Hays, R., Torous, J.: Digital phenotyping for mental health of college students: a clinical review. BMJ Ment Health **23**(4), 161–166 (2020)
31. Mohr, D.C., Shilton, K., Hotopf, M.: Digital phenotyping, behavioral sensing, or personal sensing: names and transparency in the digital age. NPJ Digital Med. **3**(1), 45 (2020)
32. Mohr, D.C., Zhang, M., Schueller, S.M.: Personal sensing: understanding mental health using ubiquitous sensors and machine learning. Annu. Rev. Clin. Psychol. **13**, 23–47 (2017)
33. Morriss, R., Vinjamuri, I., Faizal, M.A., Bolton, C.A., McCarthy, J.P.: Training to recognise the early signs of recurrence in schizophrenia. Cochrane Database of Systematic Reviews (2013)
34. Nahum-Shani, I., Smith, S.N., Spring, B.J., Collins, L.M., Witkiewitz, K., Tewari, A., Murphy, S.A.: Just-in-time adaptive interventions (JITAIs) in mobile health: key components and design principles for ongoing health behavior support. Ann. Behav. Med. **52**(6), 446–462 (2018)
35. National Collaborating Centre for Mental Health (UK and others): Psychosis and schizophrenia in adults: treatment and management. London: National Collaborating Centre for Mental Health (2014)
36. Onnela, J.P.: Opportunities and challenges in the collection and analysis of digital phenotyping data. Neuropsychopharmacology **46**(1), 45–54 (2021)
37. Patel, K.R., Cherian, J., Gohil, K., Atkinson, D.: Schizophrenia: overview and treatment options. Pharm. Ther. **39**(9), 638 (2014)
38. Perez-Pozuelo, I., Spathis, D., Clifton, E.A., Mascolo, C.: Wearables, smartphones, and artificial intelligence for digital phenotyping and health. In: Digital Health, pp. 33–54. Elsevier (2021)
39. Punja, S., Bukutu, C., Shamseer, L., Sampson, M., Hartling, L., Urichuk, L., Vohra, S.: N-of-1 trials are a tapestry of heterogeneity. J. Clin. Epidemiol. **76**, 47–56 (2016)
40. Rhemtulla, M., Fried, E.I., Aggen, S.H., Tuerlinckx, F., Kendler, K.S., Borsboom, D.: Network analysis of substance abuse and dependence symptoms. Drug Alcohol Depend. **161**, 230–237 (2016)

41. Saha, S., Chant, D., Welham, J., McGrath, J.: A systematic review of the prevalence of schizophrenia. PLoS Med. **2**(5), e141 (2005)
42. Silver, L.: Smartphone ownership is growing rapidly around the world, but not always equally (2019)
43. Torous, J., Kiang, M.V., Lorme, J., Onnela, J.P., et al.: New tools for new research in psychiatry: a scalable and customizable platform to empower data driven smartphone research. JMIR Mental Health **3**(2), e5165 (2016)
44. Wander, C.: Schizophrenia: opportunities to improve outcomes and reduce economic burden through managed care. Am. J. Manag. Care **26**, S62–S68 (2020)
45. Wang, R., et al.: Crosscheck: toward passive sensing and detection of mental health changes in people with schizophrenia. In: 2016 ACM Int. Joint Conf. Pervasive & Ubiquitous Comput., pp. 886–897 (2016)
46. Wang, R., et al.: Predicting symptom trajectories of schizophrenia using mobile sensing. Proc. ACM Interact. Mob. Wearable Ubiquitous Technol. **1**(3), 1–24 (2017)
47. Wang, W., et al.: Social sensing: assessing social functioning of patients living with schizophrenia using mobile phone sensing. In: Proceedings of the 2020 CHI Conference on Human Factors in Computing Systems, pp. 1–15 (2020)

Baseline User Calibration for Cold-Start Model Personalization in Mental State Estimation

Jaakko Tervonen[1]($\boxtimes$), Rajdeep Kumar Nath[2], Kati Pettersson[1], Johanna Närväinen[2], and Jani Mäntyjärvi[3]

[1] VTT Technical Research Centre of Finland, Tekniikantie 1, Espoo, Finland
{jaakko.tervonen,kati.pettersson}@vtt.fi
[2] VTT Technical Research Centre of Finland, Microkatu 1, Kuopio, Finland
{rajdeep.nath,johanna.narvainen}@vtt.fi
[3] VTT Technical Research Centre of Finland, Kaitoväylä 1, Oulu, Finland
jani.mantyjarvi@vtt.fi

Abstract. Robust human state detection based on analysis of physiological signals requires model personalization since physiological reactions are individual. Personalization requires prior information, which is not available for a new, unknown person, i.e. in a cold-start. To overcome this, the current study proposes user calibration, which uses easily obtainable short baseline measurements to normalize physiological variables individually. Experiments were conducted on a cognitive load detection use case to determine effectiveness of the approach, required baseline duration, and the most suitable normalization function. In addition, the behavior of the model was analyzed with Shapley additive explanations to assess its trustworthiness. The results showed that user calibration always beat the non-personalized model, the optimal baseline duration was 3–3.5 min, and there were no differences between the different normalization functions. The model paid the greatest attention to the physiological phenomena found to be indicative of cognitive load in previous studies. The results encourage further evaluation of user calibration in different use cases for smart healthcare.

Keywords: cold-start · physiology · cognitive load · personalization

1 Introduction

Recent advances in sensor technology have enabled pervasive monitoring of people's physiology, which facilitates real-time detection of stress, and mental and cognitive state of the user, to name a few. Knowledge of the user's state can be utilized in the design and implementation of novel interactive applications

The work was funded by VTT and the Academy of Finland under GrantNos: 334092, 351282, 355693.

aiming to improve user health, wellbeing, and performance. For example, a virtual physiotherapist could detect person's activities to assist in physical rehabilitation, detected stress or emotional state could trigger interaction in mental coaching or when recovering from a trauma, measuring alertness or drowsiness with interventions could help if a person has trouble sleeping, and the detected states could be used in clinical decision support as additional information.

To unlock the full potential of these applications, they should work automatically, close to real-time, and adapt to each individual, even new, unknown ones. One major drawback in current state detection approaches is that they fail to properly account for individual differences especially in a cold-start scenario. Basic physiology, reactions to external stimuli and perceptions of varying situations are individual-specific, which should be accounted for in the modelling procedure: the detection model should be personalized. Typically, the physiological features used for state detection are normalized participant-wise, using a whole dataset from each person to do so. This solution accounts for the differences in individual baselines and individual reactions to the different stimuli. However, applying it requires a complete set of data from each participant before the developed model can be applied for them. When a new user starts using the system, i.e. a cold-start occurs, completing a lengthy calibration protocol with different stimuli is burdening for them and may lead to demotivation and even giving up with the system before even properly beginning.

The current study investigates the cold-start problem in the context of cognitive load detection. Monitoring cognitive load is important in safety-critical fields such as flight control, and healthcare professionals working e.g. in the emergency room or the first aid unit, but also in everyday life like driving a vehicle, and in training and education applications for improved learning. It may also help in detecting early signs of cognitive impairments. Furthermore, it has been suggested that cognitive load of medical professionals should be monitored when considering the use of artificial intelligence assisted decision making tools in healthcare [8].

Specifically, using a few minutes of baseline data for model personalization is proposed. Different normalization functions and baseline durations are investigated, and self-reported cognitive load is detected as a continuous variable with a regression model. Additionally, model behavior is explained with a feature contribution analysis with SHAP values. The approach is evaluated on an open-source dataset ADABase [23] having several physiological signals measured in a controlled laboratory protocol consisting of simulated driving and n-back tasks. Such a dataset offers clear signals and tasks which likely results with a rather high cognitive load, making it suitable for the first evaluation of the proposed approach. The main contributions of the study are listed as follows:

- Different normalization strategies are evaluated to use short baseline period for cold-start model personalization in detecting continuous cognitive load.
- Minimal baseline duration for optimal performance is estimated.
- Feature importance and contribution analysis is provided to assess which factors increase and decrease experienced cognitive load.

2   Related Work

2.1   Methods in Cognitive Load Detection

Cognitive load or mental workload refers to the amount of mental resources used to perform a task [24]. Several approaches to measure cognitive load as a continuous variable exist, like self-report questionnaires (e.g. the NASA-TLX [13]), performance measures of cognivitely demanding tasks [30], and physiological triggers, since cognitive load is reflected to e.g. pupillary responses [36,38], heart rate variability [7,28], electrodermal activity [34,35], and facial expressions [16,41]. The link between cognitive load and physiology has led to the development of automated tools to detect cognitive load based on (wearable) sensor data. Figure 1 shows a general machine learning pipeline for the detection task based on sensor data processing.

Previous works attempting cognitive load detection with machine learning methods have primarily focused on a classification setup. Most works have detected high cognitive load from low or no load [3,9,32,37] while some have had three or more levels based on estimated difficulty of the task [18,19]. Although cognitive load can be considered a continuous measure and treating it as a continuous variable allows for a more fine grained analysis, few works attempt to detect it with a regression model. Herbig *et al.* [14,15] have recognized cognitive load in an e-learning and a machine translation task. Pejović *et al.* [25] developed a non-contact sensor to detect cognitive load during elementary cognitive tasks. Lastly, Oppelt *et al.* [23], who introduced the dataset used for experiments in this study, presented results also for regression modelling. Each work selected self-reported cognitive load as the regression target.

2.2   Cold-Start Model Personalization

Baseline physiology, physiological reactions and task perception are individual, which calls for model personalization when detecting cognitive load. Still, several previous studies aim for fully person-independent detection [3,9,19]. When personalization was considered, the most prevalent approach has been some version of participant-wise feature normalization, used in e.g. [14,15,25,32], which normalizes features separately for each person using their full dataset. In addition, it was the only personalization approach considered in a contest to detect cognitive load from wearable sensor data, applied by 5 teams from 12 [11]. Other

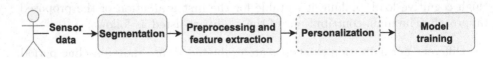

Fig. 1. A machine learning pipeline generally used for training a state detection model. Personalization is not always included, which is depicted with a dashed box and it can overlap with either preprocessing or model training.

personalization approaches include e.g. custom domain adaptation [17], where a transfer learning approach adapts the neural network to each individual. In a related context of stress detection, users have been clustered first to train the model based on similar users' data [39].

Each of these approaches require a substantial amount of data from each user, most of them a full set similar to that of the users in the training data. In a cold-start case, such data is not available, and the developed model is unapplicable for new users.

To the best of our knowledge, no earlier studies exist in cognitive load detection addressing this challenge. However, in emotion recognition, Saganowski *et al.* [27] proposed to apply transfer learning with accumulating data in real-life scenario, and in stress detection, participant-wise feature normalization has been implemented with just the baseline data [1,26]. A similar approach for stress and affect detection was examined in [31] who also analyzed the duration of baseline measurement needed. In neuroscientific research, eliminating the individual variations with baseline data is a standard procedure [20].

To set the current study apart from related work the following differences are outlined: i) continuous cognitive load is detected with a regression model as opposed to classification, ii) cold-start is addressed by personalizing based on short baseline measurement, iii) different baseline durations and normalization functions are evaluated.

3   Methodology

3.1   User Calibration

In general terms, a normalization function transforms given input data according to some normalization parameters into a representation that is better suited for a machine learning model. The normalization parameters should be computed from the training and applied for the testing data but the same parameters are used for both splits of the dataset.

In participant-wise scaling, the normalization parameters are computed separately for each participant from a full measurement protocol. Instead, the parameters could be computed from a short baseline measurement, called user calibration in this study, and applied for all subsequent data from that person. In a real-life use case, a new person should sit still and relax for a couple of minutes, allowing the collection of baseline data, which is a much less burdening option than completing the whole protocol. Figure 2 highlights the differences in the inference process between regular personalization and user calibration.

Three normalization functions are applied in this study: averaging $X_{avg} = X - mean(X)$, standard scaling $X_{std} = X_{avg}/std(X)$ and min-max transformation $X_{minmax} = \frac{X-min(X)}{max(X)-min(X)}$, for a dataset X. In participant-wise scaling, the normalization parameters (mean, std, min, max) are computed separately for each participant across the whole measurement protocol, and in user calibration they are computed separately for each participant from short baseline measurement of varying duration.

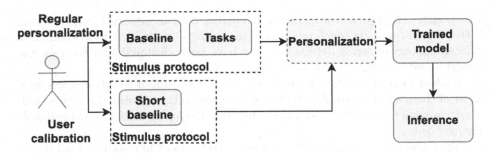

Fig. 2. The cold-start process for mental state estimation of a new user in inference mode. The boxes tagged "Stimulus protocol" display the tasks to be completed before the trained model can be personalized and applied for inferring the state of the user.

3.2 Dataset

The ADABase dataset [23] was adopted for the cognitive load detection experiments. The dataset consists of two tasks aimed at inducing cognitive load: the n-back task and a simulated driving task called k-drive. Simulators and standard cognitive tests provide a controllable and quantifiable environment and thus the induced cognitive states are more homogeneous. Thus, the dataset comprises a good basis to study algorithm development for the cold-start case.

An n-back task consists of a sequence of stimuli and the study participant must indicate when the current stimulus matches the one presented n steps earlier. The n-back task conducted in ADABase consisted of a single (visual stimulus) and a dual stimuli (visual and auditive stimuli) test with three difficulty levels (i.e. $n \in \{1, 2, 3\}$). The k-drive task consisted of watching an autonomous simulator playing a driving game and indicating, on three difficulty levels, whether the car was 1) passing another car, 2) being overtaken, or 3) accelerating or decelerating rapidly; each level was incremental and in each subsequent level the participant had to indicate the events of the previous level(s) as well. Additionally, the participant solved a secondary task of searching and adding songs to a playlist during levels 2 and 3.

The test participants' physiology was monitored with a Biopac MP160 system measuring electrocardiogram (ECG), electromyogram (EMG, trapezius muscle), electrodermal activity (EDA), respiration (RSP), skin temperature (SKT) and photoplethysmogram (PPG). In addition, video-oculography (VOG) was recorded with Tobii Pro Fusion and facial cues with a BASLER camera.

The published version of dataset contains 30 participants, 12 of whom refused the collection of facial video data. The order of n-back and k-drive was randomized, and in the public version 18 participants first completed the n-back task. The measurement set-up was the same for all participants, but it was adjusted for handedness and the time of day varied. The baseline measurement used in this study for user calibration is taken from the resting baseline that occurred before the first stimulus, whether it was n-back or k-drive.

Cognitive load was assessed after each phase of the protocol with the NASA-TLX self-report questionnaire, assessing mental, physical and temporal demand, performance, effort and frustration. Each dimension has a weighting factor to compute the final score as a sum of weighted self-report components. This final score serves as the metric for cognitive load in this study. The authors in the original paper [23] suggest transforming the score individually to a value between 0 and 1 through min-max normalisation. Since this transformation is impossible in a cold-start scenario, it was decided to opt for the unscaled metric in this study.

3.3 Data Processing

Features were extracted from each of the available data sources except for the PPG signal, which was thought redundant since ECG was available. Following the original paper [23], features were extracted with a sliding window of two minutes with a five second window slide. The physiological signals were mostly processed using the NeuroKit2 software package [22], but the heart rate variability features were extracted with the hrv-analysis library [4] and saccades, fixations, and blinks were detected from the VOG data with the PyGaze library [6]. The sum of frames with each facial activation was used as the features for the facial data; see [23] for a description of the activation units. The rest of the extracted features are listed in Table 1.

Table 1. Extracted features from each signal.

Signal	Extracted features
ECG	mean_HR, std_HR, mean_nni, sdnn, nni50, pnni50, rmssd, vlf_power, lf_power, hf_power, lf/hf ratio, total power, lfnu, hfnu, vlf_relative_power, lf_relative_power, hf_relative_power
EMG	rms, n_onsets, fraction_high_activity, max_amplitude
EDA	eda_mean, eda_std, eda_min, eda_max,eda_ slope, eda_range, tonic_mean, tonic_std, tonic_correlation_with_time, phasic_n_peaks, phasic_peak_amplitude, phasic_peak_duration, phasic_peak_area
RSP	breathing_rate_mean, breathing_rate_std, phase_ratio_mean
SKT	skt_mean, skt_std, skt_min, skt_max, skt_slope
VOG	pupil_diam_mean, pupil_diam_std, pupil_diam_slope, blink_rate, blink_duration, time_between_blinks, fix_rate, fix_duration, time_between_fix, n_fix_with_dur_>100ms, n_fix_with_dur_66-150ms, n_fix_with_dur_300-500ms, n_fix_with_dur_>1000ms, sac_rate, sac_duration, time_between_sac, sac_amplitude

ECG = electrocardiogram,   EMG = electromyogram,   EDA = electrodermal activity,   RSP = respiration,   SKT = skin   temperature,   VOG = video-oculography, diam = diameter, fix = fixations, sac = saccades

3.4 Experimental Protocol

The extracted features were used to detect cognitive load as a continuous variable using extreme gradient boosting regressor (XGBoost) [5]. The regressor was selected since extreme gradient boosting has been shown to have good performance in different domains with tabular data, and since it natively handles missing data which is prevalent in the current dataset due to some participants opting out from facial data collection.

The k-drive tasks had a duration of about five minutes and so the experienced cognitive load may have varied over the course of the task. Still, subjective ratings were given only after the task. To ensure that the physiological data is timely and best reflects the given rating, only the last two minute window from each task was used for training the model. This choice has also a balancing effect between the two task types, as the n-back tasks lasted for about two minutes.

Following the original paper [23], the adopted cross-validation strategy was leave-three-users-out, resulting in 10 folds total. For each fold, the data of three randomly selected participants was left out and the model was trained with the remaining participants data and tested on the left out fold. The model performance was assessed in terms of mean absolute error (MAE), mean squared error (MSE) and root mean squared error (RMSE). The performance was compared against a baseline of predicting the average cognitive load for each observation.

Three modelling tasks were defined: i) without feature normalization; ii) with participant-wise feature normalization; and iii) user calibration. The evaluation without feature normalization sets a baseline which user calibration should try and exceed to be useful, and participant-wise feature normalization sets an upper limit of what to expect with normalization-based personalization approaches.

In addition, the duration of the needed baseline measurement was evaluated by training the user calibration model with varying duration of baseline data, ranging from two to five minutes in 30 s increments. Shorter than two minute calibration was not considered since the used feature window length was two minutes. Moreover, three different normalization functions as specified in Sect. 3.1 were experimented with.

The statistical significance of the differences between the personalization and normalization approaches were assessed with related samples T-test, since the cross-validation errors were found to be normally distributed (Shapiro-Wilk test). P-values were corrected with the Benjamini-Hochberg method to adjust the false discovery rate for multiple testing.

4 Results

User calibration performed better than the general and the average prediction model with each normalization function tested (see Table 2) and the difference was statistically significant (Table 3). As expected, participant-wise scaling performed better than user calibration when features were normalized with standard scaling or min-max normalisation, but the two approaches performed the same when features were averaged. No statistically significant differences between the

Table 2. Regression results of predicting subjective cognitive load. Dur stands for best calibration duration in minutes.

Normalization	Personalization	Dur	MAE	MSE	RMSE
Standard scaling	Participant-wise	–	8.20 (1.12)	107.57 (31.86)	10.27 (1.47)
	Calibration	3.0	10.09 (1.69)	148.26 (51.37)	12.01 (2.02)
Averaging	Participant-wise	–	9.93 (1.34)	147.27 (42.49)	12.01 (1.72)
	Calibration	3.5	9.72 (1.54)	136.89 (35.87)	11.60 (1.56)
Min-Max	Participant-wise	–	8.57 (1.75)	114.74 (41.81)	10.52 (2.02)
	Calibration	3.5	9.78 (1.74)	146.99 (47.09)	11.95 (2.05)
No scaling	General model	–	11.03 (1.80)	175.80 (51.65)	13.11 (2.01)
Average prediction	General model	–	10.99 (1.38)	160.78 (34.89)	12.60 (1.42)

Table 3. Related samples T-test results of comparing the MAE's of the user calibration model to those of other models'. P-values were corrected with the Benjamini-Hochberg method.

Normalization	Participant-wise		No scaling		Average prediction	
	T	p	T	p	T	p
Standard scaling	−3.08	0.020	2.49	0.039	−21.64	<0.001
Averaging	0.52	0.618	3.69	0.011	−22.08	<0.001
Min-Max	−2.74	0.029	3.49	0.012	−20.67	<0.001

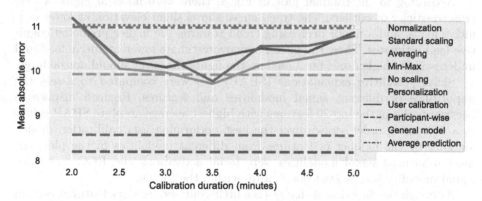

Fig. 3. Model performance at different durations of baseline measurement. The line colors refer to the normalization approach and line style to personalization approach.

three normalization functions when using user calibration were observed (test results not shown). The non-personalized model performed similarly to average prediction.

Figure 3 shows the MAE of user calibration with different baseline durations: a MAE of e.g. 10 would denote that an error of 10 units was made on average

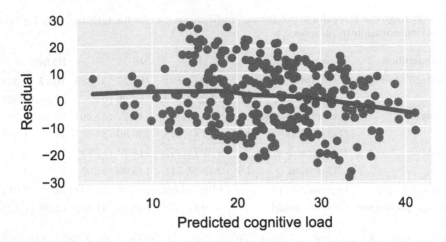

Fig. 4. Scatter plot of model residuals vs. predictions with a LOWESS trend curve, produced over test data folds of the best performing user calibration model with 3.5 min baseline with features normalized with averaging.

when predicting the load. The best performance was observed with 3 min baseline duration with standard scaling, and 3.5 min with averaging and min-max normalization. However, the differences between the different durations were not large.

According to the residual plot in Fig. 4, there were no clear signs of heteroscedasticity or outliers. The trend curve shows slight elevation at lower cognitive loads, and a minor decreasing trend towards the higher predicted cognitive load estimates. Thus, the model may overestimate lower cognitive load and underestimate higher one, but based on the figure the effect should not be large.

Shapley additive explanations (SHAP) [21] were computed to assess the importance of different signal modalities and features. Figure 5 displays a beeswarm plot of the top-20 features with highest average absolute SHAP values in a decreasing order, drawn over the best performing user calibration model. Judging by the number of features from different modalities in the plot, the most influential signal modalities were facial activations and ECG, and each signal modality had at least one feature within the top-20.

Although the direction of changes is a little confused for some features, certain conclusions can be made from the figure. The most influential feature was mean pupil diameter, with its higher values corresponding to higher cognitive load, and vice versa for lower values. Lower/higher values in AU20 (lip stretcher), AU25 (lip part), and AU05 (upper lid raiser) corresponded to lower/higher cognitive load, respectively. Moreover, higher skin temperature, variation in breathing rate, blink duration, trapezoidal EMG activity, and electrodermal activity, and lower heart rate variability all corresponded to higher cognitive load, according to the developed model. These are roughly in line with previous observations [2,7,35,36] but there was mixed evidence of skin temperature and respiration changes under cognitive load [10,12,34].

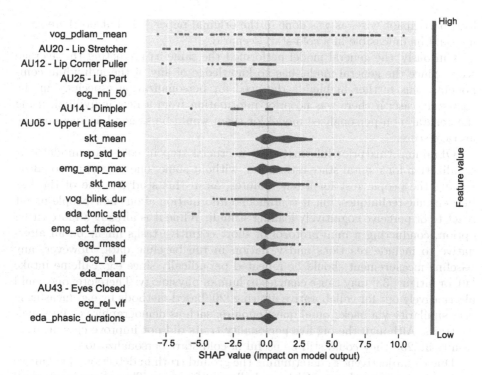

Fig. 5. Beeswarm plot of the SHAP values of the features in the user calibration model with 3.5 min baseline with features normalized with averaging.

5 Discussion

The presented analysis proved the usefulness of user calibration, since it always outperformed the general model regardless of the choice of the normalization function. Thus, collecting 3–3.5 min of baseline resting data from a new user allows making better predictions since the beginning. The proposed approach has some limitations which form the ground for future work: it only captures individual differences at the level of basic physiology, determining the correct ground truth is challenging, the used dataset was collected in a constrained environment with a large set of physiological signals, and only one modelling approach was evaluated. Each of these points are further discussed next.

The data collection protocol exhibited individual variations in three levels: basic physiology, reactions to stimuli, and self-reporting. The basic physiology between the participants differed, which was up to some extent caught by user calibration. Different people react in different ways to similar external stimuli, which in turn was caught by participant-wise normalization. Finally, different people may experience the same task in various ways: some see the task demanding while others find it enjoyable, which is reflected in the subjective reports. Such information could be included in the model by normalizing the reported load participant-wise, as was done in the original paper [23], but not here since it would be unfeasible in a cold-start scenario.

Curiously, the general model performed the same as predicting the average score. Since the general model has no knowledge of any of the individual components, this further highlights the need for personalization especially in the cold-start case: if there was no prior information from a new individual, using the general, non-personalized model for them would be as good as guessing the average score.

Obtaining this prior information is a crucial step in cold-start model personalization for mental state estimation: without some, one cannot personalize. Having the people rest for a few minutes, as in this study, is one of the less burdensome techniques, but it contains no information about how people might react to or perceive cognitively loading stimuli. While it is already a more tiring option, conducting a mini-protocol of short cognitive tasks might be an alternative to include reactions and variation in the baseline data. However, any baseline measurement should be repeated periodically since e.g. caffeine intake [40] or fatigue [33] may cause changes to human physiology. Therefore, one could alternatively opt for collaborative filtering [29] based methods by e.g. measuring user similarity via background questionnaire, such as demographics or personality traits. Although the big five personality traits did not improve classification results in [23], they could still be useful in cold-start personalization.

Due to subjectiveness, determining the ground truth in detection of cognitive load and other mental states is also a challenge of its own. The current study used non-normalized cognitive load self-reports as labels for a regression model. One could also choose to normalize the labels participant-wise (not feasible in a cold-start scenario) or choose to classify between self-reported low/medium/high load or even classify based on task labels. The latest would be an objective measure when looking at the data labelling, but still physiology would reflect subjective load and some people might not experience cognitive load in tasks labelled under high load. Ultimately the choice of the ground truth comes down to the targeted use case: what is most sensible given the context? The target used in the current study is suitable for applications where the interest is in subtle subjective changes in cognitive load. A continuous target and regression analysis applies to a more (time-wise) continuous modelling and allows developing methods to detect moments when the person is just heading towards cognitive overload, unlike classification, which provides a more definite outcome.

The dataset used in this study contained a simulated driving task and the n-back task conducted in a controlled laboratory environment. Since this was the first inspection of cold-start model personalization in cognitive load detection, such dataset with clear and likely high cognitive load periods was chosen to be able to focus on the cold-start issue. Since the results were encouraging, the method should be evaluated next on different datasets from the health domain to improve its ecological validity.

While some features showed a rather clear behavior pattern in Fig. 5, like pupil diameter and skin temperature, the behavior of other features, such as

RMSSD and maximum amplitude of EMG, was more convoluted. Here, too, there may be some individual differences. Indeed, several features are clustered around zero, meaning that for those observations the current feature had a small impact, and long tail(s) denoting observations for which the current feature had a larger impact. However, the coloring of e.g. RMSSD and EMG_max_amplitude show that higher values were related to both decreased and increased cognitive load. These may be related to some spurious events during the completion of the task, changing of cognitive load during the two-minute window, or the relation between self-reports and some physiological parameters may be unsystematic.

Investigation and understanding this relationship and finding features with systematic behavior under varying cognitive load is a necessity for robust cognitive load detection. To keep focus on user calibration and normalization options, this analysis is left for future work, together with finding the best type of a model, hyperparameter optimization, feature window duration optimization, feature selection, and signal modality selection, all of which are important steps to consider in model development. Based on Fig. 4, the developed model fit to the data reasonably well, but the described steps may help in improving the model performance.

6   Conclusions

Overcoming the cold-start situation in model personalization is a necessity for future human state detection applications. In this study, using short baseline measurements to normalize features was proposed as the solution in detecting continuous cognitive load. The experiments showed that user calibration always performed better than the general model but worse than a model with participant-wise normalization with full dataset. The optimal baseline duration was found to be 3–3.5 min and there were no differences between the tested normalization functions. A SHAP feature importance analysis revealed that the developed model found physiologically correct patterns, increasing trust to it. Future studies are needed for different mental states to further validate the proposed user calibration approach.

References

1. Albaladejo-González, M., Ruipérez-Valiente, J.A., Gómez Mármol, F.: Evaluating different configurations of machine learning models and their transfer learning capabilities for stress detection using heart rate. J. Ambient. Intell. Humaniz. Comput. (2022). https://doi.org/10.1007/s12652-022-04365-z
2. Biondi, F.N., Cacanindin, A., Douglas, C., Cort, J.: Overloaded and at work: investigating the effect of cognitive workload on assembly task performance. Hum. Factors **63**(5), 813–820 (2021). https://doi.org/10.1177/0018720820929928
3. Bozkir, E., Geisler, D., Kasneci, E.: Person independent, privacy preserving, and real time assessment of cognitive load using eye tracking in a virtual reality setup. In: 2019 IEEE Conference on Virtual Reality and 3D User Interfaces (VR), pp. 1834–1837 (2019). https://doi.org/10.1109/VR.2019.8797758

4. Champseix, R.: Heart Rate Variability analysis (2018). https://github.com/Aura-healthcare/hrv-analysis. Accessed 20 June 2023
5. Chen, T., Guestrin, C.: XGBoost: a scalable tree boosting system. In: Proceedings of the 22nd ACM SIGKDD International Conference on Knowledge Discovery and Data Mining, vol. 19, pp. 785–794. ACM, New York, NY, USA, August 2016. https://doi.org/10.1145/2939672.2939785, https://dl.acm.org/doi/10.1145/2939672.2939785
6. Dalmaijer, E.S., Mathôt, S., Van der Stigchel, S.: Pygaze: an open-source, cross-platform toolbox for minimal-effort programming of eyetracking experiments. Behav. Res. Methods **46**(4), 913–921 (2014). https://doi.org/10.3758/s13428-013-0422-2
7. Delliaux, S., Delaforge, A., Deharo, J.C., Chaumet, G.: Mental workload alters heart rate variability, lowering non-linear dynamics. Front. Physiol. **10** (2019). https://doi.org/10.3389/fphys.2019.00565
8. Ehrmann, D.E., et al.: Evaluating and reducing cognitive load should be a priority for machine learning in healthcare. Nat. Med. **28**(7), 1331–1333 (2022). https://doi.org/10.1038/s41591-022-01833-z
9. Feradov, F., Ganchev, T., Markova, V.: Automated detection of cognitive load from peripheral physiological signals based on Hjorth's parameters. In: 2020 International Conference on Biomedical Innovations and Applications (BIA), pp. 85–88 (2020). https://doi.org/10.1109/BIA50171.2020.9244287
10. Gjoreski, M., et al.: Datasets for cognitive load inference using wearable sensors and psychological traits. Appl. Sci. **10**(11) (2020). https://doi.org/10.3390/app10113843
11. Gjoreski, M., et al.: Cognitive load monitoring with wearables-lessons learned from a machine learning challenge. IEEE Access **9**, 103325–103336 (2021). https://doi.org/10.1109/ACCESS.2021.3093216
12. Grassmann, M., Vlemincx, E., von Leupoldt, A., Mittelstädt, J.M., Van den Bergh, O.: Respiratory changes in response to cognitive load: a systematic review. Neural Plast. **2016**, 8146809 (2016). https://doi.org/10.1155/2016/8146809
13. Hart, S.G., Staveland, L.E.: Development of NASA-TLX (task load index): results of empirical and theoretical research. In: Hancock, P.A., Meshkati, N. (eds.) Human Mental Workload, Advances in Psychology, vol. 52, pp. 139–183. North-Holland (1988). https://doi.org/10.1016/S0166-4115(08)62386-9
14. Herbig, N., et al.: Investigating multi-modal measures for cognitive load detection in e-learning. In: Proceedings of the 28th ACM Conference on User Modeling, Adaptation and Personalization. UMAP '20, pp. 88–97. Association for Computing Machinery, New York, NY, USA (2020). https://doi.org/10.1145/3340631.3394861
15. Herbig, N., Pal, S., Vela, M., Krüger, A., van Genabith, J.: Multi-modal indicators for estimating perceived cognitive load in post-editing of machine translation. Mach. Transl. **33**(1), 91–115 (2019). https://doi.org/10.1007/s10590-019-09227-8
16. Hussain, M.S., Calvo, R.A., Chen, F.: Automatic cognitive load detection from face, physiology, task performance and fusion during affective interference. Interact. Comput. **26**(3), 256–268 (2013). https://doi.org/10.1093/iwc/iwt032
17. Jiménez-Guarneros, M., Gómez-Gil, P.: Custom domain adaptation: a new method for cross-subject, EEG-based cognitive load recognition. IEEE Sig. Process. Lett. **27**, 750–754 (2020). https://doi.org/10.1109/LSP.2020.2989663
18. Khanam, F., Hossain, A.A., Ahmad, M.: Electroencephalogram-based cognitive load level classification using wavelet decomposition and support vector machine. Brain-Comput. Interfaces **10**(1), 1–15 (2023). https://doi.org/10.1080/2326263X.2022.2109855

19. Li, Y., Li, K., Wang, S., Li, Y., Chen, J., Wen, D.: Towards safer flights: a multi-modality fusion technology-based cognitive load recognition framework. In: 2022 IEEE 4th International Conference on Civil Aviation Safety and Information Technology (ICCASIT), pp. 525–530 (2022). https://doi.org/10.1109/ICCASIT55263.2022.9986937
20. Luck, S.J.: An Introduction to the Event-Related Potential Technique. MIT Press, Cambridge (2014)
21. Lundberg, S.M., Lee, S.I.: A unified approach to interpreting model predictions. In: Proceedings of the 31st International Conference on Neural Information Processing Systems. NIPS'17, pp. 4768–4777. Curran Associates Inc., Red Hook, NY, USA (2017). https://doi.org/10.5555/3295222.3295230
22. Makowski, D., et al.: NeuroKit2: a Python toolbox for neurophysiological signal processing. Behav. Res. Methods 53(4), 1689–1696 (2021). https://doi.org/10.3758/s13428-020-01516-y
23. Oppelt, M.P., et al.: Adabase: a multimodal dataset for cognitive load estimation. Sensors 23(1) (2023). https://doi.org/10.3390/s23010340
24. Orru, G., Longo, L.: The evolution of cognitive load theory and the measurement of its intrinsic, extraneous and germane loads: a review. In: Longo, L., Leva, M.C. (eds.) H-WORKLOAD 2018. CCIS, vol. 1012, pp. 23–48. Springer, Cham (2019). https://doi.org/10.1007/978-3-030-14273-5_3
25. Pejović, V., Matkovič, T., Ciglarič, M.: Wireless ranging for contactless cognitive load inference in ubiquitous computing. Int. J. Hum.-Comput. Interact. 37(19), 1849–1873 (2021). https://doi.org/10.1080/10447318.2021.1913860
26. Prajod, P., André, E.: On the generalizability of ECG-based stress detection models. In: 2022 21st IEEE International Conference on Machine Learning and Applications (ICMLA), pp. 549–554 (2022). https://doi.org/10.1109/ICMLA55696.2022.00090
27. Saganowski, S., Kunc, D., Perz, B., Komoszyńska, J., Behnke, M., Kazienko, P.: The cold start problem and per-group personalization in real-life emotion recognition with wearables. In: 2022 IEEE International Conference on Pervasive Computing and Communications Workshops and other Affiliated Events (PerCom Workshops), pp. 812–817 (2022). https://doi.org/10.1109/PerComWorkshops53856.2022.9767233
28. Solhjoo, S., et al.: Heart rate and heart rate variability correlate with clinical reasoning performance and self-reported measures of cognitive load. Sci. Rep. 9(1), 14668 (2019). https://doi.org/10.1038/s41598-019-50280-3
29. Su, X., Khoshgoftaar, T.M.: A survey of collaborative filtering techniques. Adv. Artif. Intell. 2009, 421425 (2009). https://doi.org/10.1155/2009/421425
30. Sweller, J., Ayres, P., Kalyuga, S.: Measuring Cognitive Load, pp. 71–85. Springer, New York (2011). https://doi.org/10.1007/978-1-4419-8126-4_6
31. Tervonen, J., Nath, R.K., Pettersson, K., Närväinen, J., Mäntyjärvi, J.: Cold-start model adaptation: evaluation of short baseline calibration. In: Adjunct Proceedings of the 2023 ACM International Joint Conference on Pervasive and Ubiquitous Computing and the 2023 ACM International Symposium on Wearable Computing. UbiComp/ISWC '23 Adjunct, pp. 417–422. Association for Computing Machinery, New York, NY, USA (2023). https://doi.org/10.1145/3594739.3610731
32. Tervonen, J., Pettersson, K., Mäntyjärvi, J.: Ultra-short window length and feature importance analysis for cognitive load detection from wearable sensors. Electronics 10(5) (2021). https://doi.org/10.3390/electronics10050613

33. Tran, Y., Wijesuriya, N., Tarvainen, M., Karjalainen, P., Craig, A.: The relationship between spectral changes in heart rate variability and fatigue. J. Psychophysiol. **23**(3), 143–151 (2009). https://doi.org/10.1027/0269-8803.23.3.143
34. Vanneste, P., et al.: Towards measuring cognitive load through multimodal physiological data. Cogn. Technol. Work **23**(3), 567–585 (2021). https://doi.org/10.1007/s10111-020-00641-0
35. Visnovcova, Z., Mestanik, M., Gala, M., Mestanikova, A., Tonhajzerova, I.: The complexity of electrodermal activity is altered in mental cognitive stressors. Comput. Biol. Med. **79**, 123–129 (2016). https://doi.org/10.1016/j.compbiomed.2016.10.014
36. Volden, F., De Alwis Edirisinghe, V., Fostervold, K.-I.: Human gaze-parameters as an indicator of mental workload. In: Bagnara, S., Tartaglia, R., Albolino, S., Alexander, T., Fujita, Y. (eds.) IEA 2018. AISC, vol. 827, pp. 209–215. Springer, Cham (2019). https://doi.org/10.1007/978-3-319-96059-3_23
37. Wu, C., Liu, Y., Guo, X., Zhu, T., Bao, Z.: Enhancing the feasibility of cognitive load recognition in remote learning using physiological measures and an adaptive feature recalibration convolutional neural network. Med. Biol. Eng. Comput. **60**(12), 3447–3460 (2022). https://doi.org/10.1007/s11517-022-02670-5
38. Xu, J., Wang, Y., Chen, F., Choi, E.: Pupillary response based cognitive workload measurement under luminance changes. In: Campos, P., Graham, N., Jorge, J., Nunes, N., Palanque, P., Winckler, M. (eds.) INTERACT 2011. LNCS, vol. 6947, pp. 178–185. Springer, Heidelberg (2011). https://doi.org/10.1007/978-3-642-23771-3_14
39. Xu, Q., Nwe, T.L., Guan, C.: Cluster-based analysis for personalized stress evaluation using physiological signals. IEEE J. Biomed. Health Inform. **19**(1), 275–281 (2015). https://doi.org/10.1109/JBHI.2014.2311044
40. Yeragani, V.K., Krishnan, S., Engels, H.J., Gretebeck, R.: Effects of caffeine on linear and nonlinear measures of heart rate variability before and after exercise. Depress. Anxiety **21**(3), 130–134 (2005). https://doi.org/10.1002/da.20061
41. Yüce, A., Gao, H., Cuendet, G.L., Thiran, J.P.: Action units and their cross-correlations for prediction of cognitive load during driving. IEEE Trans. Affect. Comput. **8**(2), 161–175 (2017). https://doi.org/10.1109/TAFFC.2016.2584042

Privacy, Ethics and Regulations

Investigating AI in Medical Devices: The Need for Better Establishment of Risk-Assessment and Regulatory Foundations

Sandra Baum[1] and Konstantinos Manikas[1,2]([✉])

[1] Computer Science Department, IT -University of Copenhagen, Rued Langgaards Vej 7, 2300 Copenhagen, Denmark
{sanb,koma}@itu.dk
[2] Accenture Consulting, Bohrsgade 35, 1799 Copenhagen V, Denmark

Abstract. Artificial intelligence (AI) has the potential to revolutionize healthcare in the EU by addressing challenges, such as shortages of healthcare personnel and more effective diagnosis and care. However, the safety concerns surrounding AI-based medical devices have been a major roadblock to the technology's wider adoption. This study aims to further investigate these concerns in the European context by analysing the AI-enabled Medical devices currently available in the European Union market along with their potential safety risks. We do this by applying a combination of three research methods: (1) a survey of the safety risks of AI-enabled Medical Devices published between 2012 and 2023, (2) an analysis of AI-based medical devices in the EUDAMED database, and (3) a survey on the perceptions of the EU Medical AI ecosystem stakeholders. Our study analyzed the state-of-the-art with a literature body of 29 papers and summarized a number of risks related to the use of AI in medical devices along with the reported mitigation strategies. Furthermore, we analyzed the approved medical devices (71 devices) that use AI in the EUDAMED database and found that there is a lack of transparency in whether the devices use AI along with the lack of crucial information necessary to asses the devices' safety risks, such information on training data. Finally, when we survey a number of medical device stakeholders (7 out of 130 respondents) we find that there is a disconnect between the industry and regulators: the medical device representatives emphasize the need for better guidance on post-market surveillance while the regulation representatives feel that they lack expertise in AI.

Keywords: Artificial intelligence · Medical device regulation · Literature survey · Medical device survey

1 Introduction

Artificial intelligence (AI) solutions, like ChatGPT are increasingly entering various aspects of our lives. This tendency is arguably also occurring in the medical

D. Salvi et al. (Eds.): PH 2023, LNICST 572, pp. 51–69, 2024.
https://doi.org/10.1007/978-3-031-59717-6_4

device area [32]. AI-based medical device software holds great promise in addressing the challenges faced by healthcare systems in the European Union, such as
the aging population, inefficient medical systems, and lack of healthcare workers.
However, these AI-enabled solutions also come with risks, from inaccurate predictions to incorporating various biases. These issues raise concerns about safety
risks, which can consequently lead to a lack of trust and pose a barrier to the
wide-scale adoption of AI into clinical practices. Lack of information about these
devices and mitigation of various risks further decreases trust. In the EU context various aspects of AI- enabled medical devices, such as their characteristics,
are unexplored. This paper aims to provide an overview of risks associated with
AI-based medical devices and describing the AI-based medical software devices
currently on the EU market, with focus on factors affecting their safety. The
core questions explored in this paper are:

1. What are the safety risks of AI-enabled medical Devices, and what strategies
   exist to mitigate them?
   Extensive focus has been put into creating frameworks for evaluating AI-
   based Medical Devices [5]. However, to the best of the author's knowledge,
   no survey of the safety risk of such devices has so far been conducted.
2. What kind of AI-based Medical Devices can be currently found on the EU
   market?
   There has been a lot of discussions and work put into regulating AI in the
   European Union. However, in comparison to the USA regulatory body (FDA),
   EU is lagging behind in terms of providing information about AI-enabled
   Medical Devices. Indeed, until the launch of EUDAMED there lacked a central
   database of Medical Devices on the EU market.
3. How do the stakeholders of the AI-enabled Medical Device ecosystem perceive
   the use, risks and regulation of AI-enabled Medical Devices?
   Analysis on stakeholders' perception of Medical AI is so far largely focused
   on healthcare specialists and their views on AI [40,43]. However, little is
   known how companies, researchers and regulators perceive the current use of
   AI various safety risks of AI-enabled Medical Devices and the regulation on
   Medical-AI in EU.

The rest of the paper is structured as follows: in Sect. 2, we analyze the
background and related works; in Sect. 3, we provide a brief overview of the
regulation of medical devices in EU; in Sect. 4, we explain the methodologies
used in various research steps; in Sect. 5, we present the findings of the research
and in Sect. 6, we provide an analysis of the research findings. Following that, we
provide a discussion section, where we delve into the implications of our findings.

This paper aims to contribute to the current discussions of legislative and
regulatory reforms intended to regulate AI/ML-based medical devices.

2   Background and Related Work

Most studies on AI-based medical devices focus on the US market and on devices
approved by the FDA. For example, Wu et al. [41] published a comprehensive

overview of medical AI devices approved by the US Food and Drug Administration, that indicated that evaluation process can mask vulnerabilities of devices when they are deployed on patients. Muehlematter et al. [28] report on a comparative study of Medical Devices approved by FDA and CE-marked in EU between years 2015–2020.

While many papers have investigated the safety risks of AI-based medical devices [15, 29, 36], we were not able to find a dedicated literature survey of the safety risks of AI-based medical devices.

3   Methodological Approach

In this study we apply a combination of quantitative and qualitative approaches to present multiple findings about AI-based Medical Devices. This mixed approach is chosen to enable triangulation in order to examine the current use and potential safety risks of AI-enabled Software as a Medical Device and from research literature, devices on the EU market and practitioner's viewpoint. The approach applied is: (a) we review the literature of safety risks associated with AI-enabled medical devices; (b) we analyze the current AI-enabled Medical Devices on the EU market achieved by the collection and manual labelling of data from the European Database of Medical Devices EUDAMED; and (c) we survey the stakeholders of the ecosystem of the European medical devices.

3.1   Literature Survey of Risks of AI-Enabled SaMD

We conduct a literature survey on the risk of AI-enabled software as a medical device (SaMD)[1]. We define a protocol based on the PRISMA methodology [30] and by leveraging our previous experience on literature surveys and systematic literature reviews [22–24, 39]. Our survey protocol includes:

Sources. The defined literature sources are: (i) Google Scholar, (ii) PubMed, and (iii) Scopus.

Search string. *((safety) OR (risks)) AND (healthcare) AND (((machine learning)) OR (deep learning)) OR (artificial intelligence)*[2].

Inclusion/exclusion criteria. In order for the paper to be included in the Literature Review the following criteria has to be met: 1) Paper discusses the safety risks of AI enabled devices in medicine; 2) The paper is from the time period 2012–2023; 3) The paper is in English;

---

[1] SaMD is defined by the International Medical Device Regulators Forum (IMDRF) as "software intended to be used for one or more medical purposes that perform these purposes without being part of a hardware medical device.".

[2] Further variation of search keywords were tested that included, among other, "AI ML & Safety & Medical Device & Medicine"; "ML & Safety Risks & Medical Device & Healthcare".

The papers are screened by title, abstract, and full text against the inclusion and exclusions criteria defined. After the papers were selected for inclusion, backwards and forward snowballing is used to find further relevant papers and gather a comprehensive and diverse set of studies that are relevant to the research question being addressed.

For all of the papers reviewed, the following information are extracted: (1)Type of article: journal, conference article or book; (2) Bibliographic data such as publication year; (3) Safety risks listed/discussed; (4) Ways of mitigating the safety risks if they were listed/discussed; (5) Reviewer notes, comments, and recommendations from surveying the article.

Although the current study focuses on medical devices limited in the EU region, geographical limitations were intentionally excluded from the literature survey to ensure an adequate literature body and variability in results.

3.2   EU AI-Based Medical Device Survey Protocol

We survey the approved software medical devices in EU and identify the devices with AI-supported functions. To do so, we survey the European database on medical devices (EUDAMED). We extract[3] all software medical devices and collect (a) Trade name, (b) Manufacturer and (c) Classification (risk class).

Having collected the initial device body, validated and cleaned the data, we process it as following. In this study we focus on medium to high risk devices, thus we exclude the low risk devices (class I and Class A) from the dataset. This group is chosen for exclusion, since the devices are subjected to a different, less rigorous approval process.

Furthermore, EUDAMED does not currently provide information on the description of the device, including whether a device is using AI or not. Thus, the resulting data are manually annotated as either AI and non-AI for filtering out non-AI devices. To validate the device data, we follow a three-source approach: FDA list of AI/ML devices, AI for Radiology database, and device publicly available data. As the first step of annotation the devices are cross-referenced with our first two sources: the FDA list of Artificial Intelligence and Machine Learning (AI/ML)-Enabled Medical Devices and the AI for Radiology database. AI for Radiology database is a database of CE-marked AI software products for clinical radiology based on vendor-supplied product specifications [18]. The FDA list of AI-enabled Medical Devices is a non-exhaustive list periodically updated by FDA based on publicly available information [6]. The rest of the devices are then manually labeled based on the publicly available data on Google. In this step, we use the device manufactures websites and press releases as primary data sources.

The resulting dataset is categorized by medical specialties using a modified version of the European Union of Medical Specialists' list, created in collaboration with two medical experts. The modified list aims to include all relevant

---

[3] We apply the Python library BeautifulSoup with extraction date 2022.09.29.

specialties while avoiding excessive granularity for the paper's purpose. Furthermore, the devices are categorized based on the risk categorization principles of the International Medical Device Regulators Forum (IMDRF) set out in Possible Framework for Risk Categorization and Corresponding Considerations [11].

Therefore the devices are further manually labeled across following dimension: the point of healthcare situation or condition the software is intended to be used in; the body part targeted and the medical speciality the device belongs to.

Furthermore, from the point of healthcare situation or condition the software is intended to be used in, the devices were classified in the following categories: critical situation or condition; serious situation or condition; Non-serious situation or condition [11]. Classifying the devices from the point of healthcare situation or condition is done by two labellers - one working in the healthcare sector and another in IT.

3.3 Medical Device Stakeholder Survey

In order to get a more complete view on the area, we conduct a survey of the EU stakeholders in AI-based medical device area. The main focus areas are the current use of AI-based medical devices in EU, potential risk factors and EU legislation regarding Medical Devices. In this survey we intend to validate the findings from the literature survey and rate the risks of using AI-based medical devices. The survey is conducted online with the survey link being sent out to the potential participants. Before launching, the survey is piloted it using a pre-screening [17]. The survey is pre-screened by four researchers with knowledge of both medical and IT field. All lists of options for multiple-choice questions, with the exception of the question about participants role, are randomized to decrease potential measurement errors [17].

The survey has four sections: *Background information* aimed at defining the role of the participant (Expert, Working in SAMD company, Regulator or Other); *AI in the EU market* aimed at defining areas with AI-enabled devices and possible overuse of them; *Safety risks of AI-enabled medical devices* focusing on rating and prioritizing the risks that are noted in the literature; and *Regulation of AI-enabled devices in EU* focusing on the largest technical challenge for ensuring the safety of AI/ML based Medical Devices in EU.

Furthermore the survey collects input in whether the participants felt that the current medical device regulation in EU is sufficient in terms of ensuring the safety of AI/ML based Medical Devices and what changes they would like to see in the medical device regulation in the EU. In this analysis we categorized the participant roles as following: *regulator*, a person working in a AI- enabled SaMD company or an expert in the area. *Expert*, a person who had published research in AI enabled Medical Devices in EU or was or had been part of an expert group or think tank such as the EU expert group on AI. *Regulator*, included in Notified Bodies in the European Union found by looking through the NANDO database for Notified Bodies. SAMD using AI companies were companies which in publicly declared using AI in their devices. Such companies were found firstly by the list of companies found on the EUDAMED database and manually labeled as AI and secondly using various online databases for companies, such as Danish startup ecosystem database or EIT health database. Experts were found by looking at speakers at relevant conferences, authors of relevant papers or looking at interest groups representing Medical-Device manufacturers. The survey was sent to 130 individuals, including 31 experts, 50 regulators, and 49 individuals from SaMD companies.

4   Findings

4.1   Literature Survey

When applying the literature survey protocol we retrieve a total of 27.073 results. 24 of the originally resulted papers are included in the final literature body. An additional five papers are added by snowballing. The literature survey process can be summarized in Fig. 1. The complete reference list can be found in the Appendix 7. Details of the included papers are also summarised in Fig. 1. The papers covered the time period 2016–2022; they came from the European Union (EU), United Kingdom (UK), United States of America (USA), and Canada; and they were primarily journal articles. Journals published in 2022 were most common.

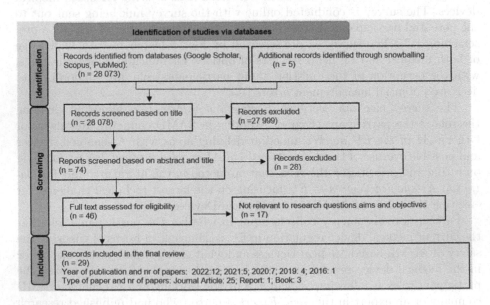

Fig. 1. Process for defining the literature body.

The risks identified in the literature survey can be classified into four categories: data-centric risks, transparency-related risks, cyber-security risks, and risks stemming from user-machine interaction. Summary of various risks and their mitigation strategies can be found in Table 1 at the end of the chapter.

Results of the survey show that data-related risks are most prevalent in the literature. These include aspects such as data drift, distributional shift or calibration drift.

Data-Centric Risks [1,3,12,13,19,21,25,34,38]. Many risks mentioned in the literature stem from the data used for the Artificial Intelligence.

Bias is a prominent topic in literature and mainly stems from disparities between training and operational data. Bias errors occur, since machine learning models do not generalize well beyond the data they were trained on [21]. Bias has different forms such as distributional shift, which arises when the underlying data distribution used for model development differs from the data where the model is deployed [34]. For instance, a skin cancer prediction model may perform poorly on dark-skinned patients [3], revealing a distributional shift due to selection bias, which can occur when marginalized populations are not adequately represented in the training data.

If not effectively implemented, evaluated, and regulated, AI solutions in the future may perpetuate and amplify systemic disparities and human biases, contributing to healthcare inequities [19].

Distributional shift can also occur due to minor difference in the radiology equipment in different hospitals [21] resulting in medical images, such as X-rays with slightly different characteristics. Another sub-type of bias is calibration drift, which can occur due to unanticipated changes in clinical practices or patient behaviour [38].

However, bias can also stem from factors beyond the shortcomings of inadequate training data. Such as measurement bias - omitting critical data-fields during model training. For example an algorithm predicting survival of postmenopausal women, that did not perform well, partly because it lacked relevant blood test results [38]. Another source for bias can be incorrect data. This is especially true in cases where data from consumer-facing health apps are merged with clinical data to create predictions. An instance is the Fitbit PurePulse Trackers' unreliable heart rate measurements [13].

Bias is further worsened by the characteristics of data-sets available. Healthcare data is often sparse and imbalanced, for example contain more samples of patients with a mild condition, due to naturally occurring distribution. This is especially prominent in fields such as pathology and mental health [1].

Further data related risks include noise and artefacts in model inputs and hidden confounders. *Noise and artefacts in model inputs* - Noise in data refers to meaningless or irrelevant data, that the model can pick up on [12]. Noisy data is often caused by the differences in or issues with medical equipment used. For example, scanning errors or differences in hospital imagining protocols [25]. Noise can also come from Imaging artifacts and poor imaging quality [25].

Hidden Confounders. are factors unmeasured in the observational data affecting both treatment and outcome. An example of hidden confounders in a clinical setting are physicians prescribing medication based on indicators not present in the health record [16]. They can reduce both model generalizability and interpretation [42].

Transparency-Related Risks   [14,19–21,34,37,42]. Risks related to the explainablility or interpretability also referred to as transparency of AI based devices were also a common topic in the literature.

Lack of Transparency: i.e. the 'black box' nature of many AI systems, like deep learning models, makes their decision-making process unclear [20,21,42]. This lack of transparency can make it difficult to determine the accuracy or reliability of the AI's output, may erode trust of patients and healthcare specialists and may make it more difficult to identify and correct errors [14,34,37]. A well-known example of a difficultly identifiable error is a case of AI models predicting pneumonia mortality risk mistakenly labeled asthma patients as lower risk of mortality, since they were treated more aggressively and quickly according to hospital protocol, which reduced their risk of death [42]. Transparency can be split into [19]: *Traceability* (clarity of AI development and usage) and *Explainability* (clarity of AI decisions).

User and System Interaction Related Risks   [7,19–21,26,31,38]. The least discussed aspect influencing the safety of the devices was User and System Interaction related risks. Examples of such risks are input errors, automation complacency, and cognitive bias of the user. Input errors can occur as a result of the user misspelling, confusing clinical terms, users employing local definitions or misrepresenting findings. This issue is further exacerbated by quickly changing medical definitions [7]. Automation complacency refers to when specialists rely too heavily on the models predictions. Research has shown that specialists tend to over-rely and delegate full responsibility to systems and lose vigilance or become deskilled [21,31]. Evidence suggests that when a clinician is uncertain, they may defer to models predictions [26]. The black box nature of many modern AI-systems will likely contribute to the worsening of this phenomenon [21,38]. Over time, automation complacency might lead to misdiagnoses and inappropriate interventions, as algorithms may lean towards overdiagnosis by detecting subclinical findings [38].

Cognitive bias of the user includes errors that are closely related to automation complacency of the users. Cognitive biases have many forms and can include to misunderstandings of statistics and mathematical rationality or be one of many forms of human cognitive biases, such as Search satisfying: Ceasing to look for further information or alternative answers when the first plausible solution is found [7].

Various User and System Interaction risks are exacerbated by healthcare specialists limited knowledge of AI. Varied studies have showed that, that healthcare specialists have received little education regarding AI and do not rate their knowledge of AI highly hidden [19].

Cybersecurity Risks [2, 38]. AI-enabled medical devices largely share common cybersecurity risks with non-AI healthcare systems, but the use of AI in healthcare increases exposure to data privacy and integrity risks, due to creating an increased need between the interconnectivity between systems and dataset [2]. Resulting attacks can compromise model accuracy, lead to harmful predictions, re-identify de-identified data, or result in data loss. Various cybersecurity risks are discussed below.

AI increases *reidentification* opportunities in anonymized patient datasets, exemplified by Liangyuan's research [2], which demonstrated that over 90% of adults' physical activity data could be reidentified using ML models.

Adversarial Attacks on AI, categorized into white-box attacks that employ subversion, such as gradient-based techniques, and black-box attacks that poison datasets [2] leading to harmful or incorrect predictions or undetectable software corruption, are not easily detectable [38].

The risks discussed can also interplay and mutually amplify each other, such as the interaction between sampling and diagnostic bias or automation complacency and lack of transparency, with the latter making it more difficult to identify bias in the training data.

Mitigation Strategies. Most papers included in the survey presented potential mitigation strategies for the risks. In this chapter mitigation strategies from the summary table warranting additional clarification are described.

Transparency. *Visualization tools for increased transparency.*

Visualization tools for ML predictions, like Local Interpretable Algorithm-Agnostic Explanations (LIME) and Shapley Values (SHAP), help visualize the key features influencing the algorithm's predictions However, a challenge remains in clinicians understanding the language of these explanations. To address this, a platform connecting medical experts with ML researchers could help establish standardized representations of explanations [35].

Cybersecurity. *Encryption* various encryption measures are usually employed for data in transfer [2].

Adversarial Training - machine learning technique, which improves models robustness and generalization ability by training it to learn data samples that are designed to be have small and often human-imperceptible differences from the original data, but, which a model misclassifies [9]. For example images, with added pixels. This technique helps the model becomes more resistant to errors and to better handle real-world inputs that may be similarly ambiguous [8].

Masking Measures. Masking techniques, such as adding random statistical noise, collapsing variables, creating synthetic data, or using ML models to generate statistically similar datasets, are commonly employed when sharing data with external stakeholders to protect sensitive information [2].

GAN-Generative Adversarial Network (GAN) is a type of machine learning model, that can be used to generate adversarial data for a model to classify to bolster a model's robustness against attacks [33].

Statistical Approaches - using statistical tests, adversarial inputs from the operational data can be detected. Statistical tests rely on the fact that adversarial examples are statistically different from other inputs [10].

Federated Learning. This technique allows the training of an algorithm on sensitive data, present at multiple decentralized sites, without the exchange of data. For example, a number of hospitals can contribute toward the training of a model, without the data itself ever leaving each hospital's data center [42].

4.2   EU AI-Based Medical Device Survey

At the time of the gathering the data of this paper[4], the EUDAMED database lists 955 medical software items, which are reduced to 765 unique devices after eliminating duplicates. Excluding lower risk devices left 327, with 5 listed in the AI Radiology database, 13 in the FDAs database for AI based medical devices The other devices are manually labeled following the protocol outlined in Chap. 3. This results in 71 AI devices. These are labeled as serious (10), non-serious (20), or critical (41). More AI devices are classified as class IIa (low to moderate risk) than non-AI devices (72% versus 68%). The most common target body parts are the heart (13 devices) and lungs (10 devices), with 13 devices targeting multiple parts. Some devices belong to two specialities. The most common speciality the device are aimed at was radiology with 28 devices, followed by cardiology with 14 devices.

4.3   Survey of Stakeholder Perceptions

The survey is send out to 130 potential respondents. Seven provided a valid response. Four of the respondents are experts and three are working in a SaMD company. The responses do not include any regulators. However, one of the regulators reports that they feel that they do not have sufficient information to fill out the survey.

The respondents report that *pathology* and *emergency* medicine are areas that AI can be used while *radiology* and *nuclear medicine* are areas where AI is underused.

Participants are requested to evaluate various aspects of AI-enabled medical devices for their potential impact on device safety. The selected characteristics are based on prominent elements from the literature survey and guidelines from the International Medical Device Regulators Forum [11].

In this question, the participant assess that whether the devices are: (a) informing of options for treatment/diagnosing, or (b) for aiding in treatment or in diagnoses. (b) had the most influence. This element received a score of 4,6

---

[4] Extraction date: 2022.09.29.

Table 1. Risks and mitigation strategies identified in the literature

Risks and Mitigation Strategies	
Risk	Mitigation Strategy
Bias [3,21]	1. Pooling of data from various countries and organisations to create large and diverse data sets,across various areas, such as race and ethnicity [3,42] 2. Verify AI technology product claims on local data set [3] 3. Comprehensive multi-location evaluation studies to identify instabilities [19] 4. Reporting performance of models across relevant subgroups [26]
Hidden Confounders	No Mitigation Strategy Suggested
Noise and artefacts in model inputs [12]	Polishing, such as relabeling of data, or filtering out the noise [12]
Adversarial Attacks	1. Adversarial training 2. Generative Adversarial Network (GAN) 3. Statistical approaches [2]
Data Privacy Attacks [2]	1. De-identification algorithms [2] 2. Federated approaches for decentralised AI [19] 3. Full disk encryption [2] 4. Masking measures [2]
Lack of Tranparency (Blackbox nature of AI) [20,21]	1. An 'AI passport' for standardised description and traceability of medical AI tools [19] 2. Auditing [21] 3. For some models, visualization software, i.e. as SHAP and LIME [27,38]
Input errors [7]	Providing the user with background information and a glossary of clinical terms used in the model [7]
Cognitive biases	Training healthcare specialists to not lose vigilance [21]
Automation Complacency [21]	1. Improving the interpretability of AI systems [21] 2. Curriculum combining medicine and engineering to allow for better understanding of the workings of models [4] 3. Training healthcare specialists to not lose vigilance [21]

(in a scale from 1-5). The aspect receiving the lowest score in terms of influence was *the medical specialisation the device is deployed in* with an average of 3. Whether it is used for critical, serious or non critical, illness/condition received an average rating of 4.1 The remaining scores were: *Testing the AI algorithm on data from the hospital where it is deployed in the launch phase* - 3.28. *How much data has been used to train the device* - 4.14. *Interaction between the user and the device* - 4.14. *The users understanding of AI/ML* - 3.28.

When examining the current regulation of AI enabled devices three participants did not feel that the current system in EU was sufficient in terms of ensuring the safety of AI/ML based Medical Devices, while two participants were unfamiliar with the system and two felt that the current system was sufficient. Reasons noted for feeling that the system was insufficient were: (i) No guidance had been published by the European authorities on surveillance following implementation; (ii) Notified Body scrutinises for safety, clinical experts review Clinical Evaluation Report; (iii) Does not sufficiently account for potential biases or oversights in the training and validation data; (iv) Re-certification of data-centric AI and learning algorithms are not fully incorporated; (v) Lack of life-cycle understanding;

Lastly, the changes the participants would like to see in the medical device regulation were: (a) more focus on post market surveillance; (b) more streamlined process, that are less dependant on the availability of notified bodies or their specific interpretations; (c) Better guidelines for post-market surveillance; (d) Better guidelines on ensuring sufficiency of data.

5 Analysis

5.1 Literature Survey

It is evident from the literature survey that the main risks stem from the AI-enabled devices reliance and interaction with data - not only during the pre-launch phase, but also during production.

This is due to the fact, that unlike traditional medical devices that function in a rather predictable, deterministic way, AI-enabled devices can evolve and change their behavior based on the data they interact with.

This means that for AI-enabled devices, post-market surveillance and real-world performance monitoring are as, if not more, important. This requires a change in regulatory frameworks, which have traditionally focused heavily on the pre-market phase where devices are tested extensively in controlled lab settings.

Second aspect, unique to AI-enabled medical devices, is risks related to the interpretability of AI-enabled Devices. Dangerous or unhelpful patterns learned by the model can be difficult to detect, as for many AI- models it is difficult and at times impossible to understand why they have reached a certain conclusion. Furthermore, the lack of transparency can exacerbate risks related to user-system interaction. To address this, regulatory frameworks need to include requirements on the level of transparency and interpretability of AI systems. A very promising direction is the use of explainable AI (XAI) techniques, that aim to make the decision-making process of AI systems more interpretable to humans.

In conclusion, the dynamic nature of AI-enabled medical devices, as well as their complexity, calls for a significant shift in thinking when designing regulatory frameworks.

5.2   AI-Based Medical Devices in EU

The current data fields available in EUDAMED point to a possible regulatory issue, as they do not contain a lot of information that would be needed to assess the safety of AI-based devices, such as information about the data - for example potential biases in the training data or amount of data used for training. As the review of the safety risks showed, having clear documentation about the design of the system, including the data used, helps mitigate risks associated with AI-enabled devices, such as the black-box nature of such devices.

Analysis of the distribution of risk classes revealed that the medical AI devices in the EUDAMED dataset had a higher proportion of "class IIa" and "class IIb" risk classes and a lower proportion of "IVD general" risk classes compared to the non-AI devices.

"Class IIa" risk classes are considered to be of low to moderate risk, while "class IIb" risk classes are considered to be of moderate risk. "IVD general" risk classes are not included in class IIa or IIb, and their risk level is not specified.

This suggests that the medical AI devices in EUDAMED are often lower to moderate risk compared to the non-AI devices. It is worth noting that this comparison is based on the proportion of devices in each risk class, and it is not necessarily indicative of the overall risk level of the medical and non-AI devices.

The second finding of the analysis of EUDAEMD is that most AI-enabled devices are dealing with critical or serious illnesses and conditions, such as stroke or cancer. Analysis of the correlation between the severity of the condition or illness targeted and the risk class of the device showed that devices targeting serious illnesses and conditions doe not necessarily get a higher risk class. This is not surprising as, the severity of the targeted condition or illness is just one factor among many considered when assigning a risk class to a medical device, with the intervention of the device carrying the most significant weight.

5.3   Survey of Stakeholder Perceptions

The low number of survey participants means that the results are not suitable for representing the medical device ecosystem as a whole, since such a small sample size can lead to sampling bias. However, the results are still useful for supplementing the literature review and for providing insights into potential safety concerns form the stakeholders perspective. Furthermore, the finding points out potential pain-points in the EU regulation of medical devices from the stakeholders perspective. Additionally, the results could potentially be used to inform future research or to identify areas for improvement in the distribution process. The fact that none of the regulators filled out the survey coupled with the fact that one of the regulators reported that he feels that they do not have sufficient information to fill out the survey, points to possible gap in regulators knowledge of AI- enabled devices. While it must be noted that since we only have one datapoint we currently have weak evidence. None the less, this is an interesting finding that could point to a future research direction. It is possible that the regulator who wrote back indicating that they did not have sufficient knowledge to fill out the survey represents a broader trend among regulators. This could point to a serious issue in the EU legislation of AI-enabled medical devices.

The concerns and pain-points pointed out by the participants show that many risks in AI -enabled medical devices are data-centric, such better guidelines on sufficient amounts of data. This feedback from actors currently active in the ecosystem indicates that EU regulators have not sufficiently addressed several data-centric risks of AI-enabled medical devices.

Furthermore the survey participants also underlined the need for better post-market guidance. This highlights another unique feature of AI that the EU might not have tackled sufficiently. Namely the changing nature of AI models and algorithms and the large amounts of risks stemming of it that can manifest in the post-market phase. Unlike many traditional medical devices such as contact lenses or pumps, AI performance can vary widely in different locations, for example in different hospitals and can also dangerously degrade when coming in contact with new data while in productions. These unique aspects would need to be clearly addressed by the EU regulators.

6   Discussion

The majority of AI devices are identified in the survey on EUDAMED were within the field of radiology or cardiology and most commonly dealt with critical conditions or illnesses, such as cancer or stroke. The fact that devices on the EU market commonly deal with critical illnesses highlights the potential severe outcomes of various risks not being properly mitigated. It was challenging for this study to identify AI in devices as the current information in EUDAMED is inadequate. EUDAMED does not contain information on whether a device is utilising AI and lacks information that would be needed to assess the safety of AI-based devices, e.g. information on the data used for the device.

In the literature survey of the risks and mitigation strategies of AI-enabled Medical Devices most papers discussed data-centric risks in various detail. Other risk categories identified were cybersecurity risks, transparency related risks and lastly user and system interaction related risks. The amount and nature of risks identified in combination with the domain mission criticality of the devices underline the importance of good praxis in the adaptation of AI and the high risks in improper adaptation.

The analysis of stakeholder perceptions found that several post-market data-related risks presented in the academic literature, such as bias, were also a concern for the stakeholders, who emphasised the need for better testing and regulatory guidance to address such risks. Some stakeholders felt that the current EU regulation on Medical-AI is inadequate, citing a lack of post-implementation guidance and guidelines on data sufficiency as examples. This points to a need for regulatory guidelines that in a larger degree take into account the dynamic and data-centric properties of AI enabled medical devices. However, there was indication that regulators feel a lack of expertise about AI.

The findings of this paper highlight lack of regulation and establishment of common understanding of safety risks of AI-enabled Medical Devices. This can be attributed in part to the immaturity of the field, however, the potential impact of risks in the medical domain are severe. The dynamic nature of AI models compared to traditional medical devices requires a stronger focus on the post-market phase from the regulators. Therefore, the study underscores the need for a more comprehensive understanding, and clear and robust regulatory guidelines to navigate through these potential hazards.

7   Conclusion

In this paper we investigate the adoption of AI in medical devices. Currently, concerns regarding the safety risks surrounding AI-based medical devices currently stand in the way of their wider adoption. In this study we conduct: (1) a survey of the safety risks of AI-enabled Medical Devices published between 2012 and 2023, (2) an analysis of AI-based medical devices in the EUDAMED database. and (3) a survey on the perceptions of Medical AI ecosystem stakeholders. Our analysis body includes 29 reviewed papers, 71 AI-based medical devices and seven responded questionnaires out of an original 130 participants. Our findings show that the presence of unique risks, such as bias or lack of transparency, in AI-enabled Medical Devices is undeniable. Looking at data available at EUDAMED we can see that it is currently hard to even pinpoint which devices in EU use AI and we have to look at company websites, press statements or published papers to discover that. We also uncovered that many AI enabled devices in EU deal with severe conditions such as arrhythmia or stroke, which further underlines the severity of potential risks manifesting. Experts and companies in the Medical AI ecosystem feel a need for guidance and regulation that covers the whole life-cycle of AI products, with more emphasis on the post-market phase, and incorporates aspects related to data-centric risks of the products. This demonstrates an openness to more structured guidelines from the industry. However, our research suggests that regulators feel that do not have expertise in AI, indicating that a gap exists between the complexities of AI technology and the understanding of those responsible for its oversight. Based on the findings we propose, that more clear and encompassing regulatory guidelines would be needed to mitigate the risks of AI-enabled Medical Devices in EU.

Appendix A - Literature Body of the Literature Survey

[21] Magrabi, F., Ammenwerth, E., McNair, J.B., De Keizer, N.F., Hyppönen, H., Nykänen, P., Rigby, M., Scott, P.J., Vehko, T., Wong, Z.S.Y., et al.: Artificial intelligence in clinical decision support: challenges for evaluating ai and practical implications. Yearbook of medical informatics **28**(01), 128–134 (2019)
[38] Scott, I., Carter, S., Coiera, E.: Clinician checklist for assessing suitability of machine learning applications in healthcare. BMJ Health & Care Informatics **28**(1) (2021)
[2] Bohr, A., Memarzadeh, K.: Artificial intelligence in healthcare. Academic Press (2020)

[35] Rasheed, K., Qayyum, A., Ghaly, M., Al-Fuqaha, A., Razi, A., Qadir, J.: Explainable, trustworthy, and ethical machine learning for healthcare: A survey. Computers in Biology and Medicine p. 106043 (2022)

[9] Goodfellow, I.J., Shlens, J., Szegedy, C.: Explaining and harnessing adversarial examples. arXiv preprint arXiv:1412.6572 (2014)

[8] Geiping, J., Fowl, L., Somepalli, G., Goldblum, M., Moeller, M., Goldstein, T.: What doesn't kill you makes you robust (er): Adversarial training against poisons and backdoors. arXiv preprint arXiv:2102.13624 1(7) (2021)

[33] Qiu, S., Liu, Q., Zhou, S., Wu, C.: Review of artificial intelligence adversarial attack and defense technologies. Applied Sciences 9(5), 909 (2019)

[10] Grosse, K., Manoharan, P., Papernot, N., Backes, M., McDaniel, P.: On the (statistical) detection of adversarial examples. arXiv preprint arXiv:1702.06280 (2017)

[42] Xing, L., Giger, M.L., Min, J.K.: Artificial intelligence in medicine: technical basis and clinical applications. Academic Press (2020)

[3] Borycki, E., Kushniruk, A.: Artificial intelligence and safety in healthcare. In: AI and Society, pp. 17–32. Chapman and Hall/CRC (2022)

[19] Lekadir, K., Quaglio, G., Garmendia, A.T., Gallin, C.: Artificial intelligence in healthcare: Applications, risks, and ethical and societal impacts. EPRS (European Parliamentary Research Service) (2022)

[26] McCradden, M.D., Joshi, S., Anderson, J.A., Mazwi, M., Goldenberg, A., Zlotnik Shaul, R.: Patient safety and quality improvement: Ethical principles for a regulatory approach to bias in healthcare machine learning. Journal of the American Medical Informatics Association 27(12), 2024–2027 (2020)

[20] Macrae, C.: Governing the safety of artificial intelligence in healthcare. BMJ quality & safety 28(6), 495–498 (2019)

[27] Moore, C.M.: The challenges of health inequities and ai. Intelligence-Based Medicine p. 100067 (2022)

[7] Galitsky, B., Goldberg, S.: Artificial Intelligence for Healthcare Applications and Management. Academic Press (2022)

[4] Briganti, G., Le Moine, O.: Artificial intelligence in medicine: today and tomorrow. Frontiers in medicine 7, 27 (2020)

[31] Paton, C., Kobayashi, S.: An open science approach to artificial intelligence in healthcare. Yearbook of medical informatics 28(01), 047–051 (2019)

[42] Xing, L., Giger, M.L., Min, J.K.: Artificial intelligence in medicine: technical basis and clinical applications. Academic Press (2020)

[37] Rubinger, L., Gazendam, A., Ekhtiari, S., Bhandari, M.: Machine learning and artificial intelligence in research and healthcare. Injury (2022)

[34] Quinn, T.P., Jacobs, S., Senadeera, M., Le, V., Coghlan, S.: The three ghosts of medical ai: Can the black-box present deliver? Artificial intelligence in medicine 124, 102158 (2022)

[14] Jia, Y., McDermid, J.A., Lawton, T., Habli, I.: The role of explainability in assuring safety of machine learning in healthcare. IEEE Transactions on Emerging Topics in Computing (2022)

[25] Martin, C., DeStefano, K., Haran, H., Zink, S., Dai, J., Ahmed, D., Razzak, A., Lin, K., Kogler, A., Waller, J., et al.: The ethical considerations including inclusion and biases, data protection, and proper implementation among ai in radiology and potential implications. Intelligence-Based Medicine p. 100073 (2022)

[12] Gupta, S., Gupta, A.: Dealing with noise problem in machine learning data-sets: A systematic review. Procedia Computer Science **161**, 466–474 (2019)

[1] Barh, D.: Artificial Intelligence in Precision Health: From Concept to Applications. Academic Press (2020)

[13] Hamid, S.: The opportunities and risks of artificial intelligence in medicine and healthcare. Apollo - University of Cambridge Repository (2016)

[16] Kallus, N., Puli, A.M., Shalit, U.: Removing hidden confounding by experimental grounding. Advances in neural information processing systems **31** (2018)

References

1. Barh, D.: Artificial Intelligence in Precision Health: From Concept to Applications. Academic Press, Cambridge (2020)
2. Bohr, A., Memarzadeh, K.: Artificial Intelligence in Healthcare. Academic Press, Cambridge (2020)
3. Borycki, E., Kushniruk, A.: Artificial intelligence and safety in healthcare. In: AI and Society, pp. 17–32. Chapman and Hall/CRC, Boca Raton (2022)
4. Briganti, G., Le Moine, O.: Artificial intelligence in medicine: today and tomorrow. Front. Med. **7**, 27 (2020)
5. Crossnohere, N.L., Elsaid, M., Paskett, J., Bose-Brill, S., Bridges, J.F.: Guidelines for artificial intelligence in medicine: literature review and content analysis of frameworks. J. Med. Internet Res. **24**(8), e36823 (2022)
6. Center for Devices and Radiological Health: Artificial intelligence and machine learning (AI/ML)-enabled medical d, October 2022. https://www.fda.gov/medical-devices/software-medical-device-samd/artificial-intelligence-and-machine-learning-aiml-enabled-medical-devices
7. Galitsky, B., Goldberg, S.: Artificial Intelligence for Healthcare Applications and Management. Academic Press, Cambridge (2022)
8. Geiping, J., Fowl, L., Somepalli, G., Goldblum, M., Moeller, M., Goldstein, T.: What doesn't kill you makes you robust (ER): adversarial training against poisons and backdoors. arXiv preprint arXiv:2102.13624 **1**(7) (2021)
9. Goodfellow, I.J., Shlens, J., Szegedy, C.: Explaining and harnessing adversarial examples. arXiv preprint arXiv:1412.6572 (2014)
10. Grosse, K., Manoharan, P., Papernot, N., Backes, M., McDaniel, P.: On the (statistical) detection of adversarial examples. arXiv preprint arXiv:1702.06280 (2017)
11. Group, I.S.W., et al.: "Software as a medical device": possible framework for risk categorization and corresponding considerations. In: International Medical Device Regulators Forum (2014)
12. Gupta, S., Gupta, A.: Dealing with noise problem in machine learning data-sets: a systematic review. Procedia Comput. Sci. **161**, 466–474 (2019)
13. Hamid, S.: The Opportunities and Risks of Artificial Intelligence in Medicine and Healthcare. Apollo - University of Cambridge Repository (2016)

14. Jia, Y., McDermid, J.A., Lawton, T., Habli, I.: The role of explainability in assuring safety of machine learning in healthcare. IEEE Trans. Emerg. Top. Comput. (2022)
15. Jiang, L., et al.: Opportunities and challenges of artificial intelligence in the medical field: current application, emerging problems, and problem-solving strategies. J. Int. Med. Res. **49**(3), 03000605211000157 (2021)
16. Kallus, N., Puli, A.M., Shalit, U.: Removing hidden confounding by experimental grounding. In: Advances in Neural Information Processing Systems, vol. 31 (2018)
17. Lavrakas, P.J.: Encyclopedia of Survey Research Methods. Sage Publications, Thousand Oaks (2008)
18. van Leeuwen, K.G., Schalekamp, S., Rutten, M.J., van Ginneken, B., de Rooij, M.: Artificial intelligence in radiology: 100 commercially available products and their scientific evidence. Eur. Radiol. **31**(6), 3797–3804 (2021)
19. Lekadir, K., Quaglio, G., Garmendia, A.T., Gallin, C.: Artificial intelligence in healthcare: applications, risks, and ethical and societal impacts. EPRS (European Parliamentary Research Service) (2022)
20. Macrae, C.: Governing the safety of artificial intelligence in healthcare. BMJ Qual. Saf. **28**(6), 495–498 (2019)
21. Magrabi, F., et al.: Artificial intelligence in clinical decision support: challenges for evaluating AI and practical implications. Yearb. Med. Inform. **28**(01), 128–134 (2019)
22. Manikas, K.: Revisiting software ecosystems research: a longitudinal literature study. J. Syst. Softw. **117**, 84–103 (2016). https://doi.org/10.1016/j.jss.2016.02. 003, https://www.sciencedirect.com/science/article/pii/S0164121216000406
23. Manikas, K.: Supporting the evolution of research in software ecosystems: reviewing the empirical literature. In: Maglyas, A., Lamprecht, A.-L. (eds.) Software Business. LNBIP, vol. 240, pp. 63–78. Springer, Cham (2016). https://doi.org/10. 1007/978-3-319-40515-5_5
24. Manikas, K., Hansen, K.M.: Software ecosystems – a systematic literature review. J. Syst. Softw. **86**(5), 1294–1306 (2013). https://doi.org/10.1016/j.jss.2012.12.026, https://www.sciencedirect.com/science/article/pii/S016412121200338X
25. Martin, C., et al.: The ethical considerations including inclusion and biases, data protection, and proper implementation among AI in radiology and potential implications. Intell.-Based Med. 100073 (2022)
26. McCradden, M.D., Joshi, S., Anderson, J.A., Mazwi, M., Goldenberg, A., Zlotnik Shaul, R.: Patient safety and quality improvement: ethical principles for a regulatory approach to bias in healthcare machine learning. J. Am. Med. Inform. Assoc. **27**(12), 2024–2027 (2020)
27. Moore, C.M.: The challenges of health inequities and AI. Intell.-Based Med. 100067 (2022)
28. Muehlematter, U.J., Daniore, P., Vokinger, K.N.: Approval of artificial intelligence and machine learning-based medical devices in the USA and Europe (2015–20): a comparative analysis. Lancet Digit. Health **3**(3), e195–e203 (2021)
29. Newaz, A.I., Sikder, A.K., Rahman, M.A., Uluagac, A.S.: A survey on security and privacy issues in modern healthcare systems: attacks and defenses. ACM Trans. Comput. Healthc. **2**(3), 1–44 (2021)
30. Page, M.J., et al.: The Prisma 2020 statement: an updated guideline for reporting systematic reviews. Syst. Control Found. Appl. **10**(1), 1–11 (2021)
31. Paton, C., Kobayashi, S.: An open science approach to artificial intelligence in healthcare. Yearb. Med. Inform. **28**(01), 047–051 (2019)

32. Powell, A.: AI Revolution in Medicine. Harvard Gazette, November 2020. https://news.harvard.edu/gazette/story/2020/11/risks-and-benefits-of-an-ai-revolution-in-medicine/
33. Qiu, S., Liu, Q., Zhou, S., Wu, C.: Review of artificial intelligence adversarial attack and defense technologies. Appl. Sci. **9**(5), 909 (2019)
34. Quinn, T.P., Jacobs, S., Senadeera, M., Le, V., Coghlan, S.: The three ghosts of medical AI: can the black-box present deliver? Artif. Intell. Med. **124**, 102158 (2022)
35. Rasheed, K., Qayyum, A., Ghaly, M., Al-Fuqaha, A., Razi, A., Qadir, J.: Explainable, trustworthy, and ethical machine learning for healthcare: a survey. Comput. Biol. Med. 106043 (2022)
36. Ross, P., Spates, K.: Considering the safety and quality of artificial intelligence in health care. Jt. Comm. J. Qual. Patient Saf. **46**(10), 596 (2020)
37. Rubinger, L., Gazendam, A., Ekhtiari, S., Bhandari, M.: Machine learning and artificial intelligence in research and healthcare. Injury (2022)
38. Scott, I., Carter, S., Coiera, E.: Clinician checklist for assessing suitability of machine learning applications in healthcare. BMJ Health Care Inform. **28**(1) (2021)
39. Seppänen, M., Hyrynsalmi, S., Manikas, K., Suominen, A.: Yet another ecosystem literature review: 10+1 research communities. In: 2017 IEEE European Technology and Engineering Management Summit (E-TEMS), pp. 1–8 (2017). https://doi.org/10.1109/E-TEMS.2017.8244229
40. Sujan, M.A., White, S., Habli, I., Reynolds, N.: Stakeholder perceptions of the safety and assurance of artificial intelligence in healthcare. Saf. Sci. **155**, 105870 (2022)
41. Wu, E., Wu, K., Daneshjou, R., Ouyang, D., Ho, D.E., Zou, J.: How medical AI devices are evaluated: limitations and recommendations from an analysis of FDA approvals. Nat. Med. **27**(4), 582–584 (2021)
42. Xing, L., Giger, M.L., Min, J.K.: Artificial Intelligence in Medicine: Technical Basis and Clinical Applications. Academic Press, Cambridge (2020)
43. Yang, L., Ene, I.C., Arabi Belaghi, R., Koff, D., Stein, N., Santaguida, P.L.: Stakeholders' perspectives on the future of artificial intelligence in radiology: a scoping review. Eur. Radiol. **32**(3), 1477–1495 (2022)

Exploring Users' Perspectives of Mobile Health Privacy and Autonomy

Thomas Starks[✉][iD], Kshitij Patil, and Aqueasha Martin-Hammond[iD]

School of Informatics, Computing, and Engineering, Indiana University – Indianapolis, Indianapolis, IN 46202, USA
{tmstarks,kshpatil,aqumarti}@iu.edu

Abstract. The increased use of mobile health (mHealth) applications and the corresponding exchange of sensitive data has underscored privacy concerns. Privacy notices are often unengaging or incomprehensible, leading to questions of informed consent and trust. While studies have focused on providing solutions aimed to simplify privacy language and reduce cognitive burden, often overlooked are the behavioral aspects of individual attitudes, norms, and perceived control that lead to dynamic intentions for engagement. In this paper, we use existing behavior models as a lens to understand users' privacy experiences, behaviors, and perspectives toward mHealth data privacy policies. In 15 semi-structured interviews with adult users of mHealth applications, participants encountered persistent challenges when engaging and articulating the value of privacy. Participants do not understand how privacy notices are designed, which leads to superficial awareness and control that does not actually support their perceptions of autonomy and trust in mHealth. As a result, users felt sub-optimal autonomy when engaging in privacy interactions. We discuss design considerations for autonomy-supporting privacy notices that may help users feel a greater sense of agency when interacting with mHealth applications.

Keywords: Human-centered computing · Human computer interaction (HCI) · Empirical studies in HCI · Security and privacy · Human and societal aspects of security and privacy · Usability in security and privacy First Section

1 Introduction

Technology-driven health solutions such as mHealth applications are both prolific and challenging for privacy policy researchers, designers, and practitioners. mHealth applications are categorized as any mobile device that captures and obtains health-related data to improve quality-of-care (Cameron et al. 2017), which span diabetes management, sleep, medication, and general health and wellness, among others. The data accompanying mHealth applications require privacy policy designers to consider both regulatory compliance and individual privacy behaviors when crafting user policies, frameworks and solutions that meet privacy goals. For example, privacy design research has shown

D. Salvi et al. (Eds.): PH 2023, LNICST 572, pp. 70–91, 2024.
https://doi.org/10.1007/978-3-031-59717-6_5

promising results for reducing users' cognitive load through limiting excessive reading and decreasing users' burden through design considerations (Schaub et al., 2017). mHealth privacy research has also examined consumer's abilities to consent to data practices, such as how their data is used and stored, which is a core component of Health Insurance Portability and Accountability Act (HIPAA), General Data Protection Regulation (GDPR), and the Common Rule, three regulations that regulate the processing of personal data, outline provisions of human subject research, and safeguards privacy of medical data and other personal data (Nurgalieva et al., (2020), Arora et al., (2014)). Practitioners have also explored technical solutions that improve users' privacy awareness and ability to comply with regulatory requirements (i.e., GDPR and HIPAA) (Iwaya et al., 2022). Yet, oftentimes existing practices and approaches emphasize obtaining consent, sometimes neglecting that people ignore, or fail to understand the risks and implications of using an application or their participation in its data usage (Degeling et al., (2018), Schaub et al., (2017)). Therefore, users are often faced with the classic tradeoff between application (i.e., app) utility and privacy which ultimately leads to a black box where users are not fully informed about their data privacy rights. This presents a chasm for users and privacy policy designers positioned at the intersection of legal compliance and usable privacy design.

The rapid emergence of connected mHealth solutions has enabled more personalized and informed care (Steinhubl et al., 2015) but the ability to understand user attitudes and behaviors towards mHealth data privacy is a known trust-related barrier to user adoption (Lynch et al., (2017), "Institute of Medicine (US) Roundtable on Value & Science-Driven Health Care", (2010), (Zou et al., 2020)) and remains a challenge. One open challenge is that these solutions often ignore other relevant factors such as dynamic intent or perceived control that might impact users' behaviors in the context of healthcare (Ruotsalainen et al., 2012). We must therefore further understand the factors beyond data control and consent that influence user behaviors in the mHealth context to identify appropriate opportunities and solutions to address users' needs when interacting with privacy policies. It is imperative to better understand the intricacies of individual data privacy behaviors when interacting with mHealth applications to derive further design considerations that can inform this ubiquitous and evolving data-driven environment of mHealth. We posit that user attitudes and behaviors have a deterministic contribution in helping to identify the strengths and limitations of current privacy policies that are designed to help motivate individual data privacy behaviors, engagement, and understanding.

In this paper, we investigate users' attitudes and self-reported behaviors when engaging with mHealth data privacy policies to understand context-specific factors and opportunities to improve mHealth privacy policy design. We conducted interviews with 15 adults that use mHealth applications to understand their attitudes and behaviors toward existing mHealth privacy policies, challenges, and opportunities for improvement of these policies. During interviews, we used a focused set of probes (Appendix Table 3) to support reflection when sharing their prior experiences with mHealth data privacy policies. We selected these applications because they covered broad reaching health domains ranging from wellness (i.e., sleep) to mission-critical healthcare management (i.e., diabetes care and medication adherence), which were believed to have unique elements in data privacy decisions. In addition, we noticed that each probe, while having some common elements, had unique user interfaces from a visualization perspective. We found that certain themes were consistent with existing usable privacy research. We also found that users' sense of autonomy, perceived control and willingness (Deci et al., 2012) in mHealth privacy policy interactions were often influenced by factors other than available data control and consent. Our work builds on usable privacy and mHealth behavioral research by extending knowledge of factors that impact users' interactions with mHealth data policies. Our work extends prior research (Atienza et al., 2015) exploring users' attitudes and behaviors toward existing privacy policies. However, we focus in the context of mHealth data exploring users' experiences engaging with applications that collect their personal health information to support them in managing their health. Our work contributes to the broader research community by merging concepts of behavioral design and usable privacy to improve language understanding, and promote trust in this environment. Specifically, we extend prior research (Audie et al., 2015) that explores users' attitudes and behaviors toward existing privacy policies.

2   Related Work

We acknowledge a few foundational domains which foreground our work. We see an evolving data collection surge where emerging questions of privacy and trust ensue. We believe health data privacy is particularly relevant at this intersection of technology and ethics, and describe these domains in detail below.

2.1   Ethics on Privacy, Trust, and Technology Acceptance

Researchers in the field of ethics have considerably investigated privacy, trust, and acceptance. In a world where pervasive automation advances significantly, AI researchers have developed frameworks to optimize personal autonomy (Calvo et al., 2020) and foreground risks (Floridi et. al., 2018). Frameworks in this space consider privacy a pillar of ethical design and essential for technology acceptance, especially in the mHealth domain (Mantovani et.al., 2017). As such, privacy as a construct has a paramount position that does not only facilitate ethical AI, but also affects utility, control, trust, and acceptance goals. Researchers recognize the broad application of AI, but ethical design must establish privacy as a basic individual right that withstands the deliverance of evolving pervasive systems (Bartoletti, 2019). The reasons consumers have a strong affinity for privacy is due to several complex factors. Researchers know that variation in demographics such as age and the type of data collected (i.e., health) can either help or hurt the trust they have in a health technology, and ultimately its acceptance or adoption (Poyner et al., (2018), Schomakers et al., (2019), Wang et al., (2019), Martin-Hammond et al., (2019), Guo et al., (2016)). While significant work has been done to improve consumers' willingness to accept health technology, some experience a sense of fatalism that is perpetuated by the evolving health system they interact with (Joo et al., (2021)). This fatalism is a sign of migrating chasms between the nature of perceived privacy and the growth at which consumers are exposed to new health promotions. Researchers explore this intersection, but many do not entirely approach grounding health privacy in a proactive tradition. It is no longer ethical to misconstrue preference and control as a sufficient end towards proactive privacy. Researchers enable preference selection and other usable privacy interactions as a means to promote control over one's health data, but control is only one variable that presupposes another integral and widely overlooked virtue of autonomy. It is this belief that motivates our work and distinguishes this research from others that focus on elderly populations (Detweiler et al., 2016). More specifically, the composition that makes up autonomy is not well understood and established within advancing interconnected health systems. We will further explore the topic in later sections.

2.2 Pervasive mHealth and Black Box Use Cases

Pervasive health through the use of sensor technology has generated broad and deep insights (Wang et al., 2022). Some mHealth sensing information architectures and functionality enable health interventions by leveraging behavioral change through different engagement techniques. Some features that drive engagement such as forums present unique privacy challenges as well (Danaher et al., 2015). Other applications such as virtual health communities' research has also explored the topic of privacy (Kordzadeh et al., 2017), yet much of this research focuses on supporting human-human communication rather than human-machine communication, which makes the domain unique. What makes this area of HCI unique is the Mobile health (mHealth) component, which is defined as, "the use of mobile devices to monitor or detect biological changes in the human body, while device management entities, such as hospitals, clinics, or service providers, collect data and use them for healthcare and health status improvement" (Park, 2016), and is similar to others' (Ruotsalainen et al., 2012) definition in the context of pervasive health. mHealth can also include self-reported health data provided by users through consumer-focused personal tracking and reporting applications (Radbron et al., 2019). Although the growing ubiquity of mHealth applications has seemingly large potential upside to improve health through innovative and connected solutions such as IoT (Bertino et al., 2016), researchers are faced with navigating the need for large amounts of data with the complex domain of opaque health privacy (Quinn et al., 2022). To this end, many mHealth technologies have the large upside potential to transform healthcare through integrated machine learning capabilities and artificial intelligence. Although many contributions have been made in this arena, health-related stigmas can influence privacy perceptions and perpetuate concerns of the technology's utility (Arora et al., 2014). Design for sharing behavioral data in social constructs as leverage of peer support for health monitoring; also establishes engagement with data privacy across a lifecycle as an interesting research avenue (Vilaza et al., 2019).

Even though policies such as HIPAA provide protections for personal health data, users often still have concerns about what data is collected about them and how it is used (Al Ameen, 2012). As such, researchers are exploring ways to reduce negative impacts and perceptions through contextualizing privacy concerns in this space (Ferreira et al., 2021). For example, some researchers note that some mHealth privacy concerns are associated with age and can be used to tailor mobile applications to these users (Ferreira et al., 2021). Significant work has been done to define regulatory frameworks and user constraints in IoT environments (Poyner et al., 2018). Other work by Irwin Altman confirms that privacy is both dynamic and subjective, and is susceptible to change over time along with different contexts, which is the basis for Privacy Regulation Theory. Irwin theorizes privacy as the control and feedback over information flow, which our work expands; however, the framework produced focuses heavily on contextualizing health environment monitoring solutions rather than mobile health, which we posit has proximal differences in interpretation (Moncrieff et al., 2009).

To address black-box perceptions in pervasive health technology, designing for transparency and choice are important in passive data sharing to reduce privacy concerns. Current design is still only accounting for upfront choice and transparency, and little with how choice and engagement are actively managed after data is shared (Kolovson et al., 2020). Some researchers posit "...the crux of modern machine learning: the reliance on powerful but intrinsically opaque models. When applied to the healthcare domain, these models fail to meet the needs for transparency that their clinician and patient end-users require. We review the implications of this failure, and argue that opaque models (1) lack quality assurance, (2) fail to elicit trust, and (3) restrict physician-patient dialogue. We then discuss how upholding transparency in all aspects of model design and model validation can help ensure the reliability and success of medical AI..." this forms the basis for not just opaque AI models in healthcare but also opaque data journeys in mHealth (Quinn et al., 2022). While regulation may be the de facto standard for ensuring privacy between interoperable devices like fitness trackers and smartwatches, device requirements subject to FDA and HIPAA are not widely acknowledged due to lack of awareness and misidentifying medical device classifications (Motti, 2019).

2.3 Privacy Control Versus Autonomy

Often, privacy behaviors appear to be dictated by technology that simply aims to provide control(s); through this lens, we see a challenge in autonomy due to a lack of self-direction, identity, and intrinsic factors (Deci et al., 2012). However, based on Self-Determination Theory (SDT), the premise of true autonomy in this context is the feeling that one is both being in control and willing to engage in good privacy-preserving behaviors – simply, we must transcend from designing controls to designing autonomy. We posit that privacy-by-design is being challenged in unique ways due to the complexity of systems that collect, process, and maintain data. While regulations such as GDPR and HIPAA exist to govern data practices and have an important role (Premarathne et al., 2015), their principles are collectively reduced to compliance-centric models, which leaves little room to improve usable mechanisms beyond 'cookies' (Degeling et al., 2018) or other usable privacy mechanisms. It is for this reason that existing privacy-preserving infrastructures are not fully capable to keep up with the needs of consumer mHealth innovations. An example of this resides in the health IoT environment where consumers value privacy over novel utilities and feel the two are somehow negotiated against each other (Zou et al., 2020). Researchers have aimed to address problems that exist between humans and ubiquitous computing, but mobile health wearables and applications in particular, have unique challenges related to secure interoperability between devices, databases, and governing infrastructures, which have created negative privacy perceptions (Ometov et al., 2021). These perceptions are perpetuated by the advancing need to continuously collect sensing and individual data to generate insights (Ometov et al., 2021). However, similar to research on mobile crowdsourcing and trust authentication, the collection and processing methods in this environment are inadequately expounded on, thus consumers are left with gaps in knowledge about their data journey and have seemingly limited trust in the wearables they use (Feng et al., 2018). While researchers explore trust and control in various privacy models, once mHealth devices begin to collect data, ultimately, users are therefore left with the belief that their data is shared in a black-box environment intended to capitalize on their use of the technology without providing sufficient awareness of their data integrity. In this research, we explore users' perceptions of privacy policies to uncover factors they perceive to influence their autonomy in privacy policy interactions beyond the existence of privacy control(s). By doing so, we aim to understand how user self-reported behaviors are influenced, or not, by their sense of perceived autonomy in those interactions and identify design considerations for future autonomy-preserving privacy interactions.

3   Methods

Our interviews aimed to answer the following research questions:

- RQ1: What are users' current experiences with mHealth privacy policies?
- RQ2: What are users' attitudes and behaviors toward privacy policies for mobile applications that collect and use personal health data and why?

3.1 Theoretical Framing

Because we wanted to understand users' behaviors when engaging with the design of privacy policies in mhealth applications, we initially started with the Fogg Behavior Model (FBM) to help frame questions in our study protocol because of its focus on user behavior and technology design (Fogg, 2009). Fogg's model describes that user behaviors can be influenced by recognizing user motivation and ability, and potentially designing triggers that characterize those relationships (Fogg, 2009). However, we later expanded our theoretical framing during the analysis phase after exploring the data and realizing that broader concepts were emerging related to the Theory of Reasoned Action (TRA). The TRA focuses on motivations such as intents and a person's ability to act or adapt to behaviors according to them (Fishbein, 1979). Within the TRA, humans are viewed as rational decision-makers that when faced with a decision of pros and cons, adequately weigh them consistently and predictably in accordance with the most optimal economic benefit (Fishbein, 1979) – this decision-making is similar to privacy calculus in our research context. We quickly realized through iterative thematic analysis that TRA would succumb to limitations about perceptions of user control, which is why we explored a similar model that allowed us to focus on that component of behavioral intent. To characterize the relationship between intention and behavior, the Theory of Planned Behavior (TPB) describes intentions as multi-faceted, which rely on perceived levels of individual behavioral control, subjective norms, and attitudes (Icek, 1991). These dimensions of intent are dynamic and inherently conflict with behavioral economics where decisions are considered rational and reliable. In our data, we began to see concerns emerging that were related to understanding health privacy language and subsequent voluntary consent to its practices. While we used FBM to design our study, we framed our analysis through the TPB to understand participant's interactions with mHealth privacy and how it relates to perceived autonomy (see Appendix Table 4 for an overview of this methodological process).

3.2 Participants

Participants were recruited from a local community in the surrounding areas of a mid-west city in the United States. They were required to be age 18 years or older, and be current users of mhealth applications and consent to privacy policies. We chose a broad age range and were not intending to compare differences based on demographics at this phase of research. No participants were excluded. Participants' ages ranged from 28–67 years old (Appendix Table 1). All participants had a smartphone or mobile phone with internet access. Participants ranged in mHealth usage and frequency of privacy notice engagements. Participants encountered the policies through a variety of devices including Apple Watch, IoMT (Internet of Medical Things), iPhone, Alexa, smart appliances, Electronic Medical Records (EMR), and Fitbits among others. To further understand participants' existing views on data and privacy, we also asked them to share what they felt data and privacy mean (Appendix Table 2).

3.3 Study Procedures

During each 60-min semi-structured interview, we asked participants about their experiences with privacy notices when using mobile applications including health related apps. Additionally, we shared with participants various mHealth privacy notice examples as probes (Appendix Table 3) to help participants reflect on their own encounters with mHealth privacy policies, their attitudes and behaviors toward them, and factors they felt influenced their attitudes and behaviors (Hutchinson et al., 2003). Finally, we asked participants to reflect on barriers and challenges they faced, if any, and to brainstorm ideas of how they feel one might improve interactions with privacy policies to improve their sense of autonomy when engaging. Each participant was asked to complete a demographic and background survey at the end of the study. These questions were gathered to understand participant characteristics and technology experiences. We conducted interviews until we stopped hearing and seeing new data (i.e., saturation) (Chun Tie et al., 2019). After completing all interviews, we began analysis of the data.

3.4 Data Analysis

We audio recorded all interviews and transcribed them prior to data analysis. We used thematic analysis situated in Grounded Theory (GT) to analyze our data. The GT research process consists of collecting qualitative data, inductively assigning codes to data to develop themes, comparing themes with external research, and building theory from these themes (Chun Tie et al., 2019). This inductive process considers data saturation and external research comparisons to iteratively refine codes and themes to support the theory (Chun Tie et al., 2019). Once we confirmed a level of support from existing literature, we generated a codebook to guide our deductive coding process.

Using the codebook, two researchers independently coded two of the transcripts to further refine the codebook and establish inter-rater reliability (McDonald et al., 2019) between the researchers. Inter-rater reliability was assessed to determine the likelihood that two independent reviews of the same participant transcript yield similar outcomes. Thus, we wanted to determine if the generated codes were interpreted similarly between independent reviewers. Pre-defined acceptance criteria for the reliability score was set at 80% or greater on an individual quotation level aligned with existing practice. The researchers defined rules prior to analysis, which established which transcripts would be coded; rationale supporting this decision was based on the participant's code distribution and nominal representation of educational background compared to other subjects (undergraduate degree). Of 41 codes and definitions, the inter-rater reliability score of 80% was exceeded after initial comparisons and a round of discussion to address agreements and disagreements. Once consensus was established, one researcher coded the entire subset of transcripts using the codebook.

4 Findings

We found a need for additional focus on autonomy in mHealth privacy interactions. Participants had mixed-attitudes about the value and usefulness of mhealth privacy policies. For instance, we found that subjective norms and perceived control (beyond actual data controls provided) uniquely contributed to users' sense of autonomy in interactions with mHealth privacy policies. Participants believed that these additional factors should be considered in privacy policy design to facilitate personalized, engaging, and meaningful interactions in highly dynamic mHealth privacy situations. Our results suggest that beyond the ability to control personal data, users' sense of autonomy in privacy interactions may also rely on the ability of designers to truly engage users to understand how the design of solutions are intended to protect them. In the following subsections, we present results of what participants told us about their unmet needs for autonomy with mHealth privacy interactions.

4.1 Incongruent Informed Consent is a Barrier to Engagement and Trust

We learned that participants felt they often had to consent to mHealth privacy policies without being fully informed about them. Participants did not attribute this problem to a lack of information, but rather the question of what it means to be "informed" and how the information presented (with the goal of informing) engages the user. For example, P14 explained consent is often a binary choice but emphasized the distinction between consenting and being informed. They stated, "Theoretically, yes…if it comes down to that binary choice and if the consumer is being informed, then that's consent. If you're signing up for something and you're not being informed, that's not informed consent. So that's a different argument and that's a different situation…" So, while participants mentioned a lack of engagement with policy information, they also challenged the notion that listing information in a policy is sufficient for engaging users and helping them understand its meaning.

Participants also encountered situations where they lacked understanding of the information presented but felt obligated to consent in order to access the services. For example,

P10 stated, "It [consent] is definitely a gray area because technically by the book I am checking the box that I read and understand the notice. But if that is the only way that I'm going to be able to use this system [a mHealth system] that I want to use, there's not really much of an option for me to get further clarification or additional resources to fully understand my data privacy rights, as far as how that company or that service is handling things." P10 also later stated, "It's sort of the ultimatum, you either use the [mHealth] system or you don't. That's the only decision that you're allowed as a user…" Another participant, P09, shared a similar sentiment, "Do I really want to access this information, or do I want to have to go through a manual way or not do anything at all? Most of the time, I just accept it because I want to be able to pay my [medical] bill online or I want to be able to access MyChart [a personal health record] information online, and in order to do that, I have to accept it. So since you don't really get a choice and you need to get to it, you pretty much have to accept it anyway." These findings are consistent with research by (Utz et al., 2019) that notes the tensions users face when weighing tradeoffs between being informed and giving consent when interacting with privacy policies more broadly. Yet, participants discuss that when in these situations they feel they have limited autonomy especially if it is necessary or critical for them to use a mHealth system.

When manufacturers require consent without ensuring that users are sufficiently informed, or when not having access to a device or service is the only alternative option to consent, users shared that they begin to experience feelings that perpetuate transactional compliance as more important than costumer feelings or expectations. For example, P01 stated, "I think it's [providing privacy notices] strictly for compliance's sake. I don't know how many people actually read the privacy notices. So I hesitate to say it protects the consumer. I mean, it should protect consumers. It should protect both parties, quite frankly, but I just don't see that actually happening. I mean, I can't imagine, or I have to imagine the percentage of people that actually read terms of service or privacy notices or anything along those lines is remarkably small." As a result, participants believed that their interests are secondary to a manufacturer's compliance requirement, and they therefore experienced mistrust. We discovered that this mistrust is tied to the institutional systems and processes that govern mHealth applications. Although participant's degree of trust was inconclusive, some participants shared that it was attributed to unclear pre-market processes and the manufacturer or governing institution's history as it relates to quality. For example, P06 stated, "if I had a suspicion…my default is that makers have been vetted through the app store and they are trustworthy. But if I felt like there was something about their quality or trustworthiness that [there were] some sort of red flag, I might go into the privacy agreements. To be honest, if it was made… [by someone] that usually doesn't have our best interests in mind…that would motivate me to look [at] trust and quality." The limited choices related to consent and transparency of institutional practices, led participants to feel they had less autonomy in their privacy decisions related to mHealth applications.

4.2   Social Influences on Privacy Perceptions Influence Decisions

We learned that the perceptions of society or others also sometimes influenced participants' privacy decisions. Akin to the influence of social norms in TPB, we found that participants sometimes see imbalances between technological advances and personal privacy on a macro socio-technical level. Some participants feared that society values the speed and convenience of mHealth technologies more than understanding their privacy implications. For example, P01 stated, "[the] balance of convenience and technology is one that's a very difficult one for me that I kind of struggle with just because I know how much you are giving up in the sense of privacy... I like to be more informed where that balance is with every individual device or piece of software, or whatever it is that I am interacting with... I like to be informed on how much of my life I am giving away or my information or my private data, or we will see how much of my soul I am selling to save eight minutes or to gain some form of convenience... I don't think that there is enough concern in the general populace for the level of information that is being collected about every individual..." Some participants therefore held a belief true privacy is hopelessly implausible due to the advancing tech market, which is consistent with attitudes of fatalism (Joo et al., (2021)). For example, P01 stated, "Unfortunately, privacy is a pipe dream that most people have given up." suggesting that they feel most users do not have autonomy in privacy decisions whether they like it or not. However, there were other users that were hopeful that future mHealth privacy research will consider these social concerns and influences and their implications.

Participants explained their privacy decisions are sometimes negatively affected by the type of health condition their mHealth device supports. Participants mentioned that mental health and addiction heighten their privacy decisions because these conditions have potential social stigmas and insurance implications. One participant was concerned about billing insurance for mental health issues. For example, P05 stated, "...when I worked in a health setting, you see a lot of patients coming in for mental health reasons or addiction reasons, and they didn't want their insurance billed, or they didn't want it to go through certain channels because they wanted to keep it highly private." Another participant was concerned about their employer receiving sensitive information about their addiction. For example, P08 stated, "...so say I had a drug problem or something, and there was an app for what I'm trying to handle that or something, I wouldn't want the fact that I was a drug addict being shared with an employer or anyone really. So, those kinds of things that could be looked on negatively..." As stated by these participants, social stigmas around sensitive health conditions have a role to play in their privacy decisions and also could impact their sense of autonomy leading to the decision not to engage with a mHealth application.

Participants also described a need for alternative modes of privacy discourse outside of traditional manufacturer notices that are typically provided. To address this, participants shared that they sometimes leverage social networks to communicate about critical mHealth privacy issues. One participant, P14 stated, "I think most people would learn through media or social media quicker than probably that a business would be notifying you that your data was compromised". Thus, participants expressed that their participation in social communication channels are needed for timely information that may affect their privacy decisions. So, participants expressed sometimes experiencing collective privacy influence. This collective influence could lead to developing apathy about privacy decisions due to perceived societal norms, more stringent views due to fear of societal stigma, or alternative paths to build confidence in their decisions through social networks affecting their autonomy when engaging with mHealth applications.

4.3 Contextual Nascence: Navigating Black Box Interoperability and Historical Preconceptions

We learned that participants' interactions with privacy notices vary significantly but may originate from unique historical preconceptions, such as black box interoperability and the evolution of health and technology. For example, interoperable mHealth environments collect and process various forms of sensor and self-reported personal health data. This data is often embedded in artificial intelligence (AI) or other personalized systems whose architecture enables health management solutions similar to those described in other work (Danaher et al., 2015). While these architectures are innovative, participants expressed privacy concerns about technologies such as proactive AI systems that continually collect their data and push untraceable targeted-marketing material. This raises broader questions about the role of emerging technologies such as IoT or voice technologies in shaping users perceptions of mHealth technologies and users interactions with health applications provided by those devices. For example, P09 stated, "…Siri and the Amazon Echo are listening all the time [and] can get information and they're going to hear private health information. If, you know, somebody's listening or they're going back and reviewing vital recordings, as they're supposedly trying to make Siri better and more interactive with better programming. There are people who hear that private information. So because it's recorded near your house, private information could also be out there if that's what happens, what was recorded at that point in time." Participants were generally uncertain about the AI black box (Lau et al., 2018), but were tangibly concerned about the inability to trace data effectively across its lifecycle, and especially when it is shared or sold for other purposes. For example, P10 stated, "…this kind of goes along the lines of sharing or understanding how my data is being shared with other companies or the service provider I am doing business with…If I start to get targeted or oddly specific targeted ads that seem to be coming from my interactions with one system in particular, that could prompt me to take a look and maybe try to get a better understanding of just how much data is being collected and how it's being used. And just kind of trying to connect the dots if I get very targeted marketing on different devices and I can try to trace it back to a certain application…".

Participants also perceived healthcare's historical evolution as a motivational factor towards privacy. Health technologies such as mHealth are burdened with negative historical connotations for various reasons such as public cases of individuals' health data rights being violated. Participants explained that the rapid prevalence of notices for various technologies is one reason why some pre-mHealth generations have negative views about mHealth technologies. For example, P07 stated, "I think at this point, I'm young enough to expect them [privacy policies] to be there and old enough to remember when they weren't." Another negative historical connotation was explained by P02, who stated, "the older cases of like Henrietta Lacks, they used her [information] and she never knew." We found that these historical references and events influenced how participants perceived privacy in certain social groups.

In summary, we learned that subjective norms around interoperable environments (e.g., wearables and remote patient monitoring) in the health context, social influences, and changing motivations each influence participants' privacy interactions, which ultimately affects their perception of autonomy and trust in those interactions. By uncovering these subjective norms, we identified unique relationships with trust that may not have been clearly articulated previously in the mHealth design space.

5 Discussion

Through the lens of TPB, our research finds that mHealth users are unengaged with privacy policies and feel there is a chasm between their individual needs and the controls provided by the privacy community. Overall, our research suggests that mHealth users generally agree that privacy policies are beneficial and crucial for mHealth applications; however, they encounter persistent challenges when engaging with those policies. Specifically, we found that not sufficiently characterizing user' perceptions of internal and external motivations may obfuscate real opportunities for making privacy language more engaging and bridging the gap to help users understand essential information. As such, one result may be that end-users do not understand how the design of these privacy solutions are intended to protect them. Thus, having superficial awareness without knowledgeable engagement does not actually support autonomy and trust in mHealth applications. Our research builds on existing literature [Cunha et al., (2020), Leon et al., (2015), Vilaza et al., (2019), Gupta, (2018)) by advocating for the development of privacy solutions to be behaviorally and contextually orientated in order to uncover real user facing problems when interacting with mHealth privacy policies. Improving users' ability to understand language and recognize dynamic mHealth privacy environments relies on systematically assessing motivational intentions that engage users beyond basic privacy awareness. Further, we found that perceived control over one's mHealth privacy is unrealized partly in fact due to the inability to tangibly see, interact, and understand what privacy means when engaging with a mHealth technology. Thus, many users feel they lack autonomy when engaging with mHealth privacy policies, but due to the criticality of the context - managing health, users feel compelled to comply or completely disengage despite their concerns. Our results show that designing for motivationally charged engagement and understanding by leveraging social factors may be one effective way to optimize autonomy-support and trust in mHealth solutions. We discuss these implications in the following sections.

5.1 More Control Does Not Equal More Autonomy

Our work considers perceived autonomy through the lens of Self Determination Theory (Deci et al., 2012), where autonomy is having the choice and will to act according to personal goals and values. For health-related technology design, (Calvo et al., 2020) distinguishes autonomy from independence and control, noting that perceived autonomy can also be influenced by individual behaviors, lifestyle or society, which in-turn impacts adoption. Significant work has been done to simplify the experience that users have with privacy policies (Acquisti et al., 2017) and provide them with more control over their data, consent, and nudging interactions (Cunha et al., (2020), Degeling et al., (2018), Schaub et al., (2017), Utz et al. (2019)). Yet, due to some of the historically untrustworthy actions that occurred that sit at the intersection of health and privacy (Grossmann et al., 2011), some users still are wary, influencing their perceptions of mHealth technologies. To address questionable trust and adoption in mHealth systems that collect and process health data, researchers and industry practitioners have seemingly held the position that providing more ways for users to access and manage personal data is a sufficient baseline for control (Schaub et al., (2017), (Atienza et al., 2015)). However, we uncovered that users' perceptions and expectations of privacy control often do not equate to the independence that is needed for autonomy. Therefore, based on our data we conclude that there is a conflated belief that control is the same as autonomy. In the design of health and well-being technologies, often autonomy extends beyond the binary concepts of control and is defined as a users' feeling of agency or their ability to act based on their goals and values (Peters et al., 2018). In the context of mHealth privacy, while it is reasonable to assume that personal responsibility is essential for consenting and using mHealth technologies, non-privacy-neutral perceptions inherently exist when users are tasked with deciding to use a service or not (binary opt-in vs. opt-out). This is further compounded by the fact that notice-choice structures present content that are likely not to be read in the first place (Meier et al., 2020). When agreements are in place with conditions that are non-negotiable to the user's existing motives or beliefs, this creates questions of perceived control over one's privacy and whether the application actually supports users' autonomy, and is deserving of trust.

Our findings highlight users' beliefs that there are not enough alternative ways of getting people to engage with their mHealth data privacy practices, specifically informed consent interactions. Further, offloading all the privacy decisions at the launch of a new app is not only contradicting the benefit of the mHealth app, but it also ignores the dynamic ways that people choose to be informed and interact with their sensitive information. In the future, it would be beneficial for usable privacy researchers and industry professionals to explore alternative strategies that focus on personalized and emotional engagements with mHealth data privacy in order to support autonomy, while also distinguishing this work from traditional views about privacy control that often focuses on actions. In similar discussions, (Christman, 2020) distinguishes basic and ideal autonomy where basic autonomy implies that users are free from influence and imply they are not under constricting conditions. We also posit that patients with health conditions who seek support from mHealth technologies are inherently constricted in autonomy and thus are forced to weigh utility-tradeoffs unfairly. While this context of autonomy relates to other work regarding "contextual integrity" (Wijesekara et al., (2015), Zimmer, (2018)), we find that meeting user expectations is not simply about control (e.g., permissions, etc.), but also recognizing the role of changing awareness and mental processing, particularly on the side of social and historical influences. Our research extends prior work that examines contextual factors related to general privacy policy design (Micinski et al., (2017), Votipka et al., (2018), Squicciarini et al., (2014)), but we extrapolate factors unique to supporting autonomy with mHealth's privacy interactions.

5.2 Balancing Perceptions of mHealth Privacy Autonomy and Automation

Privacy autonomy, through the lens of independent engagement and trust, is inherently challenged because of limited support and choices (Cunha et al., (2020), Schaub et al., (2017)). However, our examination of users' self-reported behaviors indicates that understanding mHealth privacy language is also a barrier to fully engaging with a technology. We extend the need to decouple the domains of being informed and intentional consent in order to focus research towards understanding language over simply improving consent interactions. Making information comprehensible for users reach educational and governance systems because both are needed to scale health and consumer applications, especially when data collection is essential in the user's health journey. In some mHealth technologies, such as the wearable Apple Watch, users are able to select the data that may be collected about them (i.e., biometric identifiers) conditional to the practices that are employed in a given app's functionality. Using gamification techniques may be another considerable way of building user knowledge about the personal data collected about them, which is supported in the research by (Simon et al., 2021) that describes cognitive absorption for privacy decision-making because of engaging gamification. Other research (Mavroeidi et al., 2020) also considers using gamification for engaging users about privacy. However, we also suggest that in the future, it could be useful to investigate the role of gamification in building value constructs aimed to incentivize (or motivate) learning and understanding complex mHealth data privacy.

Collective privacy influence is a unique area that emerged from our interviews because it highlights both the benefit and responsibility of understanding social contexts when developing policies about mHealth privacy. Although this finding is similar to users engaging in health-based communities for health support (Kordzadeh et al., (2017), Danaher et al., (2015)), it is unique in the sense of mHealth privacy because it exposes a gap where individuals and their social influences are not currently aligned, which affects these users' perceived privacy control, thus autonomy and trust. This is similarly discussed in research by (Gupta, 2018) that identifies external influences (e.g., such as prior experience) on older adults' general privacy behaviors, but the emerging theme from our interviews recognizes the social norms, highlighted in behavioral theories such as TPB (Icek, 1991), play a unique role in dynamic mHealth privacy behaviors. Various socially oriented topics arose from our data ranging from meta views on balancing social and personal privacy initiatives, situation avoidance for privacy discourse, data privacy footprint in social networks, balancing privacy advocacy and improving services, and providing community for individuals with stigmatized health conditions. While these topics range in variety and abstraction, they construct a basic model for the relationship between social influences and perceived individual privacy attitudes, thus extending work (Zou et al., (2020), Guo et al., (2016)) by detailing unique behavioral intentions used as a vehicle for trust in mHealth systems. It is for this reason that we suggest that future usable mHealth privacy research must continue to investigate these topics and explore opportunities to leverage and enhance these outside constructs for the development of truly autonomy-supporting privacy interactions.

Furthermore, potential design directions that strike a balance between autonomy and automation may need to focus primarily on consent, transparency, and trust. Specifically, designing preferences at the time when the user provides consent must be careful in not overwhelming the intended users with options that seemingly appear outside of the perceived guardrails. This means that while some configurable parameters may be needed, having too many options can lead to confusion or make users feel like they are completely on their own in their privacy decisions. This nuanced position is contrast to the notion of having complete awareness and control as premised in previous research (Andrews, (2019), Schaub et al., (2017)), but it more importantly must match users expectations about broadly applied privacy preference modeling across mHealth apps. Moreover, consent modeling is inherently dynamic over time and between people who share information in mHealth app environments. For example, collaborative privacy sharing models (Petronio, 2010) take into account multiple parties, but how these collaborative agreements change with participant preferences over time present uncertainty, thus designing for clear user-roles and control are critically important. Lastly, fostering trust and transparency requires a transparency about black box environments where data are collected, processed, and stored. Such transparency-enhancing tools are acknowledged as helping promote privacy and trust (Janic, et al., (2013)), but an importantThis mechanism of for this visibility must ensure traceability of data usages and clear verifiable levels of control by the user over data in those specific environments.

5.3 Limitations

One limitation of our work is that our study is retrospective of behaviors and does not actually observe behaviors with privacy policies. While the self-reported accounts provided by participants provide insights into their experiences with mHealth privacy policies, additional studies of direct user behavior may uncover additional challenges and design implications. Our work is also qualitative which is useful for providing an in-depth understanding of users' attitudes and perceptions. However, one tradeoff of qualitative work is that findings are not generalizable (Leung, 2015). We provide a rich, thick description to aid transferability, but our work like other qualitative work (Joo et al., (2021), Martin-Hammond et al., (2019), Zhang et al., (2021)) is likely limited based on the context in which it was carried out. Further, as we collected data we began to see recurring ideas, and continued until we stopped seeing new data, which. This is consistent with the processes for analyzing qualitative data., however our While our sample is small and may be limited by certain participant demographics, such as some participants that were familiar with familiarity with privacy policies, we believe this to still be a valuable step in the direction to explore this research further and look to consider age-based and other demographic perspectives in future work and therefore some users' privacy concerns may not be represented in our findings. Our N = 15 is slightly higher than other qualitative interviews (Caine, 2016) conducted by HCI researchers, however, data reached saturation at 12 participants where we noticed consistent responses with fewer new points emerging. We completed an initial review of all transcripts excluding those without response variation to determine those to include in agreement calculations. We used (McDonald et al., 2019) for determining our agreement approach. Our analysis approach was consistent with their arguments against solely using IRR for agreement. These are considerations for future research.

6   Conclusion

In this paper, we used existing behavior models as a lens to understand users' privacy experiences, behaviors, and perspectives toward mHealth data privacy policies. From 15 semi-structured interviews with adult users of mHealth applications, we extend knowledge of users' experiences and unmet needs for privacy policy design that influence users' behaviors toward mHealth applications. Through the lens of the Theory of Planned Behavior and SDT, we characterize factors beyond personal data control and consent that influence users' sense of autonomy when engaging with mHealth privacy policies. Finally, we provide unique considerations for privacy policy design that focus on improving consent preferences, transparency of privacy control statuses, and building trust on a multiple levels.

Acknowledgments. Special thanks to the participants that shared their experiences and Davide Bolchini, Ph.D., for assisting with editing.

Appendix

Table 1. Participant Demographics

P#	Gender	Age	Highest education level	OS	mHealth app usage	Privacy notice frequency
1	Male	43	Graduate degree	iOS	Daily	Weekly
2	Female	31	Graduate degree	AOS	Daily	Daily
3	Male	47	Graduate degree	iOS	Monthly	Monthly
4	Male	31	Graduate degree	iOS	Daily	Weekly
5	Female	39	Undergraduate degree	iOS	Daily	Annually
6	Male	49	Graduate degree	iOS	Monthly	Monthly
7	Female	39	Some college	iOS	Daily	Weekly
8	Female	67	Undergraduate degree	iOS	Daily	Monthly
9	Female	56	Doctorate degree	iOS	Daily	Daily
10	Male	28	Undergraduate degree	iOS	Weekly	Monthly
11	Female	57	Graduate degree	iOS	Daily	Weekly
12	Male	37	Some college	iOS	Weekly	Weekly
13	Female	32	Undergraduate degree	AOS	Daily	Weekly
14	Male	28	Undergraduate degree	iOS	Weekly	Monthly
15	Male	59	Some college	iOS	Daily	Weekly

Table 2. Preliminary Themes

Question	Answer	Theme
Meaning of "data"	Collected	Informational inputs and outputs
	Interpreted	
	Analyzed	
	Processed	
	Decision derivation	
Meaning of "privacy"	Confidentiality	Limiting exposures
	Access	
	Hopelessly implausible	Socio-technical influences
	Personal protection	Personal interventions
	Control	

Table 3. Study interview mobile health privacy policy probes (stimuli)

Apple (General)	Accu-Chek Connect (Diabetes)	Sleep Cycle (Sleep)	Medisafe (Medications)	mySugr (Diabetes)

Table 4. Methodological process

Table 5. Initial & Intermediate Thematic Codes

Emerging Themes	Privacy Challenges (Codes)
Disconnected cognition for assessing value	Modern data privacy interpretations
	Knowledge, emotional, and identity benefits
	Disconnected knowledge to propose value in pervasive environments
Challenged agency - limited freedom of choice	Incongruent consent
	Insufficient options
	Information retrieval
	Inflexible and disabled solutions
	Multivariate burdens and utilities
	Unclear privacy requirements for players
	Privacy requirements for preventing harm to organization and user
Customizable, trustworthy, and engaging solutions to build sensational experiences	UX/UI for improving privacy engagement
	Privacy volume and comprehension affecting app authenticity and trust
	Custom feature development that enable privacy interactions
Privacy awareness anticipations for the future	Balance between social and personal privacy paradigm
	Privacy competence to ensure end user interests are core

(continued)

Table 5. (*continued*)

Emerging Themes	Privacy Challenges (Codes)
	Awareness about where data exists in the wild and corrective steps to reduce its footprint
External influencers	Avoiding situations where privacy beliefs are challenged
	Knowing data footprint in connected social networks
	Balance user privacy advocacy and improving services
	Community for those with stigmatized health conditions
Unique Motivators	Mapping app's utility to types of required privacy interactions
	UX/UI not designed for diverse intended users' needs
	Robust and quality-driven app vetting to produce trust
	Privacy information designed for simple, personalized risks/controls
	Data types with high motivation
Supporting contextual autonomy through accessibility	Visual limitations persist and inhibit ability pursuant modality
	Ability dependent on environment
	Discern problem solving (self-diagnosis and resolution) VS. Seeking professional consultation
	Attention limitation
	Efficient, simple, and gratifying enable ability
Triggering autonomy through automation	Early declaration of an app intended use and relationship to your data
	Undesirable early interactions impacting attention and experience
	High frequency notices inducing questions and fatigue
	Overcoming negative historical connotations

(continued)

Table 5. (*continued*)

Emerging Themes	Privacy Challenges (Codes)
	Unclear time-value tradeoff
	Enable automatic prompts for reduced manual/mental comparisons
	App launch and preset schedule for data change notification
	Interaction and illustration for privacy change engagement
	Social risk-reward engagement
	Uncertainty in AI

References

Acquisti, A., et al.: Nudges for privacy and security: understanding and assisting users' choices online. ACM Comput. Surv. **50**(3): Article 44 (2017)

Al Ameen, M., Liu, J., Kwak, K.: Security and privacy issues in wireless sensor networks for healthcare applications. J. Med. Syst. **36**, 93–101 (2012). https://doi.org/10.1007/s10916-010-9449-4

Andrews, V.: Analyzing awareness on data privacy. In: Proceedings of the 2019 ACM Southeast Conference, pp. 198–201. Association for Computing Machinery, Kennesaw (2019)

Arora, S., Yttri, J., Nilse, W.: Privacy and Security in Mobile Health (mHealth) Research. Alcohol Res. Current Rev. **36**(1), 143–151 (2014)

Atienza, A.A., et al.: Consumer attitudes and perceptions on mHealth privacy and security: findings from a mixed-methods study. J. Health Commun. **20**(6), 673–679 (2015). https://doi.org/10.1080/10810730.2015.1018560

Bartoletti, I.: AI in Healthcare: Ethical and Privacy Challenges. Springer International Publishing, Cham (2019)

Bertino, E., et al.: Internet of Things (IoT): Smart and Secure Service Delivery. ACM Trans. Internet Technol. **16**(4): Article 22 (2016)

Caine, K.: Local standards for sample size at CHI. In: Proceedings of the 2016 CHI Conference on Human Factors in Computing Systems, pp. 981–992, May 2016

Calvo, R.A., Peters, D., Vold, K., Ryan, R.M.: Supporting human autonomy in AI systems: a framework for ethical enquiry. In: Burr, C., Floridi, L. (eds) Ethics of Digital Well-Being. Philosophical Studies Series, vol. 140. Springer, Cham (2020). https://doi.org/10.1007/978-3-030-50585-1_2

Cameron, J.D., Ramaprasad, A., Syn, T.: An ontology of and roadmap for mHealth research. Int. J. Med. Informatics **100**, 16–25 (2017). https://doi.org/10.1016/j.ijmedinf.2017.01.007

Chen, Y., et al.: Privacy games. ACM Trans. Econ. Comput. **8**(2), Article 9 (2020)

Christman, J.: Autonomy in Moral and Political Philosophy. The Stanford Encyclopedia of Philosophy (Fall 2020 Edition), Edward N. Zalta (ed.). https://plato.stanford.edu/archives/fall2020/entries/autonomy-moral/

Chun Tie, Y., Birks, M., Francis, K.: Grounded theory research: a design framework for novice researchers. SAGE Open Med. **7**, 2050312118822927 (2019). https://doi.org/10.1177/2050312118822927

Cunha, J.A.O.G.d., Aguiar, Y.P.C.: Reflections on the role of nudges in human-computer inter-action for behavior change: software designers as choice architects. In: Proceedings of the 19th Brazilian Symposium on Human Factors in Computing Systems. Diamantina, Brazil, Association for Computing Machinery: Article 56 (2020)

Danaher, B.G., et al.: From black box to toolbox: outlining device functionality, engagement activities, and the pervasive information architecture of mHealth interventions. Internet Interv. **2**(1), 91–101 (2015)

Deci, E.L., Ryan, R.M.: Self-determination theory. In: Van Lange, P.A.M., Kruglanski, A.W., Higgins, E.T. (eds.) Handbook of Theories of Social Psychology, pp. 416–436. Sage Publications Ltd. https://doi.org/10.4135/9781446249215.n21

Degeling, M., et al.: We value your privacy … now take some cookies: measuring the GDPR's impact on web privacy. Informatik Spektrum **42**(5), 345–346 (2018)

Detweiler, C.A., Hindriks, K.V.: A survey of values, technologies and contexts in pervasive healthcare. Pervasive Mob. Comput. **27**, 1–13 (2016)

Peters, D., Calvo, R.A., Ryan, R.M.: Designing for motivation, engagement and wellbeing in digital experience. Front. Psychol. **9** (2018). https://doi.org/10.3389/fpsyg.2018.00797

Schomakers, E., Lidynia, C., Ziefle, M.: Listen to my heart? how privacy concerns shape users' acceptance of e-health technologies. In: 2019 International Conference on Wireless and Mobile Computing, Networking and Communications (WiMob), pp. 306–311 (2019). https://doi.org/10.1109/WiMOB.2019.8923448

Ferreira, A., et al.: Perceptions of Security and Privacy in mHealth. In: HCI for Cybersecurity, Privacy and Trust, Cham, Springer International Publishing (2021)

Fishbein, M.: A theory of reasoned action: Some applications and implications. Nebr. Symp. Motiv. **27**, 65–116 (1979)

Floridi, L., Cowls, J., Beltrametti, M., et al.: AI4People—an ethical framework for a good ai society: opportunities, risks, principles, and recommendations. Mind. Mach. **28**, 689–707 (2018). https://doi.org/10.1007/s11023-018-9482-5

Fogg, B.J.: A behavior model for persuasive design. In: Proceedings of the 4th international Conference on Persuasive Technology, pp. 1–7, April 2009

Guo, X., et al.: The privacy–personalization paradox in mHealth services acceptance of different age groups. Electron. Commer. Res. Appl. **16**, 55–65 (2016)

Gupta, B., Chennamaneni, A.: Understanding online privacy protection behavior of the older adults: an empirical investigation. J. Inf. Technol. Manag. **29**, 1–13 (2018)

Hutchinson, H., et al.: Technology probes: inspiring design for and with families. In: Proceedings of the SIGCHI Conference on Human Factors in Computing Systems. Ft. Lauderdale, Florida, USA, Association for Computing Machinery, pp. 17–24 (2003)

Poyner, I.K., Sherratt,R.S. : Privacy and security of consumer IoT devices for the pervasive monitoring of vulnerable people. Living in the Internet of Things: Cybersecurity of the IoT - 2018, 2018, pp. 1–5 (2018). Doi: https://doi.org/10.1049/cp.2018.0043

Icek, A.: The theory of planned behavior. Organ. Behav. Hum. Decis. Process. **50**(2), 179–211 (1991)

Institute of Medicine (US) Roundtable on Value & Science-Driven Health Care. Clinical Data as the Basic Staple of Health Learning: Creating and Protecting a Public Good: Workshop Summary. Washington (DC): National Academies Press (US); 2010. 5, Healthcare Data as a Public Good: Privacy and Security. https://www.ncbi.nlm.nih.gov/books/NBK54293/

Institute of Medicine (US); Grossmann C, Powers B, McGinnis JM, editors. Digital Infrastructure for the Learning Health System: The Foundation for Continuous Improvement in Health and Health Care: Workshop Series Summary. Washington (DC): National Academies Press (US); 2011. 8, Fostering the Global Dimension of the Health Data Trust. https://www.ncbi.nlm.nih.gov/books/NBK83578/

Iwaya, L.H., Babar, M.A., Rashid, A.: Privacy Engineering in the Wild: Understanding the Practitioners' Mindset, Organisational Culture, and Current Practices (2022). arXiv preprint arXiv: 2211.08916

Joo, E., Kononova, A., Kanthawala, S., Peng, W., Cotton, S: Smartphone Users' Persuasion Knowledge in the Context of Consumer mHealth Apps: Qualitative Study. JMIR Mhealth Uhealth 9(4), e16518 (2021). https://mhealth.jmir.org/2021/4/e16518, https://doi.org/10.2196/16518

Kolovson, S., et al.: Understanding participant needs for engagement and attitudes towards passive sensing in remote digital health studies. In: Proceedings of the 14th EAI International Conference on Pervasive Computing Technologies for Healthcare, Association for Computing Machinery, pp. 347–362 (2020)

Kordzadeh, N., Warren, J.: Communicating personal health information in virtual health communities: an integration of privacy calculus model and affective commitment. J. Assoc. Inf. Syst. 18, 45–81 (2017)

Nurgalieva, L., O'Callaghan, D., Doherty, G.: Security and privacy of mHealth applications: a scoping review. IEEE Access 8, 104247–104268 (2020). https://doi.org/10.1109/ACCESS. 2020.2999934

Lau, J., et al.: Alexa, are you listening? privacy perceptions, concerns and privacy-seeking behaviors with smart speakers. In: Proc. ACM Hum.-Comput. Interact. 2(CSCW): Article 102 (2018)

Leon, P., et al.: Privacy and behavioral advertising: towards meeting users' preferences. In: PPS '15: Second SOUPS Workshop on Privacy Personas (2015)

Janic, M., Wijbenga, J.P., Veugen, T.: Transparency enhancing tools (TETs): an overview. In: 2013 Third Workshop on Socio-Technical Aspects in Security and Trust, pp. 18–25. IEEE, June 2013

Automated Decision-Making Systems in Precision Medicine – The Right to Good Administration at Risk

Sarah de Heer(✉) iD

Department of Law, Lilla Gråbrödersgatan 4, 222 22 Lund, Sweden
`sarah.de_heer@jur.lu.se`

Abstract. Automated decision-making (**ADM**) systems – whose algorithms are based on Artificial Intelligence and more specifically on machine learning and deep learning – predict the likelihood of an outcome based on profiling the input data. ADM systems, which are predominantly developed by the private sector, are a promising device for the field of precision medicine, where medical intervention is based on the patient's unique profile that consists of their genomic data, medical records data, environmental data, and lifestyle data. Such ADM systems are used when diagnosing or creating a treatment plan for patients. As these ADM systems take a bodily sample, for example from blood or human tissue, to predict which diagnosis or drug regime is most suitable, they are governed by the *In Vitro* Diagnostic Medical Devices Regulation in the European Union. However, the general features inherent to coding algorithms based on machine learning and deep learning – amongst others i) the self-learning ability, ii) the lack of a causal link, and iii) the use of intellectual property rights –, may form perils to the right to good administration that prescribes the legal norms of administrative conduct, including towards individuals. Particularly, the right to be heard, the right to access one's file, and the duty to state reasons may face considerable hurdles. Thus, this contribution aims to scrutinise these risks to the right to good administration and proposes a research agenda to overcome them.

Keywords: Automated Decision-Making System · Precision Medicine · Right to Good Administration

1 Introduction

Automated decision-making (**ADM**) systems are tools based on Artificial Intelligence (**AI**) that predict the likelihood of an outcome by means of profiling. Their developers particularly rely on machine learning and deep learning – two subsets of the more general AI. The use of ADM systems is especially alluring in precision medicine, which is a subfield of medicine that adapts medical interventions to the patient's profile. In this context, the algorithm underlying the ADM system considers, amongst others, genomic data, medical records data, environmental data and/or lifestyle data [1]. In the European

D. Salvi et al. (Eds.): PH 2023, LNICST 572, pp. 92–104, 2024.
https://doi.org/10.1007/978-3-031-59717-6_6

Union (**EU**), these ADM systems are governed by Regulation (EU) 2017/746 of the European Parliament and of the Council of 5 April 2017 on *in vitro* diagnostic medical devices and repealing Directive 98/79/EC and Commission Decision 2010/227/EU [2] (***In Vitro* Diagnostic Medical Devices Regulation**), as a bodily sample – for instance samples from blood or human tissue – serves as input data.[1] Concisely, as mentioned in its Article 1(1), the *In Vitro* Diagnostic Medical Devices Regulation governs the procedure of the ADM system from the moment they are placed on the market of the EU [2]. More concretely, as the development of these ADM systems requires expertise and ample of resources – as demonstrated by the use of machine learning and deep learning techniques –, the private sector predominantly creates them [3] and are thus to comply with the legal obligations stemming from the *In Vitro Diagnostic* Medical Devices Regulation. When interacting with the private sector, the public administration is to comply with the right to good administration, as embedded in Article 41 of the Charter of Fundamental Rights of the European Union [4] (**EU Charter**). This right to good administration includes a diverse subset of rights and principles, which all aim to safeguard the individual's right to defence during administrative proceedings [5]. However, this umbrella right to good administration may be at risk due to the generic features of the algorithm underlying ADM systems, which includes i) the self-learning ability, ii) the evidence of correlation – as opposed to causation –, and iii) the allocation of intellectual property rights.

The aim of this paper is to explore how these three general aspects of the algorithm underlying the ADM systems used in precision medicine affect the right to good administration. To this end, this contribution paints the background, which comprises the context in which these ADM systems are used (Sect. 2.1) and the legal framework that consists of the *In Vitro Diagnostic* Medical Devices Regulation with a specific focus on the principle of transparency it pursues and its transparency obligations (Sect. 2.2). After, this piece scrutinises the legal framework that comprises the right to good administration, which simultaneously consists of the legal benchmark against which the effects of the three general features of ADM systems in precision medicine are evaluated. After introducing the right to good administration (Sect. 3.1), this paper focusses on Article 41 EU Charter in which the right to good administration is embedded. In particular, this contribution dissects the three subrights that are expressly mentioned in Article 41(2) EU Charter (Sect. 3.2). Subsequently, this piece specifies the obstacles posed, caused by the characteristics of ADM systems to the right to good administration as outlined in Article 41(2) EU Charter (Sect. 4). Lastly, this paper concludes and proposes a research agenda in which the author suggests research recommendations to overcome the hurdles to the right to good administration (Sect. 5).

---

[1] The author points out that ADM systems that base their prediction on other data than those retrieved from human blood or tissue – for instance medical records or medical imagery – are not considered by the *In Vitro Diagnostic* Medical Devices Regulation but rather fall within the scope of the more generic Regulation (EU) 2017/745 of the European Parliament and of the Council of 5 April 2017 on medical devices, amending Directive 2001/83/EC, Regulation (EC) No 178/2002 and Regulation (EC) No 1223/2009 and repealing Council Directives 90/385/EEC and 93/42/EEC. For more information, see Sect. 2.2.

2 Setting the Scene

2.1 The Factual Context - Automated Decision-Making Systems in Precision Medicine

ADM systems in precision medicine use data retrieved from samples stemming from, for instance, the patient's blood or tissue to predict the likelihood that the diagnosis or the treatment plan fits the patient's unique profile [6]. As a result, ADM systems may be a useful tool for physicians in diagnosing their patients or determining a suitable treatment plan for their patients.

An example of an ADM system for the purpose of medical diagnoses in the field of precision medicine is 'CUP-AI-Dx', which identifies – by using RNA – the location of the primary cancer of patients diagnosed with the rare disease 'carcinoma of unknown primary' [7]. This type of cancer is difficult to treat since the primary cancer is unknown. As such, the ADM system may facilitate physicians to diagnose their patients by localising the primary cancer, and thereby help them to treat their patients. Another example in the field of precision medicine but focussing on treatment plans entails the identification of a suitable drug treatment for colorectal cancer by the ADM system 'IndiTreat'. This test helps decide which medicinal product is likely the most suitable for patients suffering from colorectal cancer by examining the patient's profile against a particular set of pharmaceutical products. Thus, this ADM system may help physicians to set up an effective treatment plan [8].

These ADM systems in precision medicine are characterised by three generic features, namely i) the self-learning ability, ii) the lack of a causal link, and iii) the allocation of intellectual property rights. First, *the self-learning ability* is rooted in the use of machine learning and deep learning techniques, which provides ADM systems with the ability to independently learn from its environment. Put differently, the algorithm underlying the ADM system has acquired the ability to self-evolve – that is to say without human intervention. As a result, grasping how the ADM systems reach its outcome based on the input data may be a cumbersome – if not an impossible – task. Second, these ADM systems may *lack a causal link*, since they may establish correlation between the input data and the acquired outcome. Thus, any alleged link between the input and the output may be solely a coincidence or caused by noise [9]. Third, these ADM systems largely enjoy protection rooted in *intellectual property rights*. Seeing the involvement of machine learning and deep learning techniques in the creation of these ADM systems – which requires specialised skills and competences and substantial resources –, ADM systems are mainly developed by the private sector [3]. Since the algorithm resulting from machine learning and deep learning may be the enterprise's competitive advantage, companies may opt to protect this advantage by using intellectual property rights, and more specifically the legislative framework governing trade secrets. Consequently, the protection mechanism provided by intellectual property rights may constitute an additional hurdle – and thus exacerbate – unravelling how the ADM system works.

2.2 The Legal Context - *In Vitro* Diagnostic Medical Device Regulation

General. ADM systems used to diagnose disease or to set up medical regimes are governed by Regulation (EU) of the European Parliament and of the Council of 5 April 2017 on medical devices, amending Directive 2001/83/EC, Regulation (EC) No 178/2002 and Regulation (EC) No 1223/2009 and repealing Council Directives 90/385/EEC and 93/42/EEC [10] (**Medical Devices Regulation**) or by the *In Vitro* Diagnostic Medical Devices Regulation. The Medical Devices Regulation governs medical devices in the broad sense – the main restricting factors consisting of their use having a medical purpose and the manufacturer's intended purpose, as mentioned in Article 2(1) [10]. The *In Vitro* Diagnostic Medical Devices Regulation does not merely require this medical purpose and the manufacturer's intended purpose but also – in accordance with Articles 2(1) and (2) – demands that these medical devices provide specific information in the medical context acquired by the examination of samples of the human body – which includes those originating from blood or human tissue – in a controlled environment, such as a test tube or petri dish [2]. As ADM systems in precision medicine mostly base a suggested diagnosis or a medical treatment plan on genomic data that is derived from bodily samples – be it from blood or from human tissue – and is examined in a controlled environment, these ADM systems are governed by the *In Vitro* Diagnostic Medical Devices Regulation – which will thus be the focus of this contribution. To this end, the author notes that ADM systems may solely be regulated by the Medical Devices Regulation provided they only use samples that do not come from the human body but rather from, for instance, medical imaging or data given by the patient.

Zooming in on the legal context, a distinction is warranted as regards the assessment of an ADM system in precision medicine that – on the one hand – suggests a diagnosis and – on the other hand – suggests a pharmaceutical regimen. While both these ADM systems are '*in vitro* diagnostic medical devices' under Article 2(1) [2], ADM systems that propose a diagnosis fall under Article 2(2)(a), and those that determine drug sensitivity are a specific '*in vitro* diagnostic medical device' under Article 2(2)(e), namely a 'companion diagnostic', as they i) identify which patients are likely to respond to a treatment plan, and ii) identify which patients are anticipated to suffer serious negative side-effects due to the regimen (see Article 2(7)(a) and (b)) [2].

However, to determine the applicable regime in the *In Vitro* Diagnostic Medical Devices Regulation, it does not suffice to define the ADM systems in precision medicine in these relatively general terms, they also need to be further classified in accordance with the classification rules (Article 47(1) and Annex VIII). [2] *In vitro* diagnostic medical devices are grouped in Class A to Class D, which is determined by the risks posed to the individual and to public health in general [11]. Table 1 illustrates these risks posed by *in vitro* diagnostic medical devices in order to be categorised as 'Class A', 'Class B', 'Class C' or 'Class D'.

In sum, the *In Vitro* Diagnostic Medical Devices Regulation imposes the least stringent obligations upon 'Class A' *in vitro* diagnostic medical devices, and establishes the most demanding requirements on those grouped in 'Class D'. Both ADM systems recommending a diagnosis and ADM systems proposing a treatment plan involving medicinal products are placed in Class 'C', see Rule 3(f) Annex VIII and Rule 3(h) Annex VIII, respectively [2].

The Principle of Transparency. In accordance with Recital 1, the principal purpose of the *In Vitro* Diagnostic Medical Devices Regulation is to ensure transparency, which was amongst the main aims behind the revision of the preceding legislative act [12]

Table 1. Risks of the different classes of *in vitro* diagnostic medical devices

	Risk To Individual	Risk To Public Health
Class A	Low	Low
Class B	Moderate	Low
Class C	High	Moderate
Class D	High	High

in 2017. [2] Against this backdrop, it is, thus, no surprise that the *In Vitro* Diagnostic Medical Devices Regulation places the principle of transparency in the limelight. This principle is further echoed throughout the Recitals. To this end, the European legislator acknowledges in Recital 4 that transparency was not a concern in the previous legislative act, which resulted in the introduction of this type of obligations in the current *In Vitro* Diagnostic Medical Devices Regulation [2]. Unfortunately, determining the content of the principle of transparency is no clear-cut task, as it is a multifaceted concept, whose meaning is dependent on the context in which it is used. The question then arises what entails this principle of transparency in the *In Vitro* Diagnostic Medical Devices Regulation. In this legislative act, transparency is – simultaneously with adequate access to information – crucial for, amongst others, sound regulatory decision-making procedures, as mentioned in Recital 40 [2]. Consequently, this aim is set in the transparency obligations that are permeated in the main body of the *In Vitro* Diagnostic Medical Devices Regulation. However, these transparency obligations imposed on *in vitro* diagnostic medical devices vary and are determined by their classification, and thus by the risks posed to the individual using the *in vitro* diagnostic medical device and to the general public health. Depending on its classification, which in the case of ADM systems in precision medicine for the purpose of diagnosing patients and proposing a treatment plan including pharmaceuticals is 'Class C', additional requirements are applicable to safeguard transparency.

Transparency Obligations. Focussing on the requirements to place a 'Class C' *in vitro* diagnostic medical device on the market of the EU, Article 17 stands out seeing its all-encompassing scope, as it demands to draw up the EU Declaration of Conformity that certifies that all requirements of the *In Vitro* Diagnostic Medical Devices Regulation are observed [2]. As stipulated in Articles 10(5) and 15(3)(b), this comprehensive obligation is imposed on the manufacturers of all *in vitro* diagnostic medical devices [2]. Further, by signing the EU Declaration of Conformity, the manufacturer takes full responsibility that the ADM system in precision medicine complies with the *In Vitro* Diagnostic Medical Devices Regulation (Article 17(3)) [2]. As stated in Article 48, one of the obligations to obtain an EU Declaration of Conformity is to perform a conformity assessment, [2] which – quite literally – is an assessment to affirm that the requirements of the *In Vitro* Diagnostic Medical Devices Regulation have been fulfilled (Article 2(32) [2]. This evaluation can be done with or without the involvement of a third party, the Notified Body, which is designated by the Member State to perform the conformity assessment (Article 2(33) and (34)) [2]. Specifically in the case of a 'Class C' *in vitro* diagnostic medical device, the Notified Body is to review the clinical evidence on its accuracy and verify the conclusions drawn by the manufacturer.[2]

Aiming our attention at the clinical evidence that is to be submitted by the manufacturer to the Notified Body, the clinical evidence aims to ensure that the *in vitro* diagnostic medical device is safe and produces the expected clinical benefits. Article 2(36) states that clinical evidence consists of [2].

- clinical data, and;
- results of the performance evaluation

Looking further into the results of the performance evaluation, the manufacturer is required – under Article 56(3) – to demonstrate: [2].

- scientific validity (Article 2(38)): this requires the *in vitro* diagnostic medical device to illustrate an association between the analyte and a clinical condition or physiological state [2]. Specifically in the context of an ADM system in precision medicine, this entails that the outcome produced by the underlying algorithm must indicate a link with a clinical condition or a physiological state [13];
- analytical performance (Article 2(40)): the *in vitro* diagnostic medical device is to show that the device can accurately discover and measure an analyte [2]. Looking at ADM systems in precision medicine, the output data should be accurate – as opposed to the detection and measurement of an analyte being accurate [13].
- clinical performance (Article 2(41)): here the *in vitro* diagnostic medical device must demonstrate a (medical) correlation between the results and the clinical condition or the physiological state [2]. Against the background of ADM systems in precision medicine, the output of the underlying algorithm ought to have a (medical) correlation with the clinical condition or the physiological state [13].

The above requirements linked to the EU Declaration of Conformity show that the principle of transparency, which aims to facilitate sound regulatory decision-making, is well-embedded in the *In Vitro* Diagnostic Medical Devices Regulation. During the conformity assessment procedure, the manufacturer is to submit a bulk of evidence demonstrating that the *in vitro* diagnostic medical device is safe to use and produce the anticipated clinical benefits, which requires the manufacturer to be transparent about how their *in vitro* diagnostic medical device works and their effects.

---

[2] For the review of clinical evidence during the conformity assessment of Class C *in vitro* diagnostic medical devices, which includes ADM systems in precision medicine that predict the likelihood the diagnosis fits the patient's profile, see Article 48(7), para. 1 and Annex IX, Sect. 4.4 *In Vitro* Diagnostic Medical Devices Regulation or Article 48(8), para.1 and Annex X, Sect. 3(c) *In Vitro* Diagnostic Medical Devices Regulation. For the review of clinical evidence during the conformity assessment of companion diagnostics, which encompasses ADM systems in precision medicine that predict the suitability of pharmaceuticals based on the patient's profile, see Article 48(7), para. 3 and Annex IX, Sect. 4.4 *In Vitro* Diagnostic Medical Devices Regulation or Article 48(8), para. 1 and Annex X, Sect. 3(c) *In Vitro* Diagnostic Medical Devices Regulation.

3 The Right to Good Administration

3.1 General Remarks

Before becoming a fully fledged human right within the context of the EU,[3] various elements of the – contemporary – right to good administration was already recognised by the Court of Justice of the European Union (**CJEU**) in its case law [5]. The right to good administration – in whatever form – is a pivotal human right that can hardly be overestimated. First, the right to good administration is an enabling right that facilitates individuals to effectively enjoy their fundamental rights, such as the right to an effective remedy. More concretely, the individual cannot be expected to enjoy their right to an effective remedy in case the administrative authority does not provide the underlying reasons for its decision in a clear and an intelligible manner. Put differently, the right to good administration is a vital precondition to exercise other fundamental rights [14]. Second, the right to good administration prescribes that the behaviour of public administration should be in accordance with written and unwritten law, which also includes their conduct towards individuals. Consequently, this right provides individuals with enforceable rights when interacting with public administration [14]. This demonstrates that the right to good administration is not merely a right that facilitates other human rights, but also – and perhaps more importantly – a 'stand-alone' human right [14].

3.2 EU Charter

Even though the EU Charter devotes an article to the right to good administration, much ink has been spilled about its precise status and scope. Based on its phrasing, only the Institutions, Bodies, Offices, and Agencies of the EU fall within the remit of the Charter right to good administration [15]. This reading has also been confirmed by the CJEU [16]. However, the CJEU has refined this black and white approach, and holds that general principles underlying the right to good administration are applicable to Member States when implementing EU law.

The right to good administration, as embedded in Article 41 EU Charter, is a procedural fundamental right [17] and plays a crucial role in procedures before administrative

---

[3] In some legal orders, good administration is still regarded a principle.

authorities.[4] Article 41 EU Charter is an umbrella concept[5] that contains a diverse set of rights and principles aimed at protecting the individual against the arbitrary use of power by administrative authorities. To this end, this myriad of rights and principles dictates how public administration ought to behave, especially in relation to individuals. Concentrating on Article 41's wording, the first paragraph encompasses an overall provision that entitles the individual '[...] to have their affairs handled impartially, fairly and within a reasonable time [...]' [16]. This general right is further clarified in the second paragraph, which provides a non-exhaustive list of subrights. In particular, Article 41(2) EU Charter lists three rights that – undoubtedly – fall within the ambit of the right to good administration, namely i) the right to be heard, ii) the right to access one's file, and iii) the duty to state reasons. However, apart from these three rights that are explicitly mentioned, the umbrella right to good administration may encompass other rights and principles [15].

Before delving into the three procedural subrights under Article 41(2) EU Charter, the author holds that these three subrights are vital to the contextual principle of transparency in the light of the *In Vitro* Diagnostic Medical Devices Regulation, as both pursue sound regulatory decision-making procedures. Article 41(2) EU Charter mentions the following three subrights of the right to good administration, namely:

1. the right to be heard (subparagraph a)[6] is a context-specific right, which means that its content hinges on the circumstance under which it is invoked [15]. However, in general this right requires public administration to provide the individual an opportunity to make their stance effectively known before the adoption of the administrative decision that may adversely affect the individual concerned [18, 19]. This means that

---

[4] The author is aware that Notified Bodies are not necessarily part of public administration, which means that Article 41 EU Charter is not applicable. Nevertheless, the author argues that Notified Bodies may be regarded to fall under public administration based on a case handed down by the European Court of Justice, namely *A. Foster, G.A.H.M. Fulford-Brown, J. Morgan, M. Roby, E.M. Salloway and P. Sullivan and British Gas plc*, App no C-188/89. In this case, the European Court of Justice held that any body – irrespective of its legal form – may be on an equal footing with public administration, if that body is responsible for providing a public service under the control of the State per a measure adopted by the State. The author maintains that the same holds true as regards Notified Bodies. First, Notified Bodies are responsible for providing a public service, namely they are responsible for the conformity assessment, which is a prerequisite for the placement on the market of an ADM system in precision medicine. Second, Notified Bodies are both placed under the supervision of the State (see Articles 39 and 41 *In Vitro* Diagnostic Medical Devices Regulation) and appointed by the State (see Articles 35, 36, 38 *In Vitro* Diagnostic Medical Devices Regulation). Consequently, Notified Bodies are to comply with Article 41 EU Charter.

[5] The author is aware of the debate as regards the precise content of the right to good administration, as penned in Article 41 EU Charter. However, it is not this paper's aim to exhaustively discuss its elements. For an analysis of the content of the right to good administration, see for example Kanska, K.: Towards Administrative Human Rights in the EU. Impact of the Charter of Fundamental Rights. European Law Journal 10(3), 296–326 (2004).

[6] The right to be heard is also encapsulated in the case law of the European Court of Justice, see for example European Court of Justice.: *Transocean Marine Paint Association v Commission of the European Communities* App no 17/74, [15] (1974).

this right only materialises if the foreseen administrative decision may have adverse consequences for the individual. The right to be heard, thus, enables the administrative authority to consider the individual's point of view during the decision-making process. [17] This right consists of two components: first, public administration is obliged to notify the individual about the existence of the pending administrative decision, and second administrative authorities are to ensure that the individual is given the opportunity to effectively make their point of view known before adopting the administrative decision [20]. The above is also applicable to any other individual – not being the addressee of the administrative decision –, who is adversely affected by the adoption of the decision [6].

2. the right to access one's files (subparagraph b) [21] should be given to the individual both before and after the administrative authority adopts its decision. When providing access to their file before deciding on a case, the individual can give full effect to their right to be heard, as the individual can acquaint themselves with the information related to them held by public administration. Put differently, the right to access one's file is a vital precondition to effectively enjoy the right to be heard [22]. Given the status of the right to access one's file as an essential prerequisite of the right to be heard upon which individuals can rely who are negatively affected by the administrative decision – but are not the addressee –, the right to access one's file is, thus, also applicable to such individuals. When given access after the adoption of the administrative decision, the individual has the opportunity to understand the reasoning underlying the administrative decision and can thereby decide to seek – and if needed prepare for – judicial review [15]. Public administration are to provide the individual relying on their right to access their file all relevant information in their possession, except information covered by professional secrecy or business secrets [23, 24]

3. the duty to state reasons (subparagraph c)[7] requires public administration to state the reasons for their decision in a sufficiently precise manner that would allow the individual to understand the underlying reasons of the administrative decision. This would enable the individual to decide whether to appeal the decision in front of the court, which then can adjudicate based on the stated reasons [25]. The duty to state reasons serves a threefold purpose. First, the administrative decision-making procedure becomes more transparent, as it allows the individual to comprehend why the decision is taken and to decide whether to seek judicial redress (*individual perspective*). Second, administrative authorities are now to ponder upon which reasoning their decision is based, which counters arbitrary decision-making (*public administration perspective*). Third, the duty to state reasons is a prerequisite to perform effective judicial review (*judiciary perspective*) [15].

---

[7] The duty to state reasons is not based on general principles of EU law, but rather on existing Treaty provisions, which is elaborated in the case law of the Court of Justice of the European Union. See Craig, P.: Article 41. In Peers, S., Hervey, T., Kenner, J., Ward, A. (eds), vol. 1, pp. 1125–1152. Hart Publishing, Oxford (2021).

4   Obstacles to the Right to Good Administration

The three general features of ADM systems in precision medicine – namely i) the self-learning ability, ii) the proof of correlation instead of causation, and iii) the use of intellectual property rights – is a breeding ground for perils to the subrights of the right to good administration under Article 41(2) EU Charter, namely i) the right to be heard, ii) the right to access one's file, and iii) the duty to state reasons.

While grasping how the algorithm works may already be cumbersome – since this exercise may require expert knowledge and skills – *the self-learning ability* only further hinders deciphering how the algorithm reached its outcome – or even creates an inconceivable activity. This burden to the comprehension of how the algorithm works is created due to the algorithm's ability to evolve independently based on the input of its environment. Concretely, this means that the outcomes of 'CUP-AI-Dx' predicting the location of the primary cancer and of 'IndiTreat' forecasting the suitability of medicinal products for colorectal cancer may be based on different rules than those initially programmed. Consequently, the competitors and the Notified Body may not be able to decipher how the algorithm reached its prediction. Since the competitors of the company drawing up the EU Declaration of Conformity – and thus submitting the clinical evidence for review by the Notified Body – may rely on the right to be heard, it is questionable to which extent the competitors can effectively make their points of view known before the adoption of the administrative decision due to this self-learning ability. Thus, this means that the right to be heard may be at risk. The same holds true as regards the right to access one's file. The Notified Body may provide unrestricted access to the clinical evidence to the competitors, but they will most likely not grasp what the information entails and its significance, which renders the right to access one's file meaningless. The self-learning ability also jeopardises the duty to state reasons, as the Notified Body – even though provided with the clinical evidence – may not fully understand how the ADM system has reached its outcome. Particularly, the question arises whether the Notified Body can adequately review the accuracy of the clinical evidence and verify the conclusions drawn by the manufacturer. Thus, the Notified Body may not be able to substantiate their decision as regards the review of the clinical evidence in a clear and an intelligible manner, which leaves the sound regulatory decision-making process at risk. Furthermore, the Notified Body responsible for the conformity assessment may face difficulties to pinpoint how the algorithm may evolve in the future and how this may affect the clinical evidence. In short, a sound regulatory decision-making procedure may be at risk.

The same holds true as regards the *lack of a causal link* between the input data, which consists of the patient's blood or tissue sample, and the output data, which forms the likelihood of a diagnosis or of the suitability of a pharmaceutical product. Zooming in on the ADM systems 'CUP-AI-Dx' and 'IndiTreat', this means that their outcomes may be based on correlation – as opposed to causation. As a result, the competitors and the Notified Body may not gather the right picture as to how the algorithm underlying 'CUP-AI-Dx' and 'IndiTreat' work, and whether the algorithm functions accurately. Thus, the *lack of causation* may hinder the right to be heard of the competitors. Since any alleged link may – in fact – evidence correlation, the question arises whether competitors can effectively make use of their right to be heard as they may not be able to get to the heart of the matter. This also remains true as regards the right to access one's file. The data the competitor is seeking may – in fact – not be included in the clinical evidence, as the algorithm does not demonstrate a causal link. Moreover, the duty to state reasons imposed on the Notified Body may become cumbersome. The Notified Body may be confronted with the potentially impossible exercise of verifying the clinical evidence, which may result in the Notified Body making their decision on incorrect information. Thus, this may adversely affect a sound regulatory decision-making procedure.

The use of *intellectual property rights* may worsen the hurdles posed to both the right to be heard and the right to access one's file, upon which the competitors may rely, since they may form an additional obstacle to comprehend how the algorithm underlying the ADM system in precision medicine works. Since the algorithm comprises the company's competitive advantage over their competitors, the algorithm underling 'CUP-AI-Dx' and 'IndiTreat' may be protected by the regime of intellectual property rights – most likely the regulatory framework of trade secrets. While these trade secrets are submitted to the Notified Body – which will thus not negatively impact the duty to state reasons –, they are not shared with the general public – which includes the competitors – under the right to access one's file. As a result, the competitors may also face difficulties effectively exercising their right to be heard. Therefore, a sound regulatory decision-making process may be hampered.

5 Conclusion – A Research Agenda

This contribution has demonstrated that the general characteristics of ADM systems in precision medicine – i) the self-learning ability, and ii) the lack of a causal link, and iii) the use of intellectual property rights – may very well imperil the right to good administration. In particular, this piece has illustrated the dangers to the three subrights expressly mentioned in Article 41(2) EU Charter, namely i) the right to be heard, ii) the right to access one's file, and iii) the duty to state reasons – and thereby to sound regulatory decision-making procedures.

This piece does not provide solutions to overcome the three established hurdles, rather it suggests three research lines to diminish these perils. The *first* line of recommendation is conducting more research aimed at achieving explainable AI. Specifically local explainability appears a promising field for ADM systems in precision medicine, since this field studies how AI may explain how it has reached the specific outcome based on the input data. In the meantime, however, this paper suggests focusing on creating more accurate and fairer algorithms, which is the *second* line of suggested research. Such algorithms may be achieved by ensuring that complete, representative, and accurate data are inserted both during the creation of the ADM system in precision medicine and during the input phase when the ADM system is in operation. The *third* proposal is an approach as opposed to a line of research, as this contribution calls for conducting interdisciplinary research. Consequently, not only researchers in the field of data science should explore how to overcome the established challenges to the right to good administration, but also experts in the field of law and healthcare professionals should be involved due to the interdisciplinary nature of the topic at hand, which covers all these fields of study. More importantly, these three specialisations should collaborate to achieve explainable ADM systems in precision medicine that conform to the right to good administration.

References

1. König, I.R., et al.: What is precision medicine? Europ. Respiratory J. **50**(4), 1–12 (2017)
2. The European Parliament and the Council of the European Union.: Regulation (EU) 2017/746 of the European Parliament and of the Council of 5 April 2017 on in vitro diagnostic medical devices and repealing Directive 98/79/EC and Commission Decision 2010/227/EU *OJ* [2017] L 117/176
3. Finck, M.: Automated decision-making and administrative law. In: Cane, P. et al. (eds.), The Oxford Handbook of Comparative Administrative Law, vol. 1, 657–675 (2021)
4. The European Parliament, the Council and the Commission.: Charter of Fundamental Rights of the European Union *OJ* [2012] C 326/391
5. Kańska, K.: Towards Administrative Human Rights in the EU. Impact of the Charter of Fundamental Rights. Europ. Law J. **10**(3), 296–326 (2004)
6. Borh, A., Memarzadeh, K.: The rise of artificial intelligence in healthcare applications. In: Bohr, A., Memarzadeh, K. (eds.) Artificial Intelligence in Healthcare, vol. 1, pp. 25–60. Academic Press, London (2020)
7. Zhao, Y.: CUP-AI-Dx: a tool for inferring cancer tissue of origin and molecular subtype using RNA gene-expression data and artificial intelligence. EBioMedicine **61**(103030), 1–14 (2020)
8. 2cureX, Choose the Right Treatment for Each Patient. https://usercontent.one/wp/www.2curex.com/wp-content/uploads/2023/01/IndiTreat-brochure-1.pdf?media=1676030860. Accessed 12 July 2023
9. Chen, R., Chen, C.: Artificial Intelligence. An introduction for the Inquisitive Reader. Vol 1, CRC Press, Boca Raton and Oxon (2022)
10. The European Parliament and the Council of the European Union.: Regulation (EU) of the European Parliament and of the Council of 5 April 2017 on medical devices, amending Directive 2001/83/EC, Regulation (EC) No 178/2002 and Regulation (EC) No 1223/2009 and repealing Council Directives 90/385/EEC and 93/42/EEC *OJ* [2017] L 117/1
11. European Commission.: Factsheet for Manufacturers of in vitro diagnostic medical devices. European Union (2020)
12. The European Parliament and the Council of the European Union.: Directive 98/79/EC of the European parliament and of the Council of 27 October 1998 on *in vitro* diagnostics medical devices *OJ* [1998] L 331/1
13. Müller, H., Holzinger, A., Plass, M., Brcic, L., Stumptner, C., Zatloukal, K.: Explainability and causability for artificial intelligence-supported medical image analysis in the context of the European In Vitro Diagnostic Regulation. New Biotechnol. **70**, 67–72 (2022)
14. Kristjánsdóttir, M.V.: Good Administration as Fundamental Right. Icelandic Review of Politics & Administration **9**(1), 237–255 (2013)
15. Teo, T.W., Choy, B.H.: in. In: Tan, O.S., Low, E.L., Tay, E.G., Yan, Y.K. (eds.) Singapore Math and Science Education Innovation. ETLPPSIP, vol. 1, pp. 43–59. Springer, Singapore (2021). https://doi.org/10.1007/978-981-16-1357-9_3
16. See for example European Court of Justice.: *Teresa Cicala v Regione Siciliana* App no C-482/10 (ECJ) (2011)
17. Lock, T.: Article 41 CFR Right to good administration. In: Kellerbauer, M., Klamert, M., Tomkin, J. (eds.) vol. 1, pp. 2204–2207. Oxford University Press, Oxford (2019)
18. European Court of Justice.: *Fiskano AB v Commission of the European Communities* App no C-135/92, [40] (1994)
19. European Court of Justice.: *Transocean Marine Paint Association v Commission of the European Communities* App no 17/74, [15] (1974)

20. Pranvera Beqiraj, M.: The right to be heard in the European Union – case law of the court of justice of the European Union. Europ. J. Multidisciplinary Stud. 1(1), 264–269 (2016)
21. European Court of Justice.: *Estel NV v Commission of the European Communities* App no 270/82, [13–16] (1984)
22. General Court.: *Eyckeler & Malt AG v Commission of the European Communities* App no T-42/96, [79–80] (1998)
23. European Court of Justice.: *Aalborg Portland A/S, Irish Cement Ltd, Climents français SA, Italcementi – Fabbriche Riunite Cemento SpA, Buzzi Unicem SpA and Cementir – Cementerie del Tirreno SpA v Commission of the European Communities* App no Cases C-204/00 P, C-205/00 P, C-211/00 P, C-213/00 P, C-217/00 P and C-219/00 P, [126] (2004)
24. General Court.: *Solvay SA v Commission of the European Communities* App no T-30/91, [88–92] (1995)
25. European Court of Justice.: *Club Hotel Loutraki AE, Vivere Entertainment AE, Theros International Gaming, Inc., Elliniko Casino Kerkyras, Casino Rodos, Porto Carras AE and Kazino Aigaiou AE v European Commission*, App no C-131/15 P, [46] (2016)

Datasets and Big Data Processing

HeartView: An Extensible, Open-Source, Web-Based Signal Quality Assessment Pipeline for Ambulatory Cardiovascular Data

Natasha Yamane(✉), Varun Mishra, and Matthew S. Goodwin

Khoury College of Computer Sciences and Bouvé College of Health Sciences, Northeastern University, Boston, MA 02115, USA

{yamane.n,v.mishra,m.goodwin}@northeastern.edu

Abstract. Wearable sensing systems enable peripheral physiological data to be collected repeatedly in naturalistic settings. However, the ambulatory nature of wearable biosensors predisposes them to common signal artifacts that researchers must address before analysis. Signal quality assessment procedures are time-consuming and non-standardized across research teams, and transparent reporting of custom, closed-source pipelines needs improvement. This paper presents HeartView, an extensible, open-source, web-based signal quality assessment pipeline that visualizes and quantifies missing beats and invalid segments in heart rate variability (HRV) data obtained from ambulatory electrocardiograph (ECG) and photoplethysmograph (PPG) signals. We demonstrate the utility of our pipeline on two datasets: (1) 34 ECGs recorded with the Actiwave Cardio from children with and without autism, and (2) 15 sets of ECGs and PPGs recorded with the RespiBAN and Empatica E4, respectively, from healthy adults in the publicly available WESAD dataset. Our pipeline demonstrates interpretable group differences in physiological signal quality. ECGs of children with autism contain more missing beats and invalid segments than those without autism. Similarly, PPG data contains more missing beats and invalid segments than ECG data. HeartView has a graphical user interface in the form of a web-based dashboard at https://github.com/cbslneu/heartview.

Keywords: Signal Quality Assessment · Data Pipelines · Ambulatory Cardiovascular Data · Electrocardiography · Photoplethysmography

1 Introduction

Signal quality assessment (SQA) involves detecting and evaluating outliers, artifacts, and missingness in signal-based data using expected signal morphology and dynamics. This procedure is an increasingly important step during and after data collection, as wireless ambulatory technologies are gaining popularity for their ability to monitor physiological states continuously and unobtrusively in both research and clinical settings [1–4]. Many wearable devices that capture peripheral physiological signals in free-living contexts are

D. Salvi et al. (Eds.): PH 2023, LNICST 572, pp. 107–123, 2024.
https://doi.org/10.1007/978-3-031-59717-6_8

commercially available and becoming progressively smaller and lighter. However, due to their size and ambulatory nature compared to traditional stationary systems, modern wearable system signals are more susceptible to artifacts, increasing missing or distorted data. Common sources of ambulatory signal artifacts include powerline interference, baseline wander, muscle activity, physical movement, and pressure disturbance [5, 6]. Figure 1 illustrates examples of ambulatory signal corruption by different artifacts.

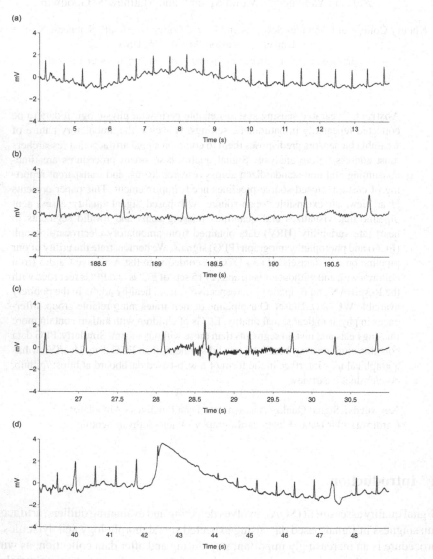

Fig. 1. Ambulatory electrocardiograph signals corrupted with (a) baseline wander, (b) powerline interference, (c) muscle activity, and (d) pressure disturbance.

Wearable devices use multiple biosensors to capture peripheral physiological signals. In the case of cardiovascular activity, photoplethysmography (PPG), to measure blood volume pulse (BVP), and electrodes, to record electrocardiograph (ECG) data, are the most common. PPG is an optical method of measuring volumetric changes in blood profusion [7]. Pulse rate, a proxy for heart rate (HR), is a function of the changes in light absorbed or reflected by blood flowing through a particular measurement site. ECG is a technique for observing and recording changes in heart electrical activity.

Before deriving summary statistics and making inferences based on PPG and ECG data, artifacts should be inspected using the expected morphological characteristics and dynamics of PPG and ECG signals. In a PPG waveform, each dominant peak represents a change in the absorption or reflection of light due to increased blood flow during systole (i.e., heart contraction). Similarly, the ECG signal contains three waveforms—the P, QRS, and T—corresponding to independent events in the cardiac cycle [8]. The most dominant wave is the QRS complex, which represents the depolarization of the heart's ventricles as a contraction begins. Correct detection of R peaks ensures that QRS complexes are captured, thus confirming valid heartbeats [9].

The primary goal of physiological SQA is to identify outliers, signal artifacts, and missingness to increase the reliability and validity of physiological measurements; however, the process varies across research teams. There is no unified approach to assessing signal quality in biosensor data [5], as standardized and transparent reporting of custom data preprocessing procedures is lacking [10]. In addition, most SQA procedures exist in closed-source pipelines, limiting reproducibility and uniformity across studies [11]. We developed HeartView to increase the reproducibility of and accessibility to SQA procedures typically performed only by trained researchers with computational backgrounds.

HeartView is a Python-based, open-source, extensible SQA pipeline and dashboard that visualizes and summarizes segment-by-segment quantification of missing and invalid beats in ambulatory cardiovascular data obtained in research contexts. SQA of a signal's basic quality and physiological feasibility is essential for making informed decisions about further data cleaning and processing procedures [5]. SQA of basic quality addresses whether beats are identifiable for reliable HR and heart rate variability (HRV) calculation. At the same time, physiological feasibility describes whether HR and inter-beat interval (IBI) values are valid. We demonstrate the utility of our pipeline in assessing the quality of physiological signals on two datasets covering different use cases: ECG data collected from children with and without autism spectrum disorder (ASD) [12], and a publicly available dataset containing PPG and ECG data collected from healthy adults [13].

2   Related Work

The level of SQA one performs depends on research integrity and clinical purpose. For instance, additional algorithmic development may be necessary in clinical contexts to assess specific waveform characteristics—e.g., whether the P, QRS, or T waves are identifiable—to diagnose conditions like myocardial ischemia [14] and heart disease [15]. Indeed, most work on SQA uses clinical datasets to derive and evaluate signal quality indices (SQIs) to detect signal artifacts. SQIs are statistical or machine learning-based measures that heuristically describe characteristics and acceptability of signal waveforms [14–17] and are thus binary in most cases (i.e., "acceptable" or "unacceptable") [5]. Statistical SQIs may include kurtosis [18], skewness [16], signal-to-noise ratio (SNR) [19], and signal power [20]. Present machine learning-based SQIs commonly include measurements derived with support vector machine classifiers [21, 22] and neural networks [23, 24].

Several open-source data processing software and libraries [25–31] are available and can be applied to SQA of cardiovascular data. Some of the most popular data processing Python packages, such as NeuroKit2 and pyphysio, also support the computation of common statistical SQIs, including kurtosis and SNR [25, 28]. Other physiological data processing libraries are available for assessing basic quality and physiological feasibility checks, including filtering and visualizing signals and deriving peaks. BioSPPy, for example, provides a library of standard biosignal processing functions and feature extraction algorithms, including filtering, QRS complex detection, and visualization [26]. NeuroKit2, a community-driven Python package, contains functions to derive different types of peaks, filter signals, and compute HR [28]. Table 1 presents several software packages and libraries and their available features and functions relevant to the SQA of ambulatory PPG and ECG data.

Table 1. Overview of popular cardiovascular data processing software and libraries.

Package	FR	CE	SF	BD	V	CA	PPG	ECG	GUI
ANSLab	◐	●	●	●	●	◐	●	●	●
BioSPPy	O	O	●	●	●	●	●	●	O
ECGAssess	●	O	●	●	●	●	O	●	O
HeartPy	O	O	●	●	●	●	●	●	O
HRVTool	●	O	O	●	●	●	O	●	●
NeuroKit2	O	O	●	●	●	●	●	●	O
pyphysio	O	O	●	●	O	●	●	●	O
HeartView	●	⊕	●	●	●	●	●	●	●

O Not existing ◐ Partially existing ● Completely existing ⊕ In development

Acronyms: *FR* = File reader; *CE* = Configuration exporter; *SF* = Signal filtering; *BD* = Beat detection; *V* = Visualization; *CA* = Code available; *PPG* = Photoplethysmography; *ECG* = Electrocardiography; *GUI* = Graphical user interface

In an informal survey of user needs distributed by one of our co-authors to 421 researchers and engineers[1] who process and analyze physiological data, 78% of respondents favored using well-documented, open-source software with user-friendly graphical user interfaces (GUIs). Based on our audit of existing popular open-source tools, only

---

[1] The survey sample comprised 31% researchers and 69% engineers from the Society of Psychophysiological Research (SPR), the IEEE International Machine Learning for Signal Processing (MLSP) workshop, and snowball sampling using personal contacts and social media.

three implement a GUI. ECGAssess is Python-based software that performs automated SQA and binary classification of the acceptability of multi-lead ECG data collected in clinical contexts for medical diagnosis [27]. ANSLab [31] provides both open-source and licensed, closed-source MATLAB-based software options through OpenANSLab and ANSLab Professional, respectively. The software suite contains modules that allow physiological data pre-processing on text files, artifact editing, and analysis. Additional functionalities in ANSLab Professional include batch processing, HRV analysis, and reading of multiple file types. To our knowledge, ANSLab is the only other GUI-based software suite with functions to process PPG data. Additionally, it is the only software suite capable of generating and exporting configuration files, a functionality that we plan to add to a future iteration of HeartView. Although open-source, OpenANSLab does not run as a standalone executable application and thus requires an installation of MATLAB, which is not free and therefore inaccessible to many outside of academia. In contrast, HRVTool is a standalone MATLAB application that performs ECG data processing and HRV feature extraction [30].

While the abovementioned open-source tools are valuable, uses are generally limited to those with programming skills. Further, some possess functionalities restricted by paywalls. In contrast, we propose a data pre-processing pipeline with an accompanying free, GUI-based solution for researchers without programming skills to perform necessary preliminary checks for basic quality and physiological feasibility of both ECG and PPG data. Our approach delivers an open-source, well-documented, and extensible web interface intended to increase efficiency and accessibility to a broader range of researchers who may not otherwise be able to conduct rigorous SQA on their ambulatory cardiovascular data.

3 HeartView Overview

We developed HeartView in Python 3.9 and its accompanying web-based dashboard using Plotly's Dash framework (version 2.8.1). Dash is an open-source Python framework built on Flask, Plotly.js, and React [32].

3.1 Data Processing Pipeline

The HeartView pipeline performs three main procedures (see Fig. 2) before outputting summary information on the dashboard: (1) data pre-processing (i.e., transformation and cleaning); (2) peak extraction; and (3) SQA metric computation.

Data Pre-processing. HeartView begins by reading and transforming raw ECG, PPG, and accelerometer data into Pandas data frames using device-specific file reading functions. Acceptable file types include European Data Format (EDF) files from the Actiwave Cardio and archive files from the Empatica E4. In addition, HeartView uses Pandas to read and pre-process comma-separated value (CSV) files generated from these devices, as well as the RespiBAN.

ECG. HeartView extracts timestamps and raw ECG values in units of millivolts from each EDF or CSV file of the Actiwave Cardio. Next, optional filters are applied to

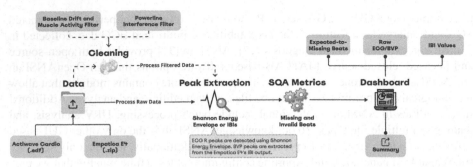

Fig. 2. HeartView pipeline architecture.

eliminate noise from the ECG data. For example, baseline wander and muscle noise can be eliminated using a bandpass filter between 0.5 and 45 Hz, and powerline interference at 60 Hz can be removed using a notch filter with a quality factor of 20.

PPG. Each archive file of the Empatica E4 comprises a set of CSV files containing raw and pre-processed data for HRV analysis. HeartView reads pre-processed inter-beat interval (IBI) values for later peak extraction and raw BVP values with timestamps for plotting and visual inspection purposes.

Acceleration. HeartView can also extract and process acceleration data from EDF, CSV, and archive files of the Actiwave Cardio, Empatica E4, and RespiBAN. The pipeline contains functions for smoothing raw data, converting from g-force to meters per second squared, and computing area under the curve (AUC) of acceleration magnitude. AUC is a commonly used proxy for movement over a given time window [33, 34], particularly when complex time or frequency-domain features are not under consideration at the SQA stage. In the present context, a higher AUC value indicates greater motion.

Peak Extraction. HeartView identifies peak locations from filtered data using the algorithm by Manikandan and Soman [35] for ECG data and from pre-processed IBI output from the Empatica E4 for PPG data[2]. R peaks from the ECG waveform are automatically detected using a Shannon Energy Envelope (SEE) estimator, peak-finding logic based on the Hilbert-transform [40], and zero-crossing point detection [35, 41]. This R peak detection algorithm has been validated using ambulatory ECG recordings from the MIT-BIH arrhythmia database [42, 43], demonstrating 99.8% average detection accuracy, 99.9% sensitivity, and 99.8% positive prediction. Peak locations in the PPG waveform are identified using timestamps from the pre-processed IBI file output provided by Empatica. Although multiple PPG peak detection algorithms exist [24, 44–46], HeartView uses the IBI time series provided by Empatica, given the device's widespread use [47] and the fact that existing algorithms have not been validated on datasets that are standardized to assess the performance of PPG peak detection algorithms.

---

[2] As our primary intent is to introduce a tool for researchers to perform initial assessment checks in their SQA, HeartView currently includes only one of several possible algorithms for ECG beat detection [36–39]. Future users could select and implement additional or alternative state-of-the-art algorithms.

Signal Quality Metrics. HeartView performs SQA on the basic quality (i.e., whether peaks are identifiable for reliable HR and IBI extraction) and physiological feasibility of a signal (i.e., whether the number of extracted peaks is valid) across segments of a user-customizable length. Thus, the pipeline measures signal quality based on the number of missing peaks per segment and invalid signal segments.

Missing Peaks. HeartView determines the number of missing peaks against an expected number of peaks. The pipeline derives this expected number of peaks by computing the median of all second-by-second HR values observed within each segment. We chose to use the median of all second-by-second HR values given its robustness to outliers. Second-by-second HR values are derived with the following steps. First, for each calculated IBI value, the pipeline computes a HR value by dividing the IBI value from 60,0000. Next, each second-by-second HR value is calculated using the harmonic mean of HRs (i.e., the reciprocal of the mean of the reciprocals of HRs) observed in a 2-s window based on Graham's approach [48].

$$\bar{x} = \frac{n}{\sum {1}/{x_i}} \tag{1}$$

In (1), n represents the number of HR values, and x_i represents a HR value at a timepoint i within the 2-s window. Thus, $\bar{x}$ represents the harmonic mean HR at one second, and the expected number is set to the median of all observed $\bar{x}$ in one segment. If the number of detected peaks is greater than the expected number of peaks in a segment, the missing number of peaks in that segment is set to zero; otherwise, the pipeline derives the number of missing peaks by calculating the difference between the number of detected peaks and the expected number of peaks.

Invalid Peaks. After peak extraction, HeartView counts invalid segments based on whether the number of detected peaks in a segment falls outside the range of [30:220] bpm. Based on prior work [2, 47, 49], the upper bound is set to the maximum human HR value, and the lower bound is set conservatively to a value close to the lower bound of the human physiological range.

3.2 Dashboard

We developed the HeartView dashboard using the open-source Dash framework, which consists of a Flask server that communicates with front-end React components [32]. Multiple callback functions with user input and state arguments are mapped to Dash core components, including a file upload component, data segmentation field, and checklist buttons corresponding to filter types (baseline wander, muscle activity, and powerline interference). These functions are then called separately to output interactive charts and a summary table. All user input components are contained within an off-canvas menu that can be toggled to appear or disappear from the left side of the screen.

As illustrated in Fig. 3, the main dashboard contains three separate panels: (1) a data summary panel, including information about the uploaded data file, computed signal quality metrics, and an export button to save all pre-processed data and signal quality information; (2) a bar chart with overlaying bars corresponding to the expected and missing numbers of beats per segment; and (3) a line chart of the raw and filtered cardiovascular data with an overlaying scatterplot of detected peak locations. Two separate buttons are provided to access additional line charts of the corresponding IBI series and raw accelerometer data. We also include a range slider tied to a callback function that takes user-selected segment values and outputs a filtered view of the line charts. For example, in the top-right view in Fig. 3, the bottom panels contain line charts displaying raw and filtered ECG data from the Actiwave Cardio with points denoting locations of detected peaks within the first 20 s of segment 5.

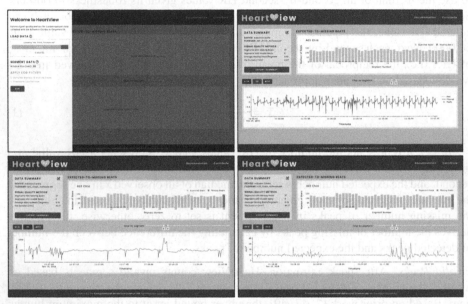

Fig. 3. Multiple panels of the HeartView dashboard. *Top left*: Launch view of the off-canvas containing user input elements; *Top right:* Dashboard view of electrocardiograph (ECG) signal quality assessment and visualization of raw and filtered ECG with peaks; *Bottom left*: Dashboard view with a visualization of inter-beat interval (IBI) series; *Bottom right:* Dashboard view with a visualization of raw acceleration data.

4   Methods

In the following subsections, we discuss the datasets and data pre-processing and analysis procedures used in our assessment of the HeartView pipeline.

4.1   Datasets

Two datasets were used to assess the utility and incipient internal and external validity of HeartView. We leverage cardiovascular data from two studies, enTRAIN and Wearable

Stress and Affect Detection (WESAD). All adult participants and children's caregivers provided written informed consent to participate in the research before data collection.

The enTRAIN study [12] was carried out to investigate socio-affective behavior in 23 typically developing (TD) children and 11 children with autism spectrum disorder (ASD) while collecting interpersonal physiological data [50] during a series of standardized social-emotional regulation tasks. Children's cardiovascular data in the enTRAIN dataset comprise a total of 82.6 h ($M = 2.4$, $SD = 0.6$) of raw ambulatory ECG recorded at 1024 Hz with the chest-worn Actiwave Cardio by CamNtech, which has demonstrated good reliability and validity with gold-standard cardiovascular measures [51]. Children in the study had a mean age of 4.0 years ($SD = 1.1$).

WESAD [13] is a publicly available dataset featuring physiological and motion data recorded from 15 healthy adults during 'neutral,' 'stress,' and 'amusement' affective states. We used 24.1 h ($M = 1.6$, $SD = 0.2$) of ECG recorded at 700 Hz with the chest-worn RespiBAN and 29.7 h ($M = 2.0$, $SD = 0.2$) of PPG simultaneously recorded at 64 Hz from the Empatica E4. Participants in the WESAD study had a mean age of 27.5 years ($SD = 2.4$).

4.2 HeartView Assessment

HeartView outputs metrics regarding the basic quality (i.e., whether beats are identifiable) and physiological feasibility (i.e., whether IBI values are valid) of cardiovascular data and visualizes them on a web-based dashboard. We evaluate the HeartView pipeline by assessing whether group differences in signal quality can be captured in each dataset. Specifically, we tested differences in the numbers of missing peaks per segment and invalid segments between TD children and children with ASD in enTRAIN and between PPG and ECG recordings in WESAD. We hypothesized the following:

H_1: **Our pipeline can capture group differences in the number of missing peaks and invalid segments between (a) ECG recordings of TD children and children with ASD and (b) PPG recordings from the Empatica E4 and ECG recordings from the RespiBAN devices.**

Our rationale for H_{1a} is based on the observation that children with ASD display increased motor stereotypies [52], wandering behaviors [53], and symptoms of attention-deficit/hyperactivity disorder [54] compared to typically developing peers. As a result, these increased movement behaviors are likely to introduce more frequent signal artifacts into data collected from this population in psychophysiological experiments [55].

Our rationale for H_{1b} is based on previous work demonstrating that ECG devices tend to provide higher-quality data than PPG devices, which are subject to motion artifact [56, 57]. This discrepancy is likened to differences in sampling rate and mechanical configuration (e.g., optical sensors versus electrodes). Thus, we expect the data quality of PPG recordings to be impacted by signal artifacts more than that of ECG recordings.

Because data distributions were found to be non-normal for all groups with quantile-quantile plots and the Shapiro-Wilk test, we tested group differences with the Mann-Whitney test in the enTRAIN dataset and with the Wilcoxon signed-rank test for paired PPG and ECG recordings in the WESAD dataset. PPG and ECG data from the WESAD dataset is time-synchronized using the timestamps recorded by the RespiBAN upon initialization. In all ECG recordings, we first apply filters to eliminate baseline wander and muscle noise, followed by powerline interference filters. All enTRAIN and WESAD recordings were segmented into 60-s windows and then trimmed to the start of the first experimental condition and the end of the last experimental condition for each participant before testing for differences.

We also present a potential use case of HeartView's signal quality metrics with data from one randomly selected participant with ASD and one randomly selected TD participant from the enTRAIN dataset. Considering previous findings [52–55] suggesting that ambulatory physiological data from children with ASD may be noisier than that of TD children due to increased physical activity, we sought to demonstrate that HeartView can reveal the relationship between ECG signal quality and physical motion in children. For each enTRAIN participant, the Actiwave Cardio device also contained a 3-axis accelerometer that collected acceleration data at 32 Hz. First, we smooth the acceleration data using a quarter-second moving average filter and then calculate acceleration magnitude values. We then compute second-by-second AUC values of acceleration magnitude using Riemann sums and normalize each value using min-max normalization so that each normalized AUC value is scaled to the range of [0, 1]. Next, we aggregate all AUC values into 60-s sliding windows with 15-s steps. Here, we use a sliding window approach to account for any time lags between physical motion and signal artifact onsets. Therefore, in each 60-s window, the AUC value of acceleration falls in the range of [0, 60]. Finally, we compute Spearman's rank correlation coefficients to evaluate correlations between AUC values and proportions of missing R peaks across all sliding windows.

5 Results

Below, we present the results of our assessment of the HeartView pipeline and demonstrate a use case of HeartView's signal quality assessment metrics with two randomly selected subjects from the enTRAIN dataset.

5.1 Group Differences

Overall, the results of our analyses substantiate our hypotheses. Among the ECG recordings of children with ASD in the enTRAIN study, we found greater proportions of invalid segments with a moderate effect size ($U = 156.0$, $p = .03$, $r = 0.32$) and average proportions of missing peaks per segment with a large effect size ($U = 210.0$, $p = .001$, $r = 0.53$) compared to the ECG recordings of TD children (see Fig. 4a).

Across all WESAD participants, Wilcoxon signed-rank tests revealed that PPG data recorded contained significantly more proportions of invalid segments ($z = -4.17$, $p < .001$, $r = 0.76$) and average proportions of missing peaks per segment ($z = -4.17$, $p < .001$, $r = 0.76$) than ECG data with large effect sizes (see Fig. 4b).

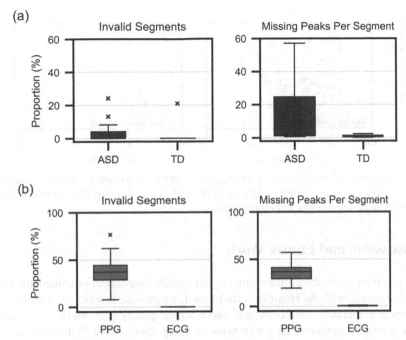

Fig. 4. Comparison of signal quality metrics between data of: (a) children with autism spectrum disorder (ASD) and typically developing (TD) children in the enTRAIN dataset; (b) photoplethysmograph (PPG) and electrocardiograph (ECG) devices in the WESAD dataset.

5.2 Cases: 'A03' and 'T10'

We randomly selected cases 'A03' and 'T10' in the enTRAIN dataset to demonstrate a use case for HeartView's signal quality metrics informing data processing procedures. Overall, across $n = 173$ sliding segments, 'A03's ECG recording contained an average of 3.47% ($SD = 6.88\%$) missing peaks per segment. Spearman's rank correlation coefficients for 'A03's proportions of missing peaks and normalized AUC values of acceleration magnitude also reveal a moderate, positive relationship between physical motion and data missingness ($\rho = .52, p < .001$). Across $n = 149$ sliding segments in 'T10's ECG recording, we found an average of 0.94% ($SD = 4.64\%$) missing peaks per segment and a non-significant correlation between physical motion and data missingness ($\rho = .12, p = .14$). Figure 5 illustrates the relationships between ECG data missingness and physical motion for 'A03' and 'T10.'

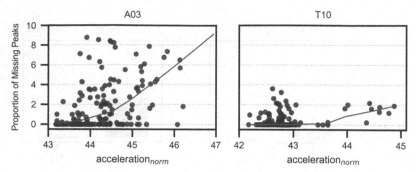

Fig. 5. Scatterplots of proportions of missing peaks per segment and normalized area-under-the-curve acceleration magnitude values in 'A03' and 'T10.' The red line represents locally weighted/estimated scatterplot smoothing curves.

6 Discussion and Future Work

HeartView is an extensible, open-source signal quality assessment pipeline with a web-based dashboard. With the HeartView dashboard, we provide researchers a tool to visually inspect ambulatory cardiovascular data's signal quality (i.e., numbers of missing beats and invalid segments) on a web browser using open-source Python libraries and frameworks. Assessments of basic quality and physiological feasibility of cardiovascular signals from wearable systems can improve the reliability of their measurements—an issue that continually precludes more widespread adoption in clinical contexts [58–60]. Our evaluation of the HeartView pipeline revealed group differences in signal quality within two datasets that support its incipient internal and external validity. We also present and discuss results from two randomly selected cases to demonstrate HeartView's ability to inform decisions about subsequent data processing procedures.

Within the enTRAIN dataset, the HeartView pipeline captured signal quality differences between ECG recordings of TD children and children with ASD. Specifically, ECG recordings of children with ASD contained significantly more invalid segments and missing peaks per segment than those of TD children. Our results are congruent with previous work by Kylliäinen and colleagues [55], who report more artifactual data collected from children with ASD or other developmental delays than from TD children, due to stereotypic behaviors and sensory differences in children with ASD. Further visual inspection of raw ECG signals with high percentages of missing and invalid data also revealed many segments containing motion artifacts and relatively weak or flat line signals. Indeed, our correlation analyses for two enTRAIN cases suggest that data missingness can be attributable to various noise sources. As observed in the case of 'A03,' data missingness can result from increased physical motion. However, it can also result from sources unrelated to physical motion, as observed in the case of 'T10.' In such instances, researchers may benefit from corroborating physiological data quality with ground truth labels, such as video-based annotations of gross motor movements (e.g., running around the observation room, fiddling with the ambulatory recording device). Additionally, researchers may decide to devote more time to cleaning data from children with ASD, as well as applying specific inclusionary and exclusionary criteria (e.g., tolerating certain fidgeting movements in the ASD group, analyzing the same number of trials and time points in both groups) to pre-processing procedures [55]. Motion and behavioral data can be used to formulate these criteria if available. Analyses of HeartView's signal quality metrics with motion data also support decision-making about excluding specific data points or applying additional signal-cleaning procedures on ambulatory cardiovascular data. Further, HeartView's signal quality metrics can support researchers during feasibility testing of experimental protocols involving young children or children with behavioral challenges and wearable cardiovascular devices in pilot studies.

Within the WESAD dataset, our pipeline captured differences in data missingness and the number of invalid segments between PPG and ECG recordings from two different devices. Compared to ECG data from the RespiBAN, PPG data from the Empatica E4 contained more invalid segments and missing peaks per segment. This finding is consistent with those of previous studies comparing the data quality of cardiovascular signals derived from ECG and PPG devices [56, 57]. However, such discrepancies in signal quality could be due to a couple of confounding reasons. First, because PPGs from the Empatica E4 were recorded using fewer inputs than ECGs from the RespiBAN (i.e., a single input versus three leads, respectively), the Empatica E4 had an inherently greater likelihood of collecting data with missing peaks or invalid segments. Second, while the RespiBAN is meant to be worn on the chest, the Empatica E4 is worn on the wrist. Differences in sensor and electrode placement sites result in different levels and types of artifacts. For example, Zhang, Zhou, and Zeng [61] found that ECG data collected from sites on the upper arm were more susceptible to motion artifacts and muscle noise than ECG data collected from the chest. While we did observe differences between wrist-derived PPG and chest-derived ECG data, a limitation of the WESAD dataset is that recordings are limited to only one placement site per signal type. Future work should evaluate HeartView based on differences in signal quality using at least two placement sites per device.

The current functions and feature set of the HeartView dashboard limit its data processing and quality assessment to cardiovascular data collected with the Actiwave Cardio, Empatica E4, and RespiBAN. To increase HeartView's functional generalizability across devices, future iterations of the pipeline and dashboard will incorporate a data transformer to streamline data pre-processing by translating data from various devices by brands commonly used in research (e.g., Polar, Bittium, Shimmer, etc.) into a single format. Further, we plan to add more data processing algorithms and SQA functions specific to different devices and sensor types. For example, researchers may benefit from various algorithmic options at different pipeline steps to evaluate their relative performance when assessing signal quality. Such algorithms may incorporate acceleration measures to corroborate cardiovascular data quality. Given differences in device capabilities to output higher-level values such as HR and IBI (or lack thereof) [62], we also plan to add an IBI detection algorithm for raw PPG data. This need for additional functionality specific to devices and sensor types highlights the importance of an extensible, community-driven approach to software development, whereby researchers and developers use their own datasets to contribute to open-source code and provide valuable feedback on usability, utility, and reproducibility.

7 Conclusion

This paper presents HeartView, an extensible signal quality assessment pipeline with a web-based visualization dashboard for ambulatory cardiovascular data. We developed HeartView using open-source libraries and frameworks in Python. We assessed our pipeline using an ECG dataset collected from children with and without autism and the publicly available WESAD dataset. Our tool has a singular advantage over most extant cardiovascular signal pre-processing and quality assessment approaches. We offer an open-source pipeline with a user-friendly web interface that summarizes signal quality metrics through interactive visualizations and a summary table. A free and well-documented user interface can increase accessibility to signal quality assessment procedures historically only available to researchers with computer science and electrical engineering backgrounds. As a result, our signal quality assessment dashboard can contribute to more methodological transparency, reproducibility, and rigor that empowers researchers from diverse methodological backgrounds to make more informed decisions about the reliability and validity of their data when ambulatory biosensor data collection systems are used.

References

1. Goodwin, M.S.: Passive telemetric monitoring: novel methods for real-world behavioral assessment. In: Handbook of Research Methods for Studying Daily Life. pp. 251–266. Guilford Press, New York (2012)
2. Mishra, V., et al.: Continuous detection of physiological stress with commodity hardware. ACM Trans. Comput. Healthcare 1, 1–30 (2020)
3. Weenk, M., et al.: Continuous monitoring of vital signs using wearable devices on the general ward: Pilot study. JMIR Mhealth Uhealth 5, 1–12 (2017)
4. Pantelopoulos, A., Bourbakis, N.G.: A survey on wearable sensor-based systems for health monitoring and prognosis. IEEE Trans. Syst. Man Cybern. Part C (Appl. Rev.) 40, 1–12 (2010)
5. Orphanidou, C.: Signal Quality Assessment in Physiological Monitoring: State of the Art and Practical Considerations. Springer, Cham (2018)
6. Fine, J., et al.: Sources of inaccuracy in photoplethysmography for continuous cardiovascular monitoring. Biosensors 11, 1–36 (2021)
7. Madhavan, G.: Plethysmography. Biomed. Instrum. Technol. 39, 367–371 (2005)
8. Kusumoto, F.: ECG Interpretation. Springer Nature, Cham (2020)
9. Elgendi, M.: Optimal signal quality index for photoplethysmogram signals. Bioengineering (Basel) 3, 21 (2016)
10. Quintana, D.S., Alvares, G.A., Heathers, J.A.: Guidelines for reporting articles on psychiatry and heart rate variability (GRAPH): recommendations to advance research communication. Transl. Psychiatry 6, 1–10 (2016)
11. Stupple, A., Singerman, D., Celi, L.A.: The reproducibility crisis in the age of digital medicine. NPJ Digital Med. 2, 3 (2019)
12. Yamane, N., Mishra, V., Goodwin, M.S.: Developing an open-source web-based data quality assessment pipeline for analysis of ambulatory cardiovascular data in individuals with autism. In: Paper presented at the International Society for Autism Research Annual Meeting (INSAR 2023), Stockholm, Sweden, 3 May 2023 (2023)

13. Schmidt, P., Reiss, A., Duerichen, R., Marberger, C., Van Laerhoven, K.: Introducing WESAD, a multimodal dataset for wearable stress and affect detection. In: Paper presented at the 20th ACM International Conference on Multimodal Interaction (ICMI 2018), New York, NY, 16 October 2018 (2018)
14. Quesnel, P.X., Chan, A.D.C., Yang, H.: Real-time biosignal quality analysis of ambulatory ECG for detection of myocardial ischemia. In: 2013 IEEE International Symposium on Medical Measurements and Applications (MeMeA), pp. 1–5 (2013)
15. Bae, T.W., Kwon, K.K.: ECG PQRST complex detector and heart rate variability analysis using temporal characteristics of fiducial points. Biomed. Signal Process. Control **66**, 1–21 (2021)
16. Clifford, G., Behar, J., Li, Q., Rezek, I.: Signal quality indices and data fusion for determining clinical acceptability of electrocardiograms. Physiol. Meas. **33**, 1419–1433 (2012)
17. Daluwatte, C., Johannesen, L., Galeotti, L., Vicente, J., Strauss, D.G., Scully, C.G.: Assessing ECG signal quality indices to discriminate ECGs with artefacts from pathologically different arrhythmic ECGs. Physiol. Meas. **37**, 1370–1382 (2016)
18. Sharma, L.N., Dandapat, S., Mahanta, A.: Kurtosis based multichannel ECG signal denoising and diagnostic distortion measures. In: TENCON 2009 - 2009 IEEE Region 10 Conference. pp. 1–5. IEEE, New York (2009)
19. Zaunseder, S., Vehkaoja, A., Fleischhauer, V., Hoog Antink, C.: Signal-to-noise ratio is more important than sampling rate in beat-to-beat interval estimation from optical sensors. Biomed. Signal Process. Control **74**, 103538 (2022)
20. Castiglioni, P., Parati, G., Faini, A.: Cepstral analysis for scoring the quality of electrocardiograms for heart rate variability. Front. Physiol. **13**, 1–13 (2022)
21. He, R., et al.: Reducing false arrhythmia alarms in the ICU using novel signal quality indices assessment method. Paper presented at the 2015 Computing in Cardiology Conference, New York, NY, 6 September 2015 (2015)
22. Orphanidou, C., Bonnici, T., Charlton, P., Clifton, D., Vallance, D., Tarassenko, L.: Signal-quality indices for the electrocardiogram and photoplethysmogram: derivation and applications to wireless monitoring. IEEE J. Biomed. Health Inf. **19**, 832–838 (2014)
23. Behar, J., Oster, J., Li, Q., Clifford, G.D.: A single channel ECG quality metric. In: 2012 Computing in Cardiology, pp. 381–384. IEEE, Kraków (2012)
24. Kazemi, K., Laitala, J., Azimi, I., Liljeberg, P., Rahmani, A.M.: Robust PPG peak detection using dilated convolutional neural networks. Sensors **22**, 1–22 (2022)
25. Bizzego, A., Battisti, A., Gabrieli, G., Esposito, G., Furlanello, C.: Pyphysio: a physiological signal processing library for data science approaches in physiology. SoftwareX **10**, 1–5 (2019)
26. Carreiras, C., Alves, A.P., Lourenço, A., Canento, F., Silva, H.P. da, Fred, A.: BioSPPy: Biosignal processing in Python (2015). https://biosppy.readthedocs.io/
27. Kramer, L., Menon, C., Elgendi, M.: ECGAssess: a python-based toolbox to assess ECG lead signal quality. Frontiers in Digital Health. **4**, 1–9 (2022)
28. Makowski, D., et al.: NeuroKit2: a python toolbox for neurophysiological signal processing. Behav. Res. Methods **53**, 1689–1696 (2021)
29. van Gent, P., Farah, H., van Nes, N., van Arem, B.: HeartPy: a novel heart rate algorithm for the analysis of noisy signals. Transport. Res. F: Traffic Psychol. Behav. **66**, 368–378 (2019)
30. Vollmer, M.: HRVTool—an open-source MATLAB toolbox for analyzing heart rate variability. In: 2019 Computing in Cardiology (CinC), pp. 1–4. IEEE, Singapore (2019)
31. Blechert, J., Peyk, P., Liedlgruber, M., Wilhelm, F.H.: ANSLAB: integrated multichannel peripheral biosignal processing in psychophysiological science. Behav. Res. Methods **48**, 1528–1545 (2016)
32. Plotly: Dash Python user guide. https://dash.plotly.com/

33. Jenkins, J.L., Valacich, J.S., Williams, P.: Human-computer interaction movement indicators of response biases in online surveys. In: ICIS 2017 Proceedings, pp. 1–16. Association for Information Systems (2017)
34. Varni, G., et al.: Interactive sonification of synchronisation of motoric behaviour in social active listening to music with mobile devices. J. Multimodal User Interfaces **5**, 157–173 (2012)
35. Manikandan, M.S., Soman, K.P.: A novel method for detecting R-peaks in electrocardiogram (ECG) signal. Biomed. Signal Process. Control **7**, 118–128 (2012)
36. Pan, J., Tompkins, W.J.: A real-time QRS detection algorithm. IEEE Trans. Biomed. Eng. BME **32**, 230–236 (1985)
37. Christov, I.I.: Real time electrocardiogram QRS detection using combined adaptive threshold. Biomed. Eng. Online **3**, 28 (2004)
38. Elgendi, M., Eskofier, B., Dokos, S., Abbott, D.: Revisiting QRS detection methodologies for portable, wearable, battery-operated, and wireless ECG systems. PLoS ONE **9**, 1–18 (2014)
39. Qin, Q., Li, J., Yue, Y., Liu, C.: An adaptive and time-efficient ECG R-peak detection algorithm. J Healthc, Eng. **2017**, 5980541 (2017)
40. Feldman, M.: Hilbert transforms. In: Braun, S., Ewins, D., Rao, S.S. (eds.) Encyclopedia of Vibration, pp. 642–648. Elsevier Ltd., Amsterdam (2001)
41. Sunami, N.: Shannon energy R peak detection (2020). https://github.com/nsunami/Shannon-Energy-R-Peak-Detection
42. Goldberger, A.L., et al.: PhysioBank, PhysioToolkit, and PhysioNet: components of a new research resource for complex physiologic signals. Circulation **101**, E215–E220 (2000)
43. Moody, G.B., Mark, R.G.: The impact of the MIT-BIH arrhythmia database. IEEE Eng. Med. Biol. Mag. **20**, 45–50 (2001)
44. Chen, L., Reisner, A.T., Reifman, J.: Automated beat onset and peak detection algorithm for field-collected photoplethysmograms. In: Paper presented at the 2009 Annual International Conference of the IEEE Engineering in Medicine and Biology Society, Minneapolis, MN, 3 Sept 2009 (2009)
45. Shin, H.S., Lee, C., Lee, M.: Adaptive threshold method for the peak detection of photoplethysmographic waveform. Comput. Biol. Med. **39**, 1145–1152 (2009)
46. Kuntamalla, S., Reddy, L.R.G.: An efficient and automatic systolic peak detection algorithm for photoplethysmographic signals. Int. J. Comput. Appl. **97**, 1–6 (2014)
47. Mishra, V., et al.: Evaluating the reproducibility of physiological stress detection models. Proc. ACM Interact. Mobile Wearable Ubiq. Technol. **4**, 1–29 (2020)
48. Graham, F.K.: Constraints on measuring heart rate and period sequentially through real and cardiac time. Psychophysiology **15**, 492–495 (1978)
49. Tanaka, H., Monahan, K.D., Seals, D.R.: Age-predicted maximal heart rate revisited. J. Am. Coll. Cardiol. **37**, 153–156 (2001)
50. Palumbo, R.V., Marraccini, M.E., Weyandt, L.L., Wilder-Smith, O., Liu, S., Goodwin, M.S.: Interpersonal autonomic physiology: a systematic review of the literature. Pers. Soc. Psychol. Rev. **21**, 99–141 (2016)
51. Kristiansen, J., et al.: Comparison of two systems for long-term heart rate variability monitoring in free-living conditions: a pilot study. Biomed. Eng. **10**, 1–14 (2011)
52. Goldman, S., Wang, C., Salgado, M.W., Greene, P.E., Kim, M., Rapin, I.: Motor stereotypies in children with autism and other developmental disorders. Dev. Med. Child Neurol. **51**, 30–38 (2009)
53. Rice, C.E., et al.: Reported wandering behavior among children with autism spectrum disorder and/or intellectual disability. J. Pediatr. **174**, 232-239.e2 (2016)
54. Sinzig, J., Walter, D., Doepfner, M.: Attention deficit/hyperactivity disorder in children and adolescents with autism spectrum disorder: symptom or syndrome? J. Atten. Disord. **13**, 117–126 (2009)

55. Kylliäinen, A., Jones, E.J.H., Gomot, M., Warreyn, P., Falck-Ytter, T.: Practical guidelines for studying young children with autism spectrum disorder in psychophysiological experiments. Rev. J. Autism Dev. Disord. **1**, 373–386 (2014)
56. McCarthy, C., Pradhan, N., Redpath, C., Adler, A.: Validation of the empatica E4 wristband. In: 2016 IEEE EMBS International Student Conference (ISC), pp. 1–4 (2016)
57. Charlton, P.H., et al.: Extraction of respiratory signals from the electrocardiogram and photoplethysmogram: technical and physiological determinants. Physiol. Meas. **38**, 669 (2017)
58. Bonnici, T., Orphanidou, C., Vallance, D., Darrell, A., Tarassenko, L.: Testing of werable monitors in a real-world hospital environment: what lessons can be learnt? In: 2012 Ninth International Conference on Wearable and Implantable Body Sensor Networks, pp. 79–84 (2012)
59. Joshi, M., et al.: Perceptions on the use of wearable sensors and continuous monitoring in surgical patients: interview study among surgical staff. JMIR Form. Res. **6**, e27866 (2022)
60. Areia, C., et al.: Experiences of current vital signs monitoring practices and views of wearable monitoring: a qualitative study in patients and nurses. J. Adv. Nurs. **78**, 810–822 (2022)
61. Zhang, Q., Zhou, D., Zeng, X.: Highly wearable cuff-less blood pressure and heart rate monitoring with single-arm electrocardiogram and photoplethysmogram signals. Biomed. Eng. Online **16**, 23 (2017)
62. Nelson, B.W., Low, C.A., Jacobson, N., Areán, P., Torous, J., Allen, N.B.: Guidelines for wrist-worn consumer wearable assessment of heart rate in biobehavioral research. npj Dig. Med. **3**, 1–9 (2020)

Heuristic-Based Extraction and Unigram Analysis of Nursing Free Text Data Residing in Large EHR Clinical Notes

Syed Mohtashim Abbas Bokhari[1]([✉]), Kriste Krstovski[2,3], Jennifer Withall[1], Rachel Lee[4], Patricia Dykes[5,6], Mai Tran[1], Kenrick Cato[7,8], and Sarah Rossetti[1,4]

[1] Department of Biomedical Informatics, Columbia University, New York, NY, USA
mohtashim_abbas@yahoo.com
[2] Data Science Institute, Columbia University, New York, NY, USA
[3] Columbia Business School, Columbia University, New York, NY, USA
[4] School of Nursing, Columbia University, New York, NY, USA
[5] Harvard Medical School, Brigham and Women's Hospital, Boston, MA, USA
[6] BWH Center for Patient Safety, Research and Practice, Boston, MA, USA
[7] University of Pennsylvania, Philadelphia, PA, USA
[8] Children's Hospital of Philadelphia, Philadelphia, PA, USA

Abstract. Free text in nurses' notes can play an important role in clinical decision-making; however, such information has not been explored to the fullest of its potential as it is hard to extract it from electronic health records (EHRs). Free text is a subset of the information recorded in nursing notes. Automated extraction of free text is challenging due to EHRs' size and structural diversity. Understanding these structural and content-level differences is essential for the extraction. Free text is embedded in other relatively structured texts, which are difficult to detect automatically. Moreover, there is no information indicating whether a note is a free text. As a first step in automating the extraction process, we explore heuristic-based algorithms with the goal of establishing a baseline and developing an annotated dataset, which could then be used for further machine learning-based extraction algorithms for a more scalable solution. In this research, we analyze over 200,000 EHR notes and extract 40,000 free text notes from them. Furthermore, we use the unigram language model to analyze the differences between free and structured texts to better understand the free text content.

Keywords: nursing documentation · health informatics · clinical notes · nursing notes · heuristics · natural language processing · information retrieval · unigram analysis

1 Introduction

Nursing documentation, including the concepts written in nursing notes, can play an integral role in healthcare prediction models to inform effective clinical decision-making [1]. Early warning scores (EWS) are one type of prediction

D. Salvi et al. (Eds.): PH 2023, LNICST 572, pp. 124–136, 2024.
https://doi.org/10.1007/978-3-031-59717-6_9

model implemented as clinical decision support tools in the inpatient setting to identify patients at risk of deterioration, including from events such as cardiac arrest and sepsis which impact approximately 330,000 inpatients per year [2,3]. Early identification of patient deterioration can allow for faster treatment and escalation of care to prevent harmful outcomes, such as inpatient mortality. EWS have had limited impact on clinical outcomes likely due to their primary reliance on vital signs, a late indicator of patient deterioration. When nurses are concerned about the potential for patient deterioration they increase surveillance of the patient and their respective nursing notes documentation in electronic health records (EHRs) [4–7]. Our team has developed an EWS named CONCERN (COmmunicating Narrative Concerns Entered by Registered Nurses) that leverages nursing surveillance and documentation patterns that reflect how nurses observe and monitor subtle changes in patients before deterioration is noted in their physiological conditions' parameters [1]. CONCERN is currently in production at 2 academic medical centers with implementation in progress at 2 more health systems [1].

The data from nursing documentation are large in volume and are structured, semi-structured, and time-varying. The large templated documentation from nursing notes also contains free text data written by nurses. These free text data can be useful as features in EWSs to predict patient health deterioration [1]. These free text data will act as an important feature in our CONCERN EWS [1]. Leveraging free text data can be challenging because of their large volume and clinical diversity [8,24,25]. Nursing EHR data are time-varying, semi-structured, and variable on a content level, which make the identification of the free text portion of notes a cumbersome task.

Nursing notes include: 1) templated documentation, which are structured data entered by nurses elsewhere in the chart, and 2) narrative (free text) information written by nurses in their own words. The free text may represent nurses' concerns about patients and can be useful in predictive modeling [1]. However, to leverage information from the free text documentation by nurses we first need to be able to identify where this free text resides within semi-structured nurses' notes and how to retrieve it. Often the narrative free text can be found embedded in other relatively structured texts, which is difficult to detect. Such data are not explicitly labeled as free text and can often be found intertwined within relatively structured texts, thereby making the detection difficult. The absence of clear distinctions between documents' information such as document headers and metadata, further adds up to the problem. This ultimately poses challenges in the automatic extraction of the free text data, which may contain important signals for improved clinical decision-making [1,9].

This research study is focused on HTML-based nursing notes from an academic medical center in the Northeastern United States. The dataset contains more than 200K notes with all free text (with no structured data in it), structured data with no free text, and free text embedded in structured data. Our study aimed to 1) identify and retrieve all narrative (free text) notes data, and 2) distinguish and retrieve the free text embedded in the nursing notes. In this regard, this research uses a heuristic-based approach to extract free text data and utilizes unigram analysis to gain deeper insights into the nursing free text. Unigrams are the elementary subset of the n-gram language models, which is a subfield in natural language processing [10,11]. Based on our prior work we know that nursing free text has signals of nurses 'concerns about a patient. Such concerns can help detect patient health deterioration early even before the vital signs start to appear [1].

While existing research [12–16] has applied machine learning and NLP algorithms directly to free text datasets, and there has been an attempt [17] to recognize tables within free text data, our research uniquely focuses on first establishing the ground truth regarding the location and nature of free text to build a training dataset. This training dataset can be used in the future by machine learning algorithms to identify the free texts dynamically independent of the heuristic-based approach, which is extremely important for the scalability of the system given the potential variation in syntax across different sites. Since we see the problem as a classification task; a training set is required, which aims to establish the foundation to use machine learning approaches for predictive modeling in the future. Moreover, the fraction of the free text in the structured portions can be less than 1%, in addition, there is no metadata to differentiate. Without an annotated dataset, machines may struggle to distinguish the relevant portions. Since the relevant free text portions are so small and as an embedded part (free text) in the structured text, all look the same. Therefore, our heuristic approach is useful for creating a training set for the supervised learning approaches to make the solution heuristic-independent in the future for scalability purposes. Moreover, this HTML format is coming from the Epic EHR which is a widely used system in many hospitals within the US which also makes our heuristic-based approach potentially generalizable across hospitals that use the Epic EHR. Furthermore, unigram analysis of both structured and free text data in this research gives us more insights into the difference in the nursing free text compared to the structured data.

This research is foundational to developing an automated framework for identifying free text containing nurses' concerns from nursing notes through machine learning approaches in the future. In addition, our framework also needs to be a scalable component of the CONCERN EWS that is already being spread to multiple sites.

2 Methods

2.1 Description of Data

In our study, we used more than 200K nursing clinical notes that originated from the Epic©EHR system. Epic is one of the most widely used EHRs in the United States. The notes were retrieved using the Fast Healthcare Interoperability Resources' standard (FHIR) document service. FHIR is a set of rules and specifications for exchanging electronic healthcare data. The notes data was stored in SQL in base64 [18] encoded format, which was decoded into HTML notes files. HTML notes files contain both free texts, as well as structured data. Figure 1 shows different stages of our dataset: notes SQL data in base64 [18] encoded format, decoded HTML notes files, retrieved text from HTML notes, and HTML text transformed into JSON documents.

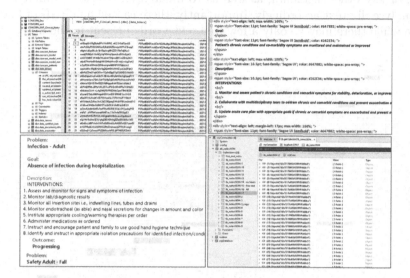

Fig. 1. Example notes originated from the Epic© EHR system: Encoded SQL notes data (top-left), HTML notes file (top-right), notes text (bottom-left), and notes JSON documents (bottom-right).

We distribute our dataset into two parts: 1) sections with structured text and 2) free text. The task is to differentiate and extract the free text. And it is important to be aware of the structural and content-level differences in the data to identify and detach free text from the structured portion. Structural differences refer to the way specific data are stored, which is important for retrieval of relevant data while the content level differences are important to uniquely identify relevant texts, which is crucial for the dynamicity of the solution.

2.2 Segregate and Retrieve the Narrative Embedded in the Nursing Notes

We started by traversing through the HTML nursing notes. We found significant variability in the formats, some of the examples are shown in Fig. 2. The figure shows different layouts of the nursing clinical notes, including plain text, different tabular and other formats, demonstrating a high level of variability. However, we observed that the independent divs in HTML notes files were primarily the place where the narrative data were stored. The 'div' tag defines a division or a section in an HTML document. In automating the extraction process, it is important to determine: 1) which div contained the relevant information (free texts), 2) how to locate the relevant divs, 3) how to differentiate the relevant divs from the other div information, and 4) where to cut and extract the information given that no nested divs exist to indicate the ideal spot to cut. Again, there were no explicit labels to differentiate parts of the notes such as document header, div name, or any other metadata, as well as to differentiate between different divs and analyze div text accordingly. Importantly, there can be hundreds of lines in a note while there may be only a few free text words present in the note.

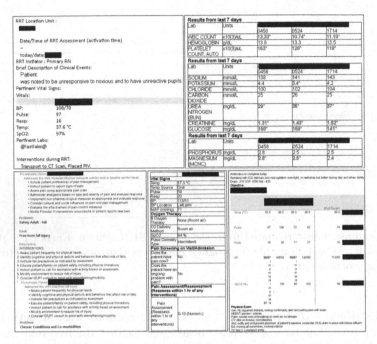

Fig. 2. Example formats of nursing notes originated from the Epic© EHR system

The approach we used was to manually review thousands of files to develop a heuristic-based algorithm, based on the identified static (prespecified) rules to retrieve the relevant portions of the data from HTML tags. For instance, we observed that if certain indicators such as tokens, formats, and headings, exist in certain locations, the data are likely to be free text. Also, it is important to determine which are the relevant and also the irrelevant tokens since token names may overlap between free text and structured portions of a note (see Fig. 3). In this case, we take into consideration other indicators to determine the relevant information, such as the location of the token in the document. The ultimate goal of this approach is to help build a free text dataset that can be used to identify such narrative texts automatically independent of the syntactical differences, which, as aforementioned, is important for the scalability of the system.

Therefore, we traverse through all the files and their respective divs and select only those divs which are relevant, i.e., div text contains specific free text tokens, e.g., 'Assessments/Comments', 'Additional Comments', 'Comments', 'Other Comments', 'Comment', 'Nursing Note', 'Progress Note', 'Treatment Note', and 'Note'. Algorithm 1 retrieves the text from the selected divs of the HTML and removes leading and trailing spaces to check if the first few words contain a heading, i.e., a title containing a colon. Having traversed through all the divs in a document, only relevant divs are selected based on the aforementioned free text tokens.

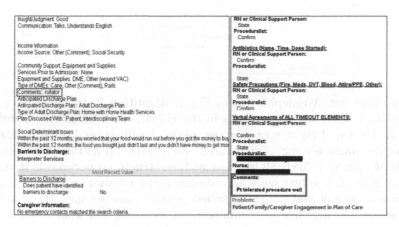

Fig. 3. Example of overlapping token: structured text (left) and free text (right)

If a relevant (containing tokens) heading is found in a div (in certain locations), the algorithm extracts the surrounding text of other divs as free text, otherwise ignores it. If the heading contains specific tokens such as 'comment' and 'comments' then it checks the location of the div within the HTML since not all comments are free text, but the comments in the later part of the documents are likely to be free text. We identified the free text nursing notes from the respective divs based on such identified static rules to build our approximate free text dataset. In the process, we ignore the divs containing the plan of care or discharge notes. The plan of care notes primarily contain structured text reflecting future plans, as opposed to immediate concerns about a patient's state. Discharge notes are documented at the end of patients' hospital stay and therefore would not be available to our algorithm because we are interested in predicting deterioration during a patient's hospital stay in real-time.

2.3   Identify and Retrieve All Narrative Notes Data

Upon examination, we observed that if no heading exists in a document, the structured text is unlikely to be present, rather, the document content is likely

---

Algorithm 1:

```
1  check_label (selected_div, div_count)
2       boolean = False
3       div_txt = selected_div.text.strip() # Remove leading and trailing empty spaces from div text

        # No 'plan of care' or discharge note'
4       if (!(div_txt.lower().contains("plan of care" or "discharge note"))):
5            words = div_txt.split()
6            for w in words[:5] # Check the first five words to check if they are heading/title
7                 if ((w.istitle() or w.isuper()) and (w.endswith(":"))):
8                      if (!w.equals("Comment" or "Comments")):
9                           boolean = True
10                          break
11            else:
                            # Only consider comments from the later divs of the document
12                     if ((selected_div.index()/ div_count)>0.95):
13                          boolean = True
14                          break
15      return boolean
```

---

to be all free text. We depict this in Fig. 4. Algorithm 2 detects all free text by checking if there are no headings in the HTML file. Overall, the algorithm works in this way if there exist relevant tokens, headings, and other indicators, then the document is a mix of structured and free text. If no tokens are present, then the document is likely all free text with no structured portions in it and we annotate it as all free text notes accordingly. If the relevant indicators (tokens) exist in a document and the pre-specified (static) rules are met, the algorithm identifies and extracts free text from relevant locations and what is left behind is merely the structured portion.

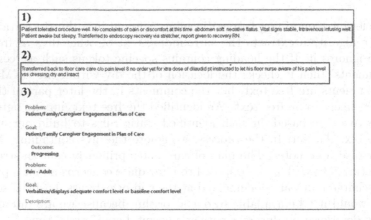

Fig. 4. Free-text examples

In this way, we extracted the relevant information and then categorized the identified free texts into different categories based on the identified tokens. For efficient analysis, the extracted information was stored in a JSON. In addition, we aimed to understand the unique characteristics of free text compared to structured text in order to inform the creation of an automated dynamic system

Algorithm 2:
1 *func_check_no_label* (all_divs):
2   check_no_label = True
3   *for* div *in* all_divs:
4   *if* (div *not* empty):
5   if (*check_label*(div) = True):
6   check_no_label = False
7   *break*
8   *return* check_no_label

that identifies free text. To do so, we conducted a thematic analysis using the unigram language model [10] to identify and compare the recurring domains with the aim to understand the clinical context in which the notes were likely written. Two registered nurses (RL, JW) who have training in informatics research and clinical experience, served as the subject matter experts and individually interpreted the unigram results in Table 1 and 2 to gain more insight about the difference between the contents of free text and structured data. They then met with the primary author (SMAB) to iteratively discuss and reach a consensus on the interpretation of the results related to clinical context and nurse documentation workflow.

3   Results

In our analysis of over 200K documents, we retrieved (based on the pre-specified rules in the algorithm) 40K free text notes in total, out of which 33K were identified as all free text records and 7K free text records found embedded in structured data. We detached free text from the structured portion through our aforementioned heuristics-based approach. A large portion (160K) of the notes consists of only the structured data while the percentage of narrative free text in a note was found to be 1–3%. We found high levels of redundancy in the structured portion of the note as compared to the narrative portion. The same words/blocks of the structured portion of the note are repeated several times. The contents of the structured and free text differed sufficiently; we detected 15K unique words in the narrative text that are not present in the structured portion of the text and 7K unique words in the structured text that are not present in the narrative portion of the text. There were 14.5K overlapping words found.

Figure 5 shows the word clouds for the free text and structured portion indicating the difference between the two where the size of each word indicates its frequency. Table 1 shows the top 20 most frequently occurring free-text terms exclusive to narrative free text while Table 2 shows the top 20 most frequently found terms unique to structured data. Tables show the frequency each of these words appears across the entire dataset (word frequency) and the number of documents in which each of these terms appears (document frequency). Again, the free text is written narratively by registered nurses while the structured

portions are generated from structured (templated) data entered by nurses elsewhere in the EHR. Therefore, our approach does not convert these words into
their respective root words in order to preserve any grammatical structures that
exist and may be helpful in the future to detect such text automatically using
machine learning approaches.

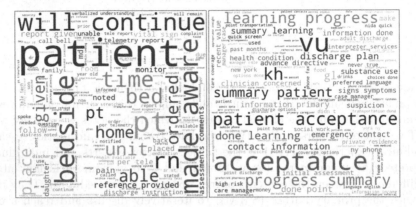

Fig. 5. Free text (left) and structured data (right) word clouds.

The free text unigrams in Table 1 revealed two primary clinical areas: 1)
wound ostomy continence (WOC) care [associated terms in yellow] and 2) cardiac
patient care [associated terms in cyan]. Interestingly, despite the existence of
specific structured fields in the EHRs to capture concepts aligned with wound
ostomy continence and cardiac care, we observed unique terms associated with
these domains captured only in the free text. There may be several reasons
that nurses choose to document this information in free text, ranging from the
usability or data granularity issues with the structured forms to a preference
for narrative forms of documentation to describe particular clinical phenomena.
Future research should seek to explain the characteristics of terms found only in
narrative text versus those found only in structured data.

As for the terms exclusive to structured text in Table 2, the most frequently
appearing word was 'VU' which is short for "verbalized understanding". The
documentation of patient verbalized understanding in structured fields indicates
the nurses' evaluation of the level of comprehension regarding the patient's education. Besides, these unigram results for the structured portion comprise the
terms primarily found in two nursing documentation templates, 1) care management assessment [associated terms in green], 2) substance use history screening
[associated terms in pink] while to a lesser extent, the others belong to templates for nursing care plans and the associated action(s) to achieve the stated
care planning goals [associated term in grey] and time-out documentation for
the operating room [associated term in peach]. This may infer that these specific
templates are more frequently used than others; further research should explore
the portion of structured documentation that are focused on these aspects of
patient care.

Table 1. Unigram analysis of the terms exclusive to narrative-free text data

Rank	Free Text Word	Word Freq.	Document Freq.
1	isol - [isolation]	599	598
2	flange	510	171
3	hollister	315	219
4	couplets	293	284
5	kpouch	279	114
6	peristomal	269	228
7	midabdominal	255	187
8	pacs [premature atrial contractions]	241	231
9	drainable	202	167
10	endo	197	177
11	budded	195	190
12	ceraring	180	159
13	urinal	171	152
14	padded	157	153
15	mf [multiform]	154	144
16	convexity	151	137
17	incont [incontinence]	149	124
18	sterility	138	138
19	phenylephrine	138	108
20	apcs [atrial premature complexes]	138	127

Also, we noticed that some aspects of the templates are not always relevant or useful in all patient cases. For instance, a prevalent term found was the word "element", which often appeared as part of a templated structured field as N/A, thereby indicating that the specific data element was not applicable. The frequent occurrences of the terms such as "element" being "N/A" in the documentation suggest that such information is continuously being recorded, even when a specific data element does not apply to the patient's situation. The need to document each aspect of patient care, even when certain data elements are not applicable, may contribute to the documentation burden specifically related to reviewing and synthesizing data, as well as "note bloat" [19,20]. This may impact the workload of clinicians, thereby affecting the time spent on direct patient care [21–23]. Furthermore, understanding the rationale of nurses regarding their decision to document certain aspects of clinical care in narrative free-text notes rather than structured flowsheet fields, could also be an area of future research. Use of our heuristic approach to detect and leverage concerning clinical concepts documented in narrative nursing notes, and subsequently incorporating this as a feature into the predictive model can help improve clinical deterioration prediction.

Table 2. Unigram analysis of the terms exclusive to structured data

Rank	Structured Text Word	Word Freq.	Document Freq.
1	vu [verbalized understanding]	192822	758
2	discipline	4632	772
3	latino	3972	1324
4	solving	3747	1100
5	element	3474	526
6	grass	3357	767
7	implement	2946	245
8	opium	2457	763
9	hydrocodone	2451	753
10	mushrooms	2394	758
11	hallucinogens	2394	758
12	ecstasy	2394	758
13	stimulants	2373	759
14	sedatives	2370	758
15	dexedrine	2361	759
16	concerta	2361	759
17	ritalin	2361	759
18	ghb	2358	758
19	serepax	2358	758
20	introductions	2352	778

4   Discussion

Literature suggests that when nurses optionally decide to write free text the contents may be a strong signal for information that the nurse wants to communicate to the rest of the healthcare team [1,9]. In this regard, this research analyzed over 200K EHR notes and extracted 40,000 free text notes from them. The problem is that such free text is often found embedded in large datasets, which are hard to retrieve given a lack of clear distinctions between the data. Furthermore, it was challenging to extract such data because of their structural diversities.

This paper describes a heuristic-based extraction and unigram analysis approach to identify as well as understand free text residing in larger EHR nursing notes. We analyzed the data by identifying the unigrams unique to free text data to determine the difference between the two datasets (structured and free text documentations). Because if there were no major differences between the two texts then it would be harder to detect such texts dynamically as both could be labeled essentially the same. Our research found the difference between free text and structured data is statistically significant; there are many clinical terms that were only recorded in the free text by nurses. The choice of nurses to exclusively document this information in the free text could be attributed to several hypotheses. It could potentially result from usability concerns or limitations with the granularity of data accommodated by structured forms. Alternatively, it may reflect a preference for narrative documentation when conveying specific clinical phenomena. Further research is needed to understand the characteristics and implications of terms present in either free text or structured data from nurses' notes. Typically, free text notes give a summarized and up-to-date picture of a patient's current state. Such free text data may be used in EWS to predict health deterioration early before changes in vital signs appear [1].

To the best of our knowledge, this is a unique contribution to the NLP literature, namely, to extract free text from the primary formats of nursing documentation (structure, semi-structured, free text) and subsequently use unigram analyses to attain deeper insights into the free text. The HTML format notes used for this research are coming from Epic which itself is a widely used system in US hospitals, implying a common HTML format. We understand the limitations of the heuristic-based approaches though; however, we see the problem as a text classification problem, which relies on annotated datasets for training purposes. Our heuristic-based approach helped annotate the data to train ML algorithms in the future for a more scalable solution CONCERN EWS system at other hospitals.

Acknowledgments. This work is supported by the National Institute for Nursing Research (NINR) CONCERN Study #1R01NR016941 and the American Nurses Foundation Reimagining Nursing Initiative (RN Initiative). JW is a postdoctoral research fellow supported by the Reducing Health Disparities through Informatics training grant (T32NR007969).

References

1. Rossetti, S.C., Knaplund, C., Albers, D., et al.: Healthcare process modeling to phenotype clinician behaviors for exploiting the signal gain of clinical expertise (HPM-ExpertSignals): development and evaluation of a conceptual framework. J. Am. Med. Inform. Assoc. **28**, 1242–51 (2021)
2. Merchant, R.M., Yang, L., Becker, L.B., et al.: Incidence of treated cardiac arrest in hospitalized patients in the United States. Crit. Care Med. **39**(11), 2401–2406 (2011)
3. Liu, V., Escobar, G.J., Greene, J.D., et al.: Hospital deaths in patients with sepsis from 2 independent cohorts. JAMA **312**, 90–2 (2014)
4. Collins, S.A., Vawdrey, D.K.: Reading between the lines of flowsheet data: nurses optional documentation associated with cardiac arrest outcomes. Appl. Nurs. Res.: ANR **25**(4), 251 (2012)
5. Collins, S.A., Fred, M., Wilcox, L., et al.: Workarounds used by nurses to overcome design constraints of electronic health records. In: NI 2012: 11th International Congress on Nursing Informatics, June 23-27, 2012, Montreal, Canada, vol. 2012. American Medical Informatics Association (2012)
6. Collins, S.A., Bakken, S., Vawdrey, D.K., et al.: Agreement between common goals discussed and documented in the ICU. J. Am. Med. Inform. Assoc. **18**, 45–50 (2011)
7. Collins, S., Hurley, A.C., Chang, F.Y., et al.: Content and functional specifications for a standards-based multidisciplinary rounding tool to maintain continuity across acute and critical care. J. Am. Med. Inform. Assoc. **21**, 438–47 (2014)

8. Kang, M.J., Rossetti, S.C., Knaplund, C., et al.: Nursing documentation variation across different medical facilities within an integrated health care system. Comput. Inf. Nurs. **39**, 845 (2021)
9. Rossetti, S.C., Dykes, P.C., Knaplund, C., et al.: The communicating narrative concerns entered by registered nurses (CONCERN) clinical decision support early warning system: protocol for a cluster randomized pragmatic clinical trial. JMIR Res. Protoc. **10**, e30238 (2021)
10. Xu, W., Xu, D., Alatawi, A., et al.: Statistical unigram analysis for source code repository. Int. J. Semant. Comput. **12**, 237–60 (2018)
11. Martin, J.H.: Speech and Language Processing: An Introduction to Natural Language Processing, Computational Linguistics, and Speech Recognition. Pearson/Prentice Hall, New Jersey (2009)
12. Afzal, Z., Schuemie, M.J., van Blijderveen, J.C., et al.: Improving sensitivity of machine learning methods for automated case identification from free-text electronic medical records. BMC Med. Inform. Decis. Mak. **13**, 1–11 (2013)
13. Zuccon, G., Wagholikar, A.S., Nguyen, A.N., et al.: Automatic classification of free-text radiology reports to identify limb fractures using machine learning and the SNOMED CT ontology. AMIA Summits Transl. Sci. Proc. **2013**, 300 (2013)
14. Wrenn, J.O., Stetson, P.D., Johnson, S.B.: An unsupervised machine learning approach to segmentation of clinician-entered free text. In: AMIA Annual Symposium Proceedings. vol. 2007, p. 811. American Medical Informatics Association (2007)
15. Koleck, T.A., Dreisbach, C., Bourne, P.E., et al.: Natural language processing of symptoms documented in free-text narratives of electronic health records: a systematic review. J. Am. Med. Inform. Assoc. **26**, 364–79 (2019)
16. Jensen, K., Soguero-Ruiz, C., Oyvind Mikalsen, K., et al.: Analysis of free text in electronic health records for identification of cancer patient trajectories. Sci. Rep. **7**, 46226 (2017)
17. Ng, H.T., Lim, C.Y., Koo, J.L.T.: Learning to recognize tables in free text. In: Proceedings of the 37th Annual Meeting of the Association for Computational Linguistics, 443–450 (1999)
18. Josefsson, S.: The base16, base32, and base64 data encodings. Tech. rep. (2006)
19. Moy, A.J., Schwartz, J.M., Chen, R., et al.: Measurement of clinical documentation burden among physicians and nurses using electronic health records: a scoping review. J. Am. Med. Inform. Assoc. **28**, 998–1008 (2021)
20. Bakken, S., Dykes, P.C., Rossetti, S.C., et al.: Patient-Centered Care Systems, pp. 575–612. Computer Applications in Health Care and Biomedicine. Springer, Biomedical Informatics (2021)
21. Tran, B., Lenhart, A., Ross, R., et al.: Burnout and EHR use among academic primary care physicians with varied clinical workloads. AMIA Summits Transl. Sci. Proc. **2019**, 136 (2019)
22. Gregório, J., Cavaco, A.M., Lapao, L.V.: How to best manage time interaction with patients? Community pharmacist workload and service provision analysis. Res. Soc. Adm. Pharm. **13**(1), 133-47 (2017)
23. Morris, R., MacNeela, P., Scott, A., et al.: Reconsidering the conceptualization of nursing workload: literature review. J. Adv. Nurs. **57**, 463–71 (2007)
24. Bokhari, S.M.A., Basharat, I., Khan, S.A., Qureshi, A.W., Ahmed, B.: A framework for clustering dental patients' records using unsupervised learning techniques. In: 2015 Science and Information Conference (SAI), pp. 386–394. IEEE (2015)
25. Bokhari, S.M.A., Khan, S.A.: Applying supervised and unsupervised learning techniques on dental patients' records. In: Emerging Trends and Advanced Technologies for Computational Intelligence: Extended and Selected Results from the Science and Information Conference 2015, pp. 83–102. Springer (2016)

A Data-Driven Methodology and Workflow Process Leveraging Research Electronic Data Capture (REDCap) to Coordinate and Accelerate the Implementation of Personalized Microbiome-Based Nutrition Approaches in Clinical Research

Hania Tourab[1] , Macarena Torrego Ellacuría[2] , Laura Llorente Sanz[2],
Arturo Corbatón Anchuelo[2] , Dulcenombre Gómez-Garre[2],
Silvia Sánchez González[2], María Luaces Méndez[2] , Beatriz Merino-Barbancho[1] ,
Julio Mayol[2,3] , María Fernanda Cabrera[1] , María Teresa Arredondo[1] ,
and Giuseppe Fico[1,3(✉)]

[1] Life Supporting Technologies, Universidad Politécnica de Madrid, Madrid, Spain
gfico@lst.tfo.upm.es
[2] Instituto de Investigación Sanitaria, Hospital Clínico San Carlos, (IdISSC-HCSC), Madrid,
Spain
[3] Departamento de Cirugía, Facultad de Medicina, Universidad Complutense de Madrid,
Madrid, Spain

Abstract. In the rapidly evolving field of precision medicine, personalized nutrition is taking over as well. As individuals respond differently to diet, personalized nutrition engages the idea of going from delivering lifestyle and nutritional recommendations from the population to the individual level, allowing thus a better adherence to the diet, an achievement of nutritional goals, and an effective behavior change. The main factor contributing to the development of personalized nutrition in healthcare is the increase in the availability of large patient data that offers the opportunity to explore and investigate the relationship between various patient features, going from integrating simple data host to metagenomics data. Therefore, using microbiome data as a component of personalized nutrition can be substantial given the close relationship of the gut microbiome with nutrition and the host's health. However, shifting recommendations from the population to the individual level requires a robust data collection and management strategy. In this paper, we aim to describe the methodology and workflow process that uses Research Electronic Data Capture (REDCap) to facilitate the implementation of personalized microbiome-based nutrition approaches in clinical research.

Keywords: personalized nutrition · microbiome data · clinical research · electronic data capture

D. Salvi et al. (Eds.): PH 2023, LNICST 572, pp. 137–147, 2024.
https://doi.org/10.1007/978-3-031-59717-6_10

1 Introduction

As stated by Van Ommen et al. [1] "Personalized nutrition tailors dietary recommendations to specific biological requirements based on a person's health status and goals". The personalized nutrition care model [2] reflects the different aspects used to allow patients to benefit from tailored interventions, with regular and continuous monitoring to reach specific outcomes. It includes: *(1)* The assessment with quantitative and qualitative host data such as diet, biochemistry, metagenomics, etc., *(2)* The interpretation of the personalized data through scientific evidence, *(3)* The intervention developed using guidance and therapeutics to design actionable interventions such as changes to diet and lifestyle factors, and *(4)* The ongoing monitoring and evaluation along the care process for regular feedback, and therapeutic interventions refinement to achieve self-efficacy and behavior change. The therapeutic intervention adherence, represented here by the adherence to an adequate diet, is an important indicator of self-efficacy and health behavior change [3]. Adherence is defined by the World Health Organization (WHO) as the degree to which a person complies with agreed recommendations from a healthcare practitioner, whether taking medication, adhering to a diet, or implementing other lifestyle changes [4]. Across all therapeutic areas, patient non-adherence represents an issue. The lack of patient treatment adherence can be associated with poorer health outcomes, lower quality of life, death, and a burden on healthcare costs [5]. In Medical nutritional therapy (MNT), we understand adherence issues as mainly poor adherence to the nutritional plan. Research indicates that individuals facing different barriers are less likely to comply with a long-term dietary plan [6]. With tailored nutritional recommendations that address patient's needs and barriers, considering the perspectives of personalized nutrition can be a great strategy for facilitating and improving nutrition adherence, and as variations in how each individual responds to diet are always present [7], personalized nutrition engages the idea of going from delivering lifestyle and nutritional recommendations from population to individual level, allowing thus a better adherence and achievement of nutritional goals, and effective behavior changes [8].

For this reason, richer data can help to achieve more targeted interventions and recommendations: from nutritional intake assessment, routine lab testing, and targeted lab testing to omics analysis, the tailored evidence-based strategies and interventions will go from generalized to more personalized for individuals [2]. As an example of the gut microbiome that is unique to each individual and can be influenced by several factors, our diet greatly impacts it, therefore, manipulating this latter with dietary approaches will consist of using gut microbiome markers to optimize dietary interventions, to modulate diet and using diet to modulate the gut microbiome [9]. Personalized nutrition is therefore considered one of the greatest advances in modern medicine, especially with the development of omics and digital technologies.

However, shifting recommendations from the population to the individual level to achieve personalized nutrition requires extensive clinical and omics data, which comes with the need for a robust data collection and management system. As defined in the FAIR (Findable, Accessible, Interoperable, Reusable) data guiding principles [10], making the data collected easily searchable, accessible, integrated, and used in combination with other data and reusable is also a crucial element for supporting personalized nutrition. Moreover, the advancement in information technologies (IT) has led to the development of health data management systems to provide to a greater extent accurate and better patient care [11]. Researchers have designed and implemented a data management system to manage patient data and support clinicians in their decision-making to diagnose genetic diseases [12]. Some worked on capturing data related to patients with inflammatory joint diseases directly from an electronic health record system and transferring them into an electronic data capture system, helping in transitioning from paper format to electronic system [13]. Another study proposed an integrated data management system to support and manage data of patients with Parkinson's disease, preventing, therefore, data loss, and offering patients clinical follow-up and monitoring [14]. In nutrition care, dietary assessment and nutritional monitoring can be challenging for healthcare professionals and nutritionists as the available methods are time-consuming and susceptible to human errors [15]. Leveraging digital health technology may now offer a new way to provide medical nutritional therapy on a more accurate, personal, and accessible level. There is evidence for example that computerized patients' data management systems can improve nutritional care and monitoring, with better data visibility and adequate nutrition delivery [16].

One of the easily accessible data collection and management systems is the Research Electronic Data Capture (REDCap) [17]. REDCap is a secure, web-based application designed for research teams as a tool to collect, manage, and store research data in a secure environment. Because of its user-friendly interface, it has been used in several domains, and more importantly in clinical research as a tool to support precision medicine in oncology [18] and support clinicians in assessing the probability of patient outcomes after surgery for pancreaticoduodenectomy [19]. The field of nutrition research is known for its huge amount and complex data, which makes it one of the healthcare fields that are advancing in the use and application of computational techniques to its important data [20]. REDCap can be an important part of data-driven projects related to nutrition, as data collected and managed using REDCap can be later processed and analyzed using various computational techniques, including machine learning (ML) and artificial intelligence (AI), evolving the field of personalized nutrition.

Therefore, given the close relationship of the microbiome with nutrition and its key role in modulating health and disease, it is important to integrate the gut microbiome as a component of a personalized nutrition intervention along with other individuals' information. With the ability to modulate the gut with diet, it is appealing to target the gut microbiome with diet-based strategies and to harness digital technologies, such as REDCap's data management features to efficiently collect and integrate data, leading to more tailored dietary interventions, which can be of interest for both healthcare professionals and patients for providing targeted and actionable nutritional approaches and receiving recommendations for achieving sustainable results, respectively. To this end, this paper aims to describe the methodology and workflow process deployed to manage and integrate data at different scales using digital health (REDCap) to advance the field of personalized nutrition and facilitate the implementation of personalized microbiome-based nutrition approaches in clinical research.

2 Materials and Methods

2.1 Ethical Statement

The study protocol was approved by the Ethics Committee of Reference of the Regional Health Service of Segovia, Spain, as well as the Ethics Committee from Hospital Clínico San Carlos of Madrid, Spain, which also approved the related data management processes (17/183-E-BS and 19/409-E).

2.2 Data Source

The Hospital Clínico San Carlos of Madrid, together with the Primary Care Centre of the province of Segovia (Autonomous Community of Castilla y León) in Spain are carrying out a collaborative study to investigate the metabolic syndrome and cardiovascular risk factors in a cohort of patients: the SEGOVIA cohort study. This study is a longitudinal population-based study with a long follow-up of 20 years involving a cohort of 809 subjects aged between 35 and 74 years, enrolled in the study between January 2000 and January 2003. Assessments were carried out at three points in time, in which the study variables are collected: a baseline visit from 2000, a second visit with a median follow-up of 7 years in 2008, and, finally, a third visit with a median follow-up of 20 years in between 2021–2023. The work presented in this paper focuses on the sub-cohort of patients with a median follow-up of 20 years, where a sub-study of metabolic syndrome, diet and characterization of the intestinal microbiota is being conducted.

2.3 Data Collection

The patient clinical information was gathered by means of a written questionnaire in a face-to-face interview with an interviewer, where an individual code was assigned to each patient. The report form includes extended questions to gather the necessary information about the patient, related among others, to his personal data, medical history, clinical data, and daily habits.

The nutritional assessment and the dietary data collection of patients were carried out using two types of evaluation tools: *(1)* a 14-item Mediterranean Diet Adherence Screener (MEDAS) [21] integrated into the general questionnaire, where the level of adherence to the Mediterranean diet is assessed using a 14-item questionnaire (12 questions on food consumption frequency and 2 questions on food intake habits considered characteristic of the Spanish Mediterranean diet), and *(2)* a Food Frequency Questionnaire (FFQ) from the University of Navarra (Spain) that consists of a list of foods and beverages with categories of response to estimate the frequency of consumption over a specified period of time. Both the patient clinical information and the nutritional data were given in a Microsoft Excel spreadsheet file in an anonymized way, with the patient ID as the identifier.

Finally, the characterization of the composition of the gut microbiota was done after the collection of feces samples provided by the patients and their analysis by the Microbiota Laboratory of the Hospital of Madrid using Next Generation Sequencing (NGC) technologies. The results were given in a tabular representation of the gut microbiome composition: Operational Taxonomic Units (OTUs) table. OTUs table summarizes the composition of the microbial communities present in each sample, where each column represents a different sample, and each row represents the taxonomic identification of the bacterial taxa from the level of phylum, class, order, family, genus to species. The abundance of each taxonomic unit in each sample is represented by the relative abundances in the cells.

2.4 Setting up the REDCap Database and Data Entry Workflow

The collected patient data was transferred to a REDCap database created on the REDCap web-based application accessed through the hospital network, with only the research team having user rights. The digitization workflow included:

Selecting the relevant variables for defining the block of variables.
Patient clinical information gathered from the general questionnaire consisted of extensive information on patient health where several types of data were collected. For now, and based on the purpose of the research team and the study, only the data of interest was captured and digitized. The selection was made by the research team based on a mapping of common variables from the different questionnaires of each of the visits at the three points of time, i.e., 2000, 2008, and 2021. The interest behind this procedure is to be able later to investigate and establish the relationship between these variables over time, in a longitudinal way, as the data of the two previous studies projects is stored in a separate REDCap repository. In the end, only the relevant data has been selected, and the block of variables has been defined and captured in REDCap, as presented in the results part.

The nutritional information to be digitized covered on one hand, the data gathered from the answers to the 14 questions of the Mediterranean Diet Adherence Screener and its total score, and on the other, the data gathered from the Food Frequency Questionnaire, that is the result of the automatic calculations of estimated daily intakes of different nutrients and food groups from the respondent-reported information.

Finally, the gut microbiome information, given the large size of the initial OTUs table and the complexity of gut microbiome data, data will be captured as the relative abundance at each phylum level for every sample (i.e., patient) to enable simple and efficient data capture.

Completing the required metadata information
The worksheet with all the defined data elements is used to complete the requirements for data entry, by filling in the specific information related to *the type of variable (field type), the field label, and the variable name in REDCap* to prepare the data entry in the software for building the environment.

Creating the environment via the Online Designer
The online designer in REDCap allows the creation of the environment via the instrument collection page, where data collection instruments, referring to the block of variables defined, can be created and the variables can be added.

Capturing the data
Once the environment has been added to REDCap, it is possible to upload the data directly into REDCap using the Data Import Tool.

3 Results

3.1 Defining the Block of Variables and Integrating Data

Our data source included 113 patients (58,4% women and 41,6% men). Overall, after the selection of variables, we were able to define five blocks of variables that represent the instruments to be created on REDCap, with their associated metadata. We integrated multiple data types, including *(1) demographic data, (2) clinical data, (3) dietary records and nutritional data, (4) analytical data, and (4) omics data*, as detailed in Table 1.

Table 1. Block of variables retrieved with the associated metadata

Demographic data
Personal ID
Gender
Clinical center
Date of interview
Age
Year of revision
The starting time of the questionnaire
Marital status
Place of residence
Professional activity
Clinical data
Medical history, including *history of diabetes, hypertension, cholesterol, cardiovascular and intestinal diseases, other diseases, birth delivery, and physical examination*
Anthropometric measurements
Weight, Height, Waist circumference, Hip circumference
Blood pressure measurements
Electrocardiogram measurements
Nutritional data
14 items questionnaire of MEDAS
Food Frequency Questionnaire
Macronutrients intake (per day)
Micronutrients intake (per day)
Vitamins
Minerals
Total intake by food groups (g/day)

(continued)

Table 1. (*continued*)

Analytical parameters
Diabetes diagnostic
Basal capillary glycemia (fasting glycemia)
Capillary glycemia 2 h after glucose tolerance test
Glycated hemoglobin HbA1c
Lipids profile: total cholesterol, LDL cholesterol, HDL cholesterol, triglycerides
Kidney and hepatic functions
Urine: microalbuminuria

Gut microbiota data (relative abundance by phylum)
Overall characterization of 26 phyla; relative abundance of each phylum for each patient

3.2 Clinical REDCap Workflow

After designing and creating the environment on REDCap, one can either import the data using the data import tool option or add records directly via the record dashboards as the surveys and the required components have been created to facilitate the capture of data. By adding a new record, we are creating a new patient profile with its personal ID. We can then start capturing the demographic data, the phenotype-based information data, including anthropometrics, clinical information and clinical biomarkers, and nutritional information by filling the dietary record related to the FFQ, as well as the survey related to the Mediterranean questionnaire that will automatically retrieve the total score of the survey. Finally, the microbiome profile will be integrated as the relative abundance of each phylum present in each sample.

Figure (1) briefly shows the clinical REDCap workflow setup to enable the deployment of the digitization of the needed data for a personalized nutrition strategy in clinical care. The data management system created on REDCap allows us to capture the data directly by filling in the information in the appropriate fields. Once capturing data is completed, reports and statistics can be accessed, as well as initiating the data export.

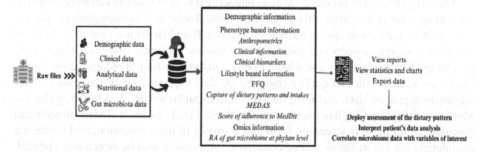

Figure. 1. Clinical REDCap workflow for supporting the implementation of personalized microbiome-based nutrition approaches in clinical research. *Abbreviation: RA. Relative abundance*

3.3 Impact of Digitization in the Clinical Setting

The digitization of the available data contributed to having an efficient process, compared to paper-based data collection, to limit the number of manual tasks and automatically capture the relevant data from capturing individual dietary records to integrating omics data and calculating the score for adherence to the Mediterranean diet. The use of the REDCap platform ensured a standardized collection of patient data, minimizing missing data and ensuring high-quality data collection. It offers hospital practitioners a practical option to easily export the data, generate reports, statistics, and charts that can help in comprehensively presenting data, as well as overviewing the included patients and the availability of their data, combining clinical and omics data, offering a support tool for clinicians to inform clinical decision making related to providing personalized nutrition strategy in a novel way that could be adopted in a clinical setting.

4 Discussion and Conclusion

The study associated with this work, the Segovia study, is a longitudinal population-based study that was at the beginning a study representative of the Segovia province resident population in urban and rural areas aiming at estimating the prevalence of the Metabolic Syndrome [22]. The present paper focuses on the sub-cohort of patients with a median follow-up of 20 years (i.e., third visit) that aims at studying the Metabolic Syndrome, diet and characterization of the intestinal microbiota. Given the importance of digital health, and to leverage the use of digital tools in clinical settings like REDCap and its advanced data storage features, we were able to create a detailed patient profile by integrating multiple data types, from dietary, and clinical data to microbial profiles. This comprehensive patient profile is important for designing nutritional recommendations that are more likely to be adhered to. The microbiome profile of the patient is provided by the relative abundance of the microorganisms at the phylum level. It gives us information on how many proportions of the microbiome are made up of bacterial taxa at the phylum level. This allows us to evaluate further if the relative abundance of the bacteria is associated with one of the variables of interest such as dietary pattern or adherence to the Mediterranean diet.

Ensuring efficient data collection and enhancing data accessibility can be relevant for supporting actionable nutritional recommendations. Tools for data management systems like REDCap have a valuable contribution and have found larger use in several domains including research projects and clinical environments. As in the study of Brauer et al., [23] where they aimed to assess whether personalized nutrition in metabolic syndrome can be associated with diet quality changes, the data capture system was used to enter the nutrition process data, including data restrictions and real-time data integrity checks. Moreover, REDCap [24] has found its use in clinical trials where included subjects can complete an online self-screening form and a survey in the application, and where the completed case report forms and demographic information will be stored and updated. Related to that, researchers [25] have designed and implemented a web-based data management system for diabetes clinical trials that had a good rating among researchers using it, showing that electronic systems can facilitate the clinical data management process in diabetes and endocrinology research. These support the extensive use of electronic data capture systems in clinical research and their ability to improve and facilitate the data management process.

Having access to data with real-time monitoring and reporting can facilitate the process of informed decision-making making, therefore be valuable for (1) achieving a proper assessment by identifying patient inputs that will help to gain a better understanding of the individual's behavior and distinctive characteristics ranging from general host data, biological data to the more advanced assessment of complex data such as gut microbiome, (2) interpreting the analysis of the patient's data gathered to derive actionable information from them and identify patterns and relationships between the different factors, (3) producing actionable interventions tailored to the specific patient's needs and goals, and (4) monitoring and evaluating to track progress and adjust recommendations as needed throughout the time, in an iterative process, and guarantee further refining in the intervention, enhancing thus patient's adherence and engagement to the personalized nutrition plan. One interesting study [26] reported the substantial contributions to patient care from using REDCap, where demographic, epidemiologic, and clinical data of HIV-positive and negative patients with or without liver and cervical cancer were accessible in REDCap, and have helped healthcare professionals in providing more personalized care, as well as promoting patients' involvement in their health care.

Overall, the data-driven methodology and workflow process leveraging REDCap has been deployed to structure the collection of data relevant for coordinating and implementing personalized nutrition in clinical practice, emphasizing the importance and value of the insights gained from data in providing efficient solutions. The digitization process and integration offer real-time accessible information to healthcare providers to inform clinical decisions for personalized nutrition purposes and improve individual health outcomes by leveraging an approach of patient-centered care, with a special focus on improving adherence to nutritional treatment plans. This study, however, has some limitations due to its design (i.e., observational) and due to the individuals lost in the follow-up assessments. Nevertheless, death causes will be available for the 20-year period of follow-up, as well as some clinical information of those subjects that were not revised during the first and second follow-up waves which will be extracted from medical registries in the coming months. Future work will eventually emphasize on making available sequenced data for genome-wide association studies (GWAS) to help achieve more targeted interventions and recommendations.

Acknowledgments. The authors wish to acknowledge the partners of the BEAMER project. This project has received funding from the Innovative Medicines Initiative 2 Joint Undertaking (JU) under grant agreement No 101034369. The JU receives support from the European Union's Horizon 2020 Research and Innovation Programme, the European Federation of Pharmaceutical Industries and Associations (EFPIA), and Link2Trials BV.

References

1. van Ommen, B., et al.: Systems biology of personalized nutrition. Nutr. Rev. **75**(8), 579–599 (2017). https://doi.org/10.1093/nutrit/nux029

2. Bush, C.L., et al.: Toward the definition of personalized nutrition: a proposal by the American nutrition association. J. Am. Coll. Nutr. **39**(1), 5–15 (2020). https://doi.org/10.1080/073 15724.2019.1685332

3. Kawamura, A., et al.: Dietary adherence, self-efficacy, and health behavior change of WASHOKU-modified DASH diet: a sub-analysis of the DASH-JUMP study. Curr. Hypertens. Rev. **16**(2), 128–137 (2019). https://doi.org/10.2174/1573402115666190318125006

4. Eduardo. Sabaté and World Health Organization., Adherence to long-term therapies: evidence for action. World Health Organization (2003)

5. Jimmy, B., Jose, J.: Patient medication adherence: measures in daily practice (2011)

6. Landa-Anell, M.V., Melgarejo-Hernández, M.A., García-Ulloa, A.C., Del Razo-Olvera, F.M., Velázquez-Jurado, H.R., Hernández-Jiménez, S.: Barriers to adherence to a nutritional plan and strategies to overcome them in patients with type 2 diabetes mellitus; results after two years of follow-up. Endocrinol. Diabetes Nutr. **67**(1), 4–12 (2020). https://doi.org/10.1016/j.endinu.2019.05.007

7. Hughes, R.L., Marco, M.L., Hughes, J.P., Keim, N.L., Kable, M.E.: The role of the gut microbiome in predicting response to diet and the development of precision nutrition models-Part I: overview of current methods. Adv. Nutr. **10**(6), 953–978 (2019). https://doi.org/10.1093/advances/nmz022

8. Tay, W., Kaur, B., Quek, R., Lim, J., Henry, C.J.: Current developments in digital quantitative volume estimation for the optimisation of dietary assessment. Nutrients **12**(4), 8–15 (2020). https://doi.org/10.3390/nu12041167

9. Kashyap, P.C., Chia, N., Nelson, H., Segal, E., Elinav, E.: Microbiome at the frontier of personalized medicine. Mayo Clin. Proc. **92**(12), 1855–1864 (2017). https://doi.org/10.1016/j.mayocp.2017.10.004

10. Wilkinson, M.D., et al.: Comment: The FAIR guiding principles for scientific data management and stewardship. Sci Data **3** (2016). https://doi.org/10.1038/sdata.2016.18

11. Ismail, L., Materwala, H., Karduck, A.P., Adem, A.: Requirements of health data management systems for biomedical care and research: scoping review. J. Med. Internet Res. **22**(7) (2020). JMIR Publications Inc. https://doi.org/10.2196/17508

12. Samra, H., Li, A., Soh, B.: G3DMS: design and implementation of a data management system for the diagnosis of genetic disorders. Healthcare (Switzerland) **8** (3) (2020). https://doi.org/10.3390/healthcare8030196

13. Olsen, I.C., Haavardsholm, E.A., Moholt, E., Kvien, T.K., Lie, E.: NOR-DMARD data management implementation of data capture from EHR. Clin. Exp. Rheumatol. **32**(5), S158–S162 (2014)

14. Folador, J.P., Vieira, M.F., Pereira, A.A., Andrade, A.D.O.: Open-source data management system for Parkinson's disease follow-up. Peer J. Comput. Sci. **7**, 1–23 (2021). https://doi.org/10.7717/peerj-cs.396

15. Zhao, X., Xu, X., Li, X., He, X., Yang, Y., Zhu, S.: Emerging trends of technology-based dietary assessment: a perspective study. Eur. J. Clin. Nutr. **75**(4), 582–587 (2021). https://doi.org/10.1038/s41430-020-00779-0

16. Berger, M.M., et al.: Impact of a computerized information system on quality of nutritional support in the ICU. Nutrition **22**(3), 221–229 (2006). https://doi.org/10.1016/j.nut.2005.04.017

17. Harris, P.A., Taylor, R., Thielke, R., Payne, J., Gonzalez, N., Conde, J.G.: Research electronic data capture (REDCap)-A metadata-driven methodology and workflow process for providing translational research informatics support. J. Biomed. Inform. **42**(2), 377–381 (2009). https://doi.org/10.1016/j.jbi.2008.08.010

18. Charles Vesteghem, A., et al.: Implementing a data infrastructure for precision oncology projects leveraging REDCap Charles Vesteghem. medRxiv preprint (2022). https://doi.org/10.1101/2022.05.09.22274599

19. Cochran, A.R., Raub, K.M., Murphy, K.J., Iannitti, D.A., Vrochides, D.: Novel use of REDCap to develop an advanced platform to display predictive analytics and track compliance with enhanced recovery after surgery for pancreaticoduodenectomy. Int. J. Med. Inform. **119**, 54–60 (2018). https://doi.org/10.1016/j.ijmedinf.2018.09.001
20. Côté, M., Lamarche, B.: Artificial intelligence in nutrition research: perspectives on current and future applications. App. Physiol. Nutr. Metab. (2021). https://doi.org/10.1139/apnm-2021-0448
21. Schröder, H., et al.: A Short screener is valid for assessing mediterranean diet adherence among older Spanish men and women. J. Nutr. **141**(6), 1140–1145 (2011). https://doi.org/10.3945/jn.110.135566
22. Martínez-Larrad, M.T., et al.: Prevalencia del síndrome metabólico (criterios del ATP-III). Estudio de base poblacional en áreas rural y urbana de la provincia de Segovia. Med. Clin. (Barc.) **125**(13), 481–486 (2005). https://doi.org/10.1157/13080210
23. Brauer, P., et al.: Key process features of personalized diet counselling in metabolic syndrome: secondary analysis of feasibility study in primary care. BMC Nutr. **8**(1) (2022). https://doi.org/10.1186/s40795-022-00540-9
24. Tang, H., et al.: Randomised, double-blind, placebo-controlled trial of Probiotics to Eliminate COVID-19 Transmission in Exposed Household Contacts (PROTECT-EHC): a clinical trial protocol. BMJ Open **11** (2021). https://doi.org/10.1136/bmjopen-2020-047069
25. Nourani, A., Ayatollahi, H., Solaymani-Dodaran, M.: A clinical data management system for diabetes clinical trials. J. Healthc. Eng. **2022** (2022). https://doi.org/10.1155/2022/8421529
26. Odukoya, O., et al.: Application of the research electronic data capture (REDCap) system in a low- and middle income country– experiences, lessons, and challenges. Health Technol (Berl) **11**(6), 1297–1304 (2021). https://doi.org/10.1007/s12553-021-00600-3

Pervasive Health for Carers

Patient-Pharmacist Interactions in Chronic Care: A Qualitative Study and Implications for Design

Ana Vasconcelos, Joana Couto Silva, Ruben Moutinho, Fernando Ricaldoni, Ana Correia de Barros, and Francisco Nunes[✉]

Fraunhofer Portugal AICOS, R. Alfredo Allen 455/461, 4200-135 Porto, Portugal
{Ana.Vasconcelos,Joana.Silva,Ruben.Moutinho,Fernando.Ricaldoni,
Ana.Barros,Francisco.Nunes}@fraunhofer.pt

Abstract. Chronic patients are often asked to perform measurements as part of their self-care. Some patients make measurements at home, but others resort to their local pharmacy for information and support. However, there is a shallow understanding of the role of pharmacists and pharmacies in chronic care management, which may hinder the development of tools to support patient care. To better understand the work carried out at community pharmacies for chronic care, and inform the design of these systems, we conducted an ethnographic informed study. We observed four community pharmacies and interviewed eleven pharmacists. Results show that pharmacists are essential in providing patients with information regarding their medication and support in health measurements. However, their work is restricted by a general lack of information about the patient and limited collaboration with other clinicians. Drawing on the insights from this work, we derived three implications for the design, including developing software for pharmacies that keeps track of patient measurements and shares them with doctors, and creating a pharmacist-doctor communication channel for enabling medication adjustments.

Keywords: chronic care · health measurements · pharmacy ·
pharmacists · chronic patients · observations · interviews

1 Introduction

Chronic conditions such as Diabetes, Hypertension, or Chronic Obstructive Pulmonary Disease (COPD) are the main causes of mortality, representing 71% of all deaths [32]. Chronic patients need to frequently monitor their condition and engage in self-care [4,9,12], however, some patients might experience difficulties transitioning to or managing autonomously, requiring the help of healthcare professionals. Given community pharmacies' proximity to patients, pharmacists can be crucial in monitoring chronic patients, releasing the burden from often overworked doctors or nurses.

© ICST Institute for Computer Sciences, Social Informatics and Telecommunications Engineering 2024
Published by Springer Nature Switzerland AG 2024. All Rights Reserved
D. Salvi et al. (Eds.): PH 2023, LNICST 572, pp. 151–165, 2024.
https://doi.org/10.1007/978-3-031-59717-6_11

Despite the recognised value that Information and Communication Technologies (ICT) bring to healthcare, there is still a gap when it comes to studies on the use of ICT in pharmacies [8]. Our work aims to contribute to understanding community pharmacists' interactions with chronic patients, including what tools they have access to, how they gather important disease-related data, and how they intervene in patient care. To this end, we conducted an ethnographic informed study in four pharmacies, performing observations and interviews with eleven pharmacists with different roles and experience levels. This approach allowed us to gain insights into the role of the pharmacy in the community and in the healthcare system, as well as the role of the pharmacist in supporting chronic care management.

This paper reports on the outcomes of this qualitative study and the derived design implications. Our results emphasise the importance of pharmacists in chronic care and detail how their role in medication management and measurements is essential to chronic patients. Moreover, it is also clear that pharmacists need improved tools to support their work and our results may better inform the development of solutions targeting pharmacies and their patients.

2   Background

2.1   The Role of Community Pharmacists

Pharmacists play a vital role in the healthcare system due to their close proximity to patients. They are experts in medication and are responsible for ensuring the safe, effective and rational use of drugs. The connection of pharmacists to medication development, supply and management is widely recognised, however, a shift in pharmacists' responsibilities is already taking place and evolving towards a more patient-centric approach [1]. In some countries, pharmacists already take roles previously exclusive to nurses or doctors, including supporting blood pressure, glucose and cholesterol measurement, pregnancy testing, or providing smoking cessation advice and diabetes guidance [1]. This shift was motivated by population ageing, an increase in number of chronic patients, shortages in healthcare professionals, COVID-19 demands, but it was also a necessary step to ensure the sustainability of the profession itself because medication dispensing can be automated [11].

Existing barriers to more patient-centred pharmacists include pharmacists' self-perception as "dispensers of medication" and not patient-centred practitioners coupled with the business-driven culture of pharmacies [25]. Other studies indicate that pharmacists are not used as public health professionals because of a negative attitude towards pharmacists' role in patient care, pharmacy education, standards, government policies [24], lack of interprofessional care, inadequate compensation models, and lack of a shared vision for pharmacy services [20]. Results from a Portuguese study with four pharmacies suggest that time management can also be a barrier to the optimal use of pharmacists' skills: while 50% of pharmacists' time was used in interactions with customers, close to 38% was spent ordering and storage of medicines, checking for errors in the dispensed prescriptions, preparing prescriptions for reimbursement issues, and meetings with vendors and salespersons [14]. A study conducted in the Netherlands [29] found similar results. The time spent with secondary tasks has burdened pharmacists and prevented them from expanding their healthcare services. Technological solutions for medicine dispensing could optimise the process thus reducing pharmacists' effort and increasing available time [14].

2.2 Technology in Community Pharmacies

The community has created several technologies for pharmacies (for a review see [7,31]). Mobile applications can be implemented in pharmacy practice for varied purposes such as clinical references, order processing, communication or patient engagement [2]. Patients with chronic conditions are one of the groups that could benefit the most from the use of these technologies and a closer relationship with pharmacists, particularly with the use of condition monitoring devices (e.g. glucometers, blood pressure monitors, etc.) that can provide valuable information to equip pharmacists to assist better patients with diabetes, COPD, or congestive heart failure [17]. Different approaches to chronic disease monitoring have been successfully explored such as telemonitoring for diabetes management and education [26], or a platform with a set of devices measuring health parameters to be positioned inside the pharmacies [3]. Another mobile solution was used for diabetic and hypertension patients connected to monitoring devices controlled by the pharmacist that store measurements taken at the pharmacy and provide patients with relevant information to manage their disease while facilitating communication between patients and pharmacists [33].

While there seems to be a consensus that a technological approach to the relationship between pharmacists and patients could benefit both, having a stronger focus on the patient and their clinical status also creates an urgent need for more and better interactions between pharmacists and physicians. Both pharmacists and physicians confirm that multidisciplinary teams can improve patient care and treatment efficacy, but there is still a need to modify infrastructures, agree upon goals and educate healthcare workers to fully take advantage of such partnership [30]. A Canadian study with 19 pharmacies and nine medical clinics observed limited communication and collaboration between primary care doctors and pharmacists, with pharmacists missing prescription data and physicians missing data on adherence [19]. Even in hospitals, where pharmacists and clinicians collaborate regularly, professionals lack agreement about their specific roles and responsibilities in the medication reconciliation process, resulting in incomplete, inefficient, and duplicate work around medication regimens [15].

Technological solutions, particularly Electronic health records (EHR) can be a potential tool to aid communication between clinicians and pharmacists [19]. Countries like Canada [10] and Australia [21] are already using these systems but there are others such as the United States where the only information available to most pharmacists when dispensing medication is essentially the prescription, which is not sufficient to make informed decisions for patients [6]. With all the advantages that EHRs could bring to pharmacy practice [13] it is then paramount to explore and understand the characteristics these solutions must exhibit to successfully implement them in a useful and sustainable way.

Pharmacists can be important in chronic care management, but little is known about how and which tools can support this. With our study we expect to better understand how pharmacists support chronic patients within the Portuguese context and derive the necessary recommendations for developing high-impact solutions that contribute to the enrichment of pharmacists' role and facilitate teamwork with physicians, ensuring the best care for their patients.

3   Methods

We conducted an observation and interview study to understand pharmacies' role in managing patients with chronic conditions. The ethnographic fieldwork was conducted between May and July 2021 by six researchers, who were grouped in pairs to observe pharmacies and interact with pharmacy workers (pharmacists and pharmacy assistants) in different settings. Notes, photographs, drawings, and interview transcripts were shared and discussed among the research team. The analysis was supported by the Affinity Mapping method [5], whereby six researchers in the team summarised, grouped, and discussed the main insights of the study individually as well as in three group sessions, around a digital whiteboard supporter by Mural [22] software.

3.1   Observations

We used non-participant observation at pharmacies [27], complemented with informal interviews with pharmacists. Observations had three main *foci*: pharmacist-patient interactions, health parameter measurement, and interactions with the existing software. Researchers did not directly interact with pharmacy clients.

The observation sessions, which ranged from 1 h to 3 h, were always conducted by two researchers simultaneously and took place in five separate locations. During observations, researchers chose different locations in the pharmacy, including being next to pharmacists, behind the counter, or standing next to shelves or near clients being attended to. In total, researchers spent 14 h in observation sessions, with some sites receiving multiple observation sessions. Data from observations were collected mainly using fieldnotes, occasionally complemented with photographs and drawings.

3.2   In-Depth Interviews

To understand pharmacists' perspectives about their role in supporting patients with chronic conditions, we conducted in-depth interviews [16]. The interviews were qualitative, and semi-structured, to touch on specific topics while giving space for participants to bring other topics to the table. We recruited pharmacists, pharmacist assistants, and technical directors, as they contacted directly with patients. We chose to involve pharmacists with different levels of experience and from different settings, to gain access to diverse experiences and backgrounds. The interview guide touched on three main topics: (1) Interactions with chronic patients, (2) Dealing with regular clients, and (3) Role of the pharmacy and pharmacist in the healthcare system. We also inquired participants about demographics, formal education, and previous experience. Before starting the interview, participants received information about the study and data privacy.

In total, 11 participants were interviewed (7 female, 4 male). Three interviews were conducted via videoconference and recorded. The remaining interviews were conducted face-to-face, inside the pharmacies, and were not recorded. Each interview lasted between 30 and 60 min, and the participants were all pharmacists, with responsibilities of customer attendance and/or technical direction of the pharmacy. Experience varied from 1 to over 30 years of experience.

3.3 Recruitment and Ethics

The four pharmacies were recruited through Associação Nacional de Farmácias, the portuguese association of pharmacies, who called potential pharmacies from a convenience sample, considering variety in terms of size, context, and innovation attitude. All pharmacies were based in Porto, Portugal, and one pharmacy had more than one physical site. Once pharmacies agreed to take part in the study, researchers called pharmacies' technical directors for arranging visits. Technical directors introduced the research team to the pharmacists, be them on site or online. In some instances, pharmacists were asked to indicate colleagues from their pharmacy to participate in the interviews. Participants were all volunteers and received no monetary compensation.

All participants provided informed consent after receiving information about the project, goals of the study, data management and security.

3.4 Portuguese Healthcare Context

In Portugal there is a national health service - Serviço Nacional de Saúde (SNS) – that is the main health service, based on universal and equal health access for people living in the country. Community pharmacies however are not part of the SNS; they are privately owned, subject to government-issued requirements (e.g. staff must be comprised of at least two pharmacists) but not directly connected to SNS entities such as hospitals or primary care clinics. There is also a national pharmacy association – Associação Nacional de Farmácias (ANF) that represents pharmacy owners, and whose mission is to support pharmacies and initiatives that value their services. In 1999, ANF created a department to develop pharmaceutical care programs that promoted the integration of pharmacists in patient care, monitoring and follow-up, thus enriching pharmacists' role. The first pilot was launched in 2001, focused on supporting the care of patients with diabetes, hypertension and COPD, and since then, more pharmacies have adhered to these programs [18].

Technology-wise, Portuguese pharmacies currently have access to software that registers the medication sold to customers, and identifies potential medication interactions. Despite its recognized usefulness to pharmacists, the system does not take into account that customers frequently buy products for members of their household, registering these under the same customer id. As such, medication interactions or dosage alerts may result from wrongful information. Moreover, customer data is separated for different pharmacies, which means that pharmacists can only act on purchase information from their own pharmacy.

4 Results: Current Practices of Managing Chronic Patients

Pharmacists are highly sought-after mediators, who repeat medical advice, listen to patients' concerns, and help them reflect on medication side-effects and interactions. They do not replace primary care services, but have a fundamental role in this ecosystem, which is sometimes underestimated. As we observed, pharmacists' role entails teaching the treatment (ongoing or about to start), explaining posology, following medical attention, considering medication interactions and medical exams, and giving advice. To exemplify the role of pharmacists, one technical director said that pharmacists often teach asthmatics how to use the expansion chamber (asthma inhaler), advise patients about a balanced diet and associated medication, or in cases of constipation to "drink water as treatment".

4.1 Support Medication Starting and Correct Usage

Pharmacists spend a considerable amount of time dispensing medication to both the general public and chronic patients. The first step is usually to understand the products that patients want to take. In a country that has adopted electronic prescription, it is common for patients to hand their smartphones to pharmacists so they can access the prescription dispensing codes (similar practices were described in [23]). We also observed patients showing medication packages or photographs of medication packages to indicate their preferred medication brand.

The most relevant chunk of the time in dispensing medication is invested in explaining how to properly take the medication. According to our participants, patients have many doubts about their medication, as doctors spend less time explaining how to take medication. As a result, patients resort to the support of their pharmacist, who seems to have more time or availability to address their doubts. An additional issue has to do with the health literacy of the patients. Clinicians often use concepts that patients do not understand which can lead to ignoring important information. For example, one pharmacist referred that clinicians sometimes ask patients to avoid anti-inflammatory medication, but that it is extremely common for patients not to know what those medications are, and thus pharmacists provide this information to support patients.

Another important task of pharmacists while dispensing medication is to screen potential medication interactions. During this search, pharmacists perform a great deal of "guessing work", as patients, which usually are older adults, lack complete information about their condition and treatments. Looking at prescriptions, pharmacists can get an idea of the reason for taking the medication, but it is not guaranteed, because, for example, a medication for diabetes could be used for losing weight. Another tool they use is the records available in the information system that can show them medication previously purchased by patients but this information is often unreliable: a patient can have on record medications that were purchased by them but not for them or they may have purchased medications in another pharmacy. The absence of data enables a lack of trust and extends the process of achieving trustworthy information, but participants argue that if they could access more data, they would have more confidence in the credibility of the information they convey to patients.

Pharmacists also supported their patients in successfully taking medication, mobilising resources that could be useful to them. One example we observed while at the pharmacy was how a pharmacist offered the patient to take a pill box for putting their medication. Noticing that the patient was having difficulties in remembering the medication they took, the pharmacist thought about potential solutions for the issue and decided to suggest the patient to try using a pill box. Even though thinking about where the patient would place the medication exceeded the pharmacist's role, she intuited that the patient would benefit from having a medication box which they could fill in daily and know when they had taken a certain medication.

The work of pharmacists is further supported by long-term relationships with their patients.

Pharmacist 3: "There are affinities with certain clients. (...) We [pharmacists] create a friendly relationship, some [pharmacists] with more, others with less, but happens with all colleagues."

A trusted pharmacist will often become the preferred professional for a specific patient, and be the person with who they share illness episodes, questions, or even the news and pictures from their family. While pharmacists try to avoid people being attended only by one pharmacist, when pharmacists have close relationships with patients they are able to pay more attention to the patient's general health and detect acute illness episodes, which can be very useful.

4.2   Performing Measurements at the Pharmacy

Pharmacies are important health parameter measurement sites for patients with chronic conditions. They possess the devices to measure blood pressure, weight, and, in some cases, blood testing equipment that can serve to understand the state of the patient's cholesterol or diabetes. In addition to equipment, making measurements at the pharmacy has the added benefit of having the pharmacist operate measurement devices or, at least, provide feedback on the values. Most patients that made measurements at the pharmacy did not have a device for performing the measurement at home. Patients who had their own device sometimes went to the pharmacy to check if the measurement of their device

158   A. Vasconcelos et al.

was correct, or because they had abnormal values and wanted to know what they could do about them. To illustrate the measurement practices occurring in pharmacies, we present a vignette of measuring blood pressure in a "self-service" blood pressure monitor machine at Pharmacy 1.

> *Pharmacist positions the patient arm in the machine and adjusts their back. Pharmacist enters the coins in the machine. Pharmacist and patient await the measurement. When the machine ends, pharmacist picks up the receipt paper with the measurement.*
> **Pharmacist 2**: "Everything is fine. Systolic is at 16; lets see if it keeps like that [or if it lowers]. Come back in 2-3 days again to see".
> **Patient**: "Is drinking coffee [before coming] bad?"
> **Pharmacist 2**: "Try avoiding coffee and then we test [to see if values change]".

As shown in the example above, pharmacists were the ones responsible for the setup of the blood pressure monitor device at pharmacy. They adjusted the position of the bench to fit the patient, they helped place the patient's arm into the inflatable cuff, and even operated the device's software. After choosing whether to perform a blood pressure measure, a weight measure, or both, pharmacists also entered the coins of the patient into the device. When asked about why pharmacists took such an active role in the setup of the blood pressure monitor device, participants explained that it was the way to obtain quality measurements. Patients were likely to have elevated blood pressure if they saw an error in the machine, so pharmacists were careful with the setup, to make sure the chances of errors by inappropriate measurement conditions stayed minimal. At the peak of COVID-19, pharmacists supported patients in performing a second measurement, adjusting the arm in the cuff or any other condition that could have caused the error in their perspective, but prior to COVID-19 they would take the patient to a separate room, sit them down, give them some minutes to relax, and only then would they perform a manual blood pressure measurement. These conditions supported the acquisition of measurements that were faithful to the patients' state and thus had clinical value.

When the machine performs the measurement, pharmacists stay close to the patient for noticing errors, might they arise. Once measurements are finished, pharmacists picked up the paper slip from the machine, read the value out loud to the patient, and explained to the patient if it was positive or negative. In case of abnormalities, pharmacists inquired patients about circumstances that could have elevated their blood pressure, including anxiety, salty food, or the recent start of a new medication. If the values obtained were concerning, they might ask the patient to return later to make a new measurement or suggest them to go see their doctor. Moreover, if values deviated considerably from standard values, they would call patients' relatives or emergency services. When asked if calling family members or emergency services was part of their responsibilities, one pharmacist explained that they had an ethical duty as healthcare professionals to care for their population, most especially in acute cases of regular clients they closely accompany. Additionally, a pharmacist shared that when communicating with emergency services, their knowledge allows them to explain patients' condition better than the patients themselves or other person outside the healthcare field. This shows a strong commitment to patients, and an active role in enabling the healthcare system to work.

Interviewed pharmacists considered that their measurement devices should save patients' values, similar to a prior study [33]. Frequently, sometimes twice a day (morning and afternoon), patients go to the pharmacy to measure blood pressure due to medical instructions and preserve a piece of paper (Fig. 1) to present to the doctor to monitor their status. However, if the machine could record and save patients' values, it could facilitate communication or collaboration with clinicians. It could also enable pharmacists to know the usual values for a specific patient. According to our participants, pharmacies could have regular patients' informed consent, for example, to save and share data within a cross-disciplinary platform accessible to both pharmacists and clinicians.

4.3   Discussing Prescription Issues with Clinicians

In some rare occasions, pharmacists spot issues with the prescription that need to be discussed with clinicians. Examples include potential interactions between medication, very high doses prescribed, or unconsidered patient characteristics that might make the prescription unsafe. In these situations, pharmacists may contact clinicians to discuss potential issues and devise an adjusted medication plan, however, communication channels are far from ideal.

> **Pharmacist 1**: "The patient needs to wait one or two hours at the pharmacy before I can get information that I need from the clinician".

Since pharmacists do not usually have direct phone numbers to healthcare units, they are usually left with general phone numbers, which may not prioritise their question. This means that, as stated by Pharmacist 1, waiting periods can be long before the pharmacist can contact the clinician, which is not desirable for neither the patient nor the pharmacist. When direct communication is not possible, pharmacists mainly give the information to their patients so they can discuss it with their clinicians. Still, pharmacists find this compromise unsatisfactory because some information can be lost, misunderstood or misinterpreted.

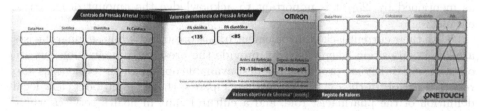

Fig. 1. Paper slip for recording blood pressure measurements currently in use in one of the pharmacies observed.

Pharmacist 1: "There could be a triangulation between clinicians, pharmacists, and patients, thinking about the benefits that those interactions could bring, even though dealing with the challenges of sensitive data protection could occur".

A more appropriate approach would be, as envisioned by Pharmacist 1, to have a more direct communication channel between clinicians, pharmacists and patients, where information could be safely shared. For this pharmacist, there are clear benefits in having access to this information despite its sensitivity and more importantly, it can avoid the long waits or misunderstandings that currently occur. As an example, they mention a mobile service connecting doctors, pharmacists and patients. Another participant referred that, in the case of patients with yearly medication subscriptions, the pharmacist could report observations about how patients are taking or reacting to the medication, which could inform medication adjustments. Another pharmacist described that, ideally, there should be an initial appointment in the pharmacy, where the pharmacist would get to know the patient's clinical conditions, medications, and medical recommendations. Currently, pharmacists only see patients when they purchase medication or perform measurements, which does not allow them to perform the role they envision. Another pharmacist emphasised that being able to accompany patients more would be ideal because pharmacists are the first healthcare professional which patients appeal to.

5 Discussion

The main goal of this study was to understand how pharmacists support patients with chronic diseases in their management, and the interactions with healthcare professionals, to inform future technology design. While performing observations in pharmacies, we noted that, in accordance to previous studies [14,29], the work carried out by pharmacists exceeds medication dispensing and includes not only contact with the public but also a significant amount of time spent with administrative tasks. It became clear that medication dispensing is a far more complex task than simply following a prescription. The process includes instructing patients, making sure they clearly understand the instructions and have the conditions to follow them while screening for possible medication interactions. As such, even when reducing the role of pharmacists as medication dispensers, as mentioned by [25], it is important to acknowledge the amount of expertise entailed.

With their current lack of involvement in the prescription phase, pharmacists are left in a position where they can provide the prescribed medication but are often unsure if they are providing the best available option for the patient, as also reported by [6]. In the opinion of our participants, there should be a clear legal definition of the pharmacist role, and a cultural shift in health services where collaboration between different services and professionals is valued in practice. These barriers and necessary changes are also mentioned in previous literature

[20,24]. Overall, pharmacists consider they should be able to have more information about the patients and their conditions, as it is their role not only to provide medication but also to check for medication interactions and support medication adherence.

Since pharmacists have a close relationship with patients, they could play an important role in communicating symptoms' evolution and adherence data to clinicians. As identified in prior work [19], clinicians often lack information that could allow them to better monitor patients, even without direct contact. Pharmacists dedicate their efforts to ensure that chronic patients have the opportunity to monitor their medication and other health parameters not only onsite at the pharmacy but also when helping patients that have difficulties performing their measurements at home an issue previously identified in prior work [28].

It became clear during this study that, as observed before [19], one of the most prominent challenges currently faced by pharmacists is the lack of direct communication with clinicians. Pharmacists envision a closer collaboration with clinicians, to support a better understanding and common agreement of the roles each will play in patient care, with doctors being in charge of the diagnosis, with pharmacists being involved in prescription and treatment adjustments.

It should be noted that our work is limited due to the localised nature of the fieldwork. We involved pharmacies from one city, and it is possible that other pharmacies in different locations (e.g. rural settings) report different practices. We compared our findings with the literature to overcome the localisation issue, but fieldwork in other locations would be required to further validate our findings.

5.1   Implications for Design

According to our fieldwork, technology can support collaboration between pharmacists, patients and clinicians to improve chronic care. As such, we derived a set of implications for the design of such technologies to ensure that they answer to the current challenges faced by pharmacists.

Enable pharmacies to keep a personalized profile of their patients. Pharmacies play a very important role in the measurement and monitoring of patients' measurements. By providing expert feedback on patients' values, pharmacists not only advise patients but also support screening of aggravations or further health issues. Having the possibility to keep track of measurements should enable pharmacists to more efficiently know the baseline of values for a specific patient, enabling them to detect minor issues before they aggravate. During the fieldwork, we also understood that pharmacists have access to the record of client purchases and use this list to screen for medication interactions. However, the list of purchases for each client may include products bought for others, which can complicate this process. With this in mind, pharmacists suggested having an individual profile for each patient, especially chronic patients taking more medication simultaneously. The data management of patient profiles will need to be carefully designed, but pharmacists already have an ethical duty to their patients and manage medication data confidentially, so having a profile for patients would be a logical next step.

Provide a direct communication channel between pharmacists and clinicians. The fieldwork showed issues in communication between pharmacists and clinicians. Without a direct communication channel, patients had to wait or come back another time to the pharmacy, each time there seemed to be a medication interaction or an error in prescription. Collaboration between pharmacist and clinician was also hindered, and there was no way for clinicians to rely on the pharmacist besides what they could intuit from a prescription. With a direct software communication channel, pharmacists would be able to: (i) support patient education and training, (ii) share observations with clinicians about patient adherence or (side)effects, (iii) recommend adjustments in medication taking into consideration health issues or the daily habits of the patient, and (iv) ask for alternative medications, e.g., when a medication is out of stock. While clearly important for patient care, having this effective communication can also be valuable in defining the role of the pharmacist as a support for doctors, helping them support patient self-care and triage of acute illness episodes.

Enable measurements made at the pharmacy to be shared with clinicians. It was clear from the fieldwork that pharmacists take a number of precautions to reach measurements with clinical quality. Currently, values measured at the pharmacy are shared with clinicians using paper slips (Fig. 1), which can be easily lost and even require additional note-taking at the clinician's office. In case the measurement process is digitised, the measurements could be uploaded directly to the patient profile or an alternative option that can be easily shared with the clinician. Having these measurements made at the pharmacy and with the support of the pharmacist ensures measurement quality, avoiding false concerns and doctor visits, or delay in care.

6   Conclusion

This study was conducted to understand current practices and challenges faced by pharmacists to inform the design of solutions that could play an important role in supporting their chronic patients. Our findings indicate that while pharmacists are a key actor in helping chronic patients manage their diseases, they lack the information and communication with clinicians to better support their decisions and provide more services and better care to their patients. Technology can be seen as a potential solution, but it needs to address these professionals' real needs, and some key features must not be left out. The derived implications for design intend to summarise these action points, which should be implemented with Participatory Design projects that involve all relevant stakeholders.

Moreover, there is a need for a change of pharmacists role in healthcare and their relationship with clinicians, patients and in particular chronic patients. While this change seems to be clear for our participants, other policy, legal and organisational aspects should be approached and discussed in future studies.

Acknowledgements. This study was funded by the project ConnectedHealth (n.º 46858), supported by the Competitiveness and Internationalisation Operational Programme (POCI) and Lisbon Regional Operational Programme (LISBOA 2020), under the PORTUGAL 2020 Partnership Agreement, through the European Regional Development Fund (ERDF).

References

1. Anderson, S.: The state of the world's pharmacy: a portrait of the pharmacy profession. J. Interprof. Care **16**(4), 391–404 (2002). https://doi.org/10.1080/1356182021000008337
2. Aungst, T.D., Miranda, A.C., Serag-Bolos, E.S.: How mobile devices are changing pharmacy practice. Am. J. Health-Syst. Pharm. **72**(6), 494–500 (2015). https://doi.org/10.2146/ajhp140139
3. Baldo, D., Benelli, G., Pozzebon, A., Sesto, R.: The fides project: a pharmacy toolbox to allow healthcare decentralization. In: 2011 E-Health and Bioengineering Conference (EHB), pp. 1–5 (2011)
4. Barlow, J., Wright, C., Sheasby, J., Turner, A., Hainsworth, J.: Self-management approaches for people with chronic conditions: a review. Patient Educ. Couns. **48**(2), 177–187 (2002). https://doi.org/10.1016/S0738-3991(02)00032-0
5. Burgess, H., et al.: The sticky notes method: adapting interpretive description methodology for team-based qualitative analysis in community-based participatory research. Qual. Health Res. **31**(7), 1335–1344 (2021)
6. Craddock, D.S., Hall, R.G.: Pharmacists without access to the EHR: practicing with one hand tied behind our backs. Innovations pharm. **12**(3), 16 (2021). https://doi.org/10.24926/iip.v12i3.4141
7. Crilly, P., Kayyali, R.: A systematic review of randomized controlled trials of telehealth and digital technology use by community pharmacists to improve public health. Pharmacy **8**(3), 137 (2020). https://doi.org/10.3390/pharmacy8030137
8. Fitzpatrick, G., Ellingsen, G.: A review of 25 years of CSCW research in healthcare: contributions, challenges and future agendas. Comput. Support. Coop. Work (CSCW) **22**(4), 609–665 (2012). https://doi.org/10.1007/s10606-012-9168-0
9. van der Gaag, M., Heijmans, M., Spoiala, C., Rademakers, J.: The importance of health literacy for self-management: a scoping review of reviews. Chronic Illn. **18**(2), 234–254 (2022). https://doi.org/10.1177/17423953211035472
10. Gheorghiu, B., Hagens, S.: Measuring interoperable EHR adoption and maturity: a canadian example. BMC Med. Inf. Decis. Making **16**(1), 1–7 (2016). https://doi.org/10.1186/s12911-016-0247-x
11. Gregório, J., Lapão, L.V.: Uso de cenários estratégicos para planeamento de recursos humanos em saúde: o caso dos farmacêuticos comunitários em portugal 2010–2020. Revista Portuguesa de Saúde Pública **30**(2), 125–142 (2012). https://doi.org/10.1016/j.rpsp.2012.12.003
12. Howard, J., et al.: Exploring the barriers to using assistive technology for individuals with chronic conditions: a meta-synthesis review. Disabil. Rehabil. Assist. Technol. **17**(4), 390–408 (2022). https://doi.org/10.1080/17483107.2020.1788181
13. Hughes, C.A., Guirguis, L.M., Wong, T., Ng, K., Ing, L., Fisher, K.: Influence of pharmacy practice on community pharmacists integration of medication and lab value information from electronic health records. J. Am. Pharm. Assoc. **51**(5), 591–598 (2011). https://doi.org/10.1331/JAPhA.2011.10085

14. Lapão, L.V., et al.: EHealth services for enhanced pharmaceutical care provision: from counseling to patient education. In: 2013 IEEE 2nd International Conference on Serious Games and Applications for Health (SeGAH), pp. 1–7 (2013). https://doi.org/10.1109/SeGAH.2013.6665308
15. Lee, K.P., Hartridge, C., Corbett, K., Vittinghoff, E., Auerbach, A.D.: Whose job is it, really? physicians, nurses and pharmacists perspectives on completing inpatient medication reconciliation. J. Hosp. Med. **10**(3), 184–6 (2015). https://doi.org/10.1002/jhm.2289
16. Lofland, J., Snow, D.A., Anderson, L., Lofland, L.H.: Analyzing Social Settings: A Guide To Qualitative Observation And Analysis, 4th edn. Wadsworth Publishing, Belmont, CA, USA (2005)
17. Martin, A., et al.: The evolving frontier of digital health: opportunities for pharmacists on the horizon. Hosp. Pharm. **53**(1), 7–11 (2018). https://doi.org/10.1177/0018578717738221
18. Martins, S., Costa, F.A.D., Caramona, M.: ImplementaÇÃo de cuidados farmacÊuticos em portugal, seis anos depois. Rev. Port. de Farmacoterapia **5**(4), 4–12 (2015). https://doi.org/10.25756/rpf.v5i4.38
19. Mercer, K., et al.: Physician and pharmacist medication decision-making in the time of electronic health records: mixed-methods study. JMIR Hum. Factors **5**(3), e24 (2018). https://doi.org/10.2196/humanfactors.9891
20. Mossialos, E., et al.: From retailers to health care providers: transforming the role of community pharmacists in chronic disease management. Health Policy **119**(5), 628–639 (2015). https://doi.org/10.1016/j.healthpol.2015.02.007
21. Mullins, A.K., et al.: Physicians and pharmacists use of my health record in the emergency department: results from a mixed-methods study. Health Inf. Sci. Syst. **9**(1), 1–10 (2021). https://doi.org/10.1007/s13755-021-00148-6
22. MURAL: Mural (2022). https://www.mural.co/
23. Murero, M.: E-prescribing: the rise of socio-tech-med micronetworks of care during the COVID-19 pandemic. Salute E SocietÀ **XX**(suppl. 2), 104–118 (2021). https://doi.org/10.3280/SES2021-002-S1007
24. Puspitasari, H.P., Aslani, P., Krass, I.: Challenges in the management of chronic noncommunicable diseases by indonesian community pharmacists. Pharm. pract. **13**(3), 578 (2015). https://doi.org/10.18549/PharmPract.2015.03.578
25. Rosenthal, M.M., Breault, R.R., Austin, Z., Tsuyuki, R.T.: Pharmacists self-perception of their professional role: insights into community pharmacy culture. J. Am. Pharm. Assoc. **51**(3), 363–368a (2011). https://doi.org/10.1331/JAPhA.2011.10034
26. Shane-McWhorter, L., et al.: Pharmacist-provided diabetes management and education via a telemonitoring program. J. Am. Pharm. Assoc. **55**(5), 516–526 (2015). https://doi.org/10.1331/JAPhA.2015.14285
27. Spradley, J.P.: Participant Observation. Holt, Rinehart and Winston (1980)
28. Storni, C.: Multiple forms of appropriation in self-monitoring technology: reflections on the role of evaluation in future self-care. Int. J. Hum. Comput. Interact. **26**(5), 537–561 (2010). https://doi.org/10.1080/10447311003720001
29. van de Pol, J.M., Geljon, J.G., Belitser, S.V., Frederix, G.W., Hövels, A.M., Bouvy, M.L.: Pharmacy in transition: a work sampling study of community pharmacists using smartphone technology. Res. Social Adm. Pharm. **15**(1), 70–76 (2019). https://doi.org/10.1016/j.sapharm.2018.03.004
30. Waszyk-Nowaczyk, M., et al.: Cooperation between pharmacists and physicians - whether it was before and is it still ongoing during the pandemic? J. Multidiscip. Healthc. **14**, 2101–2110 (2021). https://doi.org/10.2147/jmdh.s318480

31. Webster, L., Spiro, R.F.: Health information technology: a new world for pharmacy. J. Am. Pharm. Assoc. **50**(2), e20–e34 (2010). https://doi.org/10.1331/JAPhA. 2010.09170
32. WHO, W.H.O.: Non communicable diseases (2021). https://www.who.int/news-room/fact-sheets/detail/noncommunicable-diseases Accessed 14 Feb 2022
33. Zhang, H., et al.: A mobile health solution for chronic disease management at retail pharmacy. In: 2016 IEEE 18th International Conference on E-Health Networking, Applications and Services (Healthcom), pp. 1–5 (2016). https://doi.org/10.1109/HealthCom.2016.7749455

RescuAR: A Self-Directed Augmented Reality System for Cardiopulmonary Resuscitation Training

Hamraz Javaheri[1]([✉])(iD), Agnes Gruenerbl[1](iD), Eloise Monger[2](iD), Mary Gobbi[2](iD),
Jakob Karolus[1,3](iD), and Paul Lukowicz[1,3](iD)

[1] DFKI GmbH, Kaiserslautern, Germany
Hamraz.Javaheri@dfki.de
[2] University of Southampton, Southampton, UK
[3] University of Kaiserslautern-Landau, Kaiserslautern, Germany

Abstract. In recent years, the adoption of augmented reality (AR) technology for healthcare education has gained significant attention. Especially in life-critical situations, such as cardiopulmonary resuscitation (CPR) where sufficient medical training is essential and traditional methods are often limited due to availability constraints. We present RescuAR, a self-directed AR-based CPR training system enhancing CPR skill acquisition and retention by leveraging immersive AR experiences and real-time feedback using sensing modalities.

RescuAR was designed and implemented as a self-directed AR application based on survey findings with 11 healthcare professionals, incorporating both theory and practice phases. To evaluate the effectiveness of RescuAR, a randomized controlled user study was conducted involving $n = 43$ participants, including nurse students and laypeople. The experimental group used RescuAR for CPR training, while the control group underwent traditional teaching and training sessions. The results of the user study revealed that RescuAR significantly improved the overall effective CPR performance, surpassing the outcomes achieved through traditional teaching methods. In conclusion, RescuAR's self-directed and autonomous approach to CPR training shows promising results in improving CPR performance and has the potential to transform CPR education.

Keywords: Augmented-Reality · Cardiopulmonary Resuscitation · Self-Education

1 Introduction

Cardiopulmonary resuscitation (CPR) plays a crucial role in saving lives during cardiac arrest, a medical emergency with high mortality rates. The timely and effective administration of CPR significantly increases the chances of survival [9]. Therefore, it is vital to ensure that individuals are well-trained in this life-saving technique. Traditional CPR training methods, such as classroom-based instruction and mannequin practice, have been the cornerstone of CPR education for decades. However, these methods

D. Salvi et al. (Eds.): PH 2023, LNICST 572, pp. 166–185, 2024.
https://doi.org/10.1007/978-3-031-59717-6_12

have shown limitations in terms of skill acquisition, retention, and providing immediate feedback on performance.

One prominent challenge in traditional CPR training lies in the gap between knowledge acquisition and practical application. While learners may grasp the theoretical concepts, transferring that knowledge into effective hands-on performance can be challenging [6]. Research has shown that individuals often struggle to translate their theoretical knowledge into practical skills when faced with high-stress situations, such as cardiac arrest scenarios [22].

Furthermore, the ability to receive real-time feedback on performance during CPR training is critical for learners to correct errors, refine their technique, and build confidence. Immediate feedback allows learners to adjust their actions, ensuring the application of correct chest compression (CC) depth, rate, and recoil. However, traditional methods of CPR training often lack the means to provide instantaneous and accurate feedback, leaving learners uncertain about their proficiency and limiting their ability to improve their skills effectively.

To address these challenges and bridge the gap in CPR education, the combination of augmented reality (AR) technology with sensing modalities emerges as a promising solution. AR integrates virtual elements into the real-world environment, offering learners an immersive and interactive training experience, while sensing modalities provide an opportunity for the integration of real-time feedback. By leveraging computer vision and sensing technologies, these systems can analyze the learner's movements and provide immediate feedback on the accuracy and effectiveness of their CPR technique. This real-time feedback enables the learner to make adjustments on the spot, improving the quality and consistency of their compressions. This approach enhances skill acquisition, retention, and performance by overlaying instructional guidance and visual cues onto the learner's view of a CPR scenario [1, 10, 34].

While existing studies on AR-based CPR training have shown promise in enhancing training experiences and outcomes [3, 11, 13, 16], there is still a need for further research to fully explore the effectiveness of AR in addressing the current limitations of traditional CPR training methods. Although AR has demonstrated potential in providing immersive and interactive training environments, its specific impact on skill acquisition, retention, and performance during CPR training is an area that requires more investigation. Additionally, the design and implementation of AR-based CPR training systems can vary, and it is essential to evaluate the effectiveness of different approaches to optimize their educational value. Furthermore, understanding the potential benefits and challenges associated with incorporating AR technology into CPR training can inform the development of evidence-based guidelines and best practices for its integration.

In this paper, we introduce RescuAR, a self-directed AR-based CPR teaching and training system that addresses the gap between theoretical knowledge and practical applications in CPR education. RescuAR leverages AR technology to provide real-time feedback on performance during CPR training, enhancing the acquisition and retention of crucial CPR skills. We provide a comprehensive overview of the system, covering its pre-design stage, implementation process, and post-development evaluation. The design and implementation of RescuAR are carefully tailored to meet the specific needs of CPR education through survey findings from healthcare professionals. Furthermore, we conducted a user evaluation to assess the impact of RescuAR on learners' ability to acquire and retain essential CPR skills. Our study demonstrated the effectiveness of RescuAR in improving CC depth, frequency, and overall CPR performance, providing valuable insights into the potential of AR as a transformative tool for CPR education and skill development. The findings of this study will contribute to the growing body of research on AR-based medical training and inform the development of more effective CPR training programs that enhance learner performance, confidence, and ultimately save more lives.

2 Related Work

In recent years, several approaches have been investigated to improve the effectiveness of CPR training, ranging from traditional classroom-based instruction to advanced technological interventions, such as virtual reality simulations and AR applications [8,14,16,19,29,35].

In a recent study done by Balian *et al.* [3], the feasibility of an AR CPR training system (CPReality) for healthcare providers was tested. Their study results showed that the integration of AR into CPR training has the potential to be a valuable educational strategy that goes beyond simply translating knowledge and skills. However, their study has limitations, including inherent selection bias, a potential learning effect, a lack of baseline CPR performance assessment, and the absence of a control group for comparison. These limitations should be considered when interpreting the study's findings.

Leary *et al.* [21] focused on the limitations of Balian *et al.* work [3] and compared the use of CPRReality training with a standard audio-visual feedback manikin in terms of improvement in CPR quality. The findings of their study indicated that there was no statistically significant difference observed between the two groups. This implies that further, more extensive studies should be conducted to explore whether AR CPR training has the potential to enhance overall CPR quality for both new and re-certifying healthcare providers.

In another study done by Ingrassia *et al.* [13], an AR-based basic life support training system (Holo-BLSD) was proposed and evaluated in terms of feasibility and acceptability. While their study evaluates users' experiences and perceptions through a survey, it does not provide comprehensive evidence or direct comparisons of performance results in comparison to traditional CPR training methods. Therefore, the study may lack the empirical data needed to evaluate the effectiveness and efficacy of the Holo-BLSD system in terms of skill acquisition, retention, and performance outcomes.

In a related study, Johnson *et al.* [15] proposed the use of mixed reality (MR) to support time-critical emergencies. Their work introduced HoloCPR, an MR application that provided real-time instructions for resuscitation through a combination of visual and spatial cues. While their study demonstrated the potential of MR in decreasing reaction time and improving procedural accuracy, it primarily focused on the evaluation of these specific outcomes.

In this study, we aim to contribute to the existing body of research by addressing the limitations and building upon the findings of previous studies in the field. To this end, we provide insights into the design, implementation, and evaluation stages of an AR-based CPR training application suited for wearable AR devices. In addition, we introduce a unique and cost-effective solution for real-time measurement of compression depth, frequency, and recoil during CPR training. Moreover, our study strengthens the evidence supporting the effectiveness of AR-based CPR training by incorporating a control group and baseline performance measurements. By combining these efforts, we hope to enhance CPR training effectiveness and ultimately improve the outcomes of life-saving interventions.

3 Methodology

Upon reviewing the existing literature, we identified a gap in the research regarding the detailed exploration of the application design process for AR-based CPR training tools, as well as the limited availability of quantitative data for a comprehensive comparison between these tools and traditional CPR training methods. Motivated by these gaps in the existing literature, our study aims to fill this research void by answering the following research questions:

RQ1: What are the required design features and functionalities for an AR-based self-directed CPR teaching and training tool?

We answer this research question by conducting an extensive design survey among healthcare professionals and investigating their professional opinion on the required features and specifications for such training tool.

RQ2: Are the performance results of the designed system comparable with traditional teaching methods?

Our objective was to address this question by conducting an experimental trial where we compared the CPR performances of participants, who used the designed system to learn and practice CPR routine, with participants who underwent traditional teaching. We measured their performances before and after teaching sessions in terms of correct depth, correct frequency, and overall effective CPR (correct depth and correct frequency) to develop a better understanding of the efficiency of the designed system.

To this end, we employed a mixed-method design consisting of three consecutive steps: data collection for design requirements, system design and implementation, and system evaluation (Fig. 1).

Initially, a survey was conducted among a group of health professionals to gather valuable insights and identify the design requirements and constraints for an AR-based self-directed CPR teaching and training tool. The survey aimed to understand the preferences, needs, and expectations of professionals regarding CPR training, as well as their perceptions of the potential benefits and challenges of using such an interactive system.

Based on the insights and design requirements identified through the survey, RescuAR, an AR CPR self-training tool, was conceptualized and designed. The primary goal of RescuAR was to enable users to learn and improve their CPR performing skills by providing them with interactive features and real-time data visualization.

To assess the effectiveness of RescuAR, a user study was conducted involving nurse students and laypeople. The participants were randomly assigned to either the experimental group, which utilized RescuAR for CPR training, or the control group, which underwent traditional teaching methods. The CPR performances of participants were evaluated before and after the training sessions, specifically focusing on parameters such as compression depth and frequency. As various studies demonstrated the importance of hands-only CPR in bystanders [4,23], this study's primary objective was to evaluate participants' CPR performances specifically regarding hands-only CC and any effect related to breath technique was neglected.

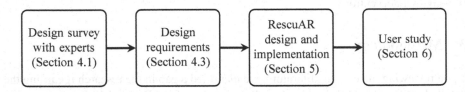

Fig. 1. The study flow process starting with the specification of design requirements based on expert survey findings and later evaluation of the designed system in a user study

4   Design Requirements for Self-directed AR-Based CPR Teaching and Training Tool

To inform the design of our interactive CPR teaching and training tool, we conducted a survey among experienced healthcare professionals. All professionals were familiarized with the AR device capabilities that will be used for the study prior to conducting the survey. The purpose of the survey was to identify the key requirements (RQ1) for developing an AR-based self-directed learning system that could effectively support CPR education. By gathering insights from these professionals, we aimed to create a tool that addresses the specific needs and challenges of learners in the context of CPR training.

4.1   Design Survey

The survey employed a combination of open-ended and multiple-choice questions. To provide a more structured approach the questions were categorized into five categories: User needs and requirements, user interface and design, instructional content, interaction and feedback, and miscellaneous.

While the questions under the user needs and requirements category focused on the participants' opinions on the features and functionalities that are considered essential for an AR-based CPR training app, the user interface and design questions focused more on the appearance and aesthetic aspects of the app.

In the instructional content section, several questions were asked to gather insights regarding the content, flow, and delivery mode of the teaching materials. Participants were asked to provide feedback on the clarity and comprehensiveness of the instructional content, as well as their preferences for the organization and sequence of the material. Additionally, participants were asked about their preferred delivery modes, such as text, images, videos, or interactive elements. Furthermore, more detailed questions focused on finding the most effective teaching methods for acquiring correct CPR skills such as correct CC depth and frequency, along with suggestions for optimization.

Under the interaction and feedback section, participants were asked to express their preferences for input methods, such as voice commands, button interactions, and gestures. Additionally, participants were asked to indicate their preferred methods of real-time feedback from app, whether visual, audio, or haptic.

Lastly, the miscellaneous section encompassed more general questions, allowing participants to share their opinions on gamification aspects of the AR-based CPR training app. Additionally, participants were given the opportunity to provide any overall suggestions or feedback they deemed relevant to the development of the app.

By capturing diverse perspectives from healthcare professionals, the survey played a crucial role in informing the design and development of an effective AR-based CPR training app.

4.2 Participants

A survey was conducted among 11 healthcare professionals. The participants' demographic characteristics, including their professional backgrounds and relevant experience, are summarized in Table 1.

Table 1. The participants' characteristic distributions

Characteristics	
Age (years), Median (IQR)	39, (32–48)
Female	2
Male	9
Non-Binary	0
Experience in healthcare (years), Median (IRQ)	20 (14–23)
Tried or Familiar with AR (yes)	6 (54%)

IQR, interquartile range; AR, augmented reality

4.3 Survey Findings

The open-ended questions in the survey were analyzed using qualitative data analysis methods to evaluate the responses and gain deeper insights into participants' perspectives. The analysis process involved systematically reviewing the open-ended responses, coding them for key themes and patterns, and organizing the data into meaningful categories. Through this approach, we were able to identify common themes, explore variations in participants' experiences and opinions, and gain a comprehensive understanding of the topics under investigation. The qualitative analysis provided valuable qualitative data that complemented the quantitative findings, allowing for a richer and more nuanced interpretation of the survey results. These results highlighted the essential design elements and interaction methods that were considered crucial for an effective CPR training application based on the professionals' expertise and daily experiences in the healthcare field.

Instructional Content, Routine, and Design Elements. The survey respondents provided valuable insights and reached a consensus on several key aspects of the CPR training application design. They emphasized the importance of incorporating a combination of audio, scripted text, and a virtual human teacher within the app to effectively deliver theoretical materials and provide personalized guidance and support. Additionally, participants strongly favored the use of animated human avatars as a demonstration tool for CC and breath techniques compared to other methods such as 2D videos of real persons performing CPR or audio instructions and verbal cues. The dynamic and interactive nature of animated avatars was perceived as more engaging and effective in conveying the correct techniques for CPR training. In terms of the teaching routine, participants suggested that it should begin with a theoretical representation of the concepts, followed by hands-on practice. They further recommended that the teaching of compression depth and frequency should be initially conducted separately before combining them in the training sessions. Lastly, participants highlighted the significance of enabling repetitive theoretical and practical sessions. They emphasized the importance of incorporating functionality to navigate through the different stages of the training. This feature would provide users with the ability to easily access previous and next steps, facilitating repetitive practice sessions. The opportunity for repetitive practice allows learners to review and reinforce their CPR skills, ultimately improving their performance and confidence.

Input and Interaction. Regarding input and interaction, the survey respondents expressed a strong preference for the integration of interaction methods through physical buttons or verbal communication via voice commands. Both methods were considered intuitive and practical for engaging with the app during training sessions. The respondents emphasized the advantages of voice commands, as they enable users to perform actions without the need for manual input, allowing them to focus on performing CPR on the manikin. This hands-free interaction was seen as a convenient and efficient way to engage with the app. On the other hand, physical buttons were identified as a suitable option for environments with high noise levels or crowded settings. Furthermore, participants expressed the belief that using virtual buttons or hand gestures for interaction would not be suitable for this task, as they would require users to have prior knowledge of how to interact with such input methods.

Methods for Frequency and Depth Acquisition. The survey respondents highlighted the crucial role of immediate and real-time feedback during hands-on training sessions for acquiring the correct frequency and depth in CPR. Among various types of feedback, the combination of audio and visual feedback emerged as the most preferred method for both frequency and depth acquisition.

In terms of frequency acquisition, healthcare professionals recommended the inclusion of audio elements to facilitate proper timing during CPR. They expressed the belief that incorporating the iconic "Stayin' Alive" sound, which aligns with the required rhythm for CPR, would enhance the training experience. However, to promote stronger muscle memory and improve precision, professionals also suggested the inclusion of a metronome sound.

For correct depth acquisition, the respondents emphasized the importance of incorporating a simple graphical visualization, similar to the devices used in traditional teaching setups to provide visual cues on the depth of CC. Participants pointed out the importance of optimizing the orientation and location of the visualization within the user's field of view to ensure clarity and accuracy during CPR training. They recommended that the depth display be positioned near the manikin's chest within the user's field of view, in a fixed position to maintain proper posture during performance. However, considering that CPR is a highly physical activity and individuals may have different preferences, participants suggested that it would be beneficial if the position of the depth display could also be adjustable by the user based on their personal preference. This customization feature would allow users to optimize their viewing experience and ensure optimal training engagement.

5   RescuAR System Design and Implementation

Based on survey findings, an AR-based system prototype was developed with the aim of creating an immersive multi-sensory CPR teaching and training tool, incorporating audio, visual, and tactile elements, to enhance the learning experience and real-time feedback to foster a comprehensive understanding of the CPR technique.

The application was designed and developed using the Unity 3D game engine [31]. Microsoft HoloLens [25] was used as a wearable AR device to run the application.

The system consisted of two main parts: RescuAR application, and a standard CPR manikin [20] covered with custom pressure sensors. The RescuAR application utilized real-time data streams from the CPR manikin to provide feedback on compression rate, depth, and recoil. A local wireless communication scheme facilitated seamless interaction between the manikin and the application, enabling accurate and immediate feedback on CPR performance.

5.1   RescuAR Application

The formulation of the CPR training app's prototype design was based on the results derived from both quantitative and qualitative data collected through the survey. According to the survey participants, a two-phase delivery of teaching material was found to be appropriate. They recognized that understanding the underlying principles and concepts of CPR is crucial in order to perform the techniques accurately and confidently. Hence the application routine was divided into two distinct phases: Theory and practice. During the initial theory phase, the application focused on imparting the fundamental principles of CPR. The subsequent practice phase emphasized hands-on practical training. The flow chart of the application routine is presented in Fig. 2.

Given that the primary objective of this study was to evaluate participants' performance specifically regarding CC, the instructions pertaining to rescue breaths were exclusively included in the theoretical section and not incorporated into the practical training. This deliberate decision allowed for a more targeted assessment of participants' proficiency in CC, aligning with the study's primary focus.

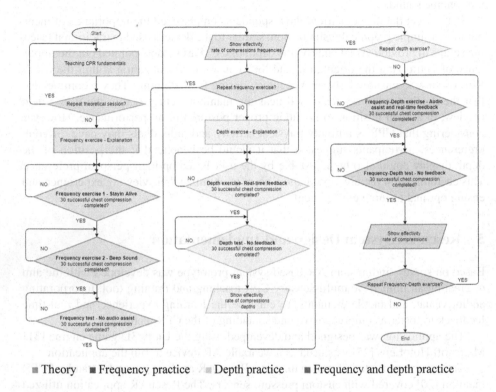

■ Theory   ■ Frequency practice   ■ Depth practice   ■ Frequency and depth practice

Fig. 2. The flowchart explaining the routine of RescuAR CPR tutorial and training application

Theory Phase. During the theoretical phase, users were introduced to the fundamentals of CPR (airway, breathing, and circulation techniques) based on European resuscitation council guidelines [26] through an engaging virtual teaching experience. A virtual teacher avatar was designed in following the survey results and served as the guide, delivering the essential CPR basics both audibly and visually. To enhance comprehension, the information was presented not only through the avatar's spoken instructions but also as easily understandable written scripts. This method was deemed to be the most suited approach for this application by survey participants. The communication between the virtual teacher and the participant was facilitated using voice commands. The virtual teacher provided the voice commands at the end of the conversation to reduce the need for memorization. For example, the virtual teacher would say, "If you

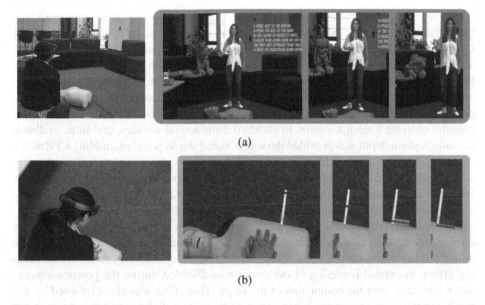

(a)

(b)

Fig. 3. Third-person and first-person (in-app) views of RescuAR application. (a) Theoretical phase. (b) Practical phase

feel like you need further practice, you can let me know at any time. Just use the word 'repeat!'"

To ensure a clear understanding of proper technique, animated 3D avatars were employed to visually demonstrate the correct posture and hand positioning during CPR (Fig. 3). By utilizing 3D virtual models and realistic placement within the room, participants were able to walk around the models and observe the CPR technique from different angles, providing a more immersive and interactive 3D training experience that cannot be achieved using 2D displays. By combining audio instruction, written scripts, and animated avatars, the theoretical phase of the training aimed to maximize participant comprehension and knowledge acquisition.

The application commenced with a calibration phase, which involved scanning the environment and room using the capabilities of the HoloLens and Mixed Reality Toolkit (MRTK) to obtain a spatial mesh of the environment. We utilized plane-finding methods to detect suitable surfaces for the placement of virtual teacher avatars and other demonstrative avatars. Colliders were added to the room mesh to create a more realistic movement area for the teacher avatar.

Practice Phase. The second phase of the application focused on practical training to cultivate the essential muscle memory required for CPR proficiency. Based on the feedback from survey participants, separate hands-on practice addressing each essential criterion of CPR was emphasized as important. As a result, two key criteria, frequency and depth, were targeted individually and then combined to ensure comprehensive learning.

To teach the correct frequency of CC, two distinct audio cues were employed. Initially, the iconic "Stayin' Alive" song, known for its rhythm matching the recommended CPR procedure (104 bpm), was utilized to encourage participants to perform CC in sync with the song's beats. Subsequently, a metronome sound with the same frequency (104 bpm) rate was introduced to enhance learner focus and synchronization.

Regarding CC depth, a trial-and-error approach was adopted to instill the appropriate technique. To align with the preferences of professionals who recognized the benefits of using a design similar to standard commercial devices, real-time feedback on compression depth was provided through a visual depth panel resembling CPRmeter devices [24]. This allowed learners to assess their performance and make adjustments accordingly (Fig. 3). The application allowed for the repositioning of the virtual depth feedback panel using the manipulation gesture of HoloLens. To address the shaking effect occurred during CPR performance, we implemented a functionality to fixate the depth feedback panel to the corner of the field of view. Participants could enable or disable this feature using a voice command. To eliminate the need and urge to look at the teacher avatar during chest compressions, which could be affected by the shaking effect, the visual rendering of the avatar was disabled during the practice session and reappeared after the completion of the stage. This effect was also explained by the teacher to the user to avoid any confusion. Additionally, a click sound reminiscent of the standard CPR dummy's internal clicker (which had been previously removed to avoid confusion) indicated the moment when the correct depth was achieved.

Upon completion of training for both frequency and depth criteria, a final session provided an opportunity for learners to combine both elements, aiming to perform CC with the correct frequency and depth in a synchronized manner. This comprehensive training approach equipped participants with the necessary skills to deliver effective CC during CPR.

5.2 CPR Manikin

To acquire information such as depth, frequency, and pressurized position of the CC on the manikin, a single FSR (Force-Sensing Resistor) was used. The sensor was attached beneath the skin layer of the CPR manikin's chest plate, precisely positioned in the center of the chest where the hands should be placed during correct CPR (Fig. 4). To facilitate seamless data acquisition and control, the pressure sensors were directly connected and managed by an Arduino Pro Mini board [2]. The analog signals generated by the embedded sensors were transformed into digital signals through the Arduino platform. Subsequently, these digital signals originating from the sensors were transmitted via a serial port to a local computer for further utilization and analysis.

To calculate the depth of chest compressions, we adopted the method proposed by Tsou et al. in their study [32]. This method utilizes Hooke's law to calculate the depth based on the pressure applied to the chest spring. We assumed the spring inside the dummy to be a linear spring due to the same diameter along its entire length. We converted the FSR readings to Newton to calculate the spring constant. Before the experiment, we measured the spring constant using the FSR force value and the spring displacement using the following formula:

$$x = \frac{F}{k}$$

Where F is the force applied to the compression spring (reading from the pressure sensor converted to Newtons, N), k is the spring constant ($\frac{N}{m}$), x is the displacement of the spring (m).

The accuracy of the employed method for calculating the depth of CC was verified against a commercial CPRmeter device [24] to ensure the validity of the measurements.

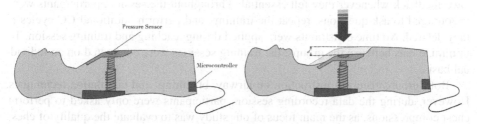

Fig. 4. Placement of Pressure sensors and controller inside the manikin. F = Applied force to the spring (N), k = spring constant ($\frac{N}{m}$), x = displacement of the spring (m)

6   User Study and System Evaluation

To evaluate the effectiveness of our designed RescuAR system, we conducted a user experiment. The study took place in two different experiment centers, Southampton University Southampton, UK, and German Research Center for Artificial Intelligence (DFKI) Kaiserslautern, Germany. The primary objective of this experiment was to assess and compare the CPR performance of participants who used the RescuAR system with those who underwent traditional CPR training methods (RQ2).

6.1   Study Design

The study utilized a randomized controlled trial design to investigate the effectiveness of different teaching methods for CPR training. Participants were randomly assigned to either the experimental or a control group.

Experimental Group. The experimental group received a self-directed CPR teaching and training session using the RescuAR system (Application and the CPR manikin). The teaching session began by calibrating the HoloLens for each individual and starting the application. Each participant completed the teaching and training session without any time limit.

Control Group. The control group underwent a traditional CPR teaching and training session, which involved classroom-based instruction and practice using the CPR manikin. The same manikin as the experimental group was used in the control group to avoid any biases. A certified teacher was recruited to provide essential information on performing CPR based on European resuscitation council guidelines [26]. The session began with a theoretical introduction to the airway, breathing, and circulation techniques, followed by a demonstration from the teacher on the correct CPR procedure using the CPR manikin. Participants were then given the opportunity to practice CPR on the same manikin under the observation of the teacher. The teacher interrupted and gave feedback whenever they felt essential. Throughout the session, participants were encouraged to ask questions, repeat the training, and perform additional CC cycles if they desired. No time constraints were applied during teaching and training session. To minimize bias between the groups, the training sessions were conducted on an individual basis.

Both groups received instruction on airway, breathing, and circulation techniques. However, during the data recording session, participants were only asked to perform chest compressions, as the main focus of our study was to evaluate the quality of chest compressions in terms of depth and frequency while neglecting the potential effects of the breath technique. No device or extra feedback method was used during data recording. The performances of participants were assessed before and after the study to measure their baseline CPR skills and the improvements achieved through the assigned teaching training method. By comparing the performance improvements between the experimental and control groups, the study aimed to evaluate the impact of RescuAR system on enhancing CPR skills.

6.2 Study Protocol

This protocol was reviewed and approved by the ethical committee of Southampton University. All of the participants were informed about being free to participate in the research and nondisclosure of personal information. They all agreed and signed written informed consent. Upon written consent, the experiment protocol was performed in five ordered stages: (1) Demographic survey, (2) baseline CPR recording (3) randomized group assignment (4) teaching and training session, and (5) post-training CPR recording. The survey collected demographic and characteristic information including age, gender, experience background in CPR, and familiarity with wearable AR devices. After completion of the survey participants were asked to perform two cycles of 1-minute hands-only CPR. Participants rested at least two minutes between each cycle. Later all participants were randomly divided into two experimental groups to receive teaching and training session. After the teaching session participants rested at least for 10 min to avoid the effect of tiredness on their performance. Later they performed another two cycles of 1-minute hands-only CPR (without usage of any feedback device or extra help) with at least two minutes rest between each cycle. As various studies demonstrated the importance of hands-only CPR in bystanders [4,23] this study only focused on the evaluation of hands-only CPR performance, and any effect regarding performing rescue breath was neglected.

6.3 Participants

Total of 44 persons volunteered to participate in this study. Among those, 43 persons' data were included and one person's data were excluded from the study due to data corruption. After exclusion, the experimental group consisted of 22 volunteer participants and the control group contained 21 participants. The participants were nurse students and laypeople who were randomly assigned to study groups. The nurse students were recruited by Southampton University and laypeople were recruited by DFKI. All participants were required to be aged above 18. Characteristics of participants are presented in Table 2.

Table 2. The participants' characteristic distributions

Characteristics	Control	Experimental
Age (years), Median (IQR)	22, (20–24)	21, (19–24)
Female	5 (23%)	9 (41%)
Male	16 (77%)	13 (59%)
Non-binary	0 (0%)	0 (0%)
Nurse Student	9 (43%)	9 (41%)
Laypeople	12 (57%)	13 (59%)
With prior knowledge	8 (38%)	11 (50%)
Tried or Familiar with AR (yes)	2 (9%)	1(4%)

IQR, interquartile range; AR, augmented reality; With prior knowledge, who is CPR certified and/or completed a first aid course

6.4 Data Collection and Analysis

Over two 1-minute cycles, two CC measurements were recorded before and after the teaching session using the same sensor-equipped CPR manikin described in Sect. 5.2 with a sampling rate of 100 Hz. The effective CPR performances of the participants were analyzed according to the latest evidence-based guidelines for resuscitation officially published by European Resuscitation Council [28]. These guidelines suggest an effective CPR as follows:

- CC in a frequency of at least 100/min but not exceeding 120/min.
- CC with a depth of at least 5 cm but not exceeding 6 cm

In this study, the percentage of effective CPR performance of a participant was calculated based on the percentage of the time that the participants complied with all the above-mentioned guidelines at the same time while doing CPR.

Statistical analysis was performed using IBM SPSS Statistics for Windows, Version 22.0 [7]. Numerical data were presented as means ± standard deviations. To compare the improvement in two groups before and after teaching sessions, Paired t-test was used. To compare the outcomes between two study groups, Chi-square test (for categorical data) and Student's t-test (for numerical data) were used. A two-sided p-value less than 0.05 was considered significant in all analyses.

6.5 Results

RescuAR Evaluation. The participants in the experimental group showed significant improvements in performing correct depth and frequency. While the calculated p-value for CC depth improvement was 0.003, the p-value for frequency improvement was below 0.0001. A comparison between both criteria before the experiment session showed that more participants had issues finding the correct frequency (39.8% ± 36.9% correct frequency) than the correct depth (58.7% ± 39.8% correct depth). Even though for most of the participants, both depth and frequency were improved after the tutorial and training session, the frequency improvement rate was higher (73.8% ± 28.2%) than the improvement rate in CC depth (84.3% ± 23.2%).

Moreover, the results showed that the overall effective CPR performance of the experimental group significantly increased ($p < 0.0001$) after teaching session with RescuAR. While the mean of participants' performance was 23.3% ± 27.2% before the teaching session, it was improved to 61.3% ± 27.4% after training with the proposed system.

Experimental Group vs. Control Group. The study analysis showed no significant difference regarding characteristics distribution between the two groups concerning sex ($p = 0.332$) and knowledge backgrounds ($p = 0.543$) of the participants. Based on the findings, RescuAR helped to achieve higher effective CPR rates compared to traditional teaching. Analyzing the final performances of both groups' participants, it was observed that, even though both groups had no significant difference in doing effective CPR before the teaching session (control = 20.3% ± 25.4%, experimental = 23.3% ± 27.2%, $p = 0.594$), the experimental group performed significantly better than the control group after the teaching session (control = 40.4% ± 28.5, experimental = 61.3% ± 27.4%, $p = 0.019$) (Fig. 5).

Moreover, performance degradation only occurred in some of the control group's participants, and all participants in the experimental group showed improvement after the teaching session (Fig. 6).

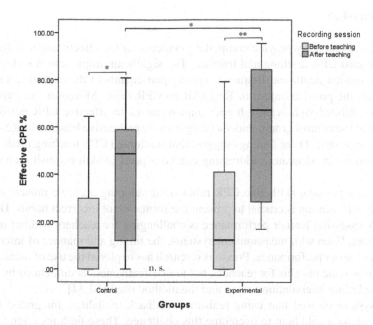

Fig. 5. The figure demonstrated the statistical analysis of control and experimental groups - n.s. = no significant difference between indicated groups ($p < 0.05$) * = Significant difference between indicated groups ($p < 0.05$), ** = Significant difference between indicated groups ($p < 0.01$)

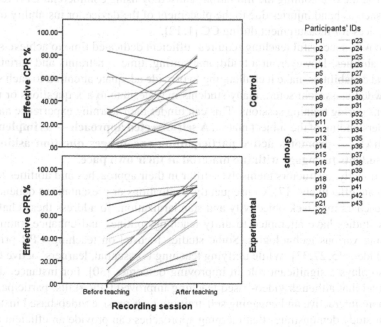

Fig. 6. Participant's performance lines before and after teaching sessions

7 Discussion

The results of our study provide compelling evidence of the effectiveness of RescuAR in self-directed CPR teaching and training. The significant improvements observed in both compression depth and frequency among participants in the experimental group demonstrate the positive impact of RescuAR on CPR skills. Moreover, the experimental group exhibited significantly higher improvements in effective CPR performance compared to the control group, underscoring the comprehensive benefits of RescuAR's AR-based approach. These findings suggest that traditional CPR teaching methods may have limitations in adequately addressing crucial aspects of skill acquisition and retention.

Acquiring physical skills like CPR relies on developing accurate muscle memory, and timely intervention is crucial to prevent the formation of incorrect habits. However, accurately assessing learner performance is challenging for teachers without measurement devices. Even with measurement systems, the timing and manner of intervention can impact learner performance. Previous research has explored the use of measurement systems to provide insights for teachers, but their effectiveness is influenced by various factors, including intervention timing and the method used [10,34].

Our system showed that using real-time feedback modalities integrated into the teaching routine could help to overcome this challenge. These findings align with previous research highlighting the benefits of audio-visual feedback in CPR education [10,18]. Furthermore, our approach for real-time detection and visualization of CC depth and frequency helped to seamlessly integrated the real-time feedback into the training routine overcoming the limitations caused by using commercial CPR feedback devices such as hand injuries due to the placement of the device, or instability of using smart devices for measurement during CC [1,12].

Moreover, successful teaching requires sufficient dedicated time to achieve specific skills or abilities. However, in a traditional setting, time constraints and variations in individual capabilities make it challenging to provide adequate attention to each student. In a crowded classroom setup, many students may hesitate to ask questions or request repetitions during training sessions. This can hinder their learning experience and limit their understanding of the subject matter. **A self-directed approach — as implemented in RescuAR — promotes active participation, encourages question asking, and allows students to engage with the material at their own pace**.

Additionally, instructors themselves differ in their approaches and abilities to teach and evaluate effectively [17]. Consequently, evaluations or presentations dependent on human teachers may lack objectivity and standardization. To address these challenges, previous studies have attempted to unify teaching routines and enhance training sessions using various technologies. Some studies focused on teaching CPR principles through videos [5,27,33]. While unifying teaching is essential, learners' active engagement also plays a significant role in improving outcomes [30]. For instance, de Sena *et al.* found that although video-based teaching improved CPR skills, participants preferred more interactive and engaging self-training over passive video-based instruction [30]. Our study demonstrates that merging approaches can provide an efficient alternative for CPR education. **By utilizing a virtual teacher with programmed curricula,** we standardized teaching routines without diminishing learners' interest, promoting verbal communication between teacher and student.

In line with the findings of Balian *et al.* [3], our study further substantiates the potential of AR in CPR training. By incorporating a control group and measuring baseline performance, we provide additional evidence to support the effectiveness of AR for CPR training. This strengthens the understanding of the benefits and possibilities that AR technology offers in enhancing CPR education through various designs and implementations.

Although Leary [21] did not find a statistically significant difference between CPRReality training and a standard audio-visual feedback manikin, our study demonstrates significant improvements in CPR performance within the experimental group, suggesting the advantages of our AR-based approach in enhancing CPR quality compared to traditional methods.

7.1 Limitations

While our system design and study results provide valuable insights, it is essential to acknowledge its limitations. Certain technical issues, such as loss of environment mapping, occasional teacher avatar misplacement, and limited field of view, were identified during the experiment indicating the need for further optimization. Additionally, the study's controlled environment and participants' awareness of evaluation may have influenced their performance, necessitating further validation of the app's real-world applicability in diverse settings with participants unaware of being evaluated. Furthermore, further research is needed to assess the long-term durability and retention of the improved CPR performance observed in our study. Lastly, our study primarily focused on compression depth and frequency as key performance indicators, future studies could consider incorporating a more comprehensive assessment, including other critical elements such as hand placement, posture, and breath technique.

8 Conclusion

In conclusion, our study provides compelling evidence of the effectiveness of RescuAR, an AR-based CPR teaching and training app, in improving compression depth, frequency, and overall CPR performance. The insights gained from our study inform the development of guidelines and best practices for incorporating AR technology in CPR training programs. Policymakers, educators, and healthcare professionals can use this information to establish standards and recommendations for the implementation and utilization of AR-based training tools. This includes considerations such as the design of instructional content and feedback mechanisms, and the integration of AR training into existing curriculum frameworks. While this study primarily focused on the fundamental teaching of CPR, our future work will delve into exploring the integration of more realistic and immersive simulation scenarios. By incorporating advanced training systems, we aim to investigate ways of providing learners with a comprehensive and realistic training experience that prepares them for a wider range of CPR situations and challenges. By doing so we aim to contribute to expanding the field of research on medical training and inform the development of more effective CPR training programs that enhance learner performance, confidence, and ultimately save more lives.

Acknowledgement. This research was supported by HumanE-AI-Net.

References

1. An, M., Kim, Y., Cho, W.K.: Effect of smart devices on the quality of CPR training: a systematic review. Resuscitation **144**, 145–156 (2019)
2. Arduino: Arduino pro mini (2018). https://www.arduino.cc/
3. Balian, S., McGovern, S.K., Abella, B.S., Blewer, A.L., Leary, M.: Feasibility of an augmented reality cardiopulmonary resuscitation training system for health care providers. Heliyon **5**(8), e02205 (2019)
4. Berg, R.A., et al.: Assisted ventilation does not improve outcome in a porcine model of single-rescuer bystander cardiopulmonary resuscitation. Circulation **95**(6), 1635–1641 (1997)
5. Braslow, A., Brennan, R.T., Newman, M.M., Bircher, N.G., Batcheller, A.M., Kaye, W.: CPR training without an instructor: development and evaluation of a video self-instructional system for effective performance of cardiopulmonary resuscitation. Resuscitation **34**(3), 207–220 (1997)
6. Brown, T.B., et al.: Relationship between knowledge of cardiopulmonary resuscitation guidelines and performance. Resuscitation **69**(2), 253–261 (2006)
7. Corp., I.: IBM SPSS statistics for windows (version 22.0) (2017). https://www.ibm.com/products/spss-statistics
8. Everson, T., Joordens, M., Forbes, H., Horan, B.: Virtual reality and haptic cardiopulmonary resuscitation training approaches: a review. IEEE Syst. J. (2021)
9. Greif, R., et al.: European resuscitation council guidelines 2021: education for resuscitation. Resuscitation **161**, 388–407 (2021)
10. Gruber, J., Stumpf, D., Zapletal, B., Neuhold, S., Fischer, H.: Real-time feedback systems in CPR. Trends Anaesthesia Crit. Care **2**(6), 287–294 (2012)
11. Higashi, E., Fukagawa, K., Kasimura, R., Kanamori, Y., Minazuki, A., Hayashi, H.: Development and evaluation of a corrective feedback system using augmented reality for the high-quality cardiopulmonary resuscitation training. In: 2017 IEEE International Conference on Systems, Man, and Cybernetics (SMC), pp. 716–721. IEEE (2017)
12. Hong, J.Y., Oh, J.H., Kim, C.W., Lee, D.H.: Hand injuries caused by feedback device usage during cardiopulmonary resuscitation training. Resuscitation **107**, e3–e4 (2016)
13. Ingrassia, P.L., et al.: Augmented reality learning environment for basic life support and defibrillation training: usability study. J. Med. Internet Res. **22**(5), e14910 (2020)
14. Issleib, M., Kromer, A., Pinnschmidt, H.O., Süss-Havemann, C., Kubitz, J.C.: Virtual reality as a teaching method for resuscitation training in undergraduate first year medical students: a randomized controlled trial. Scandinavian J. Trauma, Resuscitation Emerg. Med. **29**(1), 1–9 (2021)
15. Johnson, J.G., Rodrigues, D.G., Gubbala, M., Weibel, N.: HoloCPR: designing and evaluating a mixed reality interface for time-critical emergencies. In: Proceedings of the 12th EAI International Conference on Pervasive Computing Technologies for Healthcare, pp. 67–76 (2018)
16. Jung, C., et al.: Virtual and augmented reality in cardiovascular care: state-of-the-art and future perspectives. Cardiovascular Imaging **15**(3), 519–532 (2022)

17. Kaye, W., et al.: The problem of poor retention of cardiopulmonary resuscitation skills may lie with the instructor, not the learner or the curriculum. Resuscitation **21**(1), 67–87 (1991)

18. Kirkbright, S., Finn, J., Tohira, H., Bremner, A., Jacobs, I., Celenza, A.: Audiovisual feedback device use by health care professionals during CPR: a systematic review and meta-analysis of randomised and non-randomised trials. Resuscitation **85**(4), 460–471 (2014)

19. Kuyt, K., Park, S.H., Chang, T.P., Jung, T., MacKinnon, R.: The use of virtual reality and augmented reality to enhance cardio-pulmonary resuscitation: a scoping review. Adv. Simul. **6**(1), 1–8 (2021)

20. Laerdal: Little Anne CPR dummy. Official page (2018). https://www.laerdal.com/de/

21. Leary, M., McGovern, S.K., Balian, S., Abella, B.S., Blewer, A.L.: A pilot study of CPR quality comparing an augmented reality application vs. a standard audio-visual feedback manikin. Front. Digital Health **2**, 1 (2020)

22. LeBlanc, V.R.: The effects of acute stress on performance: implications for health professions education. Acad. Med. **84**(10), S25–S33 (2009)

23. Leong, B.: Bystander CPR and survival. Singapore Med. J. **52**(8), 573 (2011)

24. Medical, L.: CPRmeter 2 (2023). https://laerdal.com/de/products/medical-devices/cpr-feedback-devices/cprmeter-2/

25. Microsoft: Hololens. Official page (2018). https://www.microsoft.com/en-us/hololens

26. Olasveengen, T.M., et al.: European resuscitation council guidelines 2021: basic life support. Resuscitation **161**, 98–114 (2021)

27. Paglino, M., et al.: A video-based training to effectively teach CPR with long-term retention: the scuolasalvavita. it ("schoolsaveslives. it") project. Internal Emerg. Med. **14**(2), 275–279 (2019)

28. Perkins, G.D., et al.: European resuscitation council guidelines 2021: executive summary. Resuscitation **161**, 1–60 (2021)

29. Ricci, S., Calandrino, A., Borgonovo, G., Chirico, M., Casadio, M.: Virtual and augmented reality in basic and advanced life support training. JMIR Serious Games **10**(1), e28595 (2022)

30. de Sena, D.P., Fabrício, D.D., da Silva, V.D., Bodanese, L.C., Franco, A.R.: Comparative evaluation of video-based on-line course versus serious game for training medical students in cardiopulmonary resuscitation: a randomised trial. PLoS ONE **14**(4), e0214722 (2019)

31. Technologies, U.: Unity 3D game engine (version 2018.4.36f1) (2018). http://www.unity.com

32. Tsou, J.Y., Kao, C.L., Hong, M.Y., Chang, C.J., Su, F.C., Chi, C.H.: How does the side of approach impact the force delivered during external chest compression? Am. J. Emerg. Med. **48**, 67–72 (2021)

33. Wanner, G.K., Osborne, A., Greene, C.H.: Brief compression-only cardiopulmonary resuscitation training video and simulation with homemade mannequin improves CPR skills. BMC Emerg. Med. **16**(1), 1–6 (2016)

34. Yeung, J., Meeks, R., Edelson, D., Gao, F., Soar, J., Perkins, G.D.: The use of CPR feedback/prompt devices during training and CPR performance: a systematic review. Resuscitation **80**(7), 743–751 (2009)

35. Yigitbas, E., Krois, S., Renzelmann, T., Engels, G.: Comparative evaluation of AR-based, VR-based, and traditional basic life support training. In: 2022 IEEE 10th International Conference on Serious Games and Applications for Health (SeGAH), pp. 1–8. IEEE (2022)

Towards Augmenting Mental Health Personnel with LLM Technology to Provide More Personalized and Measurable Treatment Goals for Patients with Severe Mental Illnesses

Lorenzo J. James[1,2]([✉]), Maureen Maessen[1], Laura Genga[1],
Barbara Montagne[2], Muriel A. Hagenaars[3], and Pieter M. E. Van Gorp[1]

[1] Industrial Engineering and Information Systems, Eindhoven University
of Technology, Eindhoven, The Netherlands
l.j.james@tue.com
[2] Treatment Center for Personality Disorders, GGZ Centraal, Center for Mental
Health Care, Disorders, Amersfoort, The Netherlands
[3] Department of Clinical Psychology, Universiteit Utrecht, Utrecht, The Netherlands

Abstract. Mobile health (mHealth) tools are increasingly being used in various mental health domains to monitor patients with Severe Mental Illnesses (SMI), with the aim of potentially increasing patient engagement with their treatment. Patients with SMI who are prescribed Flexible Assertive Community Treatment (FACT) create a treatment plan together with their case manager, which serves as the leading document describing the goals that will be worked on during treatment. In order to incorporate the treatment plan goals of a patient in an mHealth application, the treatment plan goals need to be measurable. However, in previous work, we discovered that on average, only 25% of the available treatment plans include measurable goals. We have developed a protocol for making measurable goals with patients with SMI to address this issue. However, we anticipate low adoption of the protocol due to the potentially time-consuming nature of the steps involved. To mitigate this, we are exploring the use of AI to generate measurable treatment plan goals for patients with SMI and introduce a new workflow. In our exploratory study, we created a prototype of a system that may enable case managers and patients with SMI to generate measurable treatment plan goals using Large Language Models.

Keywords: SMI · mHealth · LLM · Gamification · Goals

1 Introduction

The impact of mental health is a growing concern for individuals and communities in our present-day society. Severe mental illnesses such as bipolar disorder,

D. Salvi et al. (Eds.): PH 2023, LNICST 572, pp. 186–200, 2024.
https://doi.org/10.1007/978-3-031-59717-6_13

PTSD, schizophrenia, and severe depression pose unique challenges for both patients and mental healthcare providers [19]. One such challenge is mental health professionals' need to dynamically scale the care for each patient diagnosed with Severe Mental Illnesses (SMI) depending on the current state of the patient. Among people with ill mental health, those diagnosed with one or more severe mental illnesses for a period of over two years, and who struggle socially from their mental illnesses, are considered patients with SMI [24]. In the last few decades, there has been a growth in the number of patients with SMI treated by mental health care institutes, increasing the workload and work pressure of healthcare professionals [11]. Many patients with SMI live independently at home or in assisted living facilities without direct help from friends or family. Due to the associated vulnerabilities experienced by patients with SMI, there is a need for long-term treatment, with the ability to scale the care to the needs of the patient. Flexible Assertive Community Treatment (FACT) is a type of treatment for patients with SMI, that treats patients within their own home environment and provides care that matches their current needs [24]. Several countries have opted to prescribe FACT to patients with SMI, in an attempt to treat patients within their home environment [22]. A case manager is a healthcare professional who is directly responsible for monitoring the effects of the treatment. During FACT treatment, patients work together with their case manager to create a treatment plan, which includes the treatment plan goals that they will work on over a one-year period [24]. The goals of the treatment plan not only target symptom recovery but also seek to empower patients, enhance their self-reliance, and provide support in addressing social issues such as employment and housing. The goals serve as guiding principles of the treatment, ensuring that the care provided to patients is in accordance with their own goals, focusing on a person-oriented and holistic approach [24].

Currently, case managers assess the functioning of their patients through direct contact with the patients or their surroundings (e.g., family, general practitioner, etc.). Outside of direct contact, case managers do not have any tools to monitor the state of their patients, which results in them not being able to assess when to scale care for patients efficiently. Previous research shows that mobile Health (mHealth) applications are promising when it comes to positively influencing and tracking the behaviors of patients with SMI [13]. Such an mHealth application could potentially also improve FACT by assisting case managers in assessing their patients' functioning and monitoring the progress that a patient is making on their treatment [13]. This could potentially be a support tool to help case managers efficiently assess when to scale care for patients.

In order to monitor patients with SMI who are prescribed FACT, an mHealth application should track the progress a patient is making on their treatment plan goals. However, in previous research in collaboration with FACT teams at a Dutch Mental Health and Addiction Care Institute, we have discovered that on average only 25% of the available treatment plans have a form of measurable goals available within them [14]. A well-defined Measurable goal is a goal that can be tracked to monitor progress [3]. The treatment plan goals were revealed to have a significant lack of structure, consistency, and difference in level of detail.

This results in the majority of the goals currently found in the treatment plans not being suitable to be used in mHealth applications [14].

To assist case managers with making measurable treatment plan goals that can be used in mHealth applications, we introduced a protocol for a structured approach to creating measurable treatment plan goals for patients with SMI. Despite case managers being positive about the protocol, due to its time-consuming nature, it will have a low adoption rate. Given the high workload of case managers, they are not always open to new time-consuming tasks. Following all the steps in the protocol is a more time-consuming process for the case manager, compared to their usual goal-setting and tracking workflow. To reduce the time case managers would spend following the protocol when creating and tracking measurable goals, we will explore ways to leverage AI to potentially automate a part of the workflow.

The recent breakthroughs of Large Language Models (LLMs), such as BERT, GPT-3, and GPT-4 have been disruptive. These LLMs have been trained on large data sets and the models available have produced impressive results when prompted by humans. When prompted correctly, these models have the ability to respond to specific queries given to them when provided a specific context [2]. Due to this technology's ability to generate relevant text responses when given a context, we will explore the potential use of LLMs to introduce a new workflow for case managers to create treatment plan goals with their patients.

This study will aim to create a prototype that explores using LLMs to create AI-generated treatment plan goals, potentially improving the workflow of creating treatment plan goals with patients. Evaluating the prototype is outside the scope of this project. Nevertheless, we will assess the goals generated by the prototype to evaluate whether the quality of generated goals can be improved through modifications to the prototype and the prompts sent to the LLM.

2   Theoretical Background

To establish how to create measurable goals, in this section, we will review relevant work in the areas of behavior change, the use of AI in mental healthcare, and the possible risks of generating goals for patients with SMI using LLMs.

2.1   Behavior Change Theories

According to behavior change theories such as the COM-B system and the Fogg behavior model, behavior is a product of three fundamental factors: capability, opportunity, and motivation [8,18]. To successfully perform a targeted behavior at a particular time, it is essential to have the capability and opportunity, including an enabling environment. The strength of motivation to engage in the behavior must be higher than any other competing behaviors. These three factors interact to produce the desired behavior [20]. Motivation can be split into intrinsic and extrinsic motivation. Where extrinsic motivation is being motivated by external factors, intrinsic motivation is motivated by an inherent interest which leads to more persistence [20].

According to the Self-Determination Theory (SDT), in the context of an mHealth tool, a tool that satisfies the need for autonomy (i.e., the desire to have control over tasks), competence (i.e., the need to acquire new skills), and relatedness (i.e., the desire to feel connected to others) can enhance intrinsic motivation [15,20]. The proposed workflow of using LLMs to generate treatment plan goals can potentially enhance the patient's intrinsic motivation, which in turn can lead to better engagement with the treatment goals. Finally, the Goal Setting Theory states that specific, challenging goals and appropriate feedback contribute to higher and better results. For engaging a person in a target behavior, goals must follow five principles: clarity, challenge, commitment, feedback, and task complexity [17]. Clear goals are Specific, Measurable, Attainable, Realistic, and Time-oriented (SMART) [4]. We will be using the SDT and Goal Setting Theory as criteria for evaluating the quality of the goals that are generated by LLMs. The generated goals will also be structured in the format of SMART goals, to the extent that we can accomplish this.

Treatment outcome goals focus on a result (e.g., losing 2 kg of weight), while treatment behavioral goals focus on an individual's action (e.g., going for a walk) [18]. For this study, we consider outcome goals as overall treatment plan goals, and behavior goals as smaller goals patients should achieve to reach their desired outcome goals. In order to track the progress toward the treatment goals, the behavior goals need to be measurable (e.g., I will go for a walk twice a week throughout the month of September). Integrating behavioral goals in mHealth interventions could potentially lead to more successful interventions [7]. An additional useful tool to motivate users in mHealth interventions is Gamification, which is the use of game design elements in non-game contexts [5].

2.2 AI in Mental Healthcare

While there has been a growing trend toward integrating AI technology in physical health applications, adopting such technology within the mental health domain has been comparatively slow [10]. Mental health practitioners emphasize patient-centered care and a hands-on approach in their clinical practice in contrast to non-psychiatric practitioners. This approach involves softer skills, including establishing strong relationships with patients and closely observing their behaviors and emotions [9]. Mental health clinical data is frequently in qualitative and subjective patient statements and written notes. Because of this, there is still much to be gained in the field of mental health practice through the incorporation of AI technology [10]. The application of AI techniques could present the opportunity to develop more accurate pre-diagnosis screening tools and risk models to determine an individual's susceptibility or likelihood of developing a mental illness [21]. AI-based LLMs have already showcased their efficacy in diverse areas, such as explainable AI, conversational agents, education, information retrieval, and text summarizing [6]. With their remarkable capabilities, LLMs can potentially transform various industries [10]. Research on LLM technology for mental health has yielded mixed results, and the enduring effects of using LLM on mental health remain unexplored [12]. The potential of LLMs in healthcare stems from the ability to process and learn from massive amounts of free-text data. In theory, LLMs could generate measurable treatment goals based on data available on the web. Currently, much of the responsibility of creating treatment plan goals falls under the workload of the case manager [24]. In previous work, we created measurable goals for patients with SMI together with case managers [14]. Even when provided with a protocol for creating measurable goals, case managers found creating measurable goals for their patients a time-consuming and difficult task. Generating measurable goals using LLMs, could potentially alleviate some of the workload from case managers to patients, as it could empower patients to easily formulate measurable goals for their treatment. To the best of our knowledge, no literature is available that discusses the use of LLMs to generate treatment goals for patients with SMI.

The recent LLMs that have been released for public use usually strictly abide by the relevant laws and regulations of the countries in which they are released [16]. The LLMs usually do not mention anything offensive, violent or criminal in their conversations, and do not give any unethical medical advice. However, it is known that LLMs are known to hallucinate [1]. Hallucinations in the context of LLMs are when the system generates information not found in its training set [1]. This could potentially cause the generated goals to contain harmful elements. It is important to note that case managers are responsible for ensuring the safety of the goals within the patient's treatment plan. If patients are allowed to generate treatment plan goals unchecked using LLM technology there could be potential risks associated with that. Therefore it is recommended for both patients and case managers to assess the generated plan goals before adding them to the treatment plan.

Currently, electronic treatment records are utilized by mental health institutes to keep records of patients, including their treatment goals. However, these systems lack the inclusion of measurable goals. In our prototype, we explore features that can possibly add measurable goals to these systems.

3   Methods

To explore the feasibility of using LLMs to generate treatment plan goals for patients with SMI, a prototype of such a system was built. The functioning prototype was built using the GPT-3 LLM, the prototyping tool Mendix, and the gamification engine Gamebus. The architecture of the system can be seen in Fig. 1. The goals generated by the prototype were then evaluated using behavior change theory guidelines by a group of students. To evaluate a prototype with patients with SMI, a prerequisite entails securing the approval of the study by at least three ethical committees. In addition to obtaining ethical approval from the university, the mental health institute mandates an external committee to ascertain whether the study qualifies as medical-scientific research before conducting its own ethical review. Considering that the study is in the exploratory phase, evaluating the basic capabilities of LLMs and prompt engineering strategies to evaluate if generated goals could possibly be improved upon, it was deemed

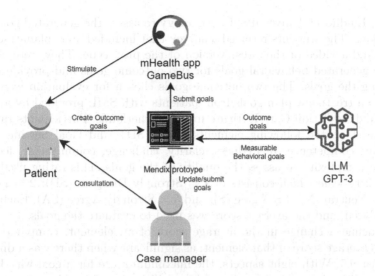

Fig. 1. The architecture of the prototype.

appropriate to first evaluate the goals with students before entering the ethical procedures. Once the basic capabilities have been established we will again involve patients and case managers in the process.

3.1 Prototype

Mendix. Mendix is a low-code development platform that was chosen to develop the prototype of the new goal-setting workflow, because of its ease of use built-in capabilities with REST API architectures, and ability to facilitate rapid prototype development. GPT-3 was accessed using the available API. The responses were formatted and directly implemented in both Mendix and the GameBus system. As the new workflow is being constructed, specific milestones were identified for evaluating the goals. For this purpose, behavior change theories were utilized. While three main theories were outlined in the theoretical background, in the scope of this study we focus on SDT and goal-setting theory.

GameBus. GameBus is a digital platform that promotes a healthy lifestyle by hosting and facilitating healthy challenges and competitions. Users are motivated to continue working on the challenges available to them through the use of gamification elements such as leaderboards and points [23]. For this study, we configured the GameBus platform as an mHealth application. The GameBus application can use measurable goals as input for challenges.

3.2 Measurable Goals

To assess if it is possible to improve the quality of the measurable goals that GPT-3 generates, by prompt engineering. We recruited a group of 8 students from the Eindhoven University of Technology to assess the generated goals, over 5 iterations. The students received a survey that included an explanation of the project and a video of the latest version of the prototype. They were asked to rate the generated behavioral goals for two outcome goals and provide tips for improving the goals. The two outcome goals chosen for evaluation were based on data on treatment plan goals from patients with SMI, provided by a Mental Health and Addiction Care Institute in the Netherlands. Participants rated the goals based on the following elements of the SDT and Goal Setting theory: autonomy, competence, relatedness, clarity, challenge, commitment, feedback, and task complexity to assess the quality of the goals. This rating used a five-point Likert scale which consists of 1 = Strongly Disagree (SD); 2 = Disagree (D); 3 = Neutral (N); 4 = Agree (S); and 5 = Strongly Agree (SA). Each aspect was analyzed, and the average score was used to evaluate the goals.

We define a change in the average score of an element, compared to the previous average score of that element, as significant when there was a difference of at least 0.5. With eight aspects, the maximum score for a goal was 35. This approach allowed participants to provide specific ratings for each aspect, ensuring an assessment of their perceptions. By implementing the dimensions within the goal-setting theory and SDT frameworks into the goals, we increase the potential intrinsic motivation a person has to complete the goals. The group of students was also given a plain text field to provide feedback.

The information gathered, along with the provided feedback, guides the areas for improvement. The prompt in the prototype was revised according to the chosen improvements. Once these changes were implemented, the group was requested to complete the updated survey again. This iterative process aims to use prompt engineering to refine the goals based on participant feedback. By incorporating this, the prompt sent to GPT-3 can be improved and the quality of the generated behavioral goals can potentially be increased.

4   Results

4.1   Prototype

Mendix. The created Mendix prototype allows users to log in as patients or case managers. Patients can create, edit, and delete treatment outcome goals. For each treatment goal, the system generates 3 behavioral goals using GPT-3's API. Patient information and goal format instructions are included in the prompt sent to GPT-3. GPT-3's response is mapped and stored in the data model created in Mendix, and the goals are assigned to the patient. Patients can view and modify their behavioral goals. They can also remove or regenerate specific behavioral goals. After finalizing their treatment outcome goals, patients submit them to their case manager for approval before adding them to the treatment plan in the Mendix prototype. Patients have an overview page displaying all their approved and non-approved treatment outcome goals along with associated behavioral goals, each with a step-by-step guide. Case managers can also generate, edit, and remove goals for their assigned patients. Case managers are able to see all the submitted goal requests, requests for goal changes, and goal edit requests by their patients. Case managers can also accept or reject these requests, save the treatment plan in the Mendix prototype, and ultimately submit the treatment plan to the GameBus application.

GameBus. The GameBus application has been extended to receive the treatment plan goals of the Mendix prototype, through the API. The Mendix prototype sends an API request to the GameBus application, sending a patient's approved treatment plans to the GameBus application in JSON format. The GameBus application converts the treatment plan it receives into GameBus challenges and saves the treatment outcome and behavioral goals within the treatment plan, in the GameBus data model. The patients using the Mendix prototype to create the treatment plan goals, also have access to the mHealth configuration of the GameBus application. The GameBus mHealth application supports multiple modular gamification and personalization options that have been designed to increase the intrinsic motivation of GameBus users. GameBus can personalize the challenges of users by tailoring the elements within them such as adjusting the frequency of the tasks needed to be completed within the challenge, adjusting the time and date a challenge should be completed or tracked, and allowing challenges to be done in groups. The GameBus application can be configured to use gamification such as giving points to users when they complete tasks within challenges, displaying a leaderboard displaying user scores, and awarding users loot boxes. The system administrator of the GameBus application can easily configure these personalization and gamification elements to be visible to any of the GameBus users. Each of the patient accounts in the Mendix prototype has a GameBus account assigned and can log into the GameBus application. Due to the challenges in the GameBus application now deriving directly from the treatment plan of the patients the challenges present in the application are even more relevant to the patient's treatment.

We extended the GameBus application to include the gamification element of levels. The relevant Mendix treatment plan goals of the patients are mapped into a level structure where each outcome goal is separated into different levels with increasing difficulty. The levels can be unlocked by completing the relevant behavior goals associated with the outcome goal. This level extension showcases the potential for patients to be more engaged with their treatment through this mHealth application, as the gamification and personalization elements are designed to maximize intrinsic motivation to the challenges in the application. The GameBus application also makes it possible to monitor which challenges each user is taking part in and track the progress users made on each of their challenges. Case managers can use this data to track which challenges their patients are making progress on, when their patients work on tasks within their challenges, and when patients have completed their challenges. The data could then potentially be used as a proxy for user engagement with their treatment.

4.2 Evaluating Generated Measurable Goals

The group of 8 students that was enlisted to fill in the 5 rounds of surveys to assess the behavioral goals rated the LLM-generated behavioral goals formulated for the following two outcome goals: 1) I want to learn how to deal with negative thoughts about events that have happened in the past. 2) I want to learn to discuss my fears, but I especially want to understand my fears.

In the following section, we describe the results of each evaluation phase and the overall changes that were made to the prompts and goals based on the results of the previous phase. An overview of the survey results can be seen in Table 1.

Table 1. Displays the average scores assigned by the participants to goals 1 (G1) and 2 (G2) based on how the goals scored on the elements of the SDT and Goal Setting Theory. Scores for evaluation phases 1–3 and 5 are presented, including total and combined average scores (AS) for both goals in each phase.

Evaluation phase	1			2			3			5		
	G1	G2	AS	G1	G2	AS	G1	G2	AS	G1	G2	AS
Autonomy	4.125	4	4.063	3.625	3.125	3.375	3.375	3.25	3.313	4	4.125	4.063
Competence	3.375	3.625	3.5	4.5	3.75	4.125	3.75	3.625	3.688	4.25	4.25	4.25
Relatedness	1.875	4.5	3.188	1.5	4.5	4	3.375	3.25	3.313	4	3.875	3.938
Clarity	3.625	4.125	3.875	4.5	3.75	4.125	3.375	3.875	3.625	4.625	4.5	4.563
Challenge	3.875	3.875	3.875	3.25	4.125	3.688	4.25	4.25	4.25	4.5	4.25	4.375
Commitment	3.75	3.5	3.625	4.25	3.5	3.875	4	3.125	3.563	4	4	4
Feedback	1.75	3.875	2.813	2	3.375	2.688	2.625	3.25	2.938	3.625	3.75	3.688
Task complexity	3.375	3.375	3.375	3.625	3.625	3.625	3.75	4	3.875	4.25	4.125	4.188
Total score	25.7	28.375	28.313	27.25	29.75	28.5	28.5	28.625	28.563	33.25	32.875	33.063

Evaluation Phase 1

The first version of the prototype features a user interface where patients can input their outcome goal and receive a corresponding behavioral goal. Additionally, the case manager also has the option to enter treatment goals for their assigned patients. The prompt used in this first iteration to generate a goal from GPT-3, only includes asking for one behavioral goal based on an outcome goal.

In the evaluation, based on the survey, participants felt a high level of autonomy in pursuing both behavioral goals, with an average score of just above 4. They clearly understood the behavioral goals and found them moderately challenging. Commitment and competence to the behavioral goals were strong across both goals. However, there were differences in relatedness and feedback. Through the open text field, participants claimed to have felt stronger social support in goal 2 than in goal 1, this may be because goal 1 is carried out alone whereas goal 2 involves others. Clarity and task complexity were consistent across both goals, indicating a similar understanding of the goals and tasks' complexity. The average total score: 28.313 out of 35 points.

Despite clarity receiving a relatively high average score of 3.875, there is still room for improvement. There were several comments that the participants did not understand the goals well. It is important that goals are clearly defined. Therefore, the goals in the next evaluation phase will be presented in a more structured manner, in the format of SMART goals.

Instead of goals being generated in standard text form, each goal will now include the following attributes which are based on the SMART goal structure: goal, duration, frequency, frequency scale, and time period. An example of a structured goal can be seen in Fig. 2. This structured approach also facilitates an easier transformation to JSON format.

Evaluation Phase 2

In this version of the prototype, the patient is now able to modify the goals at the attribute level. Case managers now also have the ability to evaluate the goals of their patients, by allowing them to approve, modify, or reject goals. Once a goal is evaluated and approved by a case manager, the patient will receive a notification and be able to view the approved goals in their treatment plan.

The prompt has been modified for GPT-3 to respond in a more structured manner. To ensure conciseness, it is emphasized that only a subject, verb, and object are allowed in the generated goal.

The main goal of this evaluation phase was to improve clarity, which increased significantly for goal 1 but decreased for goal 2. Overall clarity increased by 0.25. For goal 1 the dimensions of competence and commitment significantly increased, whereas the dimensions of autonomy and challenge saw a significant decrease. For goal 2, autonomy and feedback significantly decreased. For the average score, autonomy was significantly reduced, but competence significantly increased. The average total score: is 28.5 out of 35 points. This is a slight increase of 0.187 compared to the previous evaluation phase.

As autonomy is currently one of the lower-scoring aspects, this improvement area will be investigated. Providing three behavioral goals instead of one has the potential to increase autonomy. Combined with the ability to modify attributes, this can lead to greater personalization and foster a stronger sense of ownership. This decision also may indicate that a single behavioral goal as a response per outcome goal may not be sufficient to achieve the desired outcome.

Evaluation Phase 3

In this version of the prototype, goals have the same structure as in evaluation phase 2, however, patients now receive three behavioral goals per outcome goal, instead of one. Initially, for outcome goal 2, three identical behavioral goals were generated. Although, the goal attributes varied. This occurred despite configuring GPT-3 to maximize the randomness of its responses.

The main goal of this evaluation phase was to improve autonomy. This slightly increased for goal 2, but decreased for goal 1. Overall there was a slight decrease in autonomy. The other results also varied from the last round. The biggest changes were found for goal 1. The dimensions of relatedness, challenge, and feedback significantly increased, whereas competence and clarity significantly decreased. For goal 2, there was a significant decrease in relatedness. For the average score, clarity significantly decreased. Average total score: 28.563 out of 35 points. A slight increase compared to the previous evaluation phase.

So far, the prompt has remained general without specifying the target group for whom the goals are intended. The next direction is to explore if giving the context that the generated behavioral goals are for patients with SMI would impact the response. Additionally, it would be interesting to investigate how including specific diagnoses would influence behavioral goals. This could potentially lead to more tailored results.

Evaluation Phase 4

The prompt has undergone two modifications. Firstly, by explicitly stating in the initial sentence that the treatment goals are intended for patients with a severe mental illness and emphasizing the goal's suitability for this individual. Secondly, an additional sentence has been included to specify the patient's diagnosis with an emphasis that the goal should be attainable for someone with this diagnosis.

Tests were conducted on these two scenarios, however, the behavioral goals did not show a significant change compared to the results from the previous evaluation phase. Modifying the attributes of the goal also yielded similar responses as before. As a result, this version will not undergo further surveys since the behavioral goals did not exhibit significant changes. It remains uncertain whether this new prompt would impact other goals.

In the earlier surveys, respondents expressed uncertainty about how to carry out the goal effectively and desired additional support through guidelines or a step-by-step plan that would enable them to pursue the goal effectively. As a result, addressing this issue will be the focus of the next evaluation phase.

Evaluation Phase 5

Attributes were added to the prompt to also include a step-by-step plan on how to achieve the behavioral goals, supportive tips to aid progress, and an explanation of the goal.

The behavioral goals have the same structure as in evaluation phase 4, with these three attributes added. As occurred in evaluation phase 3 the generated goals appeared to be very similar. In the case of goal 1, three separate behavioral goals were initially generated, but two were highly familiar, and therefore one was modified by the researcher using the edit function. The main goal was to improve clarity, which increased significantly in both goals. The other survey results also varied quite from the last evaluation phase. The most important changes were for goal 1. The dimensions of autonomy, competence, relatedness, feedback, and task complexity significantly increased. For goal 2, there was a significant increase in autonomy, competence, relatedness, commitment, and feedback. For the average

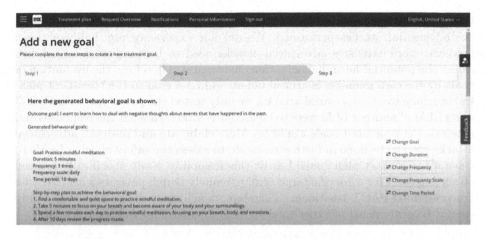

Fig. 2. Screenshot of the working prototype, showing one of the generated treatment plan goals and the option to edit the goal and its attributes.

score, autonomy, competence, relatedness, clarity, and feedback increased. Average total score: 33.063 out of 35 points. This is an increase of 4.5 compared to the previous evaluation phase.

5 Discussion

Study Limitations

In this study, it is important to note that the evaluation of the prototype itself fell outside the scope of the study. Consequently, aspects related to user-friendliness, UI, and UX elements were also outside the scope of the study. It is also worth highlighting that no testing was conducted with case managers or patients with SMI. Our primary focus was centered on determining whether modifications to the prototype and prompts could lead to improvements in the quality of the generated goals. In the evaluation phase, only the behavioral goals of two outcome goals were evaluated by students, the quality of the generated goals may differ depending on how outcome goals are structured and the type of outcome goals provided. The goals were also not evaluated by case managers on their quality, it is possible that they could consider other elements.

A major risk of using LLMs to generate goals for patients with SMI is that LLMs may hallucinate and could potentially generate goals that may not align with standard FACT treatment which may result in further complications for the patient. Accordingly, we performed some exploratory adversarial attacks on the prototype to expose potential vulnerabilities in the system when it comes to generating goals that may potentially not be in line with FACT treatment. A list of 26 treatment outcome goals that were deemed potentially harmful by the researchers, was used as input in the latest version of the prototype. The treatment behavioral goals given as output by the prototype were then inspected by the researchers. Upon analysis of the generated behavioral goals resulting from the adversarial attacks performed. We did not experience any hallucinations, however, more extensive adversarial attacks need to be conducted in order to assess the potential harm hallucinations may cause. Therefore, the evaluation of goals by the case manager is crucial before adding a goal to the treatment plan. In the exploratory adversarial attacks, we only tested the prototype with GPT-3 as its LLM, if another LLM were to be used it is unknown what the responses and how safe the generated goals would be. More elaborate and in-depth adversarial attacks need to be done in further research, to assess the safety of using LLMs to generate treatment plan goals. Lastly, this feasibility study specifically focused on setting goals for a specific target group, namely Dutch patients with SMI who are prescribed FACT treatment. Therefore, conclusions drawn from this study cannot be generalized to other (non) SMI groups without further research.

Future Work

In future work, we should recruit case managers, and patients with SMI to evaluate the goal-setting workflow and the quality of goals, as the results from healthy participants cannot be generalized to people with SMI. It is worth evaluating and tracking the progress patients with SMI are making toward the generated goal, through an mHealth application like GameBus, compared to non-LLM generated goals. The integration of SDT and Goal-setting has proven valuable in this research, but including other behavior theories, such as the COM-B, could enhance the assessment. COM-B is a valuable tool to address instances where individuals lack the necessary preconditions for certain behaviors. For example, if the generated goal says to 'ride a bicycle' it becomes an unfeasible goal if the patient does not possess a bicycle. Incorporating the COM-B model into an interactive goal-setting approach can address these situations more effectively and take the prerequisites needed to complete a goal into consideration. Mental healthcare professionals could also be given a hands-on session with the system in a usability study. An addition to the user interface that could potentially make it easier for case managers and patients to select treatment plan goals that are relevant to the treatment is to create an interface that allows users to easily swipe irrelevant goals away, and save relevant ones. Another interesting direction to explore is to investigate the willingness and privacy concerns of patients with SMI regarding using such technology in their treatment. Given the current level of distrust among patients with SMI, understanding their attitudes and perceptions toward AI-based tools and data privacy implications would provide valuable insights. Such research is essential for ensuring the ethical and effective integration of such technology in the treatment journey of patients with SMI.

6   Conclusion

This feasibility study aimed to explore the use of LLMs in enabling patients with SMI and case managers to easily create measurable treatment goals for treatment plans. The study suggests that it is feasible to develop a system that utilizes LLMs to allow users to generate measurable treatment plan goals. Using the prototype to create measurable goals, does make it possible to directly add meaningful goals to gamified mHealth systems like GameBus, which could potentially intrinsically motivate patients further to work on their treatment goals. Although the quality of the generated goals was not assessed by healthcare professionals or patients with SMI, the evaluation process with students indicated that incremental improvements in behavior goals were attainable. Furthermore, the study revealed that the application of SDT and Goal-Setting theory could enhance the quality of behavioral goals. However, improving a certain aspect and maintaining a consistent appreciation of all other aspects can be challenging. Now that it has been established that the proposed workflow has the potential to improve the process of case managers creating goals with their patients with SMI. We can now evaluate the system within the treatment process, and gather patient and case manager feedback. It is important to acknowledge that the results of this research should be considered preliminary, as there are currently no comparable findings in the existing literature for appropriate comparisons. These preliminary findings provide a foundation for further investigation and highlight the need for future research in this area.

References

1. Alkaissi, H., McFarlane, S.I.: Artificial hallucinations in ChatGPT: implications in scientific writing. Cureus **15**(2) (2023)
2. Arora, A., Arora, A.: The promise of large language models in health care. Lancet **401**(10377), 641 (2023)
3. Bovend'Eerdt, T.J., Botell, R.E., Wade, D.T.: Writing smart rehabilitation goals and achieving goal attainment scaling: a practical guide. Clin. Rehabil. **23**(4), 352–361 (2009)
4. Chase, J.A., Houmanfar, R., Hayes, S.C., Ward, T.A., Vilardaga, J.P., Follette, V.: Values are not just goals: online act-based values training adds to goal setting in improving undergraduate college student performance. J. Contextual Behav. Sci. **2**(3–4), 79–84 (2013)
5. Cheng, V.W.S., Davenport, T., Johnson, D., Vella, K., Hickie, I.B.: Gamification in apps and technologies for improving mental health and well-being: systematic review. JMIR Ment. Health **6**(6), e13717 (2019)
6. Dale, R.: GPT-3: what's it good for? Nat. Lang. Eng. **27**(1), 113–118 (2021)
7. Eckerstorfer, L.V., et al.: Key elements of mhealth interventions to successfully increase physical activity: meta-regression. JMIR Mhealth Uhealth **6**(11), e10076 (2018)
8. Fogg, B.J.: A behavior model for persuasive design. In: Proceedings of the 4th international Conference on Persuasive Technology, pp. 1–7 (2009)
9. Gabbard, G.O., Crisp-Han, H.: The early career psychiatrist and the psychotherapeutic identity. Acad. Psychiatry **41**, 30–34 (2017)
10. Graham, S., et al.: Artificial intelligence for mental health and mental illnesses: an overview. Curr. Psychiatry Rep. **21**, 1–18 (2019)

11. van Greuningen, M., Borgs, B.: Feiten en cijfers over mensen met een ernstige psychiatrische aandoening (2022). https://www.vektis.nl/intelligence/publicaties/factsheet-ernstige-psychiatrische-aandoeningen
12. Hamdoun, S., Monteleone, R., Bookman, T., Michael, K.: AI-based and digital mental health apps: balancing need and risk. IEEE Technol. Soc. Mag. **42**(1), 25–36 (2023)
13. Jameel, L., Valmaggia, L., Barnes, G., Cella, M.: mHealth technology to assess, monitor and treat daily functioning difficulties in people with severe mental illness: a systematic review. J. Psychiatric Res. **145**(2021), 35–49 (2022). https://doi.org/10.1016/j.jpsychires.2021.11.033
14. James, L.J., et al.: Evaluation of personalized treatment goals on engagement of smi patients with an mhealth app. In: 2022 IEEE International Conference on Bioinformatics and Biomedicine (BIBM), pp. 1568–1573. IEEE (2022)
15. Litvin, S., Saunders, R., Maier, M.A., Lüttke, S.: Gamification as an approach to improve resilience and reduce attrition in mobile mental health interventions: a randomized controlled trial. PLoS ONE **15**(9), e0237220 (2020)
16. Liu, B., et al.: Adversarial attacks on large language model-based system and mitigating strategies: a case study on ChatGPT. Secur. Commun. Netw. **2023** (2023)
17. Locke, E.A., Latham, G.P.: Building a practically useful theory of goal setting and task motivation: a 35-year odyssey. Am. Psychol. **57**(9), 705 (2002)
18. Michie, S., et al.: The behavior change technique taxonomy (v1) of 93 hierarchically clustered techniques: building an international consensus for the reporting of behavior change interventions. Ann. Behav. Med. **46**(1), 81–95 (2013)
19. Organization, W.H., et al.: World mental health report: transforming mental health for all (2022)
20. Ryan, R.M., Deci, E.L.: Self-determination theory and the facilitation of intrinsic motivation, social development, and well-being. Am. Psychol. **55**(1), 68 (2000)
21. Shatte, A.B., Hutchinson, D.M., Teague, S.J.: Machine learning in mental health: a scoping review of methods and applications. Psychol. Med. **49**(9), 1426–1448 (2019)
22. Svensson, B., Hansson, L., Markström, U., Lexén, A.: What matters when implementing flexible assertive community treatment in a Swedish healthcare context: a two-year implementation study. Int. J. Ment. Health **46**(4), 284–298 (2017)
23. Van Gorp, P., Nuijten, R.: 8-year evaluation of GameBus: status quo in aiming for an open access platform to prototype and test digital health apps. Proc. ACM Hum.-Comput. Interact. **7**(EICS), 1–24 (2023)
24. Van Veldhuizen, J.R.: FACT: a Dutch version of ACT. Community Ment. Health J. **43**(4), 421–433 (2007). https://doi.org/10.1007/s10597-007-9089-4

Fanima! Pervasive Serious Game for Phonetic-Phonological Assessment of Children Towards Autonomous Speech Therapy

Inês Antunes[1], André Antunes[1,2], and Rui Neves Madeira[1,2]

[1] NOVA LINCS, NOVA School of Science and Technology, NOVA University
of Lisbon, Caparica, Portugal
ig.antunes@campus.fct.unl.pt
[2] Sustain.RD, Escola Superior de Tecnologia de Setúbal, Instituto Politécnico de
Setúbal, Setúbal, Portugal
{andre.antunes,rui.madeira}@estsetubal.ips.pt

Abstract. Many children have difficulties with speech and language,
sometimes even both. Speech therapy for children is usually a tedious
process where one of the drawbacks of traditional solutions is the repetition of exercises. A known strategy to increase engagement is to deliver
speech therapy through mobile games. A serious game-based diagnosis
tool for phonetic-phonological assessment of speech disorders focused on
the European Portuguese language was designed with therapists' participation. The integration with a web platform allows real-time therapist
interaction to control the game based on the classification of vocalisa-
tions made by the child in response to the gameplay, which follows the
therapeutic structure for the intended diagnosis. One first user study was
made with five speech therapists to validate the tool's concept and the
system's usability for responding to the therapeutic requirements. The
results are positive, validating the tool and suggesting its acceptance
by the community of therapists, allowing us to move on to a thorough
second study with therapists in a therapeutic context with children.

Keywords: Serious Games · Speech Therapy · Phonetic-Phonological
Assessment · Mobile Computing · Interaction Design and Children

1 Introduction

Children at a very young age learn to use devices like smartphones, controllers, or
tablets. Many children feel excited about using mobile devices [20]. The growing
popularity of smart mobile devices among young children, driven by their unique
characteristics and the rapid development of age-appropriate applications, has
been highlighted in previous research, emphasizing these devices as the preferred

This work was supported by NOVA.ID.FCT/NOVA LINCS (UIDB/04516/2020).

technological tool due to their advantages over older technologies [17,30]. More-over, games are a prominent tool of entertainment for children [4]. Games offer a valuable avenue for enhancing various skills, including logic, dexterity, memory, and motor skills, among others. By strategically integrating games into educational or therapeutic contexts [7,32], we can leverage the interactive engagement between individuals, especially children, to foster skill development and learning. For instance, they can be used to help children with speech or language development [33].

Speech is one of the most important forms of communication. Unfortunately, the diagnosis of speech sound disorders (SSD) in children has been common. Approximately 5% to 8% of children have difficulties with speech and language, sometimes even both [19]. There are not many studies in Portugal that provide information on the prevalence of SSD [29,34]. In a cohort of 630 children, Oliveira et al. reveal that the prevailing issue, affecting 68% of the sample, is rooted in phonological challenges, highlighting a shared concern within the broader collective. [29]. This type of problem makes it difficult to generate or understand phonemes, which frequently causes mistakes with substitutions, syllable structure, and phoneme distortions.

Children with SSD may face some challenges, which can have a major negative effect on their adult life [21]. One of them is the social impact. The child may begin to feel shame and frustration in talking to other children, so s/he may become more insecure and anxious, which can lead to self-isolation. These can also interfere with the child's academic path, also having a negative effect concerning education. Some problems in this domain can cause difficulties in reading, spelling, and other fields, such as mathematics. It has been estimated that about 50% to 70% of children with SSD show general academic difficulty throughout secondary education. This may be one of those negative impacts on their adult life. If these problems are not detected early and treated properly, they may permanently impact depending on the severity level. However, speech therapy plays an important role in the early detection of the type of speech disorder and in adapting an appropriate therapy.

A speech-language pathologist (SLP) conducts sessions that are usually based on illustrative card-based exercises where children are asked to answer some questions about what they see on the cards, thus promoting spontaneous speech. One of the drawbacks of these so-called traditional solutions is the repetition of exercises/tasks. Vocal apparatus exercises tend to be dependent on repetition. A child having some difficulties in the correct production of a phoneme makes the therapist to be more focused on repeating words where that phoneme is and asking the child to repeat it until reaching a correct production. These types of methodologies for children at young ages can be monotonous and demotivating, making the child lose interest and concentration in the proposed exercise/task.

Motivation is an important factor since if a child is motivated, and enjoying sessions, the treatment will be much more efficient, and it will accelerate the treatment process of the child. At times when the SLP/therapist feels that the child is unmotivated, s/he resorts to tablet games and uses them intending to make her talk. The drawback of these games is that they are not intended for the context of speech therapy and end up serving merely for the child's amusement. At the same time, the therapist needs to make her/his assessment, which leads to recording the necessary data to be able to analyze it later.

For the research presented in this paper, we are teaming up with the clinic *Cresce com Amor*[1], which challenged the research team according to the needs mentioned before. Our research focuses on the diagnostic phase through exercises of visualization, interpretation, and description of images present in a serious game (SG) based tool for tablets. To develop the solution, a participatory design approach and design guidelines were explored to create a game design suitable for children. It was essential to create a tool based on a game environment that was appealing and fun for the child, in order to motivate him/her to play. During the period when the child is playing, the therapist is in real-time validating the child's process throughout the game. Through this approach, it will be possible to create a motivating, challenging, and more autonomous environment for the child under pervasive direct supervision. The idea is for the therapist to be able to intervene in the session in the same way but in a non-intrusive way. Therefore, the therapist's interface response time was worked on so that it would not affect the game flow, avoiding dead times as much as possible. Since this is the diagnosis phase of therapy, it is very likely that it is one of the first contacts that the child has with the therapist, which may feel more withdrawn, affecting the diagnosis assessment.

The paper is organized as follows. Section 2 contextualizes the background and related work. Afterwards, in Sect. 3, we present our participatory design approach towards developing the Fanima prototype. A first user study is described and results presented in Sect. 4, and conclusions and further work are summarized in Sect. 5.

2 Background and Related Work

The evolution of technology has facilitated some tasks in people's daily lives. Computer technology has been relevant in promoting some educational activities in schools. All children have benefited, but especially children with disabilities. This makes it possible for them to have an education suited to their needs [15]. Moreover, pervasive computing technologies can make play-based occupational therapy more effective by embedding digital technology into playful activity [23]. In occupational therapy, an effective means to motivate a change in a child's behavior is by designing playful activities that leverage the child's desire to play. Video games designed specifically for rehabilitation can do the work without adding significant costs to both the healthcare system and patients [5].

SGs are basically games that aim to promote the learning of a skill beyond the fun of playing it. A serious game is much more than an application with some game elements and game concepts, as there is a whole content and immersive game environment used for purposes other than mere entertainment [27]. SGs constitute a subgenre of serious storytelling, wherein narrative elements

---

[1] https://www.cresce.pt.

are utilized beyond the realm of entertainment. The storytelling unfolds as a sequence of high-quality patterns, integral to a purposeful progression [24]. SGs can be inserted in different contexts such as military, government, educational, corporate, and healthcare. According to Nasiri et al., SGs are a great approach to the education and entertainment of children with disabilities. Children who play educational games learn quickly and more easily a skill in comparison to the ones who do not play them [28]. SGs are experiencing great growth in terms of solutions in the therapeutic context [35]. Therapeutic serious games (TSG) is estimated to be the area where the concept will grow more over the years. Games can benefit an individual on both a psychological and physical level, which meets the goals of SGs for healthcare. TSG have been identified as a valuable tool for enhancing health through therapy and rehabilitation, as highlighted by studies such as Durango et al. [8] and Horne-Moyer et al. [16]. Integrating therapeutic content with gaming elements and aligned objectives can forge innovative, motivating, and immersive therapeutic environments [38].

Regarding speech therapy, children who suffer from psychological problems, like autism, have difficulties with communication, so it is normal that they have problems communicating with the therapist and get tired of the treatment really quickly [9]. Adults with speech disorders have an intrinsic motivation for the treatment, as they know by doing treatment, they will eventually get better. This factor does not have the same effect on children since they get bored too easily, which can slow their treatment. Thus, the field of speech therapy is no exception to the incorporation of serious games, where different studies have developed games specifically within this domain to address and treat speech disorders [33]. As these games prove to be beneficial, they should extend beyond basic mobile applications. For instance, they should possess the capability to compare a child's pronunciation of a word, who has a speech disorder, with the correct pronunciation, providing necessary feedback to encourage continued engagement [33].

There have been several research regarding the use of technology (e.g., mobile apps [10] and Automated Speech Analysis [26]) or SGs (e.g., [13] and [3]) in speech therapy. Hajesmaeel-Gohari et al. conducted an insightful study reviewing articles that have used digital games for speech disorders therapy [14]. In another interesting research, Saeedi et al. conducted a study based on a systematic and comprehensive review of the games in this area, aiming to answer several questions and ambiguities about the games they found [33]. Many TSG fell short of meeting children's expectations, especially when compared to traditional games [36]. Therefore, it is important to follow state-of-the-art sets of guidelines for the design of solutions based on games for children. Guidelines are high-level statements ranging from various cases to low-level declarations limited to specific contexts [36]. Valenza et al. evaluated a set of 40 guidelines for designing SG for children. Fifty-nine experts concluded that the majority of the guidelines hold high relevance, with all of them warranting attention when developing SG for children [36]. On the other hand, Zaki et al. conducted a study focused on finding the set of design guidelines for developing TSG in speech therapy, specifically on cognitive stimulation [1]. The guidelines were derived through the study of relevant literature and best practices gained from interviews with experts in speech therapy [1]. While studies have shown a positive impact of digital serious games on addressing speech disorders, it is important to incorporate personalized speech therapy elements into the design of these games for optimal effectiveness [14].

Read et al. carried out a study of participatory design activity with children to design a SG. This study shows how the participation of children during the development phase can contribute to a successful SG. The game is focused on communicating the importance of hand-washing, the educational content is health, the target user is children in elementary school, and the SG platform is a mobile tablet. For the game design, some analyses were made on children's drawing activities. In terms of fun and gameplay, five criteria were determined: the SG should have a goal, fun add-ons (fun sound), rewards (to show the game progress and the feel of success), desirable child-centred content and randomness to provide a surprise. For learning, the criteria were organization of the learning material, formative feedback on learning, appropriate language (including images), consistency of learning presentation, interactivity (to increase engagement), and knowledge (imparted through the game) [31].

Finally, it is important to consider the stakeholder's intervention in the design phase of a project. Introducing stakeholders into an early phase can bring other perspectives of the problem or, perhaps, even the solution to the problem, leading to more advantageous outcomes. Co-creation and co-design are two very similar terms, almost synonymous. It is common to call participatory design to co-design in the design community [37]. Co-design focuses more on the interaction between designers, stakeholders, and end-users. It is crucial that all parts agree with decisions made in a given situation, and it is also important to create design ideas that may increment a positive change in some situations [11].

3   Participatory Design of Fanima

In this research, our emphasis was on developing an SG within the realm of speech therapy. The design process of this system had a strong component of participatory design by *Cresce com Amor*, following the design thinking methodology, which consists of five different stages: Empathize, Define, Ideate, Prototype and Test [6]. Figure 1 illustrates how we organized the working workshops (detailed in the following subsections) according to the stages of the design process. We are counting on the active collaboration of therapists (experts) with deep experience working with children with different disabilities. The final solution should be the result of an iterative process involving, as much as possible, different actors, such as therapists, children, parents, designers and developers.

3.1   First Workshops - Empathize and Define Problem

In the first workshop, discussions with therapists provided insights into the clinic's environment and methodologies employed during therapy sessions. It

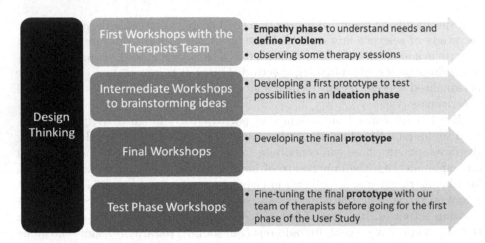

Fig. 1. Design thinking approach for the development of Fanima.

allowed to gather some essential insights that helped to understand what was important to have in the intended SG-based solution. The only decision already made before that workshop was that we would apply the SG concept.

The concern during a therapy session is how the feeling of being evaluated may affect the child's performance. By having the SLP guiding the session, some of the behaviours and interactions of the child may change. They may not feel very comfortable and get more intimidated during practice. Therefore, the intention was to have a relaxed environment where the child would feel motivated and not under pressure during practice, leading to more natural behaviour. One of the main objectives was to create a playful, motivating, challenging and comfortable environment for the child so that it is possible to maintain the child's interest and focus during the therapy session. It was imperative to craft a visually engaging and age-appropriate design tailored for children undergoing diagnosis, aged 3 to 7 years old.

It was also decided we needed to delve into the specificity of the field, particularly discerning the needs of therapists during diagnostic sessions. In speech therapy, there are two major dimensions, phonetics and phonology, and Fanima aims to cover both dimensions, being a phonetic-phonological diagnostic assessment tool. In Portuguese language, there are 33 phonemes, that can be grouped into vowels, nasal vowels, semivowels, and consonants [25]. For this study, in collaboration with therapists, the decision was made to concentrate on consonants, which are categorized into four distinct groups:

- Oclusives - produced when the air coming from the lungs encounters an obstacle, resulting in an explosion. They are the phonemes /p/, /b/, /t/, /d/, /k/, /g/, /m/, /n/, /nh/
- Fricatives - pronounced from the friction of the air on an obstacle such as the tongue or lips. For example, /f/, /v/, /s/, /z/, /ch/, /j/

- Vibrants - pronounced from the vibration of one of the elements of the vocal apparatus. For example, /r/, /rr/
- Laterals - pronounced from the air passage through the mouth's corner. For example, /l/, /lh/

Follow-up workshops and informal discussions with the team of therapists facilitated the clarification of needs and led to the creation of a first set of guidelines (see Table 1), which emphasized the incorporation of feedback elements to enhance the child's motivation and commitment to the proposed tasks. Additionally, the suggestion of subsequent game chapters based on incorrectly produced phonemes emerged as a key consideration.

Table 1. First set of guidelines for the Fanima design.

ID	Description	Type
G1	Create appealing and age-appropriate design	Fanima UI
G2	Provide phoneme classification	Validation
G3	Provide feedback	Fanima UI
G4	Suggest specific chapters based on wrong phonemes	Validation

In this first design phase, the team recognized the therapist's need to conduct assessments and record essential data for later analysis. Typically, therapists commonly record sessions using mobile phones and document data either in Excel tables or notebooks. These notes are usually related to which phonemes the child shows more difficulties, in which phoneme position the child has more problems (in the beginning, middle, or at the end of the word), for instance. This process can bring some problems for the therapist concerning keeping up with the treatment and evolution of each patient. Therefore, the therapist would need a game control interface for configuration before the session, real-time control as the game progresses, and a support platform for analyzing the data collected during the session.

3.2 Intermediate Workshops - Ideate

This phase was focused on the co-creation of an initial concept based on a first set of ideas (Fig. 2 illustrates the first concept). A multi-chapter game concept was suggested to run on mobile devices, such as tablets, where the initial phase involved the child reproducing sentences. If inadequately produced sounds were detected (e.g., the phoneme —r—) the subsequent task would focus on repeating that specific phoneme to promote accurate reproduction. In the first phase, the phonemes were grouped by age groups, which would facilitate the choice of the levels by age group and within that age group in which phonemes are intended to work in a session. This model also facilitates the process of choosing the following levels suggested by the system after the end of a level.

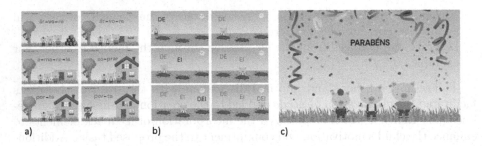

Fig. 2. First prototype: a) Example of a level with a repeating sound task, b) Example of the most basic level of isolation of a phoneme, and c) Full-level feedback example.

The game consisted of several levels where provoked speech was promoted in an initial phase. After that, the therapist would use the real-time control interface to identify the errors. Based on the therapist's input, the system would suggest a set of levels. In these levels, the child was asked to reproduce some sounds that have been found to be incorrect in spontaneous speech. If difficulties prevail in the same phoneme, the idea was to play a mini-game (Fig. 2b) where the isolated production of this phoneme is carried out. This was the idea for the level cycle, but the game period ends when the therapist decides. As mentioned before, as a guideline, in order to keep children collaborative during the session, each task had feedback so that they could have the feeling of success.

After showing the first proposal of the solution, a new workshop was held where it was possible to validate the proposed ideas and brainstorm around them. A second set of guidelines was defined (see Table 2), where we can highlight that the error should not be transmitted to the child since Fanima is just a diagnostic assessment rather than a treatment intervention. Moreover, the therapist must be able to enter the type of error that s/he detects throughout the test (SODA - Substitution, Omission, Distortion, and Addition/simplification) [12].

Table 2. Second set of guidelines for the Fanima design.

ID	Description	Type
G5	Do not transmit the error to the child	Fanima UI
G6	Prevent negative feedback (could lead to child disinterest)	Fanima UI
G7	Allow therapist to classifiy error	Validation
G8	On substitution error, register the substitute phoneme	Validation
G9	An x number of mandatory stimuli must appear in each test	Game structure
G10	Perform error consistency test for detected error phonemes	Fanima UI

Additionally, the game model structure (see Fig. 3) was approved by the research team and the therapists, having been a facilitating model and adequate to the needs identified previously.

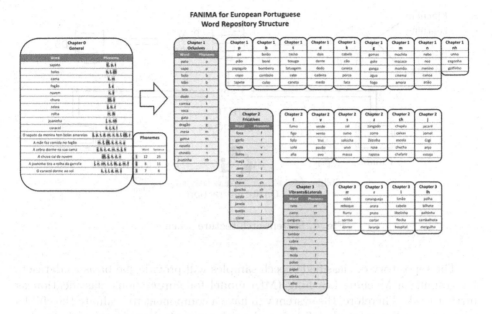

Fig. 3. Game model using a multi-chapter structure.

In this phase, the system's architecture (Fig. 4) was also defined, being composed of the child's mobile interface (the Fanima game), the therapist's game control interface, a web server and its database, both provided by the PLAY platform [2], which also provides additional interfaces to the therapist in order to analyse results and configure the game. Communication between Fanima and PLAY is achieved using an API, allowing user authentication, game structure and content retrieving, and game results and sample submission. PLAY provides a bidirectional channel for real-time interaction between the two interfaces, allowing to follow the current state of the exercise and interact with the patient session (e.g., receive the sampled speech and classify it, validating or assigning an error state).

The therapist's pervasive control interface is simple and straightforward with just a few controls, where the therapist can make the child repeat the level/chapter, choose the next chapter, and introduce some notes or issues detected in the child's performance. This way, the therapist can pervasively control the course of the session, manipulating the chapters and phonemes to work on, and the child feels total control and autonomy over the tasks to be performed. The PLAY platform supports the recording of each patient's sessions as well as level settings. The therapist can then follow the evolution of the sessions for each patient. Another positive point is that the results of each task can be accessed by other health professionals or clinics, depending on permissions. Therefore, patients may have a better follow-up in treatment across different therapists and clinics.

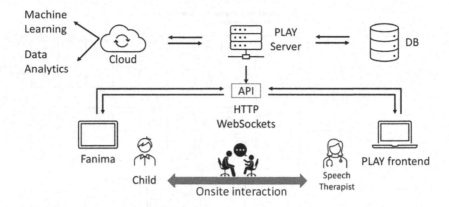

Fig. 4. System architecture scheme.

The repository of classified speech samples will provide the basis as datasets for training a Machine Learning (ML) model for autonomous classification as further work. Therefore, the system will have a component to evaluate the child's performance based on classification algorithms, replacing the therapist as the controller of the gameplay and letting the child to play without supervision. or giving additional support.

3.3   Final Workshops - Prototype

The prototype stage was an iterative process that involved implementing the Fanima concept, adding new features, correcting/improving existing features, and validating each new prototype's version through workshops and meetings. Meanwhile, multiple versions were discussed after the first design idea shown in Fig. 2 and a new game design and mechanics were defined. It was decided to have an animal-based theme for the game based on the recommendation given by the clinic's team since children enjoy animals and exploring. The scenarios of each chapter were focused on a childish theme with bright colours. The main requirements/challenges for the child are: recognize an image and name it; encourage spontaneous speech; repetition of a phoneme at different positions in a word (begin, middle, or final); when needed, use speech by repetition.

During this iterative design process, a third set of implementation guidelines focusing on validation, game structure, and user interface (UI) were devised, which helped achieve the current prototype. The final third set of guidelines is displayed in Table 3 and includes aspects such as adjustment of the type of evaluation and an increment on the type of errors, for instance. The Fanima game provides a login UI and four chapters (from 0 to 3), according to the structure presented in Fig. 3, which are detailed as follows.

Login. The therapist uses it to input the child's username and password so it is possible to identify which patient is logged in on the PLAY platform. Meanwhile, the therapist logged into the web platform and entered the patient activity area. If the play button in Fanima is pressed and the therapist is not already logged in, then the game does not proceed; which only happens when the therapist is logged in and in the right area of the platform.

Table 3. Third set of guidelines for the Fanima design.

ID	Description	Type
G11	Adjust type of evaluation and increase type of errors	Validation
G12	Play extra games right after a chapter	Game structure
G13	Use chapter zero just for error detection	Validation
G14	Do not put captions on pictures that the child has to name	Fanima UI
G15	Allow therapist to provide word hints	Validation
G16	Provide child capability to ask for hint	Fanima UI
G17	Provide possibility to identify errors in different phonemes	Validation
G18	Allow therapist to select to play sentences section	Validation
G19	Give therapist capability to ask for word repetition	Validation
G20	Repeat same word 3 times for error consistency	Game structure
G21	Be able to save the recordings of all repetitions	Results
G22	Have an indication to when the game is recording	Fanima UI

Chapter 0. Once both the child and therapist successfully log in, the game initiates, and the first chapter unfolds. Every participant begins with Chapter 0, wherein the child is prompted to articulate what they observe in the displayed frame. To introduce an extra challenge, at the outset, the child must click on the branch when it shakes. Subsequently, the frame evolves, transitioning to the scenario depicted in Fig. 5a). After identifying all frames, Chapter 0 centres on words. If the child demonstrates proficiency in producing sentences, the subsequent scenario shifts the focus to sentence construction. In such instances, there are no additional tasks beyond mentioning what is depicted on the paper, as illustrated in Fig. 5b). This streamlined approach is intentional, given the fewer sentences than words in the prior exercise, aiming to maintain the child's concentration on the targeted sentences. Redirection to the next chapter is determined at the therapist's discretion if the child struggles to produce sentences.

Chapter 1. If the child encounters challenges with occlusive phonemes in Chapter 0, Chapter 1 is introduced. In this segment, the child aids a frog in recovering coins by vocalizing the contents of the coin; when the coin shakes, the child taps it to prompt the frog to jump and catch it, as depicted in Fig. 6a). Importantly, even if the phoneme is not produced correctly, the intention is to proceed, recognizing that this SG is designed for diagnostic sessions where the child may exhibit difficulties with certain phonemes. This approach is consistent across all chapters, including Chapter 0, aligning with the recommendations of

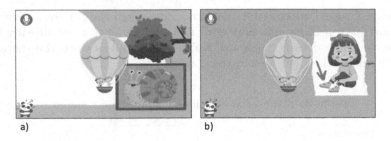

Fig. 5. Fanima interface: a) Chapter 0 focusing words, b) Chapter 0 focusing sentences

the *Cresce com Amor* team. If errors are identified in this chapter, an additional chapter is introduced. In this supplemental chapter, the child identifies and repeats the presented word three times, as illustrated in Fig. 6b). Following the repetition, an extra task is assigned—locating and touching a monkey (Fig. 6c)).

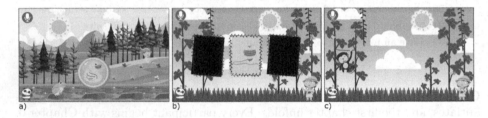

Fig. 6. Fanima interface: a) Chapter 1, b) Chapter 1 Extra, c) Chapter 1 Extra (task)

Chapter 2. If the therapist identified issues with fricative phonemes in the child while playing Chapter 0, the child proceeds to Chapter 2. The objective of this chapter is to assist the owls in popping all the balloons. When a balloon appears, the child must touch it to pop it and then identify and name what is inside the balloon, as illustrated in Fig. 7a). Again, as in Chapter 1, if errors were detected, the child plays an extra chapter. In the extra chapter, the child is challenged to say what is in the square figure as seen in Fig. 7b) and then find and touch (or click depending on the device that the game is being played) the missing chameleon as seen in Fig. 7c). These exercises play on a loop until all the words in the game structure are used.

Chapter 3. If the therapist identified issues with vibrants and laterals in the child in Chapter 0, the child proceeds to Chapter 3. In this underwater-themed chapter, the child is tasked with feeding the fish. To accomplish this, the child must first vocalize what is depicted on the food container. When the container starts to shake, the child touches it, prompting the fish to swim towards the

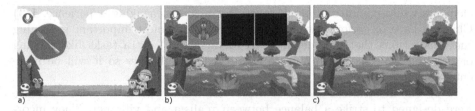

Fig. 7. Fanima interface: a) Chapter 2, b) Chapter 2 Extra, c) Chapter 2 Extra (task)

food and eat, as depicted in Fig. 8 a). After completing all the tasks, if there are any mispronounced phonemes, an additional chapter is again introduced. The dynamics remain similar to the previous two chapters, but with a distinct theme, as depicted in Figs. 8b) and 8c). The child's task is to assist the octopuses in locating their misplaced items by matching them with the paint of their colour. After repeating the object's name three times, the child must drag the object to the corresponding octopus once the black ink disappears.

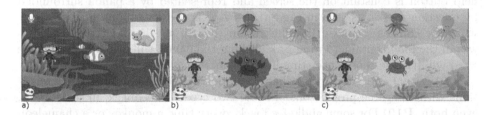

Fig. 8. Fanima interface: a) Chapter 3, b) Chapter 3 Extra, c) Chapter 3 Extra (task)

3.4   Test Phase Workshops - Validate Fanima Design Principles

The Fatima design was based on the set of 22 guidelines produced throughout the previous stages and on the guidelines provided by [36]. All these guidelines worked as the essential principles for Fanima. Hence, as the initial step in the Test stage of the design process, we validated the prototype against those principles with our therapists team and implemented refinements to the final version through a fine-tuning intervention before progressing to the first phase of the User Study (Sect. 4). The main principles in the game design of Fanima are summarized as follows.

P1) In all chapters except for Chapter 3 extra, the proposed tasks are done through simple touches on the screen, such as in Chapter 0 touching the branches, in Chapter 1 touching the coins, and in extra Chapters of 1 and 2 in which the child has to touch the monkey and the chameleon, respectively, as soon as they find them. **P2)** Unique scenarios were crafted for each chapter, aiming to evoke surprise and motivation throughout the game. Each scene was richly adorned with themes such as forest, jungle, ocean, or river, incorporating related elements while minimizing blank spaces for a more engaging experience. **P3)** Children have to perform two types of tasks: a) the most important is naming the illustrations that are presented to them, and b) extra tasks like clicking or dragging objects, which help to create extra challenges so it will be more entertaining.

P4) The illustrations chosen to depict the words within the game structure were designed to strike a balance between realism and vibrancy. They incorporate images that closely resemble reality, yet maintain a colorful and slightly cartoonish aesthetic. **P5)** Initially, illustrations included subtitles, but this extra information proved to be distracting for children. Since the game's users are not expected to know how to read, each time a new chapter begins, the story and goals are narrated to facilitate the child's understanding of the tasks. The primary focus is on ensuring swift and efficient response/feedback to maintain the child's concentration during gameplay.

P6) The size of the interactive items was considered to be big enough and have a reasonable spacing between them so that it is easy for children to touch the item they want. **P7)** An avatar is always present on all screens to act as an intermediary-friendly character between the therapist and the child. **P8)** The help button is constant on the screen and represented by a panda surrounded by question marks, as seen in Fig. 8a). Its goal is to provide information about what the child is seeing in the illustration (e.g., if she/he did not know what was in the food container in Fig. 8a), clicking the panda will give a hint, and the child will have to repeat the stimulus right after).

P9) Visual and auditory feedback is important so all of the child's interactions with the game provide one of these two types of feedback, in some cases, even both. **P10)** For some audio feedback, every time a monkey or a chameleon appears in Chapter 1 Extra and Chapter 2 Extra, a sound is produced, indicating to the child that a new item has appeared on the screen and can be searched for. Audio is used in other moments. **P11)** A microphone icon is present to ensure accurate sound capture and indicate when the child should speak. It is red when not recording and turns green upon successful sound recording.

4   User Study

For the second part of the Test stage of our design process, we designed a study composed of three main phases: 1- tests with SLPs to validate the concept, system integration, and theoretical background, as the basis for the achievement of therapeutic requirements; 2- thorough tests with children and therapists (recruited from the first phase) to assess Fanima regarding usability and user experience of children; 3- effectiveness study during three months in the wild to assess the tool under therapy contexts.

Here, we present the initial results from the first phase of the second part, which is focused on the end users.

4.1   Design and Participants

After a brief introduction, the test protocol required participants to: a) consider a user profile of a child; b) play chapter 0 considering that profile; c) choose only one between Chapters 1, 2 and 3; d) signal a single phoneme in the selected chapter to play the extra one; and e) answer a post-test questionnaire, composed of six sections.

The first section gathers some basic demographic information about the therapist. The second section refers to the Fanima concept and its main features and principles (see Table 4). The third section is about the therapist's interface in the web platform. The fourth section requires therapists to evaluate the word repository and structure used in the application. Section five assesses system usability using the standard System Usability Scale (SUS). As all therapists answering this questionnaire are Portuguese, we are using the European Portuguese version of SUS [18]. The sixth section is a generic final remarks section for extra feedback. Statements based on a seven-point Likert scale were mostly used in sections 2 to 5. Long text answers are also used for some questions where therapists are asked to give feedback/suggestions and demographic information.

Table 4. Domain-specific statements of section 2.

Q	Question
9	I think the game has an appealing design for children
10	I think this game will be a useful tool for children to feel more motivated during the therapy session
11	It is interesting to have a tool that makes it possible to "control" the game in real time (while the child is playing)
12	The game flow supports a proper diagnostic assessment of the user, so you can check the set of phonemes where the user has difficulties
13	I think that the "Repeat", "Help", "Error" and "Submit" options are adequate to be able to manipulate the course of the game
15	It is useful to be able to listen again to the recorded audios in consolidation with the evaluation made during the session
16	I can carry out a full evaluation after visualising the data collected during the course of the game
17	I would use this system to diagnose speech problems in children, specifically phonetic-phonological disorders

The study participants included five (1 male, 4 female) SLPs, and all of them have specialization in SLT for children. They all use games in interventions with children, being familiar with the SG concept and considering that games help children stay interested during a session.

4.2 Results and Discussion

We are summarizing the outcomes of this preliminary evaluation, primarily focusing on responses from sections 2 and 5 of the questionnaire, supplemented by additional insights derived from comments and observations made during the tests. Results of the domain-specific questionnaire related to the Fanima solution are displayed in Fig. 9.

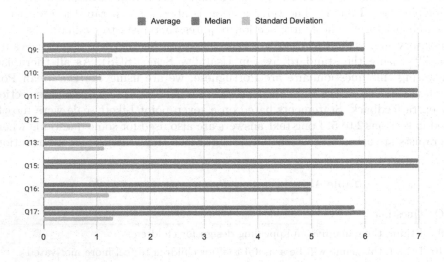

Fig. 9. User Study: questionnaire's section 2 results.

The majority found the Fanima design appealing towards children, drawing from their individual experiences. All participants found interesting the possibility of having a real-time control interface and being able to listen again to samples captured during a session. All participants found the Fanima concept interesting, with the game flow supporting an adequate diagnostic assessment of the user, allowing verification of the set of phonemes where the user has difficulties. One suggestion is the ability to state which phoneme was replaced for, in case of a phoneme substitution error. One specialist was concerned about the Internet connection because it is common to have some problems in public schools, which can interfere with the game flow.

Divergent opinions arise when examining the game's collected data due to therapists employing varied methodologies and approaches in utilizing metrics. However, it is crucial to note that in this phase, the emphasis was not on evaluating data visualization but rather on scrutinizing the specific information that each therapist deems essential to retain and observe in the results.

Summarizing SUS results, they show that all participants consider Fanima easy to use, with the majority of them not considering it too complex. All agree that Fanima functionalities are well integrated, with the majority not considering it to have significant inconsistencies. Most participants do not consider it complicated to use the Fanima tool, and they feel they did not have to learn much to use it, with all of them agreeing that most people would quickly learn to use it. All participants felt confident when using Fanima and were willing to use it frequently. Regarding the overall SUS score until now, it was 85 on the SUS Scale, meaning the results can be interpreted as being in the 96th to 100th percentile range, which is already within the range of a "Best Imaginable" usability rating and an A+ grade [22].

The small number of participants in the study prevents it from being statistically representative so it is not possible to assert definitive conclusions. Nevertheless, considering the obtained results, we observe a tendency to validate the Fanima concept, system integration, and theoretical background. SUS results demonstrate that system usability is progressing in the right direction.

5   Conclusions and Future Work

This research focused on the participatory design process of Fanima, a serious game-based tool for phonetic-phonological assessment in speech therapy with children. The goal is to use this tool in a clinical environment, with the presence of a therapist, and create a relaxed and motivating environment for the child to carry out the proposed tasks. The overall goal of this solution is to create various environments, challenges, and playful illustrations so the child will be immersed on the game and less aware of the assessment under a therapeutic context, but also having the therapist around and able to control the gameplay when needed.

The research needed to cope with the following main challenges: a) design a persuasive tool based on serious games and mobile devices; b) create a game model suitable for the therapy session that meets the needs of a heterogeneous group (based on age, gender and motivations for the sessions); c) provide an adequate assessment of the phonemes produced by the child; and d) integrate a game control interface to allow the therapist to guide the session, having a direct intervention in the flow of the game.

Fanima can be regarded as a novelty, standing apart from existing tools without direct comparisons. It features an interface for the therapist that allows her/him to control the game in real-time for personalised therapy in a pervasive non-intrusive way. Fanima also allows to building a dataset for training an automatic classifier based on audio captured from vocalizations made by children and classifications made by therapists in real-time (they can reclassify afterwards and update). As of today, there is no dataset available. The design study contributed with a set of 22 guidelines. Moreover, Fanima can be easily adapted to be used with other languages.

Positive results are taken from the first phase of the user study, which also provided room for improvement: changing some images; the errors list presented to the therapist; a.o. aspects we are discussing. Future work includes completing tests with therapists, initiating the second evaluation phase with children to assess Fanima within therapy contexts, and subsequently advancing to the effectiveness study. Another future task is adding the ML classification model aiming at an automated version of Fanima where the therapist is not needed to control the gameplay.

References

1. Ahmad Zaki, N.A., Tengku Wook, T.S.M.T.W., Ahmad, K.: Therapeutic serious game design guidelines for stimulating cognitive abilities of children with speech and language delay. J. Inf. Commun. Technol. **16**, 284–312 (2017). https://doi.org/10.32890/jict2017.16.2.5
2. Antunes, A., Madeira, R.N.: PLAY - model-based platform to support therapeutic serious games design. Procedia Comput. Sci. **198**(2018), 211–218 (2021). https://doi.org/10.1016/j.procs.2021.12.230
3. Anwar, A., Rahman, M.M., Ferdous, S., Anik, S.A., Ahmed, S.I.: A computer game based approach for increasing fluency in the speech of the autistic children. In: 2011 IEEE 11th International Conference on Advanced Learning Technologies, pp. 17–18 (2011). https://doi.org/10.1109/ICALT.2011.13
4. Auxier, B.Y.B., Anderson, M., Perrin, A., Turner, E.: Parenting children in the age of screens. Technical report July, Pew Research center (2020). https://www.pewresearch.org/internet/2020/07/28/parenting-children-in-the-age-of-screens/
5. Barrett, N., Swain, I., Gatzidis, C., Mecheraoui, C.: The use and effect of video game design theory in the creation of game-based systems for upper limb stroke rehabilitation. J. Rehab. Assist. Technol. Eng. **3** (2016). https://doi.org/10.1177/2055668316643644
6. Brown, T.: Change by Design: How Design Thinking Transforms Organizations and Inspires Innovation. Harper Collins, New York (2009)
7. Dias, L.P.S., Barbosa, J.L.V., Vianna, H.D.: Gamification and serious games in depression care: a systematic mapping study. Telematics Inform. **35**(1), 213–224 (2018). https://doi.org/10.1016/j.tele.2017.11.002, https://www.sciencedirect.com/science/article/pii/S0736585317305865
8. Durango, I., Carrascosa, A., Gallud, J.A., Penichet, V.M.R.: Using serious games to improve therapeutic goals in children with special needs. In: Proceedings of the 17th International Conference on Human-Computer Interaction with Mobile Devices and Services Adjunct, MobileHCI 2015, pp. 743–749. Association for Computing Machinery, New York (2015).https://doi.org/10.1145/2786567.2793696
9. Frutos, M., Bustos, I., Zapirain, B.G., Zorrilla, A.M.: Computer game to learn and enhance speech problems for children with autism. In: Proceedings of CGAMES'2011 USA - 16th International Conference on Computer Games: AI, Animation, Mobile, Interactive Multimedia, Educational and Serious Games, pp. 209–216 (2011). https://doi.org/10.1109/CGAMES.2011.6000340
10. Furlong, L., Morris, M., Serry, T., Erickson, S.: Mobile apps for treatment of speech disorders in children: an evidence-based analysis of quality and efficacy. PLOS ONE **13**(8), e0201513 (2018). https://doi.org/10.1371/journal.pone.0201513, http://dx.doi.org/10.1371/journal.pone.0201513
11. Gazulla, D., Bauters, E., Hietala, M., Leinonen, I., Kapros, T.: Co-creation and co-design in technology-enhanced learning: innovating science learning outside the classroom. ID&A Interact. Design Archit. 202–226 (2020)
12. Hadław-Klimaszewska, O., Jankowska, A., Laskowska, J., Woldańska-Okońska, M.: Using the soda scale to assess the effectiveness of neurological speech and language therapy on improving language functions in post-stroke patients. Wiadomości Lekarskie **75**(5), 1229–1233 (2022). https://doi.org/10.36740/wlek202205201, http://dx.doi.org/10.36740/WLek202205201
13. Hair, A., Monroe, P., Ahmed, B., Ballard, K.J., Gutierrez-Osuna, R.: Apraxia world: a speech therapy game for children with speech sound disorders. In: Proceedings of the 17th ACM Conference on Interaction Design and Children, IDC 2018,

pp. 119–131. Association for Computing Machinery, New York (2018). https://doi.org/10.1145/3202185.3202733

14. Hajesmaeel-Gohari, S., Goharinejad, S., Shafiei, E., Bahaadinbeigy, K.: Digital games for rehabilitation of speech disorders: a scoping review. Health Sci. Rep. **6**(6) (2023). https://doi.org/10.1002/hsr2.1308, http://dx.doi.org/10.1002/hsr2.1308

15. Hasselbring, T.S., Glaser, C.H.W.: Use of computer technology to help students with special needs. Future Child. **10**, 102–122 (2000). https://doi.org/10.2307/1602691

16. Horne-Moyer, H.L., Moyer, B.H., Messer, D.C., Messer, E.S.: The use of electronic games in therapy: a review with clinical implications. Curr. Psychiatry Rep. **16**(12) (2014). https://doi.org/10.1007/s11920-014-0520-6, http://dx.doi.org/10.1007/s11920-014-0520-6

17. Hosokawa, R., Katsura, T.: Association between mobile technology use and child adjustment in early elementary school age. PLOS ONE **13**(7), e0199959 (2018). https://doi.org/10.1371/journal.pone.0199959, http://dx.doi.org/10.1371/journal.pone.0199959

18. Isabel, A., Filipa, A., Queirós, A., Silva, A.: European Portuguese validation of the system usability scale (SUS). Procedia - Procedia Comput. Sci. **67**(Dsai), 293–300 (2015). https://doi.org/10.1016/j.procs.2015.09.273, http://dx.doi.org/10.1016/j.procs.2015.09.273

19. Law, J., Dennis, J.A., Charlton, J.J.: Speech and language therapy interventions for children with primary speech and/or language disorders. Cochrane Database Syst. Rev. **2017** (2017). https://doi.org/10.1002/14651858.CD012490

20. Lawrence, A., Choe, D.E.: Mobile media and young children's cognitive skills: a review. Acad. Pediatr. **21**(6), 996–1000 (2021). https://doi.org/10.1016/j.acap.2021.01.007, https://www.sciencedirect.com/science/article/pii/S1876285921000085

21. Lee, A.S., Gibbon, F.E.: Non-speech oral motor treatment for children with developmental speech sound disorders. Cochrane Database Syst. Rev. **2015** (2015). https://doi.org/10.1002/14651858.CD009383.PUB2

22. Lewis, J.R., Sauro, J.: Item benchmarks for the system usability scale. J. Usabil. Stud. **13**, 158–167 (2018)

23. Lo, J.L., Chi, P.Y., Chu, H.H., Wang, H.Y., Chou, S.C.T.: Pervasive computing in play-based occupational therapy for children. IEEE Pervasive Comput. **8**(3), 66–73 (2009). https://doi.org/10.1109/MPRV.2009.52

24. Lugmayr, A., Sutinen, E., Suhonen, J., Sedano, C.I., Hlavacs, H., Montero, C.S.: Serious storytelling – a first definition and review. Multimed. Tools Appl. **76**(14), 15707–15733 (2016). https://doi.org/10.1007/s11042-016-3865-5, http://dx.doi.org/10.1007/s11042-016-3865-5

25. Marques, R.: Língua portuguesa e assuntos linguísticos: Os fonemas da língua portuguesa (2008). http://linguaportuguesabyrogeriomarques.blogspot.com/2008/12/os-fonemas-da-lngua-portuguesa.html. Accessed 15 July 2022

26. McKechnie, J., Ahmed, B., Gutierrez-Osuna, R., Monroe, P., McCabe, P., Ballard, K.J.: Automated speech analysis tools for children's speech production: A systematic literature review. Int. J. Speech-Lang. Pathol. **20**(6), 583–598 (2018). https://doi.org/10.1080/17549507.2018.1477991, http://dx.doi.org/10.1080/17549507.2018.1477991

27. Michael, D.R., Chen, S.L.: Serious Games: Games That Educate, Train, and Inform. Muska & Lipman/Premier-Trade (2005)

28. Nasiri, N., Shirmohammadi, S., Rashed, A.: A serious game for children with speech disorders and hearing problems. In: 2017 IEEE 5th International Conference on Serious Games and Applications for Health (SeGAH), pp. 1–7 (2017). https://doi.org/10.1109/SeGAH.2017.7939296
29. Oliveira, C., Lousada, M., Jesus, L.M.: The clinical practice of speech and language therapists with children with phonologically based speech sound disorders. Child Lang. Teach. Ther. **31**(2), 173–194 (2015). https://doi.org/10.1177/0265659014550420
30. Pereira, Í.S.P., Ramos, A., Marsh, J.: The digital literacy and multimodal practices of young children: engaging with emergent research: proceedings of the first training school of cost action is1410, University of Minho, Braga, Portugal, 6–8 June 2016 (2016). https://api.semanticscholar.org/CorpusID:78251270
31. Read, J., Sim, G., Gregory, A., Xu, D., Ode, J.: Children designing serious games. EAI Endors. Trans. Game-Based Learn. **1**, e5 (2013). https://doi.org/10.4108/TRANS.GBL.01-06.2013.E5
32. Roxo, G., Nóbrega, R., Madeira, R.N.: Dance mat fun - a participatory design of exergames for children with disabilities. In: Tsanas, A., Triantafyllidis, A. (eds.) PH 2022. LNICS, vol. 488, pp. 513–527. Springer, Cham (2023). https://doi.org/10.1007/978-3-031-34586-9_34
33. Saeedi, S., Bouraghi, H., Seifpanahi, M.S., Ghazisaeedi, M.: Application of digital games for speech therapy in children: a systematic review of features and challenges. J. Healthc. Eng. **2022**, 1–20 (2022). https://doi.org/10.1155/2022/4814945, http://dx.doi.org/10.1155/2022/4814945
34. Silva, C., Peixoto, V.: Rastreio e prevalência das perturbações da comunicação num agrupamento de escolas. Rev. Fac. Ciências Saúde (5), 274–282 (2008). https://bdigital.ufp.pt/handle/10284/969
35. Susi, T., Johannesson, M., Backlund, P.: Serious games: an overview (2007). https://api.semanticscholar.org/CorpusID:13561855
36. Valenza, M.V., Hounsell, M.D.S., Gasparini, I.: Serious game design for children: validating a set of guidelines. In: Proceedings - IEEE 19th International Conference on Advanced Learning Technologies, ICALT 2019, pp. 110–112 (2019). https://doi.org/10.1109/ICALT.2019.00034
37. Weiler, M., Weiler, A., McKenzie, D.: Co-design: a powerful force for creativity and collaboration (2016). https://medium.com/@thestratosgroup/co-design-a-powerful-force-for-creativity-and-collaboration-bed1e0f13d46. Accessed 15 July 2022
38. Wrzesien, M., Alcañiz, M., Botella, C., Burkhardt, J.-M., Lopez, J.B., Ortega, A.R.: A pilot evaluation of a therapeutic game applied to small animal phobia treatment. In: Ma, M., Oliveira, M.F., Baalsrud Hauge, J. (eds.) SGDA 2014. LNCS, vol. 8778, pp. 10–20. Springer, Cham (2014). https://doi.org/10.1007/978-3-319-11623-5_2

Pervasive Health in Clinical Practice

A Decentralized Clinical Trial of a Digital Intervention with Multiple Health Trackers for Heart Failure: Early Learnings and Practical Considerations

Rachel Tunis[1]([✉]), Tom Baranowski[2], Angelica Rangel[3], James Custer[4],
Edison Thomaz[5], Paul Rathouz[4], Jay Bartroff[6], Christine Julien[5], Grace Lee[5],
Matthew O'Hair[7], Miyong Kim[3], and Kavita Radhakrishnan[3]

[1] School of Information, The University of Texas at Austin, Austin, USA
rtunis@utexas.edu
[2] Children's Nutrition Research Center, Department of Pediatrics, Baylor College of Medicine, Houston, USA
[3] School of Nursing, The University of Texas at Austin, Austin, USA
[4] Department of Population Health, Dell Medical School, The University of Texas at Austin, Austin, USA
[5] Department of Electrical and Computer Engineering, The University of Texas at Austin, Austin, USA
[6] Department of Statistics and Data Sciences, The University of Texas at Austin, Austin, USA
[7] Good Life Games, LLC, Austin, TX, USA

Abstract. DT4HF (Digital Tools for Heart Failure) is carrying out, to the best of our knowledge, the only fully decentralized randomized clinical trial assessing an intervention for heart failure self-management. Participants in the study use a smart scale and activity tracker to monitor important self-management behaviors, and those in the Intervention Group also play a digital game to help further motivate adherence to these behaviors. All study activities take place remotely. In this paper, we describe our experiences recruiting and enrolling participants during the first six months of the study. We also discuss themes and challenges that are unique to decentralized trials and contribute to existing literature by describing how we have dealt with these issues and what considerations might be relevant to other researchers executing decentralized trials. While completing screening, enrollment, and installation entirely remotely presents challenges, we have already begun to see some of the benefits of the decentralized design and the positive impact the study is having on participants.

Keywords: Heart Failure · Self-Management · Remote Monitoring · Decentralized Trials · Digital Health

D. Salvi et al. (Eds.): PH 2023, LNICST 572, pp. 223–234, 2024.
https://doi.org/10.1007/978-3-031-59717-6_15

1 Introduction

1.1 Background and Related Work

More than six million Americans live with heart failure (HF), a chronic condition which is the leading cause of hospitalization among older adults in the U.S. [5] HF is expected to increase in prevalence, incurring tens of billions of dollars in costs in the coming years [1]. Furthermore, there are widening geographical [2, 3] and racial [4] disparities in the HF patient population. For example, Mujib et al. [2] found evidence of a "heart failure belt" spanning the southeast United States, with age-adjusted mortality rates 69% higher than the national rate. Given the chronic nature of HF, diligent self-management is required to improve outcomes, involving adherence to a regimen of medication, regular physical activity, weight management, and monitoring of diet and fluid intake. Self-management may be aided by digital health technologies that allow for continuous monitoring and measurement, track important information, and provide feedback directly to users.

The increasing uptake of novel digital health tools for managing and monitoring many elements of one's health has coincided with a trend towards decentralized clinical trials (DCTs), or trials where activities "occur at locations other than traditional clinical trial sites," such as virtually or in participants' homes [8]. The Clinical Trials Transformation Initiative (CTTI), which was co-founded by the U.S. Food and Drug Administration (FDA) and Duke University, released recommendations for the conduct of DCTs in 2018, citing possible improved retention, greater control for participants, and increased participant diversity [6]. In 2020, the Decentralized Trials and Research Alliance was launched by the FDA and more than 50 other health-focused organizations, from pharmaceutical companies to patient advocacy groups [7]. In May 2023, the FDA released draft guidance on DCTs, stating that, "by enabling remote participation, DCTs may enhance convenience for trial participants, reduce the burden on caregivers, and facilitate research on… diseases affecting populations with limited mobility or access to traditional trial sites" [8].

Indeed, many clinical trials have incorporated elements of remote participation in their design, aided largely by digital health devices such as wearable sensors and mobile apps which can both collect data passively to be shared with research teams and can serve as elements of health interventions for patients managing chronic health conditions. Tools like Apple's ResearchKit [23] have made it possible for researchers to set up studies that can easily access and integrate the rich data collected through or synced with the devices people use every day. Trials focusing on HF or cardiovascular health more broadly have provided participants with step counters/activity trackers [9–13], weight scales [10], blood pressure monitors [10, 11], sleep trackers [11], and ECG sensors [13], among others. While embracing elements of remote trial participation, these studies are not completely decentralized. Nearly all of them are still tethered to some primary clinical site through which they recruit participants. A few notable exceptions are the MyHeart Counts study [22], which participants can join by downloading the app and going through an eConsent process, and Health eHeart [14], which recruits participants online. However, these studies are focused on heart health broadly, not just HF.

To the best of our knowledge, our study, DT4HF (Digital Tools for Heart Failure), is the first fully decentralized trial for HF patients. DT4HF assesses the efficacy of a sensor-controlled digital game (SCDG) for helping older adults with HF improve adherence to key self-management behaviors, i.e., daily physical activity and weight monitoring. We recruit participants entirely remotely, with a focus on the seven southern states that have higher rates of HF, in hopes that the decentralized approach may target a portion of the patient population that is of high need and are underserved [2, 3].

1.2 Research Aims

In this paper, we discuss major themes that have emerged six months after beginning enrollment. We build upon prior work by describing screening, enrollment, and installation processes as one of the first fully decentralized trials testing a digital intervention for HF self-management. We contribute to existing literature by providing detailed descriptions of the unique challenges and benefits of decentralized studies that we have seen firsthand in DT4HF, as well as strategies used to address these issues. We also discuss our early experiences with recruitment and compare our recruitment rate with those of similar centralized studies. As clinical studies increasingly move towards decentralization, we hope our findings and reflections may be useful to others planning or executing similar studies.

2 Methods

2.1 Study Procedure

DT4HF is a randomized clinical trial that aims to assess the efficacy of a SCDG for helping older adults with HF improve adherence to important self-management behaviors (weight management and physical activity). In total, the study will recruit two-hundred participants with HF, each randomized to either the Intervention (IG) or the Control Groups (CG). All participants are 45 years of age or older, have been hospitalized for HF within the past 12 months, and live in one of the seven southern U.S. states (Alabama, Arkansas, Georgia, Louisiana, Mississippi, Oklahoma, and Texas). Participants in both groups receive a Withings smart scale and activity tracker in the mail to regularly track their daily weight and steps. The IG also plays the SCDG, Heart Health Mountain, developed and tested by the study team [15], which collects data from the scale and tracker and provides personalized feedback to continually motivate participants to actively engage in important behaviors. In the game, participants progressively climb a mountain by adhering to their self-management behaviors and completing mini-games and challenges containing educational information related to HF. The game was designed using behavior change theoretical frameworks, specifically the Fogg Behavioral Model and self-determination theory, as described in detail elsewhere [21]. Our study protocol, which describes the methods in greater detail, is also available elsewhere [16].

The first participant was enrolled in the study in November 2022. As of May 2023, twenty participants have been enrolled across five of the seven eligible states.

Recruitment. For the first six months, our primary method of recruitment has been through TrialFacts, an online recruiting company [20]. TrialFacts distributes advertisements through social media to people who appear to meet our inclusion criteria. Potential participants then complete a survey demonstrating interest and indicating a time that works for them for a screening call with the study team.

Screening and Enrollment. Once a potential participant has demonstrated interest and been referred through TrialFacts, a member of our team conducts a screening call to confirm eligibility (i.e., age, ability to walk independently, willingness to install apps with remote support, WiFi status at home). During this call, our team informs potential participants that they need to provide a hospital discharge summary showing that they were hospitalized for HF within the past 12 months. If they are not able to do this, they may provide written confirmation of their HF diagnosis and recent hospitalization from their healthcare provider with a list of current medications. Potential participants also complete a brief mini-cognitive screening [17] to assess cognitive eligibility for the study. If a potential participant is confirmed as eligible and has shared their discharge summary, a study team member calls the participant and goes through the Informed Consent document, which the participant electronically signs.

Installation of Apps and Devices. After a participant has consented to participate, their devices (Withings Body scale and Pulse HR activity tracker) are sent by mail. All participants receive printed instructions for installing these devices, the accompanying Withings Health Mate app, and the digital game app (for participants in the IG). Participants in the CG receive printouts of standard evidence-based HF educational content [18] which IG participants receive through playing the game. All participants are instructed not to install their devices until a study team member calls to walk them through the installation, which can take place either on Zoom or over the phone (depending on the participant's preference). Installation calls have taken anywhere between twenty minutes and two hours.

2.2 Assessment of Early Learnings and Practical Considerations

To reflect upon the major themes and issues that have arisen during the initial months of enrollment, our team extracted data from the project management platform, Trello, to glean information related to participant recruitment, such as the amount of time between first contact and enrollment in the study and the average number of touchpoints with each potential participant. We reviewed all data in Trello[1] on the progress of participants from the time they initially expressed interest, continuously as they progressed through the 24 weeks of data collection. We also reviewed notes taken by the technical support team

---

[1] Trello is used systematically by the study team to log notes following any touchpoint with participants during the initial phases of the study (recruitment, enrollment, and installation) and to track their progress over the course of the study. If 3 days elapse where no data is synced from a participant's study apps or devices, the study team contacts them to address any issues (whether technical, such as installing a new WiFi router at home, or logistical, such as going on vacation). These incidents are then logged as official "protocol deviations" and are out of the scope of this paper.

from installation calls with newly enrolled participants. Additionally, we discuss four qualitative interviews which informed us directly about participants' experiences in the study. By reporting on the unique challenges and benefits that come with decentralized studies and sharing how our team has addressed these issues, this paper contributes to existing literature on conducting decentralized clinical trials that leverage digital tools.

3   Results

3.1   Overview

Six months after our first participant was enrolled (from November 2022 to May 2023), we enrolled twenty participants, including nine IG and eleven CG participants (see Table 1), which is 27.8% of the 72 patients who completed the pre-screening survey through TrialFacts. Of the twenty enrolled participants, five have dropped out (25% attrition was allowed in the study design [16]). The average age of participants is 58.5, and seventy percent of the currently enrolled participants are male. Eighty percent are White, fifteen percent are Black or African American, and five percent are American Indian or Alaskan Native. The participants live in five of the targeted seven states. Fourteen of the twenty live in Texas; two participants live in each of Georgia and Oklahoma; and one participant lives in each of Louisiana and Alabama. The average distance (in miles) of participants' zip codes from the UT Austin campus zip code is 310.4 (min: 8.4, max: 928). From the time of first contact until the date of installation of the participant's study apps and devices, the average elapsed time was 15.4 days. During this time, our study team had an average of 3.4 contacts with each participant (e.g., a follow-up on missed calls or a reminder to send discharge summaries).

Table 1. Recruitment data for enrolled participants

Participant number	Points of contact before enrollment	Days between first contact and equipment installation	Distance from UT Austin (miles)	State	Dropped since enrollment?
1	6	16	88.8	TX	Yes
2	3	23	149.5	TX	No
3	3	11	140.7	TX	No
4	2	11	307.4	TX	No
5	4	37	730.3	AL	No
6	3	17	913.1	GA	No
7	3	7	239.3	TX	Yes
8	4	27	211.1	TX	Yes

(*continued*)

Table 1. (*continued*)

Participant number	Points of contact before enrollment	Days between first contact and equipment installation	Distance from UT Austin (miles)	State	Dropped since enrollment?
9	6	12	149.2	TX	No
10	2	10	20.7	TX	No
11	3	13	397.9	OK	No
12	4	21	104.9	TX	No
13	1	9	126	TX	No
14	3	12	8.4	TX	No
15	2	14	511.4	LA	No
16	2	14	223.1	TX	No
17	6	N/A	928	GA	Yes
18	3	9	480	OK	No
19	5	14	373	TX	No
20	2	16	104.9	TX	Yes
Average	3.4 ($\sigma = 1.42$)	15.42 ($\sigma = 7.07$)	310.39 ($\sigma = 269.04$)		

3.2 Themes and Challenges

Screening. A potential participant's completion of an initial screening questionnaire is far from an automatic indicator that they will be willing and able to enroll in the study. Even though the screening questionnaire asks potential participants to commit to answering their phones at the time they designate, many do not. The screening call requires potential participants' full attention for ten to fifteen minutes, as it includes a brief cognitive screening, so the call cannot take place while they are doing something else, such as driving or shopping. Of the potential participants that can be reached for a screening call, some turn down participation in the study (see Table 2) upon realizing that some effort will be required of them (e.g., completing surveys, installing digital tools). Since participation in the study comes with a small financial incentive, some participants are enticed by this prospect without realizing what is necessary on their part. Nine of the seventy-two initially screened potential participants ultimately declined participation; an additional twenty-two were lost to follow-up. Finally, the biggest barrier to enrollment has been not meeting inclusion criteria. Even though it is a part of the initial screening questionnaire, potential participants often do not meet the criteria of having a hospitalization related to HF in the past 12 months. Twenty-one of the seventy-two initially screened potential participants were ultimately not eligible for the study—twelve of these had not had a hospitalization in the past 12 months, eight did not have a HF diagnosis or related hospitalization. This discrepancy between the information the patient provides through their initial screening questionnaire and the facts of their medical diagnoses and hospitalizations is a challenge for decentralized trials, as traditional clinical trial sites would be able to verify and screen for this information internally.

Table 2. Outcomes for all potential participants screened in first 6 months

Not eligible: No HF diagnosis or related hospitalization	8 (11.1%)
Not eligible: Hospitalization was not in previous 12 months	12 (16.7%)
Not eligible: Age	1 (1.4%)
Turned down participation	9 (12.5%)
Lost to follow-up	22 (30.6%)
Enrolled in study	20 (27.8%)
Total	**72**

Enrollment. Once a potential participant is deemed eligible from the screening call, a big hurdle is receiving a copy of their discharge summary from their recent hospitalization and validating the diagnosis of HF. Participants can either scan or photograph a hard copy of their discharge summary or download it electronically through their patient portal, and then upload the file to the study's secure platform. Given an older study population, uploading and transferring files can be intimidating or discouraging to some participants. It is common for the study team to follow up several times to assist participants with locating and/or uploading the correct file.

Additionally, some potential participants have had a recent hospitalization but not a HF diagnosis; they might have had, for example, a heart arrhythmia or a cardiac arrest. Health literacy can be a relevant factor, as potential participants might think they are eligible for a HF study given some kind of cardiac-related hospitalization. This is also a challenge traditional trials would not face, as they are generally connected to a hospital or clinic that can automatically access discharge summaries and verify diagnoses; patients are not usually in the position of vouching for their own diagnoses.

While the process of obtaining and validating potential participants' discharge summaries is the most time-consuming part of the enrollment process and requires the most effort on the part of the patient, the study team believes it is the best way to rigorously assess an important inclusion criterion, especially given that the study is not tied to any clinical site.

Installation of Apps and Devices. Once a participant has been enrolled in the study after completing Informed Consent, they receive their study devices (Withings Body scale and Pulse HR activity tracker) by mail. A member of the study team conducts a telephone or Zoom call to walk them through the installation of the devices, as well as the Withings app and, for game group participants, the Heart Health Mountain app. While installation calls with Control Group participants are typically shorter given that there is one less thing to install and explain, the length of all installation calls vary considerably depending on the participant's familiarity with apps and sensor-connected devices, WiFi or syncing issues, or communication challenges due to being remote.

Technical issues while syncing the scale or activity tracker to the Withings app on the participant's phone happen fairly frequently and are generally not due to user error or communication issues. The scale had consistently more issues syncing to the Withings app on participants' phones than the watch. Troubleshooting steps available through the Withings website often helped, such as taking out batteries and restarting the scale, holding the phone near to the scale, making the phone "forget" the device, or attempting the installation on a different device such as a tablet. Slow WiFi was also occasionally the cause of syncing issues. When troubleshooting efforts still did not resolve syncing or other technical issues, the issues usually resolved themselves over the course of a few days or through a troubleshooting call at a later time. We were able to progressively foresee and address certain technical issues; for example, activity trackers could not be successfully installed with a low battery, so as the study progressed and our stock of activity trackers began to lose battery charge, the team began plugging the trackers in to charge prior to mailing them to participants.

Outside of technical issues, installation calls varied in that participants themselves ranged significantly in their familiarity with digital health devices, technological literacy, and confidence in navigating the installation. Typically, the study team member completing the installation began by asking participants whether they had ever used similar devices before; some regularly used Fitbits or Apple Watches, others had never used any kind of health tracker before. Some participants came into the call having already prepped and charged devices and downloaded the required apps, while others required step-by-step instruction and were more unsure and tentative during the installation. For participants who were less experienced with health trackers and more easily discouraged, consistent encouragement was vital. When roadblocks arose with these participants (such as having clicked the wrong button and being unable to return to the right screen), the remote design of the study proved difficult as the study team was not able to intervene except through verbal guidance, and while some sort of remote administration tool may have helped address this issue, this was not something we considered for privacy reasons. Instead, strategies such as having the participant send a screenshot or verbally describe every option visible on the screen was helpful. All participants were ultimately able to install their devices and apps with the remote support provided by the study team.

4 Discussion

As previously mentioned, one of the elements of the study that presents added challenges given the decentralized design is the recruitment of participants, as DT4HF has no primary study site tied to a clinical database and large group of patients. After the first six months of the study, however, our recruitment rate stands at 27.8% (twenty participants enrolled out of seventy-two who completed our initial screening questionnaire). Despite being a fully decentralized study, our recruitment rate may be comparable to and, in some cases, higher than, similar studies with traditional trial sites. A comprehensive review of recruitment, consent, and retention rates of hundreds of trials found that the median recruitment rate (participants per trial site, per month) was 0.95 [19]. Having recruited twenty patients in six months, our recruitment rate is 3.33, which would put us just below the 80th percentile (3.70) of studies in the review. Of course, this review encompasses a wide range of study types and focus areas; it serves as just one reference point for trial recruitment rates. As for studies focused on HF specifically, while we did not complete a comprehensive review, we found recruitment rates to range significantly, from less than 1% [13] to about 40% [10]. While there is no single reliable metric to serve as a reference point for clinical trial recruitment rates, this study's rate certainly does not seem to be significantly lower than traditional clinical studies (in some cases it may even be higher), despite the additional challenges in screening and enrolling patients that have arisen from the study's decentralized design. Thus, while it may be a good idea to plan for the possibility of lower recruitment rates and make sample sizes estimates accordingly, the prospect of lower recruitment rates in decentralized trials should not dissuade researchers from this study design. Regardless of the circumstances, it is important for researchers to analyze recruitment rates early on in trials to inform their strategies. As such, our team is currently pursuing additional avenues for recruitment in an effort to raise our recruitment rates over the course of the 24 months of recruitment that remain. For example, the strategies we are currently pursuing include (1) expanding from working with only social media marketing-based recruitment partners to Internet-search based recruitment partners (allowing us to advertise our study to people who are actively searching for information, resources, or research opportunities related to HF), (2) utilizing word-of-mouth and networking at local clinical settings to solicit interest, (3) radio advertising in areas that correspond to the zip codes with the highest concentration of HF cases in the U.S.

A final strategy that we used to boost our recruitment rate was reexamining the inclusion criteria with a focus on what was causing the most interested participants to be ineligible. For example, initially, our inclusion criteria required having been hospitalized for HF within the past 6 months, but this was causing a large number of interested participants to be ineligible. To address this, we discussed the topic with clinical experts and submitted an IRB update proposing to adapt our inclusion criteria to include those hospitalized within the past 12 months, which allows us to maintain our focus on HF patients with recent hospitalizations while being inclusive of more potential participants. We advise other researchers who may be assessing their recruitment rates and strategies to ask themselves where it might be possible to expand either their inclusion criteria or the places they are looking to recruit.

While our study is in its early stages, initial assessments of participants' experiences have begun to shed light on the potential benefits of the study's decentralized design. To date, four qualitative interviews have been completed with participants.[2] Two of the four interviewees had used health self-tracking devices prior to the study, and they both reported positive experiences in the study; they felt that regular use of their devices helped them keep tabs on their HF and feel confident that they were on the right path. The other two interviewees had never used such devices previously, but they also reported extremely positive experiences. One of these interviewees shared that prior to the study,

---

[2] One out of every five participants will be interviewed when they reach the 12-week mark (the halfway point in the study).

he thought "that stuff was for treehuggers." This participant has had a life-changing experience in the study, claiming that using health trackers for the first time has helped him care about his health again; his devices have become "integral and paramount" to his daily routine, leading to him having more energy, motivation, and even better relationships with those around him. The second interviewee who also had never used any digital trackers before stated that he "just never thought about it," but now says that he "will not be without some sort of monitor, even after the study is over." This participant lives in a remote area more than one hundred and fifty miles from the nearest large city (more than a quarter of participants in the study live more than fifty miles from the nearest large city). The study's decentralized design may thus allow participants like these to be more engaged and derive more value from the study, as they are not required to make regular visits to a central clinic, which are usually found in larger cities. Given that two of the four interviewees did not use or were not interested in using digital tools prior to the study, their motivation to participate in a study on digital tools for self-management may not have been sufficient to travel long distances multiple times to a central research site. However, with a small sample size given the study is still in its early stages, it remains to be seen whether we will continue to see this trend.

On a final, related note: an important aspect of our study is the personalization of both our approach to working with participants and the digital tools themselves. Participants come into the study with very different backgrounds, self-management preferences, and experiences with technology. Participants' motivations for joining the study (as reported in their initial screening questionnaires) range from looking for knowledge and educational resources, to looking for accountability, to just wanting to participate in research. Some were newly diagnosed and looking to learn the ropes of self-management, while others have lived with HF for years, even decades. With the variation in participants' levels of familiarity with technology and comfort using new digital tools, the study team can quickly adapt over the course of the installation (i.e., by simplifying explanations, taking things more slowly, etc.) What really shapes participants' experiences in the study, however, is the digital tools themselves, and this is even more true in a decentralized study where the in-person element is removed, and the focus is fully on the digital tools. As such, it is critical for decentralized studies testing digital tools to ensure that they can be adaptable, encompassing a range of participants' potential contexts and preferences. Future research should seek to explore additional ways that patients' unique circumstances, goals, and/or health management preferences could be incorporated into health interventions.

5 Conclusion

The first six months of DT4HF have demonstrated both the challenges and the potential advantages of a decentralized design for a clinical trial. Screening and enrollment in particular come with the challenge of potential participants having to vouch for their own diagnosis, which they may not be aware is not a fit for the study's eligibility criteria. For patients who are indeed eligible, the study faces the challenge of not being able to verify a potential participant's diagnosis without a hospital discharge summary, which can be difficult for participants to locate and transmit virtually. Remote installations of digital tools often come with technical issues, but remote support from the study team has been sufficient to ensure that all study participants are able to get their equipment set up properly. While the study is still in its early stages, we have seen some advantages of the decentralized design in that we have successfully enrolled multiple participants who live in remote areas who may not have been able to participate in a centralized trial as easily. Our early assessments of participants' experiences have indicated that some participants have come to view the digital tools as crucial in their self-management routines, despite having never used anything similar before the study. As our study progresses and as other studies testing digital health interventions evolve, it is vital to ensure that interventions can adapt to variations in patients' health-related preferences and circumstances in order to create meaningful, positive change in their lives.

References

1. Benjamin, E.J., Muntner, P., Alonso, A., Bittencourt, M.S., Callaway, C.W., et al.: Heart disease and stroke statistics—2019 update: a report from the American Heart Association. Circulation **139**(10), e56–e528 (2019). https://doi.org/10.1161/CIR.0000000000000659
2. Mujib, M., Zhang, Y., Feller, M.A., Ahmed, A.: Evidence of a "Heart Failure Belt" in the southeastern United States. Am. J. Cardiol. **107**(6), 935–937 (2011). https://doi.org/10.1016/j.amjcard.2010.11.012
3. Liu, L., Yin, X., Chen, M., Jia, H., Eisen, H.J., Hofman, A.: Geographic variation in heart failure mortality and its association with hypertension, diabetes, and behavioral-related risk factors in 1,723 counties of the United States. Front. Public Health **6**, 132 (2018). https://doi.org/10.3389/fpubh.2018.00132
4. Lewsey, S.C., Breathett, K.: Racial and ethnic disparities in heart failure. Curr. Opin. Cardiol. **36**(3), 320–328 (2021). https://doi.org/10.1097/HCO.0000000000000855
5. Virani, S.S., Alonso, A., Benjamin, E.J., et al.: Heart disease and stroke statistics—2020 update: a report from the American Heart Association. Circulation **141**(9), e139–e596 (2020). https://doi.org/10.1161/CIR.0000000000000757
6. Clinical Trails Transformation Initiative. Decentralized Clinical Trials, September 2018. https://ctti-clinicaltrials.org/wp-content/uploads/2021/06/CTTI_DCT_Recs.pdf
7. Decentralized Trials & Research Alliance. Dtra.org
8. Food and Drug Administration. Decentralized Clinical Trials for Drugs, Biological Products, and Devices: Guidance for Industry, Investigators, and Other Stakeholders. Draft Guidance, May 2023. https://www.fda.gov/media/167696/download
9. Deka, P., Pozehl, B., Williams, M., Norman, J., Khazanchi, D., Pathak, D.: MOVE-HF: an internet-based pilot study to improve adherence to exercise in patients with heart failure. Eur. J. Cardiovasc. Nursing **18**(2), 122–131 (2019). https://doi.org/10.1177/1474515118796613
10. Thorup, C., Hansen, J., Gronkjaer, M., Andreassen, J., Nielsen, G., et al.: Cardiac patients' walking activity determined by a step counter in cardiac telerehabilitation: data from the intervention arm of a randomized controlled trial. J. Med. Internet Res. **18**(4), e69 (2016). https://doi.org/10.2196/jmir.5191
11. Habibovic, M., Broers, E., Piera-Jimenez, J., Wetzels, M., Ayoola, I., et al.: Enhancing lifestyle change in cardiac patients through the Do CHANGE System ("Do Cardiac Health: Advanced New Generation Ecosystem"): randomized controlled trial protocol. JMIR Res. Protoc. **7**(2), e40 (2018). https://doi.org/10.2196/resprot.8406
12. Nagamoti, Y., Ide, T., Higuchi, T., Nezu, T., Fujino, T., et al.: Home-based cardiac rehabilitation using information and communication technology for heart failure patients with frailty. ESC Heart Fail **9**(4), 2407–2418 (2022). https://doi.org/10.1002/ehf2.13934

13. Steinhubl, S.R., Waalen, J., Edwards, A., Ariniello, L., Mehta, R., et al.: Effects of a home-based wearable continuous ECG monitoring patch on detection of undiagnosed atrial fibrillation: the mSToPS randomized clinical trial. JAMA **320**(2), 146–155 (2018). https://doi.org/10.1001/jama.2018.8102

14. Guo, X., Vittinghoff, E., Olgin, J., Marcus, G., Pletcher, M.: Volunteer participation in the health eHeart study: a comparison with the US population. Sci. Rep. **7**, 1956 (2017). https://doi.org/10.1038/s41598-017-02232-y

15. Radhakrishnan, K., Julien, C., Baranowski, T., et al.: Feasibility of a sensor-controlled digital game for heart failure self-management: randomized controlled trial. JMIR Serious Games **9**(4), e29044 (2021). https://doi.org/10.2196/29044

16. Radhakrishnan, K., Julien, C., O'Hair, M., Tunis, R., Lee, G., et al.: Sensor-controlled digital game for heart failure self-management: protocol for a randomized controlled trial. JMIR Res. Protoc. **12**, e45801 (2023). https://doi.org/10.2196/45801

17. Borson, S., Scanlan, J., Brush, M., Vitaliano, P., Dokmak, A.: The Mini-Cog: a cognitive "vital signs" measure for dementia screening in multi-lingual elderly. Int. J. Geriatr. Psychiatry **15**(11), 1021–1027 (2000). https://doi.org/10.1002/1099-1166(200011)15:11%3c1021::aid-gps234%3e3.0.co;2-6

18. Heart Failure Society of America. Heart Failure Educational Modules. https://hfsa.org/heart-failure-educational-modules

19. Jacques, R., Ahmed, R., Harper, J., Ranjan, A., Saeed, I., et al.: Recruitment, consent and retention of participants in randomized controlled trials: a review of trials published in the National Institute for Health Research (NIHR) Journals Library (1997–2020). BMJ Open **12**, e059230 (2022). https://doi.org/10.1136/bmjopen-2021-059230

20. TrialFacts. Trialfacts.com

21. Radhakrishnan, K., Julien, C., O'Hair, M., Lee, G., DeMain, A.S., et al.: A sensor-controlled digital game for heart failure self-care based on behavioral change frameworks. In: 2022 IEEE 10th International Conference on Serious Games and Applications for Health, pp 1–6 (2022). https://doi.org/10.1109/SEGAH54908.2022.9978594

22. Hershman, C., Bot, B., Shcherbina, A., Doerr, M., Moayedi, Y., et al.: Physical activity, sleep, and cardiovascular health data for 50,000 individuals from the MyHeart Counts Study. Sci. Data **6**(24) (2019). https://doi.org/10.1038/s41597-019-0016-7

23. Apple. ResearchKit and CareKit: Empowering medical researchers, doctors, and you. https://www.apple.com/lae/researchkit/. Accessed 9 Oct 2023

Activity Recognition of Nursing Tasks in a Hospital: Requirements and Challenges

Fenja T. Bruns(✉) [iD], Alexander Pauls [iD], Frauke Koppelin [iD],
and Frank Wallhoff [iD]

Jade University of Applied Sciences, Oldenburg, Germany
fenja.bruns@jade-hs.de

Abstract. In nursing, the documentation of the nursing activities carried out plays an important role. However, the shortage of nursing staff and the resulting increasing lack of time means that the documentation is often not filled out completely. Human activity recognition (HAR) could assist with documentation by automatically recognising the services performed and entering them into the documentation system. For this purpose, data from different wearable and stationary sensors have to be processed. This paper will describe the requirements to develop such an activity recognition system. These are both functional and non-functional requirements. These requirements have been developed both from a review of current literature and after discussions with nursing students and representatives of nursing management of local hospitals and nursing science. In addition, activities in nursing that frequently need to be documented are listed. The results should therefore serve as a basis for the implementation of a system for the HAR of nursing activities.

Keywords: Activity Recognition · Requirements · Nursing Documentation · Nurse Care Activity Recognition

1 Introduction

In nursing care, both short- and long-term care, it is essential to have information on the patient's activities and nursing records. Nursing documentation contains information about activities that have been carried out as part of the nursing process. This includes aspects of care education, diagnosis, planning, implementation and duration of care. The increasing demands for quality assurance and transparency lead to additional obligations with regard to the documentation. One study confirms a time expenditure of 13% of working time for care documentation, while employees estimate the effort at 20–30% [1,2].

Studies show that employees in nursing suffer from burnout comparatively often. In 2017, a survey showed that almost 40% of nurses suffer from burnout, compared to only 28% in the rest of the population [3]. Dall'Ora et al. have shown that a high workload in particular can lead to burnout. This is also due to staff

D. Salvi et al. (Eds.): PH 2023, LNICST 572, pp. 235–243, 2024.
https://doi.org/10.1007/978-3-031-59717-6_16

shortages in nursing. Higher patient-to-nurse ratios as well as high time pressure are associated with emotional exhaustion and dissatisfaction [4]. In addition, dissatisfied patients can also lead to this. In combination with low usability of the electronic health record, this is a source of stress and frustration among nurses [5].

Germany's Federal Ministry of Health is planning the digitalisation of the health care system. Digitally supported care documentation should lead to a reduction in the workload of caregivers. Automatic documentation of vital parameters can take place through networked monitoring systems. In addition, a major goal of the digitisation strategy is to increase the syntactic and semantic interoperability of nursing documentation [6].

An examination of existing digitisation projects has shown that the majority of projects (48.4%) relate to the support of people in need of care. These include projects on coping and dealing with illness- or therapy-related stress, projects on social participation and mobility. Only 14% of the work examined is directed at professional carers, with just under half of the projects focusing on documentation, especially the (further) development of documentation systems and the networking and automation of staff and route planning. It is noticeable that most of the work focuses on the outpatient sector (49%), while only 7% of the work is related to stationary care [7].

2 Related Work

To facilitate nursing documentation, digital products in particular are distributed to make documentation clearer and to enable immediate availability of the patient's record. Based on text entries from the assessment and nursing reports, nursing diagnoses and a nursing care plan are automatically suggested. However, text-based entries are tedious and can be error-prone, and in the case of voice-based entries, incorrect entries can occur due to lack of text comprehension and background noise [8].

An alternative to manual documentation, whether typed or by voice input, is the automatic recognition of the performed activity and the automatic documentation in the system afterwards. Both cameras and wearable sensors are used for Human Activity Recognition (HAR). Mainly activities of daily life, such as walking, climbing stairs, or fall detection are recognised [9].

Initial research work is dealing with the HAR of nursing activities. Kaczmarek et al. use accelerometers on the upper body to record activities such as repositioning, transfer and mobilisation. However, the accuracy of the classification was only about 55%, but could be improved with additional information about the caregiver's location [10]. Konak et al. combine accelerometer and image data to record nursing activities, such as helping with dressing or preparing medication. Video recordings are also used to determine the optimal sensor placement for the accelerometer. It is stated that optimal sensor placements are at the wrists and pelvis. However, results for other body regions are not described. With the multimodal approach, recognition difficulties occur when the camera is obscured [11].

Lago et al. use a motion capture system, but they use body markers tracked by infrared cameras. In addition, the acceleration sensors of a smartphone and sensors for localisation are used. Activities such as measuring vital parameters, oral care or washing were recorded. The result shows that only the use of acceleration data is unsuitable for tracking activities. Instead, the other modalities should be used [12]. However, a motion capture system and the application of body markers are impractical. This is because several cameras are needed and several body markers have to be placed all over the body or upper body. This is not user-friendly for everyday use. Carrying a smartphone during working hours also often does not correspond to reality. The acceleration data is provided as part of the Nurse Care Activity Recognition Challenge [13].

3   Aim and Methods

In order to relieve the nursing staff, nursing activities will therefore be tracked and stored in the documentation software as part of the "Data-driven Health (DEAL)" project. It should not be a tracking of the person being cared for or the patient by checking whether he or she has fallen or how much has been drunk. Instead, the system should recognise the activities of the nurse, e.g. whether medication was given or whether vital signs were checked. This should be done in order to automate the nursing documentation and thus give the nursing staff more time for the care and the patients. In contrast to the related work presented, which for the most part have not specified a setting, we want to focus specifically on the clinical setting. The specification is necessary because the scope of the documentation and the activities to be documented depend on it. In addition, the clinical setting is characterised by a more dynamic daily routine than, for example, the outpatient setting [14].

In order to develop a user-oriented technology, nursing professionals are to be involved in the development. By actively involving nursing students in the development process, acceptance problems and barriers to innovation can be reduced [15]. In the context of a World Café with twelve nursing students, initial ideas were developed about which nursing activities need to be documented frequently and which critical aspects need to be taken into account in an automatic activity recognition system. The participants were divided into two groups and discussed the questions for about 30 min each. In addition, representatives of the nursing management and nursing science of regional hospitals were invited as part of a project advisory board. This advisory board will support the realisation of the project and advise on any questions that may arise. In a first meeting, expert feedback was given on which organisational and technical aspects should be considered in the development of a system for activity analysis. The resulting requirements for the system from the World Café and the advisory board will be described in the following.

4   Results

At this point, the requirements for the system should be described first. These are divided into functional (FR) and non-functional requirements (NR). This is followed by a description of possible activities and scenarios that often need to be documented in the clinical setting.

4.1   Functional Requirements

The main task of the system is to recognise activities of a nurse in a clinical setting (FR1). If the system has recognised an activity incorrectly or not at all, it must be possible to correct or supplement the entries (FR2). An activity often consists of several steps. For example, wound care involves removing the dressing, photographing and measuring the wound for documentation, cleaning the wound and applying a new dressing. The system must therefore know the regularly performed activities that are to be recognised, as well as the individual intermediate steps that belong to the activity (FR3). For this, an activity inventory must be defined and relevant data must be collected. The system must make it possible to interrupt an activity and continue it at a later time (FR4). It must also be possible to swap the order of intermediate steps, depending on the nurse's routine. The system should be able to identify the care activity despite the changed sequence (FR5).

The system should also remind the nurse of missing actions (FR6). An example of this would be closing a window on bedridden people when the room cools down. For this, it is important that the system has knowledge of the patient's care plan and diagnoses (FR7). Feedback on the identified activities and ticking off of the care plan must be available (FR8), so that the nurse has an overview of the activities that still need to be carried out.

Often there are several patients in one room in a hospital. The system must therefore be able to distinguish between the individual patients and assign the activities that have been carried out and recognised to the respective patient (FR9).

4.2   Non-functional Requirements

As feedback is important for caregivers, the system must recognise the activities in near real time (NR1). In addition, the recognition rate for identifying the activities must be high (NR2). If the recognition rate is too low, the system will not provide any added value, but will require a lot of time due to the correction of the entries. Therefore, the recognition accuracy should be above 80%. This accuracy was achieved on average in related work [10–12,16]. Good recognition must also be available under changing influences, such as changing light conditions, and it must be independent of gender, body shape and ethnicity (NR3). It is important in detection that no fraudulent activities are recorded. By this is meant that no simulated activities should be detected.

In order for the system to support the nurse in her daily work, the system must be easy to use. Nursing professionals are usually not familiar with IT. The use of this system should not be more complicated than the method used so far (NR4). Sensors used to detect the activities must be easy to attach and not hinder the caregiver in their exercise (NR5). For example, sensors on wrists should be avoided for reasons of hygiene and possible risk of injury. An important aspect of the implementation of such a system is the consideration of ethical, legal and social implications, such as data protection, as patient data is collected. Therefore, the system should be GDPR compliant (NR6). When using cameras for activity analysis, no image data should be stored or processed. The nursing staff should not get the impression of surveillance. Instead, only features read from the data should be used, ideally standardised to prevent later misuse (NR7). Particular attention must be paid to sensitive areas, e.g. in the bathroom, when using video recordings.

There is no uniform standard for nursing documentation, i.e. each facility records it in a different format. Therefore, the data must be standardised or the data model must be flexible and transferable to different application programmes (NR8). In the event of a transfer to another hospital, the care measures carried out must be fully accessible to the new facility. This is possible through the use of two of the most important international standards for the semantic interoperability of clinical information. One is the HL7 Clinical Document Architecture (CDA), which is a widely used standard for representing clinical information in the form of XML documents. The other is the combination of CEN/ISO 13606 and openEHR, which is based on the use of a reference model to represent data instances and an archetype model to represent clinical concepts [17].

It may be possible that the internet is not fully covered in the hospital. This means that captured data cannot be uploaded immediately. Therefore, the system must also be usable offline (NR9). The collected information from the sensors must therefore be temporarily stored so that it can be sent to the database as soon as the system is online again. Since a nurse often works an 8- or even 12-hour shift, it is important that the battery of the hardware used lasts at least one shift without needing to be charged in the meantime (NR10).

4.3   Possible Activities and Scenarios

In collaboration with the nursing students, the activities that often need to be documented in a clinical setting were identified. These are activities that take place within the scope of a given care plan. These include checking vital signs and measuring blood sugar and body weight. But also the mobilisation of the patient and personal hygiene are frequent activities. Other medical interventions include wound care and changing wound bandages, medication management, which also includes intravenous infusions and subcutaneous injections, and nutritional monitoring. Other relevant activities are the preparation of a care plan, patient observation and documentation of the patient's condition and the taking of a social history.

Derived from the requirements and the possible activities, one imaginable scenario is the recognition of nursing activities during the morning routine. This reflects a large part of the activities mentioned (measuring vital parameters, administering medication, personal hygiene, etc.). Inertial measurement units (IMU), such as the xSens DOT, could be used to collect movement data. These consist of acceleration sensors and gyroscopic sensors. It must be investigated at which positions the IMUs must be placed in order for them to provide meaningful data and be suitable for activity detection. In doing so, the NR5 requirement must not be disregarded. The Microsoft Azure Kinect is also conceivable for the recognition of nursing activities. At this point, however, the requirements NR6 and NR7 must be observed so that both the caregiver and the patient are protected. In combination with information about the location, i.e. in which patient room the nurse is and at which patient bed, and further information about the care plan (FR7) and the activities (FR3), the activities can be recognised. This is reflected in Fig. 1, which shows the general architecture. The requirements indicate that, in addition to sensors and location information, background information is also necessary for recognizing and classifying nursing activities. This background information includes the activity inventory with the intermediate steps (FR3) as well as information about the nursing plan or the patient (FR7) and knowledge about the nurse. The recognized informations must then be presented (FR2) so that the nurse can correct them, if necessary.

5   Discussion

The listed requirements show that the detection of nursing activities is a challenging task. The requirement that the activities can be interrupted or that the sequence of the individual intermediate steps of an activity can be changed leads to a high degree of complexity in the detection of nursing activities. The requirement that the sensors must not disturb the caregiver (NR5) is also relevant in consideration of related work. Konak et al. have indicated the wrists as the optimal sensor placement [11], and yet these are not suitable for sensor attachment for injury and hygiene reasons. A critical approach to public datasets and related work considering sensor locations is therefore necessary. Data protection is also an important aspect that must not be neglected in the development of the system. Aspects such as privacy and security must be taken into account here, both in relation to the caregiver and in relation to the person being cared for. Especially when using video or image data, these must be processed to the extent that a human observer cannot draw any conclusions. However, this also increases the complexity of activity recognition, since not all features can be used. Questions about how to both identify and distinguish the caregiver from the patient in a camera-based evaluation need to be answered.

When working with the nursing students, often documented activities were elaborated. These refer to the clinical setting. However, during the inventory, no distinction was made between different departments in a hospital. A possible distinction would be between surgical and non-surgical wards.

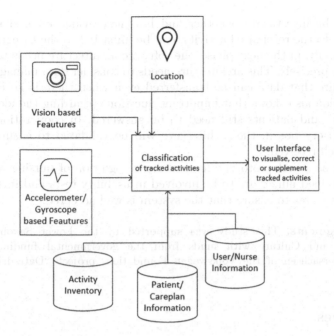

Fig. 1. The general architecture for the recognition of nursing activities. Sensors, location, and background information on activities, patients, and caregivers are used to classify activities. The detected activities are then visualized.

6   Conclusion and Future Work

Nursing documentation is a quality indicator as well as important for achieving good patient care and safety. In this paper we have introduced and collected the requirements necessary for the recognition of nursing activities in the clinical setting. For this purpose, we looked at the current literature, as well as conducted a World Café with students of nursing science and invited representatives of the nursing management and nursing science of regional hospitals as part of a project advisory board. The sensors needed for recognition could be IMUs worn on the body as well as camera-based hardware. However, safety must always be a focus when using them, both physically and in terms of the privacy of the nurse and the patient.

In the next phases of the project, the activities to be recognised are to be narrowed down further and recorded with the help of sensors in a skills lab. For this purpose, it is important to find out which individual steps these activities consist of. In addition, domain-dependent background knowledge must be collected for the recognition. Online surveys and expert interviews will be conducted for these purposes. A more detailed survey could provide results on whether there are ward-dependent differences between the activities that are frequently documented and whether there are activities on which the application should focus.

It can also be investigated whether and how new evidence-based knowledge, appropriate to the recognised activity, can be imparted to the caregivers.

Additionally, in the next phase, the software architecture needs to be determined more precisely. This architecture needs to consider data management and how to ensure that data can be transferred even when there is no connection. The discussion also shows that important questions regarding the identification of caregivers and patients still need to be answered. In cooperation with the project advisory board, the architecture will be validated to ensure that the system is well received.

As soon as a first prototype for activity recognition of nursing activities is available, trained nurses are to be involved in usability tests and further evaluations. This serves to ensure that the system is well accepted.

Acknowledgments. This study was supported by the Lower Saxony Ministry for Science and Culture with funds from the governmental funding initiative zukunft.niedersachsen of the Volkswagen Foundation, project "Data-driven health (DEAL)".

References

1. Joukes, E., Abu-Hanna, A., Cornet, R., de Keizer, N.F.: Time spent on dedicated patient care and documentation tasks before and after the introduction of a structured and standardized electronic health record. Appl. Clin. Inform. **9**(1), 46–53 (2018). https://doi.org/10.1055/s-0037-1615747
2. Statistisches Bundesamt (Destatis): Erfüllungsaufwand im Bereich Pflege: Antragsverfahren auf gesetzliche Leistungen für Menschen, die pflegebedürftig oder chronisch krank sind, pp. 160–161 (2013)
3. Shanafelt, T.D., et al.: Changes in burnout and satisfaction with work-life integration in physicians and the general US working population between 2011 and 2017. Mayo Clin. Proc. **94**(9), 1681–1694 (2019)
4. Dall'Ora, C., Ball, J., Reinius, M., et al.: Burnout in nursing: a theoretical review. Hum. Resour. Health **18**(41) (2020) https://doi.org/10.1186/s12960-020-00469-9
5. Melnick, E.R., et al.: The association between perceived electronic health record usability and professional burnout among US nurses. J. Am. Med. Inform. Assoc. **28**(8), 1632–1641 (2021). https://doi.org/10.1093/jamia/ocab059
6. Bundesministerium für Gesundheit: Gemeinsam Digital: Digitalisierungsstrategie für das Gesundheitswesen und die Pflege, pp. 25–30. Berlin (2023)
7. Roland Berger GmbH: ePflege: Informations-und Kommunikationstechnologie für die Pflege, pp. 18–21, Berlin, Vallendar, Köln (2017)
8. Avendano, J.P., et al.: Interfacing with the Electronic Health Record (EHR): a comparative review of modes of documentation. Cureus **14**(6), e26330 (2022)
9. Wang, Y., Cang, S., Yu, H.: Survey on wearable sensor modality centred human activity recognition in health care. Expert Syst. Appl. **137**, 167–190 (2019)
10. Kaczmarek, S., Fiedler, M., Bongers, A., Wibbeling, S., Grzeszick, R.: Dataset and methods for recognizing care activities. In: Proceedings of the 7th International Workshop on Sensor-Based Activity Recognition and Artificial Intelligence. Association for Computing Machinery (2022)

11. Konak, O., et al.: Nurses on the edge: an on-device human activity recognition framework that optimizes the sensor placement, Preprint (2022). https://doi.org/10.36227/techrxiv.20532060.v1

12. Lago, P., et al.: Nurse care activity recognition challenge: summary and results. In: Adjunct Proceedings of the 2019 ACM International Joint Conference on Pervasive and Ubiquitous Computing and Proceedings of the 2019 ACM International Symposium on Wearable Computers, pp. 746–751. Association for Computing Machinery (2019)

13. Nurse Care Activity Recognition Challenge. https://abc-research.github.io/challenge2022/. Accessed 7 July 2023

14. Hanson, J.L., Stephens, M.B., Pangaro, L.N., Gimbel, R.W.: Quality of outpatient clinical notes: a stakeholder definition derived through qualitative research. BMC Health Serv. Res. **12**(407) (2012)

15. Compagna, D., Kohlbacher, F.: The limits of participatory technology development: the case of service robots in care facilities for older people. Technol. Forecast. Soc. Chang. **93**, 19–31 (2015)

16. Ijaz, M., Diaz, R., Chen, C.: Multimodal transformer for nursing activity recognition. In: IEEE/CVF Conference on Computer Vision and Pattern Recognition Workshops (2022)

17. Moner, D., Moreno, A., Maldonado, J.A., Robles, M., Parra, C.: Using archetypes for defining CDA templates. Stud. Health Technol. Inform. **180**, 53–57 (2012)

Exploring How Telephone Triage Nurses Support Older People with Multimorbidity to Engage in Digital Self-management

Patricia McAleer[1]([✉]) [iD], Julie Doyle[1] [iD], and John Dinsmore[2] [iD]

[1] NetwellCASALA, Dundalk Institute of Technology, Dundalk, Co Louth, Ireland
patricia.mcaleer@dkit.ie
[2] TCPHI, Trinity College Dublin, Dublin, Ireland

Abstract. In the European Union (EU), 50 million people live with multimorbidity (two or more chronic diseases), which increases in prevalence with age. As a result, a significant burden is placed on those who live with multimorbidity and on health care systems that manage it. Hence, solutions to support people aged 65+ years to self-manage their illnesses are necessary, and digital health technologies hold promise. However, human support may also be necessary, particularly for those managing multiple complex chronic conditions. A nurse-led telephone triage monitoring service offers a potential solution. The aim of this study was to explore the role of a nurse-led telephone triage service in supporting older peoples' engagement with digital health technology. One focus group was conducted via Zoom with three telephone triage nurses (TTNs), and six telephone interviews were conducted with a sub-set of older people with multimorbidity (PwMs). Qualitative data were thematically analysed using Nvivo 12 software. PwMs reported being motivated to engage in self-management by knowing their readings were being monitored. Looking at data over time and observing trends helped the TTNs to make accurate assessments of the PwMs' needs. Both PwMs and TTNs spoke about the warmth of their relationship even though it was conducted remotely. In conclusion, triage nurses play an important role in supporting older people to engage in self-management of multimorbid health conditions.

Keywords: Digital health technology · Multimorbidity · Older people · Telephone Triage Nurse

1 Introduction

With life expectancy increasing exponentially and showing little sign of slowing down [1], the number of older people (people aged 65 years+) is also growing significantly and is forecast to accelerate more quickly in the coming decades [2]. The number of people aged 80 years+ is increasing faster than the number of older people overall. It is estimated that by 2050 this age cohort will number 434 million, tripling the 2015 figure of 125 million [2].

D. Salvi et al. (Eds.): PH 2023, LNICST 572, pp. 244–255, 2024.
https://doi.org/10.1007/978-3-031-59717-6_17

Although one of the greatest achievements of the modern age is the increase in life expectancy, whilst people are living longer, they are not necessarily living *well* for longer [1]. The prevalence of chronic health conditions such as cancer, cardiovascular disease (CVD), chronic obstructive pulmonary disease (COPD), dementia and diabetes is increasing as a result of an ageing population, and it is asserted that this may become the norm rather than the exception [3]. Multimorbidity is the presence of two or more chronic diseases and it places a large burden on health services who struggle to manage it. The cost of care places a considerable financial burden on EU health services, with €700 billion or 70% to 80% of the total spend on health care being spent on chronic illnesses annually [4]. Further, according to Bähler et al. [5], multimorbidity is associated with twice as many contacts with health care professionals and those contacts increase in number with each additional illness. People with multimorbidity (PwMs) are not only high users of health care resources but are also some of the costliest and most difficult to treat patients, with the cost of care increasing with each additional condition [6].

To alleviate the effects of multimorbidity and hence, to improve health outcomes, PwMs need to engage with the self-management of their illnesses. Barello and Graffigna [7] characterise engagement in health management as being a process in which a fully engaged patient emerges from a series of emotional, cognitive, and behavioural adjustments of their health, and that their success in completing this process depends on how they fared in previous phases of the process. One way that patients can engage effectively with their health and well-being management is through the use of digital health technologies (DHTs). DHTs are shaping the future of health care delivery, driven by the shift towards a knowledge-based economy. The emergence of DHTs has arisen from an urgent need to address the growing burden of chronic diseases [8], Moore's law – the increasingly rapid growth in computer power resulting in the development of smaller and cheaper electronics [9], and finally, health care models becoming more patient focused [10]. Technologies used in health care include email, electronic heath records, clinical decision support software (CDSS), mobile health (m-health) systems (e.g., smartphones, mobile phone apps and tablets), telemedicine (the delivery of medical advice using technology to patients at a distance), wearable devices and monitoring sensors, which play an important role in helping people to make better-informed decisions about their health [11–15].

However, engagement levels with technology-based health interventions are concerning, with limited participation and high attrition rates being common [16, 17]. For example, digital health applications are abandoned by more than 25% of people after only one use which implies that users are not gaining real health benefits from achieving their health goals [18]. Chaudhry et al. [19] reported on an app used by 20 community based older people to set health and wellness goals. Challenges faced by PwMs included time constraints, a lack of technical knowledge and doubts about goal setting. This points to the need to potentially provide support for older people to help them how to use DHTs, e.g., set health goals, input readings, troubleshoot issues, understand their data and know how and when to respond to high readings [19–23]. Moreover, older people when engaging with DHTs face additional difficulties related to the ageing process, with Wilson et al. [24] reporting that age related physical health barriers to technology engagement, such as visual acuity, hearing difficulties and dexterity issues, are prevalent.

Other health problems such as the presence of cognitive impairment can affect attention span, executive functioning and memory, in particular remembering passwords and acquiring new information [22, 25].

Further, older people perceive technology as being impersonal and lacking empathy which results in them feeling little more than a statistic; they lack confidence and the ability required to try new things; and, they also feel the need to retain control over personal information, expressing a lack of trust in sharing that information with others [20]. Another important barrier to engagement with DHTs for older people is the lack of supports, both technical and social, i.e., support received from either HCPs, peers or family members [24]. Difficulties experienced by PwMs in their relationships with their HCPs include limited access to health care, a lack of time during consultations, poor communication between them leaving patients feeling unheard, a lack of trust making it difficult to share information with them, and contradictory information from multiple HCPs leading to a lack in knowledge in how to self-manage [26–29].

One solution to this issue may lie in providing older people with support from a nurse-led telephone triage service. Telephone triage is a procedure in which telephone calls from ill members of the public are received by trained staff who assess and manage the calls by either giving advice or referring them to a more appropriate service [30]. It is a way for people to avoid needless visits to an HCP and to save unnecessary expenditure on health care [31, 32]. According to Vaona et al. [33], telephone triage services have become an integral part of modern medicine with almost a quarter of all care consultations being conducted by telephone. One of the main reasons for implementing such a service is to lessen the burden of care on General Practitioners (GPs) and emergency departments [34]. Jácome et al. [35] found that Telephone Triage Nurses (TTNs) were effective in directing adults aged 65+ years who presented with chronic conditions to a telephone triage service, to the appropriate type of care, thus reducing the overall demand for care.

In this paper, we report on qualitative findings from a study whereby six older people with multimorbidity used a digital health platform, ProACT, to self-manage their health (each of their chronic conditions and related parameters) and well-being (e.g., sleep and physical activity) at home while being monitored and supported by a team of TTNs. The findings reveal the importance of the relationship with the TTNs and its potential impact on PwMs' engagement with the platform.

2 Methods

Semi-structured interviews were conducted with older people (aged 65 years and over) who had two or more of the following conditions: chronic heart disease (CHD); chronic heart failure (CHF), chronic obstructive pulmonary disorder (COPD); diabetes; and, HTN (hypertension) and who had been using the ProACT digital health platform for approximately eight to 10 months as part of a wider clinical programme SMILE (Supporting Multimorbidity self-care through Integration, Learning and e-Health) being coordinated by a clinical triage company. A sub-set of six PwMs from SMILE, as well as three TTNs who provided them with support to manage their conditions were recruited for this PhD project. PwMs were referred to the trial by their respective GPs across three counties in the South-East of Ireland. The TTNs had between 11 and 17 years' experience of working as triage nurses, and also had one year's experience providing triage support to PwMs in a previous study in which the ProACT CareApp was developed. Due to restrictions imposed by the COVID-19 pandemic, the semi-structured interviews with the PwM participants were conducted by telephone and a semi-structured focus group was conducted over Zoom with the TTNs. The PwMs were asked a series of questions that related to the challenges they faced in managing their conditions, their use of the DHT, their relationships with the TTNs, the supports given to them by the triage nurses and finally, the impacts (if any) of COVID-19 on their self-management and access to health care. The focus group with the TTNs covered topics such as their relationships with the PwMs, the supports they provided to them, the advice given, and how they cared for the PwMs during the COVID-19 pandemic.

At the beginning of the SMILE programme, PwMs were given a suite of digital devices for symptom monitoring depending on their conditions (e.g., blood pressure monitor, blood glucometer, pulse oximeter) as well as a weighing scales and an activity watch for measuring steps and sleep. An iPad with the ProACT CareApp was also provided on which the PwMs could view their symptom readings over time, self-report on their health and well-being, set activity goals and view personalised educational content. Further detail on the ProACT CareApp used by PwMs can be found in [36]. The triage platform used by the TTNs (Sims-triage) is a custom-designed application through which the triage nurses viewed and responded to alerts generated by data collected from the PwMs. In the event of an alert, the TTNs would call the PwMs to check on their health status. These alerts occurred when the thresholds set for different conditions in the system were outside the normal range for the participant. For example, a reading for high blood glucose was anything over 14 mmol/L (which was configured for each participant). The app's dashboard also allowed the nurses to see if alerts were new, under review or resolved. PwMs' health and well-being data were also available, providing the triage team with a holistic picture of the PwMs' health before they called them to discuss an alert. Finally, technical support was provided to the PwMs by the clinical triage company.

All interviews and the focus group were audio recorded and transcribed verbatim. The data were thematically analysed using Nvivo 12 software and followed Braun and Clark's [37] protocol for analysing qualitative data. Ethical approval for the study was obtained by the School of Health and Science Research Ethics Committee at Dundalk Institute of Technology.

3 Findings

Participants were all aged 65 years and over with two or more of the conditions of interest and 60% were male. Five themes were identified relating to the relationship between the PwMs and TTNs and the impact of that relationship on PwMs' engagement with technology. For identification purposes, at the end of PwM participant quotes respondents are identified thus: (ID, age, gender, conditions).

3.1 Supports Provided by the TTNs

The PwMs spoke about the practical supports provided to them by the TTNs, which included getting advice and educational tips about their medications or health conditions or about when to contact their GP, help with the technology, and monitoring of their readings. They were asked if they always followed the advice given and the majority said they did for reasons such as the triage nurses being professional, having expertise, having knowledge and also because they believed that the advice worked for them: *"Like they're professionals, so they know what they're doing, you know what I mean, what they're saying. If they give me advice on something, I certainly will do it, you know"* (P08, 65, F, CHD + HTN).

Several PwMs said that they would be foolish if they ignored the advice, however one participant reported that she had ignored the advice given about contacting her GP and consequently regretted that decision: *"You know, like when they say to me 'oh well go to the doctor and get this and do this' and I think 'oh well, I won't bother' and then a couple of days later I think that I should have done it when they said it to me"* (P03, 86, F, CHD + COPD).

The TTNs spoke about the approach they took in giving support to the PwMs. They talked about tailoring the advice they gave, according to the person they were dealing with and not taking a 'one-size fits all approach'. Using previous conversations held with the PwMs, knowing about the PwMs' backgrounds, understanding their environmental impacts, looking at the data over time and observing trends were all important in helping them to make accurate assessments of the PwMs' needs. They also spoke about keeping the advice simple so that the PwMs understood it and took it on board: *"It's very gradually bringing it absolutely down to a level of education that you know that they'll understand and take it on board. If you give them too much too quickly, they'll do nothing. It's like baby steps"* (TTN03). The TTNs were asked whether the PwMs always followed their advice. The majority did because they were invested in improving their health and so were willing to take the advice on board. Humour, encouragement and not 'telling the PwM off' were strategies used by the TTNs to prevent the PwMs from ignoring the advice. In cases where the advice was not taken, the triage nurses persisted until the advice was listened to: *"But like I mean as I say we're like a stone in the shoe. We keep ringing you know. There's a lot of very gentle cajoling and you know, and then when they do it, and they do it well, we're full of praise, you know what I mean"* (TTN03).

When asked whether COVID-19 had changed the supports they were giving the PwMs, the TTNs responded that they were giving much more emotional support and reassurance than they had prior to the pandemic: *"Allaying fears isn't it again? It comes back to fear of the unknown, how much was unknown for us all really. The news was always harping on about chronic conditions and chronic conditions. You know that was a difficult thing"* (TTN02). This was because they found the PwMs to be very fearful and anxious. They were also experiencing loneliness and depression because of not being able to see their families, but even after the lockdowns were lifted, the PwMs were isolating themselves from family members through fear of contracting COVID-19. Their advice also changed to advising the PwMs how to keep safe during the pandemic by wearing face masks, proper handwashing and telephoning their GPs first rather than visiting them: *"It was just talking them through good practice, letting them open up again and trying to learn to live with it rather than live in fear all the time, keeping safe at the same time"* (TTN01).

3.2 The Nature of the Relationship

The PwMs appeared to have formed a close bond with the triage nurses, with several of them saying that they felt they knew them, even though they had never met: *"No matter who came on the line I knew who it was. I knew who it was from their voice. I always felt as if I knew them – as friends as well as nurses"* (P01, 78, F, CHD + COPD). The friendliness of the TTNs was commented on by several PwMs who noted that conversations were more than just about health-related matters which they appreciated, with P04 (69, M, COPD + HTN) saying that he *"had craic"* (an Irish slang word for fun) while speaking to them, although he also noted how professional they were in dealing with him: *"They are marvellous. Like, they've done their job with the utmost professionalism all the way down"* (P04, 69, M, COPD + HTN). Finally, P10 (66, M, Diabetes + HTN) reported that he wanted to maintain contact with the nurses after the SMILE project because of the relationship he had built with them.

TTNs shared this perception of the friendliness of their relationship saying: *"I mean we've built up some extraordinary relationships with these people. We haven't even met them, it's phenomenal really"* (TTN01). They spoke about discussing everyday topics such as the PwMs' families or what was happening in their lives, for instance. They felt that it was important to create a holistic relationship because it enabled the PwMs to benefit more from the triage service. The nurses spoke about taking time to talk to the PwMs and the importance of getting to know them on a deeper level. It helped them to 'pick up on cues', something that was vital to treating the PwMs appropriately because they were not dealing with them face-to-face. As one triage nurse noted: *"Our ears are our eyes"* (TTN03).

3.3 The Quality of the Relationship

All PwMs described the TTNs positively, with terms such as 'professional', 'kind', 'caring', 'helpful', 'supportive', and 'encouraging' used throughout the interviews. The PwMs felt confident to be able to contact the TTNs with any issues they had, mentioning that they would do so at any time and as often as they needed, because they did not feel that they were an inconvenience. One participant spoke about the nurses taking the time to talk to him for as long as he needed them, compared to the amount of time afforded to him by his HCPs. The PwMs also felt that they could be open and frank or 'be themselves' with TTNs. For instance, P04 (69, M, COPD + HTN) felt comfortable enough to speak to them if he was feeling depressed:

I did feel that over the period of time, the relationship I built up with the different [nurses], that I could have said anything to them. If I was in the pits of depression here and needed someone, that I could have said 'listen, have you five minutes, I need to talk to someone?' You know I felt that at ease and comfortable with them (P04, 69, M, COPD + HTN).

The TTNs also acknowledged this: *"A lot of them say 'we know you have our backs; we know you're minding us' and that in itself is hugely comforting"* (TTN03). The nurses reported that they had very few difficulties with the PwMs, attributing this to the fact that they had wanted to participate in the project and engaged with it well from the outset. The main issue was needing to be persistent with some PwMs in getting them to attend the GP, something they were reluctant to do because of COVID-19.

3.4 The Important Aspects of the Relationship

The PwMs were asked what they felt were the most important aspects of their relationship with the TTNs. One factor that was mentioned as important for the PwMs was the advice on health issues and being advised on what course of action to take, such as contacting their GP. In fact, one participant P10 (66, M, Diabetes + HTN) stated that he would contact the triage nurses before he contacted his GP or diabetes clinic.

The type and consistency of the contact was also important to the PwMs who felt it important that the nurses were at the end of the telephone and would contact them if there was any issue with their readings: *"Knowing that I can contact them at any time and they can contact me if there's any problems whatsoever"* (P08, 65, F, CHD + HTN). She believed that having this level of contact with the TTNs had increased her confidence in her health and well-being. For P03, (86, F, CHD + COPD), having the triage nurses there to talk to and provide her with advice made a big difference to her well-being given that she was cocooning during COVID-19. P10 (66, M, Diabetes + HTN) felt that being able to communicate with people who were trained and could spot if there was anything wrong was important for him. Further, he also appreciated the amount of time the triage nurses spent advising him, in comparison to the time he was given when visiting his GP.

Being consistent and conveying warmth in their tone of voice when talking to the PwMs was also important to the TTNs because it helped them to build a rapport and consequently develop a high level of trust in their relationship. This was important because occasionally PwMs were afraid or frustrated because of their readings, and it helped to reassure them. Rapport was fundamental to building trust with the PwMs, so that they followed the advice that they were being given. The nurses also spoke about using their conversations as a way of assessing the PwMs' health, which was important for knowing what advice to give:

It's not even just about the chitchat. It allows us to, we use it as an assessment tool as well so you're talking about patients with COPD. They're telling you they're well because they're very fearful of going to the doctors a lot of the time. But in actual fact you know whether or not they're unwell whether they're talking to you in sentences or it's just one-word answers, whereas you know that the last time N03 spoke to them they were full of the chat (TTN01).

3.5 The Role of the TTNs in Supporting Engagement in Self-management

There were several factors which influenced the PwMs' motivation to engage in their self-management, which included their health conditions – P02 (76, M, COPD + Diabetes) for example mentioned his health conditions as the reason he kept engaging with his self-management – and their interactions with the TTNs. The PwMs felt a sense of loyalty to the triage nurses, noting that if they were concerned enough to phone them then they should also engage: *"Well, like when they're going to the bother of ringing me and keeping an eye out, well I have to play my part as well"* (P01, 78, F, CHD + COPD). However, the most frequently mentioned factor to explain their sustained engagement was knowing that the TTNs were monitoring them. In fact, some PwMs perceived that they would not be able to continue using the DHT without the support of the TTNs who were able to help them understand why a reading was high, for example.

Further, PwMs felt that knowing the TTNs were looking at their readings and would phone them if a blood pressure reading was high for example, was motivation for them to take action to avoid it recurring. This would have been by keeping a better watch on their own readings, changing when they were taking them (for example, waiting for a period of time after exercising when their pulse would have returned to normal), or taking a walk. Further, two PwMs mentioned that without being monitored they would not be inclined to take exercise. For others, knowing that they were going to receive a phone call if they did not take their readings was an incentive to do so.

When discussing continued engagement with the technology, a sense of responsibility to the TTNs was acknowledged by P10 (66, M, Diabetes + HTN) who stated that he did not want to let them down as a reason for engaging with his self-management. He felt that the TTNs were a complement to the DHT and they were another reason for sustaining his engagement: *"Without them, I don't know if I would have stuck it out"* (P10, 66, M, Diabetes + HTN).

4 Discussion

There is a proliferation of literature related to PwMs' engagement in the self-management of their health [26, 38–40]. Indeed, in order to achieve better health outcomes, it is imperative that PwMs are successful in the self-management of their multimorbidity. This necessitates them to set priorities and make decisions on a daily basis [41]. It is described in the literature as being an 'iterative process' that requires patients to learn effective techniques to manage their illness, and cope over time through trial and error [42]. This process is viewed as a component of living with chronic conditions within the range of personal, social, spiritual contexts and daily life specific to each person [42]. Yet there is little extant literature related to how older people can be supported to use DHT to self-manage their health with the support of TTNs. Indeed, the type of telephone nurse monitoring described herein was created for the studies detailed here and has not been identified in the literature to the best knowledge of the authors. Hence, this is the first study to examine the phenomenon. It must be noted that the TTNs with their many years working as telephone triage nurses, had acquired listening skills that allowed them to holistically assess patients, taking into account any background cues, illness history, how they were able to respond to questions, and what they weren't saying in order to make informed decisions.

DHT plays an important role in the effective self-management of chronic diseases, having the potential to overcome some of the difficulties patients face in the health care system such as expensive health care which may be difficult to access and poorly synchronised [26, 43]. However, Yardley et al. [44] warn that dropout rates and "non-usage attrition" are higher when there is no human support system in place for users. This factor is also mentioned by Lupton [45] who asserts that the abandonment of wearables for instance, results from a lack of community support as well as users not being provided with what they require. Lupton also posits that issues such as users perceiving their health goals to be unattainable or irritating reminders and alarms also contribute to low engagement rates. Indeed, patients frequently prefer support from their HCP with their self-management, rather than managing their conditions alone [46,

47]. Moreover, Pichon et al. [46] argue that a lack of HCP support can be damaging to the patient. However, HCP support is not always available, for reasons such as time constraints, HCPs feeling burdened by having to monitor patient data, and the conflict between what a patient expects from their HCP and what the HCP can provide [48].

A lack of support from HCPs, family members and friends [24] is one of the barriers that older people face when using technology. Further, having to rely on family who often show a lack of patience and understanding for older relatives trying to learn the technology is far from ideal, and in fact may be a barrier to engagement [49]. Further, Pywell et al. [21] report that a lack of face-to-face engagement is a major deterrent in engagement with technology, and that the absence of interpersonal communication reduces the therapeutic effect of the technology they use. Nevertheless, the findings of this study demonstrate that older people are motivated to use technology to self-manage their health through having the support of the remote TTNs. PwM PwMs on the SMILE study had been engaged in using the technology for between eight and 10 months at the time of interview. This motivation appears to have been driven by the nature and the quality of their relationship which was described as friendly by both the PwMs and the TTNs in spite of the relationship being conducted remotely. Indeed, one participant wanted to remain in contact with the TTNs because of the rapport he had built with them. Further, the PwMs were confident enough in their relationship with the TTNs to feel able to contact them whenever they needed to. They also felt able to open up to the triage nurses in the event of feeling depressed. They perceived that the triage nurses took time to talk to them, something not encountered when dealing with their HCPs. From the TTNs' perspective, getting to know the PwMs by discussing family or life events was a way of creating a holistic relationship which ultimately led to better treatment for the PwMs and enabled them to benefit more from the triage service.

It was important to the PwMs that the TTNs would contact them if their readings were outside their normal range. The level of contact with the triage nurses led to increases in confidence in their health and also relieved their anxiety about their health. In addition, having trained people monitoring their symptoms was important as they could identify if there was anything wrong. The TTNs felt that the high level of trust they had built with the PwMs meant that they had a rapport with them, resulting in the advice they gave being followed. This was important in view of the fact that this research was conducted during the COVID-19 pandemic, when the PwMs were reluctant to attend their GPs.

One of the limitations of the study was the small sample size which makes generalisation of the findings difficult. Another limitation was conducting the interviews by telephone which meant that the PwMs' body language and cues could not be read. However, this method of data collection was made necessary because it took place during the COVID-19 pandemic.

5 Conclusion

This research study contributes to a greater understanding of how PwMs using digital health technologies for health self-management can be supported by TTNs to remain engaged in the process. The findings in this paper are important for future health care service delivery, which aims to decentralise care to the community and support older adults to better self-manage, given the rapidly ageing global population with health care systems struggling to meet the demand for care. This paper's findings demonstrates that older people will use technology to self-manage their conditions and will keep using it if they have support to do so.

Acknowledgements. Funding for this PhD project was granted by Landscape Funding from the Higher Education Authority, Ireland. This work was part-funded under the SEURO project which received funding from the European Union's Horizon 2020 research and innovation programme under grant agreement no. 945449. We would like to sincerely thank all the participants who gave their time to take part in this PhD research project.

References

1. Jagger, C.: Trends in life expectancy and healthy life expectancy. Foresight, Government Office for Science. https://www.gov.uk/government/uploads/system/uploads/attachment_d ata/file/464275/gs-15-13-future-ageing-trends-life-expectancy-er12.pdf. Accessed 15 Apr 2020
2. United Nations, Department of Economic and Social Affairs, Population Division.: World Population Ageing 2015. http://www.un.org/en/development/desa/population/publications/ pdf/ageing/WPA2015_Report.pdf. Accessed 04 Feb 2020
3. Feather, A.: Managing patients with multimorbidity. Medicine (United Kingdom) **46**(7), 397–401 (2018)
4. European Commission. Digital Agenda for Europe. http://eur-lex.europa.eu/legal-content/ EN/ALL/?uri=CELEX%3A52010DC0245R(01). Accessed 20 Jan 2020
5. Bähler, C., Huber, C.A., Brüngger, B., Reich, O.: Multimorbidity, health care utilization and costs in an elderly community-dwelling population: a claims data base observational study. BMC Health Serv. Res. **15**, 1–12 (2015)
6. Xu, X., Mishra, G.D., Jones, M.: Evidence on multimorbidity from definition to intervention: an overview of systematic reviews. Ageing Res. Rev. **37**, 53–68 (2017)
7. Barello, S., Graffigna, G.: Patient engagement in healthcare: pathways for effective medical decision making. In: Balconi, M. (ed.) Neuropsychological Trends, pp. 53–61. LED, Milan (2015)
8. Bhavnani, S.P., Narula, J., Sengupta, P.P.: Mobile technology and the digitization of healthcare. Eur. Heart J. **37**(18), 1428–1438 (2016)
9. Moore, G.E.: Cramming more components onto integrated circuits. Electronics **38**, 114–117 (1965)
10. Topol, E.J.: Transforming medicine via digital innovation. Sci. Transl. Med. **2**(16) (2010)
11. The American Telemedicine Association. ATA Policy Principles. https://www.americantele med.org/policy/. Accessed 22 Feb 2020
12. Calthorpe, R.J., Smith, S., Gathercole, K., Smyth, A.R.: Using digital technology for home monitoring, adherence and self-management in cystic fibrosis: a state of the art review. Thorax **75**(1), 72–77 (2020)
13. US Food and Drink Administration. What is Digital Health? https://www.fda.gov/medical-devices/digital-health-center-excellence/what-digital-health. Accessed 14 Sept 2020
14. Fadahunsi, K.P., et al.: Protocol for a systematic review and qualitative synthesis of information quality frameworks in eHealth. BMJ Open **9**(3) (2019)
15. Widmer, R.J., Collins, N.M., Collins, C.S., West, C.P., Lerman, L.O., Lerman, A.: Digital health interventions for the prevention of cardiovascular disease: a systematic review and meta-analysis. Mayo Clin. Proc. **90**(4), 469–480 (2015)

16. Yeager, C.M., Benight, C.C.: If we build it will they come? Issues of engagement with digital health interventions for trauma recovery. mHealth **4**(37) (2018)
17. Lie, S.S., Karlsen, B., Oord, E.R., Graue, M., Oftedal, B.: Dropout from an eHealth intervention for adults with type 2 diabetes: a qualitative study. J. Med. Internet Res. **19**(5), e187 (2017)
18. Todd, G.: App user retention: less than 25% of new App users return the day after first use (here's what to do about it). https://www.braze.com/blog/app-customer-retention-spring-2016-report/. Accessed 14 Mar 2022
19. Chaudhry, B., Dasgupta, D., Chawla, N.: Formative evaluation of a tablet Application to support goal-oriented care in community-dwelling older adults. In: Proceedings of the ACM on Human-Computer Interaction 2022, vol. 6, No. MHCI, Article 208. ACM (2022)
20. O'Reilly, P.M., Harney, O.M., Hogan, M.J., Mitchell, C., McGuire, B.E., Slattery, B.: Chronic pain self-management in middle-aged and older adults: a collective intelligence approach to identifying barriers and user needs in eHealth interventions. Digital Health **8**, 1–15 (2022)
21. Pywell, J., Vijaykumar, S., Dodd, A., Coventry, L.: Barriers to older adults' uptake of mobile-based mental health interventions. Digital Health **6**, 1–15 (2020)
22. Nymberg, V.M., Bolmsjö, B.B., Wolff, M., Calling, S., Gerward, S., Sandberg, M.: Having to learn this so late in our lives: Swedish elderly patients' beliefs, experiences, attitudes and expectations of e-health in primary health care. Scand. J. Prim. Health Care **37**(1), 41–52 (2019)
23. Cajita, M.I., Hodgson, N.A., Lam, K.W., Yoo, S., Han, H.-R.: Facilitators of and barriers to mHealth adoption in older adults with heart failure. CIN (Comput. Inf. Nurs.) **36**(8), 376–382 (2018)
24. Wilson, J., Heinsch, M., Betts, D., Booth, D., Kay-Lamb, F.: Barriers and facilitators to the use of e-health by older adults: a scoping review. BMC Public Health **21** (2021)
25. Borg, J., Lantz, A., Gulliksen, J.: Accessibility to electronic communication for people with cognitive disabilities: a systematic search and review of empirical evidence. Univ. Access Inf. Soc. **14**, 547–562 (2015)
26. Villalobos, N., Serna Vela, F., Morales Hernandez, L.: Digital healthcare intervention to improve self-management for patients with Type 2 diabetes: a scoping review. J. Sci. Innov. Med. **3**(3), 1–11 (2020)
27. Doyle, J., et al.: Managing multimorbidity: identifying design requirements for a digital self-management tool to support older adults with multiple chronic conditions. In: Proceedings of the 2019 CHI Conference on Human Factors in Computing Systems (CHI 2019), pp. 1–14. (2019). https://doi.org/10.1145/3290605.3300629. Accessed 30 June 2022
28. Lim, C., et al..: "It just seems outside my health": how patients with chronic conditions perceive communication boundaries with providers. In: Proceedings of the 2016 ACM Conference on Designing Interactive Systems (DIS 2016), pp. 1172–1184 (2016). https://doi.org/10.1145/2901790.2901866. Accessed 03 July 2023
29. Maneze, D., et al.: Multidisciplinary care: experience of patients with complex needs. Aust. J. Prim. Health **20**(1), 20–26 (2012)
30. Mulcahy, D., O'Callaghan, D., Hannigan, A.: Nurse triage in an Irish out-of-hours general practice co-operative. Irish Med. J. (2017)
31. Onubugu, U.D., Earp, J.K.: Telephone nursing practice: how do telenurses perceive their role? J. Best Pract. Health Profess. Diversity: Educ. Res. Policy **6**(1), 891–902 (2013)
32. Andersson Bäck, M.: Conceptions, conflicts and contradictions: in the introduction of a Swedish health call centre. https://pdfs.semanticscholar.org/99fe/161dab171a0e2354476ac cd6de2268b3261d.pdf. Accessed 10 Mar 2020
33. Vaona, A., Pappas, Y., Grewal, R.S., Ajaz, M., Majeed, A., Car, J.: Training interventions for improving telephone consultation skills in clinicians. Cochrane Datab. Syst. Rev. **2017**(2), 1 (2017)

34. Lake, R., et al.: The quality, safety and governance of telephone triage and advice services - an overview of evidence from systematic reviews. BMC Health Serv. Res. **17**(1) (2017)

35. Jácome, M., Rego, N., Veiga, P.: Potential of a nurse telephone triage line to direct elderly to appropriate health care settings. J. Nurs. Manag. **27**(6), 1275–1284 (2019)

36. Doyle, J., et al.: A digital platform to support self-management of multiple chronic conditions (ProACT): findings in relation to engagement during a one-year proof-of-concept trial. J. Med. Internet Res. **23**(12), e22672 (2021)

37. Braun, V., Clark, V.: Using thematic analysis in psychology. Qual. Res. Psychol. **3**, 77–101 (2006)

38. Yang, H., Du, H.S., Wang, L., Wu, T.: The influence of social support networks on health conditions via user engagement: gender as a moderator. J. Electron. Commer. Res. **20**(1), 35–54 (2019)

39. D'Agostino, T.A., et al.: Promoting patient participation in healthcare interactions through communication skills training: a systematic review. Patient Educ. Couns. **100**(7), 1247–1257 (2017)

40. Ibe, C., et al.: Intensity of exposure to a patient activation intervention and patient engagement in medical visit communication. Patient Educ. Couns. **100**(7), 1258–2167 (2017)

41. Bratzke, L.C., Muehrer, R.J., Kehl, K.A., Lee, K.S., Ward, E.C., Kwekkeboom, K.L.: Self-management priority setting and decision-making in adults with multimorbidity: a narrative review of literature. Int. J. Nurs. Stud. **52**, 744–755 (2015)

42. Miller, W.R., Lasiter, S., Bartlett Ellis, R., Buelow, J.M.: Chronic disease self-management: a hybrid concept analysis. Nurs. Outlook **63**(2), 154–161 (2015)

43. Chien, I., et al.: A machine learning approach to understanding patterns of engagement with internet-delivered mental health interventions. JAMA Netw. Open **3**(7), e2010791 (2021)

44. Yardley, L., et al.: Understanding and promoting effective engagement with digital behavior change interventions. Am. J. Prev. Med. **51**(5), 833–842 (2016)

45. Lupton, D.: Wearable devices: sociotechnical imaginaries and agential capacities. In: Pedersen, I., Iliadis, A. (eds.) Embodied Computing: Wearables, Implantables, Embeddables, Ingestibles, pp. 49–70. The MIT Press, Cambridge, MA (2020)

46. Pichon, A., Horan, E., Massey, B., Schiffer, K., Bakken, S., Mamykina, L.: Divided we stand: the collaborative work of patients and providers in an enigmatic chronic disease. Proc. ACM Hum.-Comput. Interact. **4**(CSCW3), 1–24 (2021). https://doi.org/10.1145/3434170. Accessed 03 July 2023

47. Chewning, B., Bylund, C.L., Shah, B., Arora, N.K., Gueguen, J.A., Makoul, G.: Patient preferences for shared decisions: a systematic review. Patient Educ. Counsel. **86**(1), 9–12 (2012)

48. Doyle, J., et al.: The role of phone-based triage nurses in supporting older adults with multimorbidity to digitally self-manage – findings from the ProACT proof-of-concept study. Digital Health **8**, 1–17 (2022)

49. Zibrik, L., Khan, S., Bangar, N., Stacy, E., Novak Lauscher, H., Ho, K.: Patient and community centered eHealth: exploring eHealth barriers and facilitators for chronic disease self-management within British Columbia's immigrant Chinese and Punjabi seniors. Health Policy Technol. **4**(4), 348–356 (2015)

Remote Monitoring

Mobile Application for Remote Monitoring of Peripheral Edema

Aaron John Bernante(✉) ⓘ, Khristine Joie Recto ⓘ,
and Jhoanna Rhodette Pedrasa ⓘ

Electrical and Electronics Engineering Institute, University of the Philippines
Diliman, Quezon City, Philippines
aaron.john.bernante@eee.upd.edu.ph

Abstract. The prevalence of heart disease continues to become a relevant issue globally. One of the most common symptoms in heart failure (HF) patients is peripheral edema. Peripheral edema can be caused by various underlying conditions. Thus, early detection and consistent monitoring are vital for its appropriate treatment. Several studies have explored the use of telehealth for a more accessible remote monitoring of HF patients. With the current gap in monitoring patients remotely, the proposed solution is a mobile application that detects the presence and severity of peripheral edema in HF patients. It allows patients to take a video of their extremities and a deep learning model in the application will evaluate the presence and severity of peripheral edema. The dataset collected consists of 150 photos for each edema stage. Transfer learning was utilized on a MobileNetV3 model with pre-trained weights from ImageNet. The model yielded an accuracy of 95.24% and recall of 0.96 on the test dataset, and an accuracy of 86.67% and recall of 0.95 during the field testing of the application. The high accuracy indicates that the model performs well in classifying different peripheral edema severity. Moreover, the high recall value shows that the model is able to accurately detect the presence of edema by minimizing false negatives.

Keywords: Peripheral edema · MobileNetV3 · mHealth ·
Convolutional neural networks · Deep learning

1 Introduction

Edema is the accumulation of fluid in the tissues [23]. Peripheral edema, more specifically, is a kind of edema that occurs in the legs, making them swollen. Due to the lack of blood circulation in arteries and veins, excess blood and fluids accumulate in the capillaries and eventually leak onto the tissues in the legs or arms, causing peripheral edema [6]. Peripheral edema is assessed by conducting a pitting test on the affected area. The pitting test is administered by applying

Supported by the Department of Science and Technology - Science Education Institute and Ms. Jennifer Cua.

pressure on the affected area, and classified into grade 1 (mild edema), grade 2, grade 3, or grade 4 (severe edema) depending on the indentation depth. A more severe peripheral edema would have a deeper indentation [20]. This type of assessment produces a burden and increased workload on physicians, requiring them to conduct the pitting test several times a day for optimal patient care. Thus, this project developed an offline mobile application for the early detection of peripheral edema and remote monitoring of patients who are prone to it. The deep learning model in the application was designed and trained using the Keras framework. The built-in libraries in Keras were used to do transfer learning and fine-tuning on a MobileNetV3-Large model with pretrained weights from ImageNet. The mobile application that hosts the deep learning model for on-device inference was developed using Android Studio.

The collection of the dataset was conducted on a Life/Form® Pitting Edema Trainer [1]. Due to the limitation of using edema simulators, nuances in actual human skin such as complexion, body hair, body marks, and other relevant variables were not taken into account during the dataset collection. The variables that were considered in the data collection were lighting, i.e., indoor or outdoor, the phone used to capture the images, and the phone operator. As for the mobile application, all features and functionalities would not require internet connection as the processing of the images will be done on the user's hardware. Thus, the user's hardware specifications can limit the application's performance.

2   Related Work

2.1   Peripheral Edema and Its Causes

Edema is the accumulation of fluid in tissues in different parts of the body. This occurs when capillary filtration exceeds its drainage limits, and fluid builds up in the tissues [23,25]. There are two types of edema: pitting (with indentation) and non-pitting edema (lack of indentation) [25]. Peripheral edema can be attributed to various medical conditions. It is crucial to determine the cause of peripheral edema, as specific therapeutic approaches are to be done based on its underlying cause [16]. Severe peripheral edema may be indicative of a severe heart condition, thus, a mild peripheral edema should be consulted to a physician for its appropriate treatment to be determined immediately.

2.2   Assessment of Edema and Current Challenges

The traditional way of differential diagnosis of peripheral pitting edema is through physical examination [21]. A pitting test is done, where the severity of pitting edema will be classified according to the indentation depth and/or rebound time of the skin [3]. While the pitting test is a widely used technique, this method of assessing the severity of peripheral edema is primarily qualitative due to the highly variable technique of applying the pressure [3,20]. The most widely known quantitative assessment in edema testing is water displacement volume-try [18]. The results of the study by Petersen et al. show that water displace-ment volumetry is a reliable way of measurement specifically in lower-extremity swelling. However, this method is considered time-consuming and inapplicable to postoperative conditions [8]. Another proposed quantitative way of detect-ing peripheral edema is through bioelectrical impedance vector analysis (BIVA), where the conductivity of electrical current in the body is normalized by the subject's height and plotted in a nomogram [15]. This study shows that BIVA is a semi-quantitative volume assessment method which produces highly accurate results. However, this process was proven to be inconvenient for immediate test-ing of patients and requires equipment that is expensive and not easily accessible. Finally, the assessment of peripheral edema puts extra workload on the medical staff who are already burdened due to inadequate staffing and poor workforce planning [10]. Thus, this issue has to be emphasized as this burden on hospital staff affects many aspects, including quality of care and patient outcomes [14].

2.3 Telehealth Monitoring

Implementing a system that allows patients to monitor their condition remotely will help promote active patient participation in taking care of their health and reduce the workload of hospital staff onsite. Such systems can be described as telehealth or telemedicine which are means of providing healthcare services remotely with the use of technology [11]. Monitoring the condition of heart failure (HF) patients remotely via telehealth will be highly beneficial since the majority of their treatment costs are allotted to hospitalizations. Moreover, the treatment of chronic HF patients also consists of frequent outpatient visits to monitor their current health status. Thus, several advanced monitoring means and devices are being introduced to lessen both the patients' mortality rate and financial burden [2]. Information and Communication Technology (ICT) has potential in improving the healthcare system, specifically in monitoring at-risk patients without requiring any in-person health consultations [22]. Due to the increased risk of HF patients to develop peripheral edema [17], the challenge is to utilize existing technologies that will aid in monitoring the presence and severity of peripheral edema remotely with telehealth.

2.4 Deployment of Telehealth Services via Mobile Applications

Global mobile technology usage has significantly increased in the past decade. With this trend, the use of mobile phones in healthcare, also known as Mobile Health (mHealth), has proven to be beneficial for patients and healthcare providers. Mobile health assists patients through various means, such as follow-up appointments and adherence to treatments [4]. Studies have shown the effec-tiveness and acceptability of patients on the usage of mobile applications for their health-related treatments [7]. Thus, mobile applications have the potential to be an ideal medium to deliver telehealth services that will remotely monitor the presence and severity of peripheral edema.

2.5   Potential Application of Deep Learning in the Assessment of Peripheral Edema

Due to the qualitative nature of peripheral edema assessment through the pitting test and low accessibility to other methodologies, there is a need for a more quantitative and accessible approach. The application of machine learning and deep learning in monitoring the presence of peripheral edema has already been explored in previous studies. Chen et al. evaluated the accuracy of machine learning using linear support vector machine (SVM) trained on histogram of oriented gradients (HOG) to classify the severity of edema (no edema, grade 1, grade 2, grade 3, grade 4+) based on images and videos taken right after a pitting test [5]. The performance of AlexNet with pretrained weights from ImageNet was compared to the performance of the HOG+SVM method. The dataset used in their model training consisted of two sets: single-frame images showing the indentation depth of the skin and three-frame stacked images which include temporal information on the skin's rebound time. Their dataset was obtained from pitting edema simulators which are tissue pads used to emulate the tissues of humans with different edema grades. Their results showed that the HOG+SVM approach has an accuracy of 87.33% when trained on single-frame images and 94.22% when trained on three-framed stacked images. The deep learning model proved to be a more accurate model regardless of the dataset used with 97.33% accuracy on single-frame images and 98.77% accuracy on three-frame stacked images. However, the paper lacked testing on actual human skin so there is uncertainty on whether the accuracy of the model will hold when it is used with inputs from actual human skin.

2.6   Limitations in the Integration of Deep Learning and Mobile Application Development

Deploying a deep learning model on mobile applications that will assess peripheral edema will be advantageous in telehealth monitoring because the patients will be able to do it with just their handheld devices. However, there are issues that need to be addressed regardless of the infrastructure being used. Web-hosted deep learning models are vulnerable to adversarial attacks and data privacy issues such as reverse engineering of the model and recovery of sensitive user data used for training [13]. Deploying the model on the client's device is one solution to address these issues since no data has to be transmitted over the internet. However, with the increasing complexity of deep learning models, there is also an increase in the demand of hardware resources that are needed to run the model. Since mobile phones are resource-constrained in terms of computing power, memory, and storage due to its form factor, the complexity of the model poses a challenge in its deployment [24]. Therefore, there is a need for the use of deep learning models that are mobile friendly in terms of efficiency while also maintaining good accuracy.

2.7   Use of the MobileNetV3 CNN Model for Image Classification in Mobile Devices

MobileNetV3 was developed in a bid to optimize the deployment of deep learning models in mobile and embedded devices. Qian et al. compared the performance of MobileNetV3-small and MobileNetV3-large to AlexNet, InceptionV3, ShuffleNetV2 and concluded that MobileNetV3 uses less floating point operations than other models. The training and validation accuracy of MobileNetV3 was also comparable to the accuracy of the other models that are more complex and designed for more powerful devices [19]. Hussain et al. also evaluated the performance of MobileNetV3 on image classification of plants through handheld devices. Their results showed that the accuracy of MobileNetV3 is comparable to existing leaf recognition CNN algorithms with the training time being significantly lower while also keeping the model size as small as less than 5 megabytes [12].

3   Methodology

3.1   Dataset Collection

The Life/Form® Pitting Edema Trainer was used in collecting the dataset for the deep learning model. The pitting edema trainer simulates human tissue to demonstrate edema from grades 1 to 4. It is a medical grade equipment that adheres to a standardized criteria specific to its use, and is often used for training clinicians in assessing pitting edema. Upon conducting a pitting test on the Life/Form® Pitting Edema Trainer, the grades 1 and 2 edema simulator pads did not show distinguishable indentations because of their toughness. Due to these issues, only grades 3 and 4 were used to represent mild and severe edema, respectively. Furthermore, the edema trainer pad for grade 1 edema was used to represent grade 0 (no edema), as it more closely resembles the effect of pitting test on a normal skin. For each edema grade, 150 closeup images of the trainer pad were collected right after the finger was lifted from the pitting test (see Fig. 1). This amount of data collected was based on the experiment of Chen et al. where they used 150 single-frame images per peripheral edema grade as their dataset for training an AlexNet model [5]. Moreover, the temporal information in the edema pads' rebound time was omitted since the results of Chen et al. showed only a 1.44% increase in Alexnet's accuracy in three-framed stacked images compared to single-framed images. This was also done to reduce the computational size and resources needed to train the model. The mobile phones used had a resolution of at least 1080p, and the images were captured under unregulated environmental conditions, i.e., varying lighting conditions.

3.2   Deep Learning Model Design

To determine the severity of peripheral edema (normal, grade 3, or grade 4), the convolutional neural network (CNN) must be suited for multiclass classification.

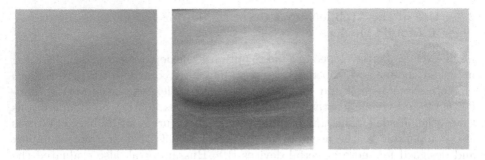

Fig. 1. Sample images of grade 3 (left), grade 4 (middle), and no edema (right) from the dataset

Given the small dataset for this application, training a CNN model from scratch to evaluate the presence and severity of edema will likely yield poor accuracy due to overfitting [27]. Thus, transfer learning was utilized to reduce the effects of overfitting from small datasets since the ability of the model to distinguish features has already been pretrained on a larger dataset [28]. A MobileNetV3-Large model with pretrained weights from ImageNet was used for this application.

The convolutional layers of the model were frozen to retain their weights during the training of the model on the edema dataset. This allowed the model to keep the general feature extraction and recognition capabilities that it has already learned from training on millions of images on ImageNet. To use the pretrained model for the specific purpose of classifying the severity of peripheral edema, the fully connected layers were designed accordingly and appended to the frozen convolutional layers (see Fig. 2). First, an average pooling layer was added to help the model accurately predict the classification of an object regardless of the positioning of its features in the input while also cutting the computation cost by reducing the number of parameters and weights [9]. Three dense layers with rectified linear units (ReLU) as their activation function and 512, 256, and 128 neurons at their outputs, respectively, were then appended. These layers are responsible for the prediction of the edema classification. Finally, the output layer is a softmax layer with three neurons to represent the three edema stages and their probability distribution. The neural network hyperparameters that helped improve the accuracy of the model were also specified. A dropout of 0.5 was used. Dropout is a form of regularization that reduces overfitting by dropping random neurons in the fully connected layers. The optimizer used was the Adam optimizer with a learning rate of 0.001. Moreover, categorical cross entropy loss was used as the loss function for the training. During training, the dataset was also augmented to further improve the generalization of the model. Particularly, the brightness of the images was randomly varied from 20% to 100%. The images were also rotated within the range of -90∘ to 90∘. These hyperparameter configurations that yielded the best-performing model were determined empirically.

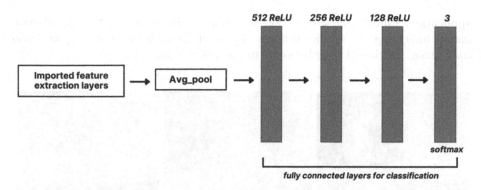

Fig. 2. MobileNetV3-Large model for peripheral edema classification

3.3 Deep Learning Model Validation Strategy

Due to the small dataset that was used for this project, it was not ideal to split the dataset into training and validation sets because there are some useful information that might be excluded from the model training. To address this limitation, the K-Fold Cross Validation technique was used [26]. This technique splits the dataset equally into an arbitrary value of k partitions or folds, each with equal class distribution. In particular, the proponents set the number of folds to five. The training was done five times where for each iteration, one fold was used as the validation set while the others were used for training. This technique allows every fold to be used as the validation set, thus, leaving no data unused for training. Moreover, 42 test images were collected which consist of seven images for each edema grade in certain lighting environments, i.e., indoor or outdoor. The accuracy of the model on images outside the dataset was evaluated in these test images.

3.4 Mobile Application Development

The mobile application developed aims to provide a medium for peripheral edema assessment which would allow patients to monitor their condition remotely without the supervision of medical practitioners. This would effectively reduce the workload of medical practitioners as they will only need to attend to their patients if the application detects the presence of peripheral edema. Since the application is targeted for the use of patients using their own mobile phones, it is ideal for the design of the application to be clear and straightforward. The application's main feature is a camera to capture a close-up video of the pitting test. The user will be instructed to capture the moment the finger is lifted during the pitting test (see Fig. 3). After the video is taken, the application will divide it into frames. The user must then select the first frame without a visible finger or shadow. A cropping feature will then allow the user to crop the frame such that only the indentation occupies the whole image (see Fig. 1). This cropped image will be used as the input to the deep learning model hosted inside the application. Finally, the application will display the results of the model evaluation indicating the predicted edema grade along with the model's prediction confidence, which will then be saved to the phone's gallery.

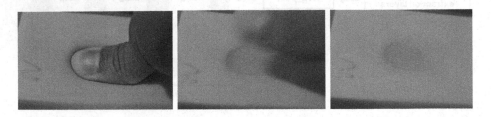

Fig. 3. Sample frames from a captured video

3.5   Integrated Testing of Mobile Application

The performance of the integrated mobile application and deep learning model was tested on images not included in the dataset. The proponents used the application to take 10 images of each peripheral edema stage from the edema simulator for a total of 30 images. The real-life accuracy of the model was then computed.

$$\%Accuracy = \frac{Number\ of\ Correct\ Predictions}{Total\ Number\ of\ Tests} \times 100\% \tag{1}$$

Moreover, it was determined if the model can accurately assess the presence of peripheral edema, i.e., if it can distinguish no-edema class from the other two classes using a metric called recall. Recall is the measurement used to compute the fraction of actual positives that were correctly classified. This metric needs to be maximized because it is important to avoid false negatives, i.e., images with peripheral edema being classified as normal. Regardless of the model's accuracy in distinguishing grade 3 from grade 4 edema, having a high accuracy on the detection of presence of edema will provide useful information for medical intervention since the patients would need to be treated regardless of severity.

$$Recall = \frac{True\,Positive}{True\,Positive + False\,Negative} \tag{2}$$

3.6   User Satisfaction Survey

After the completion of the mobile application, a user testing was held to evaluate the functionality and user interface of the application. The mobile application was used and evaluated by five users who were selected through convenience sampling. The selected users are aged 22–23 years old students at the University of the Philippines Diliman. They had no prior knowledge on the purpose of the mobile application and edema classification. Thus, the users were given a brief background of the study and its objectives. The pitting test was demonstrated using the Life/Form® Pitting Edema Trainer pads, in order to show the users how to properly use the tool. A single Android phone was used by all the test users to explore the functions and flow of the application on their own without any external help.

A survey questionnaire on Google Forms was given to the users in order to understand their perspective and consider their suggestions to improve the mobile application. Criteria such as ease of use, mobile application design and user experience were asked in the survey, asking the respondents to provide their thoughts on the specific criteria. Lastly, the respondents were asked for any improvements and feedback on the application.

4   Results

4.1   Deep Learning Model

The training and validation accuracy and loss of the model during the k-fold cross validation were collected (see Fig. 4). This shows the performance of the best model derived after hyperparameter tweaking and data augmentations. It can be seen that the accuracy and loss of both training and validation sets flatten out at around the 10th epoch.

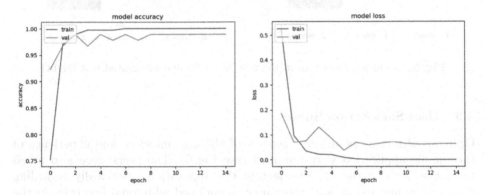

Fig. 4. Training and validation accuracy and loss

From the test dataset, a confusion matrix was generated to see how the model misclassifies each edema grade (see Fig. 5). From this, the recall can be calculated. Both grades 3 and 4 served as the positive variables, whereas the normal class served as the negative variable. This means that even if a grade 3 was misclassified as grade 4, it was still counted as a true positive as long as they were not misclassified as normal. This essentially measures the performance of the model in predicting the presence of peripheral edema regardless of its accuracy in detecting the specific severity. It can be seen that there are 27 true positives and one false negative. Therefore, the recall is 0.96. Moreover, the total accuracy of the model is computed to be 95.24%.

4.2   Integrated Testing of Mobile Application

The performance of the deep learning model was also evaluated once it was hosted in the mobile application. A confusion matrix was generated to summarize the model's performance in the integrated testing (see Fig. 5). Similar to the test dataset, the integrated testing yielded a high recall measurement of 0.95 with only one out of 20 positives being classified as a false negative. The total accuracy of the mobile application is 86.67%. It is also notable that all misclassifications in both test dataset and integrated testing involve grade 4 edema and normal classes being misclassified as grade 3 edema, and vice versa.

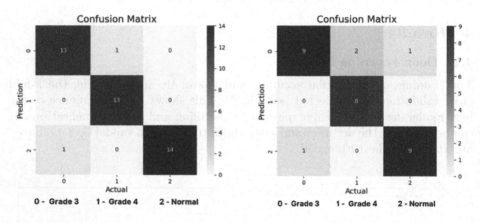

Fig. 5. Confusion matrix from the test set (left) and integrated test (right)

4.3   User Satisfaction Survey

Opinions of test users on some aspects of the user interface and experience of the mobile application were obtained (see Fig. 6). The users were also asked for suggestions on the improvement of the application, specifically regarding its functionality and design. Some users mentioned additional functions in the application that could aid them in the video recording and frame selection to maximize their chances of getting accurate results. First, a function that would detect the angle of the video recording, which would also state if the current angle is optimal or needs to be adjusted. Another functional improvement would be an automatic selection and cropping of a frame from the recorded video. Having these additional features would improve the ease of use of the application.

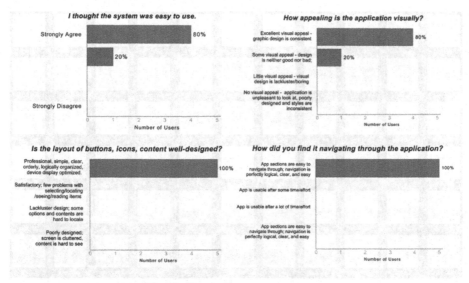

Fig. 6. Survey response summary

5 Discussion

It was shown that there was a quick stabilization of the deep learning model's accuracy to its maximum performance and a steep decline of the loss after just a few epochs. These results can be attributed to the nature of the dataset used. Since the dataset is small and the images generally have the same image composition with just the lighting and angle of capture varying (see Fig. 7), the model was able to easily distinguish the feature, i.e., the indentation depth, that defines the different edema grades. The high validation accuracy and low validation loss even at the earlier epochs can be explained by the fact that even the validation set had similar image composition as the training set. These results may be indicative of model overfitting as the model only performs well on new images outside the training and validation set that have the same image composition as the dataset.

To address the problem of overfitting, more images must be added to the dataset for training. Moreover, the composition of the new images should deviate from those that are already in the existing dataset. Having new images with more noise, i.e., background objects, shadows, etc., will negatively affect the training and validation accuracy and loss due to the model having to deal with random features and objects aside from the indentation. However, this will improve the model's generalization.

It was also shown in the confusion matrices that grade 3 edema was always involved in the model's incorrect predictions. These misclassifications are due to the fact that grade 3 edema may look similar to both normal and grade 4 edema depending on the lighting of the image. In the integrated testing, more factors involving human error could explain the lower accuracy compared to the

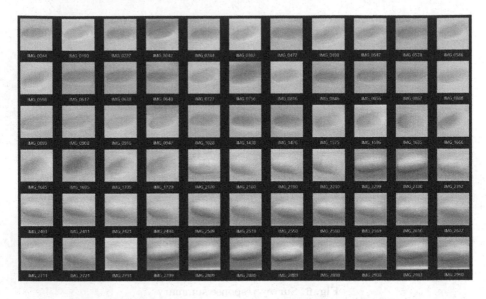

Fig. 7. Sample grade 4 edema images from the dataset

model's evaluation on the test dataset. This involves the angle at which a user took the video, the force they applied on the edema simulator pads, and the distance between the camera and the pad.

As for the mobile application, the users mostly found the application to be easy to navigate and understand, despite it being their first time using the application. The aesthetic design of the application was well received and the logical flow of the application was found to be cohesive. Some improvements need to be implemented to improve the application's ease of use to allow patients to capture the optimal image for edema prediction.

The results obtained in this study show that the performance of MobileNetV3-Large, a lightweight deep learning model specifically designed for mobile and embedded devices, is comparable to those of more complex and computational resource-heavy models such as AlexNet and SVM+HOG model [5]. The model's accuracy of 95.24% on the test dataset and 86.67% during the field testing of the application comes close to the 87.33% accuracy of HOG+SVM approach and 97.33% accuracy of AlexNet. This further enables the use of mobile devices in remote assessment of peripheral edema as there would be less reliance on expensive and inaccessible equipment used in water displacement volumetry and BIVA assessment [15,18]. Moreover, this will lessen the burden on clinicians as the application can be used by patients to monitor their condition remotely without their supervision.

6   Conclusion and Recommendations For Future Work

6.1   Conclusion

It was demonstrated in this paper the development of a deep learning model, particularly the MobileNetV3-Large, using transfer learning to predict the presence and severity of peripheral edema. A dataset which contains images of different edema severities was collected from an edema simulator due to the lack of publicly available dataset and the difficulty of obtaining images from actual patients with peripheral edema. The resulting model accuracy is comparable with the performance of SVM+HOG and Alexnet models, trained on both single-frame and three-frame images [5]. Moreover, both tests yielded a recall value of at least 0.95 which indicates that the model performs well in detecting the presence of peripheral edema. However, it was also observed that the model experiences overfitting on the dataset. This entails that new images to be fed to the model for prediction must also have the same image composition as the images in the dataset to get an accurate result. Thus, the mobile application was specifically designed to guide users on how to take images that will closely resemble how the images in the dataset look to aid the model in making correct predictions.

6.2   Recommendations

For the application to be viable for use in the medical field, a larger dataset with thousands of images of peripheral edema in actual human skin has to be collected. This dataset should take into account factors such as skin complexion, body hair, body marks, different lighting environments, and others that might be relevant to further improve the generalization of the model. Subject to ethical and technical review of concerned institutions, this would require a pilot study to assess the feasibility of obtaining the dataset from actual patients and testing of the application in hospital setting. To ensure correct labeling of the dataset and fair evaluation of the application's performance in assessing peripheral edema, a medical practitioner must verify the severity of the patients' peripheral edema using conventional methods of assessment such as the pitting test. Several improvements in the mobile application can also be done in terms of functionality and design. An automatic selection of the most optimal frame for use in edema prediction may be implemented to lift the burden of choosing from the users. The application may also employ an online infrastructure to allow real-time updates and communication between patients and medical staff.

References

1. Life/form® Pitting Edema Trainer [SKU: LF00947]. https://nascohealthcareglo bal.com/products/lf00947
2. Braunschweig, F., Cowie, M.R., Auricchio, A.: What are the costs of heart failure? Europace: European Pacing, Arrhythmias Cardiac Electrophysiology: J. Working Groups Cardiac Pacing, Arrhythmias Cardiac Cellular Electrophysiol. Europ. Soc. Cardiol. 13 (Suppl 2), ii13–17 (2011). https://doi.org/10.1093/europace/eur081

3. Brodovicz, K.G., McNaughton, K., Uemura, N., Meininger, G., Girman, C.J., Yale, S.H.: Reliability and feasibility of methods to quantitatively assess peripheral edema. Clin. Med. Res. **7**(1–2), 21–31 (2009). https://doi.org/10.3121/cmr.2009. 819
4. Cannon, C.: Telehealth, mobile applications, and wearable devices are expanding cancer care beyond walls. Semin. Oncol. Nurs. **34**(2), 118–125 (2018). https://doi. org/10.1016/j.soncn.2018.03.002
5. Chen, J., Mao, T., Qiu, Y., Zhou, D., Masterson Creber, R., Kostic, Z.: Camera-Based Peripheral Edema Measurement Using Machine Learning. In: 2018 IEEE International Conference on Healthcare Informatics (ICHI), pp. 115–122 (Jun 2018).https://doi.org/10.1109/ICHI.2018.00020
6. Clark, A.L., Cleland, J.G.F.: Causes and treatment of oedema in patients with heart failure. Nat. Rev. Cardiol. **10**(3), 156–170 (2013). https://doi.org/10.1038/ nrcardio.2012.191
7. Coorey, G.M., Neubeck, L., Mulley, J., Redfern, J.: Effectiveness, acceptability and usefulness of mobile applications for cardiovascular disease self-management: Systematic review with meta-synthesis of quantitative and qualitative data. Eur. J. Prev. Cardiol. **25**(5), 505–521 (2018). https://doi.org/10.1177/2047487317750913
8. Fallahzadeh, R., Ma, Y., Ghasemzadeh, H.: Context-aware system design for remote health monitoring: an application to continuous edema assessment. IEEE Trans. Mob. Comput. **16**(8), 2159–2173 (2017). https://doi.org/10.1109/TMC. 2016.2616403
9. Gholamalinezhad, H., Khosravi, H.: Pooling Methods in Deep Neural Networks, a Review (Sep 2020) https://doi.org/10.48550/arXiv.2009.07485
10. Greaves, J., Goodall, D., Berry, A., Shrestha, S., Richardson, A., Pearson, P.: Nursing workloads and activity in critical care: a review of the evidence. Intensive Critical Care Nursing **48**, 10–20 (2018). https://doi.org/10.1016/j.iccn.2018.06.002
11. Howard, I.M., Kaufman, M.S.: Telehealth applications for outpatients with neuromuscular or musculoskeletal disorders. Muscle Nerve **58**(4), 475–485 (2018). https://doi.org/10.1002/mus.26115
12. Hussain, A., Barua, B., Osman, A., Abozariba, R., Asyhari, A.T.: Performance of MobileNetV3 transfer learning on handheld device-based real-time tree species identification. In: 2021 26th International Conference on Automation and Computing (ICAC), pp. 1–6 (Sep 2021) https://doi.org/10.23919/ICAC50006.2021. 9594222
13. Liu, X., et al.: Privacy and security issues in deep learning: a survey. IEEE Access **9**, 4566–4593 (2021) https://doi.org/10.1109/ACCESS.2020.3045078
14. Magalhães, A.M.M.d., Costa, D.G.d., Riboldi, C.d.O., Mergen, T., Barbosa, A.d.S., Moura, G.M.S.S.d.: Association between workload of the nursing staff and patient safety outcomes. Revista Da Escola De Enfermagem Da U S P **51**, e03255 (2017) https://doi.org/10.1590/s1980-220x2016021203255
15. Massari, F., et al.: Accuracy of bioimpedance vector analysis and brain natriuretic peptide in detection of peripheral edema in acute and chronic heart failure. Heart Lung: J. Critical Care **45**(4), 319–326 (2016). https://doi.org/10.1016/j.hrtlng. 2016.03.008
16. Michelini, S., et al.: Peripheral Edema: differential diagnosis. In: Inflammation in the 21st Century. IntechOpen (Oct 2020) https://doi.org/10.5772/intechopen. 82400
17. Navas, J.P., Martinez-Maldonado, M.: Pathophysiology of edema in congestive heart failure. Heart Disease and Stroke: J. Primary Care Phys. **2**(4), 325–329 (1993), https://pubmed.ncbi.nlm.nih.gov/8156185/

18. Petersen, E.J., et al.: Reliability of water volumetry and the figure of eight method on subjects with ankle joint swelling. J. Orthop. Sports Phys. Ther. **29**(10), 609–615 (1999). https://doi.org/10.2519/jospt.1999.29.10.609

19. Qian, S., Ning, C., Hu, Y.: MobileNetV3 for Image Classification. In: 2021 IEEE 2nd International Conference on Big Data, Artificial Intelligence and Internet of Things Engineering (ICBAIE), pp. 490–497 (Mar 2021) https://doi.org/10.1109/ICBAIE52039.2021.9389905

20. Sanderson, J., Tuttle, N., Box, R., Reul-Hirche, H.M., Laakso, E.L.: The Pitting test; an investigation of an unstandardized assessment of Lymphedema. Lymphology **48**(4), 175–183 (2015), https://pubmed.ncbi.nlm.nih.gov/27164763/

21. Schroth, B.E.: Evaluation and management of peripheral edema. JAAPA: Official J. Am. Acad. Phys. Assistants **18**(11), 29–34 (2005) https://doi.org/10.1097/01720610-200511000-00005

22. Sparks, R., Celler, B., Okugami, C., Jayasena, R., Varnfield, M.: Telehealth monitoring of patients in the community. J. Intell. Syst. **25**(1), 37–53 (2016). https://doi.org/10.1515/jisys-2014-0123

23. Trayes, K.P., Studdiford, J.S., Pickle, S., Tully, A.S.: Edema: diagnosis and management. Am. Fam. Physician **88**(2), 102–110 (2013), https://pubmed.ncbi.nlm.nih.gov/23939641/

24. Wang, Y., et al.: A survey on deploying mobile deep learning applications: a systemic and technical perspective. Digital Commun. Netw. **8**(1), 1–17 (2022). https://doi.org/10.1016/j.dcan.2021.06.001

25. Whiting, E., McCready, M.E.: Pitting and non-pitting oedema. Med. J. Aust. **205**(4), 157–158 (2016). https://doi.org/10.5694/mja16.00416

26. Yadav, S., Shukla, S.: Analysis of k-Fold cross-validation over hold-out validation on colossal datasets for quality classification. In: 2016 IEEE 6th International Conference on Advanced Computing (IACC), pp. 78–83 (Feb 2016).https://doi.org/10.1109/IACC.2016.25

27. Ying, X.: An overview of overfitting and its solutions. J. Phys. Conf. Ser. **1168**(2), 022022 (2019). https://doi.org/10.1088/1742-6596/1168/2/022022

28. Zhao, W.: Research on the deep learning of the small sample data based on transfer learning. AIP Conf. Proc. **1864**(1), 020018 (2017). https://doi.org/10.1063/1.4992835

Pervasive Glucose Monitoring: A Non-invasive Approach Based on Near-Infrared Spectroscopy

Maria Valero$^{(\boxtimes)}$ ⓘ, Katherine Ingram ⓘ, Anh Duong ⓘ, and Valentina Nino ⓘ

Kennesaw State University, Marietta, GA, USA
mvalero2@kennesaw.edu

Abstract. With more than 12% of Americans living with diabetes and more than 30% suffering from metabolic syndrome, the United States is facing the need for more technology for easy and non-invasive blood glucose monitoring. The current pervasive technologies can be leveraged as the foundation for new sensor devices and intelligent models to monitor and manage glucose. This paper presents an approach for monitoring glucose concentration with a pervasive device. The device capture and processes spectroscopy images of a body's extremity using a powerful machine learning model. The spectroscopy or spectral image is based on the theory of light intensity data from the spectrum. Using light absorption, the proposed sensor executes a model that permits glucose estimation. The procedure is noninvasive as no blood or needles are required. The device also pairs the information to a mobile application for real-time monitoring. Preliminary studies show an accuracy of 90.78% compared with traditional blood glucose estimation.

Keywords: Glucose Monitoring · Non-invasive Spectroscopy · Diabetes · Sensors · Machine Learning

1 Introduction

Pervasive computing has an essential role in healthcare applications [37]. Glucose monitoring, required for the successful management of diabetes, is enhanced by pervasive devices with the capacity of insitu computation [23]. Conventional glucose monitoring devices use an electrochemical method [13] to sample glucose concentration directly from blood or tissues. These require using a finger-prick to collect a droplet of blood or implanting a thin lancelet under the skin. The former provides a snapshot of the blood glucose concentration, while the latter provides continuous monitoring of glucose within the subcutaneous tissues. These minimally invasive methods involve inherent risks, including tissue damage and infection [49].

Non-invasive estimation of blood glucose concentrations with pervasive devices has emerged as an exciting alternative to collecting blood samples.

Supported by the University of Pennsylvania (NIA/NIH). Sub-Award # 587764.

D. Salvi et al. (Eds.): PH 2023, LNICST 572, pp. 274–289, 2024.
https://doi.org/10.1007/978-3-031-59717-6_19

However, current non-invasive technologies for estimating blood glucose are inaccurate, complicated to use, and/or expensive. methods using *Surface Plasmon Resonance (SPR)* [30] require a metal surface, typically gold, and is dependent on the refractive index of the medium. In addition, this method is sensitive to motion, requires a long calibration process, and involves carrying a large, inconvenient device [58]. Methods based on *fluorescence* [16] are more robust to variations in glucose concentration but are susceptible to interference from changes in pH and oxygen levels and carry a high risk of infection from contamination within the biological media [58]. *Optical Polarimetry (OP)* uses light transmitted through the retina of the eye to determine blood glucose concentration [34,44]. This technology benefits from good resolution, however the method is prone to interference from temperature changes, motion, and optically active compounds [58]. *Near-infrared Spectroscopy* [2] is becoming increasingly utilized as an alternative method to estimate blood glucose for its relatively low cost, minimal sample preparation, and its robustness to interference from substances, such as glass or plastic [58].

In this paper, we compare current methods of glucose estimation and describe our approach, including a detailed evaluation of a novel, non-invasive approach to pervasively monitor blood glucose using near-infrared spectroscopy. The glucose sensor is a small, intelligent device that can be fitted to a finger or ear. It is paired with a mobile application and smart voice assistant to deliver real-time blood glucose results. Our work contributes:

- Real-time non-invasive blood glucose monitoring based on near-infrared spectroscopy and machine learning.
- Rapid glucose detection suitable for pervasive devices and executed on a single-board computer.
- A device with 90.78% accuracy that has been validated against a popular commercial-grade glucometer in a racially-diverse population.

2   Related Works

Diabetes and metabolic disease are considered a silent epidemic in the United States [46]. Monitoring blood glucose is critical for the successful management of diabetes, though it involves either extracting blood several times per day or implanting subcutaneous needles. Both of these can be invasive, uncomfortable, and associated with risk of infection. Non-invasive methods to estimate blood glucose have been proposed and are summarized in Fig. 1.

Noninvasive technology for monitoring blood glucose has limitations, and each approach carries a unique set of challenges. Electrical approaches [19,35, 47,54] are overly sensitive to environment temperature, causing serious errors in the detection of the glucose level [22,58]. Thermal approaches [8,12,52,53] are susceptible to interference by skin conditions making the sensors very sensitive to sweat, leading to inaccuracies. This technology integration time is long and expensive, making it a poor choice for disadvantaged population [58]. Nanotechnology approaches [5,9,28,41], introduce issues with potential toxicity in

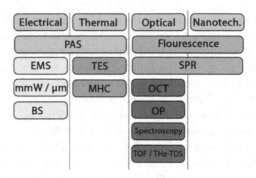

Fig. 1. Non-invasive approaches for blood glucose estimation. Photoacustic Spectroscopy (PAS), Electromagnetic Sensing (EMS), mmW-milimeter wave (mmW/μm), Bioimpedance Spectroscopy (BP), Termal Spectroscopy (TES), Metabolic Heat Conformation (MHC), Optical Coherence Tomography (OCT), Optical Polarimetry (OP), Time of Flight (TOF), Terahertz Time Domain Spectroscopy (THzTDS), Surface Plasmon Resonance (SPR).

addition to poor lifespan, poor photostability, and poor accessibility due to the need for expensive materials [58].

Optical technologies are becoming increasingly adopted for use in noninvasive glucose estimation in response to these challenges, though they are not completely free of limitations. *Mid-Infrared Spectroscopy* [15, 31, 32] is a vibrational spectroscopy technique that has provided the capacity to obtain signals from skin regions. However, this approach is expensive and has poor penetration in deep skin, which limits its effectiveness in glucose estimation [58]. *Raman Spectroscopy* [33, 38, 59] provides a way to measure molecular composition through inelastic scattering, but it is prone to interference by other molecules such as hemoglobin and has a lengthy collection time [58]. *Far-Infrared Spectroscopy* [53] has less scattering than Raman approaches, but has strong water absorption that makes extremely difficult the identification of molecules in the sample [58]; the *Time of Flight* and *Terahertz Time-Domain Spectroscopy* [11, 20] uses short and ultrashort laser pulses to measure the travel time of the reflected signals, but have long measurement time and low spatial and depth resolution [58].

Finally, the *Near-Infrared Spectroscopy (NIR)*, which relies on the absorption and scattering of wavelengths, has the advantage of being low cost, the signal intensity is directly proportional to the concentration of the analyte, requires minimal sample preparation, and works in the presence of interfering substances such glass and plastic [58]. Monte-Moreno et. al [36] used this method to estimate blood sugar, obtaining a Clarke error grid placed 87.7% of points in zone A, 10.3% in zone B, and 1.9% in zone C. Yamakoshi et al. [60] also use NIR for estimating glucose, obtaining a Clarke error grid placed 90.05% of points in zone A, and 9.95% in zone B. Also, Alarcon-Paredes et al. [3] used this technology to estimate blood sugar with a Clarke error placed 90.32% of points in zone A, and 9.68% in zone B. For information about Clarke error and zones, refer to Sect. 6.4.

While previous studies exhibit promising results, our proposed work is novel because (1) we incorporate a machine learning statistical approach that has not been used before for glucose estimation; (2) we develop a light method that can be run in pervasive devices and present results in real-time, and (3) we exhibit better results with more rigorous evaluation, including Parkes error grid [40], a more robust method to evaluate glucose estimation devices.

3 Principles of Near-Infrared Spectroscopy for Glucose Estimation

Near-infrared spectroscopy (NIR) illuminates the target tissue with a near-infrared light to visualize the organic composition of the material or tissue of interest [56]. NIR light waves contain a broad spectrum of wavelengths and frequencies, which are then absorbed, transmitted, reflected, or scattered by the sample of interest [42]. In our model, a polychromatic light source (Light Emitting Diode (LED)) is radiated through the sample. A diffraction grating then splits the transmitted radiation into its constituent wavelengths to a camera (sensor) and the images are analyzed by a computer board (detector). Figure 2 illustrates this absorption mode. Our prototype uses image capture via camera for its superior speed, replicability, and accessibility, in comparison to other forms of spectroscopy measurement, such as light intensity and Photoplethysmography (PPG) signals.

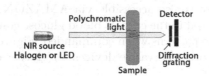

Fig. 2. Foundation of Near-Infrared Spectroscopy.

Our approach is based on the Beer-Lambert law of absorption that is shown in Eq. 1 [48].

$$I = I_0 10^{(-l.\epsilon.c)} = I_0 10^{(-l.\mu_a)}, \qquad (1)$$

where I_0 is the initial light intensity (W/cm^2), I is the intensity of the ith at any depth within the absorption medium in W/cm^2, l is the absorption depth within the medium in cm, ϵ is the molar extinction coefficient in $L/(\text{mmol cm})$, and c is the concentration of absorbing molecules in mmol/L. The product of ϵ and c is proportional to the absorption coefficient (μ_a).

The concentration of absorbing molecules is based on the above equation. However, the effect of other blood components and absorbing tissue components affect the amount of light absorbed. As a result, the total absorption coefficient is the summation of the absorption coefficients of all the absorbing components [26]. Then, to minimize the absorption due to all the other components, the wavelength of the light source should be chosen so that the light source is highly absorbed by glucose and is mostly transparent to blood and tissue components.

4   Approach Overview

Our prototype uses a clip attached to a finger or other accessible extremity and irradiates a NIR laser light of 650 nm and 5 mW voltage. On the other side of the clip, a Raspberry PI camera captures the diffraction grating images. A small computer board extracts data from the images and applies a machine learning model to generate estimates of blood glucose concentration. The data is saved to an InfluxDB time-series database [24] for continuous data collection. Figure 3(a) illustrates the prototype and approach.

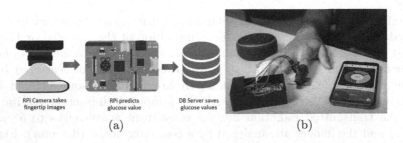

RPi Camera takes   RPi predicts   DB Server saves
fingertip images   glucose value   glucose values

(a)   (b)

Fig. 3. (a) General overview of the proposed approach. (b) Prototype structure and external communication with other devices of the proposed approach.

The associated mobile application displays real-time results from the database. The database is also accessible via AMAZON ALEXA, which will reply to commands related to the current blood glucose concentration and recent history of blood glucose patterns when commanded. Figure 3(b) depicts the prototype compared with other pervasive devices for glucose estimation.

5   System Design

5.1   Data Gathering and Cleaning

Images are collected using a KY-008 laser transmitter with a 5 mW voltage and a wavelength of 650 nm. The size of the laser is 24×15 mm/0.94×0.59 inch(L*W). A 640×480 resolution was selected to preserve small details without sacrificing computing time and resources. The standard RGB (red, green, and blue) color format was used. An average of 15 measures for each sample was used to minimize the influence of random errors such as the noise of the spectrometer and variations in humidity within the laboratory. A set of 4 fingertip images is shown in Fig. 4.

5.2   Features Extraction

Each image is analyzed by three color channels (red, green, and blue) and also in grayscale. For each channel, the image is first converted into numerical tensors with 3-dimensional matrices. The tensors are then converted into

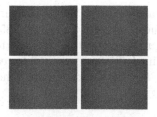

Fig. 4. Example of spectroscopy images collected from a finger at 8 s (top left), 16 s (top right), 24 s (bottom left), and 32 s (bottom right) after comparison blood draw.

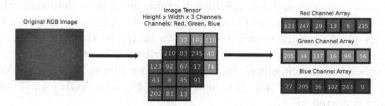

Fig. 5. Demonstration of Measurement Dataset Creation

a one-dimensional array and pixel statistics are calculated including center of mass, minimum, maximum, mean, median, standard deviation, and variance, as depicted in Fig. 5.

Values for each channel were compiled into the same dataset with the comparison blood glucose value and repeated for each image. The resulting "Measurement Dataset" consisted of seven measures from each of the four channels plus one measure of the blood glucose, for a total of 29 distinct measures. Next, the 29 measures from the image are merged with the intensity values of the image. The intensity values are calculated as follows: for each possible value of red, green, and blue (0–255), the number of pixels with that same value in an image can be counted and recorded in a histogram [21]. Through this process, a histogram with RGB values on the x-axis (256 possible values for red, green, and blue) and the number of pixels on the y-axis can be created, as shown in Fig. 6.

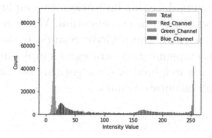

Fig. 6. Histogram of RGB Intensity Values in an Image.

The merge of the 29 measures from each of the four channels and the intensities estimated via the image's histogram, produce four new datasets: "Red-

Measurement", "Green-Measurement", "Blue-Measurement", and "RGB- Measurement". The first three new datasets contained 285 features: 256 for the pixel intensities, 28 for the measurement features, and one for the blood glucose value. The last new dataset contained 797 features: 256 for each color channel, 28 measurement features, and one for the blood glucose value.

5.3 Model Selection

In our previous works [55], we use a Convolutional Neural Network (CNN)to estimate glucose from spectroscopy images reaching only 72% accuracy. Then, we decide to compare multiple machine learning models to determine the best one for our type of images and data. We selected the AdaBoost classifier trained with KNN for its accuracy and its ability to adapt to the limited computing resources of the computer board [51], as described in Sect. 6. It was evaluated against other popular classifiers, including Random Forest [17], Elastic Net [57], Support Vector Machine [43], Bayesian Ridge [45], and XGBoost [7] and the results are reported in [27].

AdaBoost is a meta-estimator regressor that fits multiple copies of the model in layers onto the original dataset using adjusted weights of instances based on the error of the current prediction [1]. The layers are versions of the same model that tackle different sections of the training data, which results in reduced error overall. Due to the large number of varying estimators created by AdaBoost, the model is much less prone to overfitting than other models.

In contrast, KNN classifies a data point based on its nearest neighbors in the graph. It is a non-parametric supervised learning method used for classification and regression [29]. The regression algorithm uses the average values from a specified number of the nearest data and does not make assumptions. Therefore the algorithm handles outliers and minimizes error better in many cases than other algorithms, such as decision trees and linear regression. This model was selected for our approach due to its novel approach to ensemble learning, high training speed, and high performance.

AdaBoost is known as an effective method for improving the performance of base classifiers [10], though previous studies have shown that it is prone to overfitting [18]. To accommodate this limitation, we employ the KNN algorithm for its simplistic method of pattern classification. When KNN is combined with prior knowledge, it often yields competitive results. In our model, we combine AdaBoost and KNN as complementary strategies, employing AdaBoost for training the data and adding a weighted KNN algorithm on the classifiers produced by AdaBoost to generate accurate results.

6 Experiments

6.1 Experiment Ethics

The study was approved by the Institutional Review Board at Kennesaw State University (IRB-FY22-318). All participants provided written consent before participating.

6.2 Data Collection

A racially-diverse cohort of 43 individuals (23F/20M) between 18 and 65 years old participated in this study. Only 1 participant had diabetes, while the rest were normoglycemic. Participants were instructed to fast for at least four hours prior to testing and to remove any dark nail polish to minimize its potential impact on light absorption.

Glucose data were collected in two rounds: one at baseline and the other 1 h later, after eating a self-selected snack containing carbohydrates to modify glucose levels. Each round provided a set of 15 images collected from the finger and a finger prick blood draw to estimate blood glucose from the FORA 6 Connect BG50 glucometer per manufacturer instructions. After data cleaning, the final dataset consisted of 1128 sample images. Data collection and the glucometer are depicted in Fig. 7.

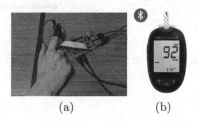

(a)   (b)

Fig. 7. (a) Example of data collection. (b) Glucometer used for comparison purposes.

6.3 Training of the Model

Data were divided into subsets for training (75%) and evaluation (25%). The training data is used to train the models to identify patterns, while the evaluation data is used to evaluate the predictive quality of the trained model.

6.4 Evaluation Rigor

Error Grids. Both Clarke and Parkes error grids were used to test the accuracy of our method in comparison to estimates from our referent device, the FORA 6 Connect glucometer [6]. For the Clarke Error Grid, data collected from the two devices are plotted and compared according to the degree of risk that an erroneous measurement would represent [58]. The degree of risk is divided into five regions, as depicted in Fig. 8. RData in Region A is considered "clinically accurate", while those in Region B are considered "clinically acceptable". Data found in Regions C, D, and E are considered clinically inaccurate and dangerous due to the potential for misdiagnosis [14]. The Parkes error grid similarly uses five risk levels for comparative analysis [39] and represents a new set of innovative error grids based on the proficiency of a big group of medical experts.

ISO 15197 Standard. The International Standards Organization (ISO) defines specifications for the reliability of medical devices, including glucometers [25]. The ISO standard (2013) requires that 95% of the results are within a glucose concentration of pm 15 mg/dL, compared with the reference method, for concentrations less than 100 mg/dL, or pm15% of zones A and B of the Parkes (Consensus) Error Grid [50].

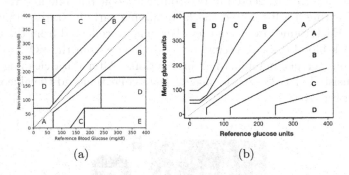

(a)   (b)

Fig. 8. Error grids (a) Clarke. (b) Parkes.

6.5 Data Analysis

The model performance was compared using the Mean Average Error (MAE) and the percent of data that falls into Zone A of the Clarke Error Grid, indicating "clinically accurate". Mean Average Error (MAE) and Root Mean Square Error (RMSE) were calculated. Models were further trained, tuned, and tested against the testing data. Findings are displayed in Table 1.

Table 1. Model Testing Results from Measurement Datasets - MAE and Zone A percentages from Clarke error grid analysis

	RM	GM	BM	GBM
Random Forest	12.85–87.23%	12.63–86.52%	13.91–85.82%	12.74–88.65%
Elastic Net	15.68–84.04%	16.89–85.11%	15.55–81.56%	14.41–83.69%
KNeighbors	9.55–90.78%	14.3–86.17%	15.81–84.4%	12.43–87.59%
Support Vector	14.3–87.94%	15.02–89.01%	14.58–87.23%	13.28–87.94%
Bayesian Ridge	15.52–84.04%	17.43–85.46%	15.52–82.62%	14.3–83.33%
XGBoost	13.03–86.88%	12.86–88.3%	13.6–86.52%	12.89–87.59%
AdaBoost	9.4–90.78%	12.74–86.88%	13.41–87.59%	13.18–86.52%

AdaBoost with KNeighbors trained on the Red-Measurement dataset provided the most accurate blood glucose estimates among all of the dataset models tested (MAE, 9.4 mg/dl; RMSE, 16.72 mg/dl). As shown in Fig. 9(a), all data were located in Zones A and B, with 90.72% of the measures in Zone A ("clinically accurate") and 9.22% in Zone B ("clinically acceptable"). No values were outside of these categories.

The Parkes Error Grid, was also used to evaluate our model. As shown in Fig. 9(b), 87.2% of the values were in Zone A, while 11.7% were in Zone B. Two measures (1.1%) narrowly extended into Zone C, and were classified as "clinically inaccurate - likely to affect the clinical outcome".

We used the Parkes Error Grid to further evaluate our model. Figure 9(b) shows the results based on this error. In this case, 87.2% of the values fell into Zone A or "clinically accurate", 11.7% fell in Zone B or "clinically acceptable", and 1.1% fell in Zone C or "clinically inaccurate – likely to affect clinical outcome".

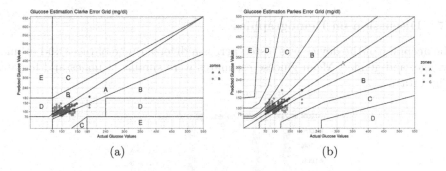

(a)   (b)

Fig. 9. (a) Clarke Error Grid. (b) Parkes Error Grid.

Table 2. Sample comparison of results of the proposed approach and the ground truth

	Demographics			Glucometer Readings		Proposed Approach Readings		Errors (mg/dL)		
	Age	Gender	Race	First	Second	First	Second	Error 1	Error 2	Av. Error
1	43	Female	White	83	85	83	88	0.0	3.53	1.77
2	21	Male	Black	113	120	113	115	0.0	4.17	2.09
3	24	Female	White	98	98	99	99	1.02	1.02	1.02
4	33	Female	Latino	92	95	93	96	1.09	1.05	1.07
5	24	Male	Latino	100	124	96	125	4.0	0.81	2.41
6	18	Female	Asian	82	84	83	87	1.22	3.19	2.21
7	18	Female	Black	95	100	98	94	3.16	6.0	4.58
8	31	Female	White	108	131	105	123	2.78	6.11	4.45
9	41	Male	Latino	84	105	89	102	5.95	2.86	4.41
10	24	Female	Latino	87	96	89	95	2.3	1.04	1.67
11	29	Female	Black	80	102	82	101	2.5	0.98	1.74
12	39	Male	Asian	80	102	80	102	2.5	0.98	1.74
13	27	Female	White	80	106	84	105	5.0	0.94	2.97
14	29	Male	Asian	83	101	85	99	2.41	1.98	2.2
15	28	Male	Asian	87	140	86	133	1.15	5.0	3.08
...	...	...	...	...	...	...	...	...	...	...

6.6 Discussion on Accuracy

A comparison between glucose estimates from our model and from the FORA6 Connect for 15 individual participants is shown in Table 2. The average deviation between the actual value and the estimated value is within ±1.02 mg/dL and ±4.5 mg/dL. Our prototype and model meet the ISO 15197 standard requiring ±15% of data to be within Zones A and B.

We further compared the accuracy of our approach with published findings of other noninvasive approaches using the Clark Error method only. Figure 10 illustrates our accuracy compared with these approaches [36,60], and [3]. None of these studies had Parkes Error grid data available, and therefore we cannot make comparisons with these data. Our findings indicate that the accuracy of our approach is as strong as, or superior to, other approaches that have been introduced.

6.7 Discussion on Demographics

The accuracy of the device was tested across a diverse range of races and ethnicity, age, and gender. Mean glucose estimates were similar in males and females (Fig. 11(a)).

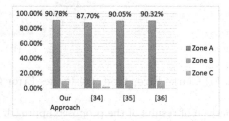

Fig. 10. Clarke error accuracy comparison with other research approaches.

No significant difference in average error was observed in mean glucose concentration when data was stratified and analyzed by mean age (30 years) or sex, as shown in Fig. 11(b) We found no significant difference in the average error between both groups.

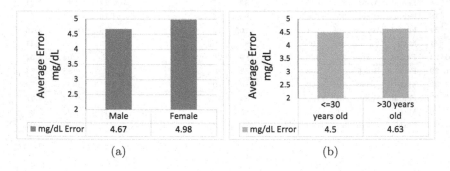

Fig. 11. Comparison of average error in mg/dL based on (a) gender, (b) age.

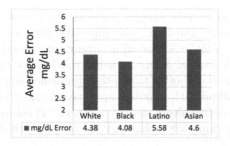

Fig. 12. Comparison of average error in mg/dL based on race.

Finally, glucose estimates were compared by differences in skin pigmentation to test our hypothesis that darker skin tones would yield less accurate results than lighter tones. In Fig. 12 the results of the average error in terms of race are presented. Glucose estimates for Latino and Asian participants were less accurate than those for the other participants, while estimates for black individuals were more accurate than the white participants. These findings suggest that measures taken on lighter skin tones are less accurate than those taken on darker skin tones, counter to our original hypothesis. More research is needed to study the effect of skin pigmentation on the accuracy of these models.

7 Limitations

The following limitations were identified. We have created a strategy to overcome these issues in our future work:

- External Factors: Depending on the radiation used, a viable noninvasive optical sensor must consider skin pigmentation, surface roughness, skin thickness, breathing artifacts, blood flow, body movements, and ambient temperature [4]. We plan to address all these factors in future enhancements of the model. Currently, we are not analyzing the impact of these factors, but our vision is to add some of these features into account to understand the reliability of the prototype and the technique.
- Prototype enclosure design: Our prototype design is in development with the goal of maximizing usability.

8 Conclusion

In this paper, we presented a non-invasive pervasive glucose monitoring approach for diabetes management that is based on near-infrared spectroscopy and machine learning techniques that leverage sensor device computation power. This approach uses images collected through the skin on a finger or ear and does not require blood samples. After testing several machine learning models, we have determined that AdaBoost trained with KNeighbors is the best model for estimating blood glucose from images collected by spectroscopy. Furthermore, the red channel provides the best color intensity data for training the model. Our final model had a 90.78% clinical accuracy rate based on the Clark Error Grid. and had 87.2% clinical accuracy using the Parkes Error Grid. Our approach performed as well or better than other published approaches. The ability to connect our prototype with a mobile application and a voice assistant makes this approach an attractive alternative to current methods of glucose monitoring and a potentially life-changing technology for people with diabetes.

Acknowledgments. Research reported in this publication was supported by the National Institute On Aging of the National Institutes of Health under Award Number P30AG073105. The content is solely the responsibility of the authors and does not necessarily represent the official views of the National Institutes of Health.

Conflict of Interest. All authors declare that they have no conflicts of interest.

References

1. Sklearn.ensemble.adaboostregressor. https://scikit-learn.org
2. Agelet, L.E., Hurburgh, C.R., Jr.: A tutorial on near infrared spectroscopy and its calibration. Crit. Rev. Anal. Chem. **40**(4), 246–260 (2010)
3. Alarcón-Paredes, A., Francisco-García, V., Guzmán-Guzmán, I.P., Cantillo-Negrete, J., Cuevas-Valencia, R.E., Alonso-Silverio, G.A.: An iot-based non-invasive glucose level monitoring system using raspberry pi. Appl. Sci. **9**(15), 3046 (2019)
4. do Amaral, C.E.F., Wolf, B.: Current development in non-invasive glucose monitoring. Med. Eng. Phys. **30**(5), 541–549 (2008)
5. Barone, P.W., Strano, M.S.: Single walled carbon nanotubes as reporters for the optical detection of glucose. J. Diabetes Sci. Technol. **3**(2), 242–252 (2009)
6. Boren, S.A., Clarke, W.L.: Analytical and clinical performance of blood glucose monitors. J. Diabetes Sci. Technol. **4**(1), 84–97 (2010)
7. Brownlee, J.: Xgboost for regression (Mar 2021). https://machinelearningmastery.com/xgboost-for-regression/
8. Buchert, J.M.: Thermal emission spectroscopy as a tool for noninvasive blood glucose measurements. In: Optical Security and Safety, vol. 5566, pp. 100–111. SPIE (2004)
9. Chen, L., Hwang, E., Zhang, J.: Fluorescent nanobiosensors for sensing glucose. Sensors **18**(5), 1440 (2018)
10. Chen, Y., Dou, P., Yang, X.: Improving land use/cover classification with a multiple classifier system using adaboost integration technique. Remote Sens. **9**(10), 1055 (2017)
11. Cherkasova, O., Nazarov, M., Shkurinov, A.: Noninvasive blood glucose monitoring in the terahertz frequency range. Opt. Quant. Electron. **48**(3), 1–12 (2016)
12. Cho, O.K., Kim, Y.O., Mitsumaki, H., Kuwa, K.: Noninvasive measurement of glucose by metabolic heat conformation method. Clin. Chem. **50**(10), 1894–1898 (2004)
13. Clark, L.C., Jr., Lyons, C.: Electrode systems for continuous monitoring in cardio-vascular surgery. Ann. N. Y. Acad. Sci. **102**(1), 29–45 (1962)

14. Clarke, W.L., Cox, D., Gonder-Frederick, L.A., Carter, W., Pohl, S.L.: Evaluating clinical accuracy of systems for self-monitoring of blood glucose. Diabetes Care 10(5), 622–628 (1987)
15. Coates, J.: Vibrational spectroscopy: instrumentation for infrared and raman spectroscopy. Appl. Spectrosc. Rev. 33(4), 267–425 (1998)
16. DiCesare, N., Lakowicz, J.R.: Evaluation of two synthetic glucose probes for fluorescence-lifetime-based sensing. Anal. Biochem. 294(2), 154–160 (2001)
17. Donges, N., Contributor, E., entrepreneur, N.a.: Random forest algorithm: a complete guide. https://builtin.com/data-science/random-forest-algorithm
18. Gao, Y., Pan, J.y., Gao, F.: Improved boosting algorithm through weighted k-nearest neighbors classifier. In: 2010 3rd International Conference on Computer Science and Information Technology, vol. 6, pp. 36–40. IEEE (2010)
19. Gourzi, M., et al.: Non-invasive glycaemia blood measurements by electromagnetic sensor: study in static and dynamic blood circulation. J. Med. Eng. Technol. 29(1), 22–26 (2005)
20. Gusev, S., et al.: Application of terahertz pulsed spectroscopy for the development of non-invasive glucose measuring method. In: 2017 Progress In Electromagnetics Research Symposium-Spring (PIERS), pp. 3229–3232. IEEE (2017)
21. Guzmán-Guzmán, I.P., Cuevas-Valencia, R.E.: An iot-based non-invasive glucose level monitoring system using raspberry pi (Jul 2019). https://www.mdpi.com/2076-3417/9/15/3046/htm
22. Haller, M.J., Shuster, J.J., Schatz, D., Melker, R.J.: Adverse impact of temperature and humidity on blood glucose monitoring reliability: a pilot study. Diabetes Technol. Therapeut. 9(1), 1–9 (2007)
23. Hartz, J., Yingling, L., Powell-Wiley, T.M.: Use of mobile health technology in the prevention and management of diabetes mellitus. Curr. Cardiol. Rep. 18(12), 1–11 (2016)
24. Influxdata Inc: InfluxDB (2019). https://www.influxdata.com/
25. International Organization for Standarization (ISO). https://www.iso.org
26. Jacques, S.L.: Optical properties of biological tissues: a review. Phys. Med. Biol. 58(11), R37 (2013)
27. Kazi, T., Ponakaladinne, K., Valero, M., Zhao, L., Shahriar, H., Ingram, K.I.: Comparative study of machine learning methods on spectroscopy images for blood glucose estimation. In: for Innovation, E.A. (ed.) EAI PervasiveHealth 2022 - 16th EAI International Conference on Pervasive Computing Technologies for Healthcare, Tessaloniki, Greece (December 2022)
28. Klonoff, D.C.: Overview of fluorescence glucose sensing: a technology with a bright future. J. Diabetes Sci. Technol. 6(6), 1242–1250 (2012)
29. Kramer, O.: K-nearest neighbors. In: Dimensionality Reduction with Unsupervised Nearest Neighbors, pp. 13–23. Springer (2013). https://doi.org/10.1007/978-3-031-02363-7_6
30. Li, D., et al.: Glucose measurement using surface plasmon resonance sensor with affinity based surface modification by borate polymer. In: 2015 Transducers-2015 18th International Conference on Solid-State Sensors, Actuators and Microsystems (TRANSDUCERS), pp. 1569–1572. IEEE (2015)
31. Liakat, S., Bors, K.A., Huang, T.Y., Michel, A.P., Zanghi, E., Gmachl, C.F.: In vitro measurements of physiological glucose concentrations in biological fluids using mid-infrared light. Biomed. Opt. Express 4(7), 1083–1090 (2013)
32. Liakat, S., Bors, K.A., Xu, L., Woods, C.M., Doyle, J., Gmachl, C.F.: Noninvasive in vivo glucose sensing on human subjects using mid-infrared light. Biomed. Opt. Express 5(7), 2397–2404 (2014)

33. Lundsgaard-Nielsen, S.M., Pors, A., Banke, S.O., Henriksen, J.E., Hepp, D.K., Weber, A.: Critical-depth raman spectroscopy enables home-use non-invasive glucose monitoring. PLoS ONE **13**(5), e0197134 (2018)
34. Malik, B.H., Coté, G.L.: Real-time, closed-loop dual-wavelength optical polarimetry for glucose monitoring. J. Biomed. Opt. **15**(1), 017002 (2010)
35. Melikyan, H., et al.: Non-invasive in vitro sensing of d-glucose in pig blood. Med. Eng. Phys. **34**(3), 299–304 (2012)
36. Monte-Moreno, E.: Non-invasive estimate of blood glucose and blood pressure from a photoplethysmograph by means of machine learning techniques. Artif. Intell. Med. **53**(2), 127–138 (2011)
37. Orwat, C., Graefe, A., Faulwasser, T.: Towards pervasive computing in health care-a literature review. BMC Med. Inform. Decis. Mak. **8**(1), 1–18 (2008)
38. Pandey, R., et al.: Noninvasive monitoring of blood glucose with raman spectroscopy. Acc. Chem. Res. **50**(2), 264–272 (2017)
39. Parkes, J.L., Slatin, S.L., Pardo, S., Ginsberg, B.H.: A new consensus error grid to evaluate the clinical significance of inaccuracies in the measurement of blood glucose. Diabetes Care **23**(8), 1143–1148 (2000)
40. Pfützner, A., Klonoff, D.C., Pardo, S., Parkes, J.L.: Technical aspects of the parkes error grid. J. Diabetes Sci. Technol. **7**(5), 1275–1281 (2013)
41. Pickup, J.C., Hussain, F., Evans, N.D., Rolinski, O.J., Birch, D.J.: Fluorescence-based glucose sensors. Biosens. Bioelectron. **20**(12), 2555–2565 (2005)
42. Prieto, N., Pawluczyk, O., Dugan, M.E.R., Aalhus, J.L.: A review of the principles and applications of near-infrared spectroscopy to characterize meat, fat, and meat products. Appl. Spectrosc. **71**(7), 1403–1426 (2017)
43. Raj, A.: Unlocking the true power of support vector regression (Oct 2020)
44. Rawer, R., Stork, W., Kreiner, C.F.: Non-invasive polarimetric measurement of glucose concentration in the anterior chamber of the eye. Graefes Arch. Clin. Exp. Ophthalmol. **242**(12), 1017–1023 (2004)
45. Rothman, A.: The bayesian paradigm & ridge regression (Dec 2020). https://towardsdatascience.com
46. Sherling, D.H., Perumareddi, P., Hennekens, C.H.: Metabolic syndrome: clinical and policy implications of the new silent killer. J. Cardiovasc. Pharmacol. Ther. **22**(4), 365–367 (2017)
47. Siegel, P.H., Tang, A., Virbila, G., Kim, Y., Chang, M.F., Pikov, V.: Compact non-invasive millimeter-wave glucose sensor. In: 2015 40th International Conference on Infrared, Millimeter, and Terahertz waves (IRMMW-THz), pp. 1–3. IEEE (2015)
48. Singh, K., Sandhu, G., Lark, B., Sud, S.: Molar extinction coefficients of some carbohydrates in aqueous solutions. Pramana **58**(3), 521–528 (2002)
49. So, C.F., Choi, K.S., Wong, T.K., Chung, J.W.: Recent advances in noninvasive glucose monitoring. Med. Dev. (Auckland, NZ) **5**, 45 (2012)
50. for Standardization, I.O.: In vitro diagnostic test systems: requirements for blood-glucose monitoring systems for self-testing in managing diabetes mellitus. ISO (2003)
51. Suja, P., Tripathi, S., et al.: Real-time emotion recognition from facial images using raspberry pi ii. In: 2016 3rd International Conference on Signal Processing and Integrated Networks (SPIN), pp. 666–670. IEEE (2016)
52. Tanaka, Y., Tajima, T., Seyama, M.: Differential photoacoustic spectroscopy with continuous wave lasers for non-invasive blood glucose monitoring. In: Photons Plus Ultrasound: Imaging and Sensing 2018, vol. 10494, pp. 494–498. SPIE (2018)
53. Tang, F., Wang, X., Wang, D., Li, J.: Non-invasive glucose measurement by use of metabolic heat conformation method. Sensors **8**(5), 3335–3344 (2008)

54. Tura, A., Sbrignadello, S., Cianciavicchia, D., Pacini, G., Ravazzani, P.: A low frequency electromagnetic sensor for indirect measurement of glucose concentration: in vitro experiments in different conductive solutions. Sensors **10**(6), 5346–5358 (2010)
55. Valero, M., et al.: Development of a noninvasive blood glucose monitoring system prototype: Pilot study. JMIR Formative Res. **6**(8), e38664 (2022)
56. Van Kempen, T.: Infrared technology in animal production. Worlds Poult. Sci. J. **57**(1), 29–48 (2001)
57. Verma, Y.: Hands-on tutorial on elasticnet regression (Aug 2021). https://analyticsindiamag.com/hands-on-tutorial-on-elasticnet-regression/
58. Villena Gonzales, W., Mobashsher, A.T., Abbosh, A.: The progress of glucose monitoring-a review of invasive to minimally and non-invasive techniques, devices and sensors. Sensors **19**(4), 800 (2019)
59. Xu, Y., et al.: Raman measurement of glucose in bioreactor materials. In: Biomedical Sensing, Imaging, and Tracking Technologies Ii, vol. 2976, pp. 10–19. SPIE (1997)
60. Yamakoshi, K.i., Yamakoshi, Y.: Pulse glucometry: a new approach for noninvasive blood glucose measurement using instantaneous differential near-infrared spectrophotometry. J. Biomed. Opt. **11**(5), 054028 (2006)

Co-design of a Data Summary Feature with Older Adults as Part of a Digital Health Platform to Support Multimorbidity Self-Management

Sarah Tighe⬤, Julie Doyle(✉)⬤, and Séamus Harvey⬤

NetwellCASALA, Dundalk Institute of Technology, Dublin Road, Dundalk 91 K584, Co. Louth, Ireland
Julie.doyle@dkit.ie

Abstract. The ProACT digital health platform helps older people living with multimorbidity (PwMs) to measure symptoms and activities related to their health and well-being, while also allowing them to share this information with their care networks. This paper describes the co-design process used to develop a 'Data Summary' (DS) feature within the ProACT platform. Participants were 7 PwMs aged ≥65 years living with ≥2 chronic conditions. Activity-based workshops took place where participants and researchers worked collaboratively to design the DS feature. Interactive activities and guided discussions were inspired by participatory design techniques to promote proactive involvement of participants who may not be familiar with design research. This process revealed that a concise DS displaying a self-selected month of data could help older PwMs to communicate key health information to their healthcare professionals, optimising time-constrained appointments. A colour-coded priority list within the DS would also highlight important health issues that an older PwM could utilise for goal-setting. In conclusion, the rigorous co-design process led to a clear design brief for the new DS feature, guided by 7 individuals who shared their lived experiences of navigating multimorbidity-related health challenges. The contribution of this work lies in an understanding of how to visualise complex data across multiple conditions, that will ultimately support enhanced self-management for older PwMs. A further contribution is the detailed presentation of co-design activities and prompts that may be of use to other researchers.

Keywords: Multimorbidity · Digital Health · Co-Design · Older Adults

1 Introduction

An estimated 50 million people in the European Union live with multiple chronic conditions or multimorbidity [1–3], which is typically defined as the presence of two or more chronic conditions in the same individual [4]. For people with multimorbidity (PwMs), services are often inconvenient and burdensome [5–7]. Diminished quality of

D. Salvi et al. (Eds.): PH 2023, LNICST 572, pp. 290–308, 2024.
https://doi.org/10.1007/978-3-031-59717-6_20

life is often a result of negotiating burdensome care pathways, as time and energy spent managing multiple conditions reduce their opportunity to engage in social or personal activities [8]. In response, there has been a necessary shift toward flexible and convenient home-based services [9–14], offering an evidence-based alternative to existing services while also reducing the distance of care [15]. One way this has been achieved is through the empowerment of PwMs to use digital health technology to play an active role in the self-management of their health and wellbeing.

In recent years, a small number of researchers have examined how to design digital health for multimorbidity self-management, and older adults in particular [16–19]. These studies showed that it is imperative to consider how such technologies can be designed to deal with the complexities of multimorbidity, as the management of various self-care tasks can be cumbersome. A previous requirements gathering study carried out for the ProACT platform [20] highlighted that the PwM is often the coordinator of their own care, given the lack of integration among healthcare professionals. Thus, it is imperative that the design of a comprehensive digital health platform is centred around the PwM, creating opportunities for them to actively participate in the development process.

1.1 Overview of the Design of the ProACT Platform

The ProACT platform - designed, developed and trialled during the ProACT Horizon 2020 (H2020) project[1] - aims to ease older PwMs' (hereafter referred to as PwMs) treatment burden by facilitating a number of complex multimorbidity self-management tasks including symptom monitoring, managing medication, inter-stakeholder communication, information management and coordination. People with more than one chronic health condition sometimes find it difficult to keep track of the different symptoms, medications, and tasks that are needed to manage their health and well-being. PwMs and members of their care network were involved in the design and development process of the first version of the ProACT digital health platform as part of the ProACT H2020 project. This involved an extensive requirements gathering process [20] that included semi-structured interviews and focus groups, co-design workshops, and usability testing. The output of this process was the ProACT platform, consisting of a suite of off-the-shelf devices for measuring symptom and wellbeing parameters and the ProACT App for viewing and reflecting on data, answering daily questions, receiving education content, and setting goals [21]. The iterative, user-centred design process aimed to ensure that the user interface and the information it presents were understood by, met the needs of, and fit into the daily lives of PwMs with varying cognitive capacities, health literacy and digital literacy.

Findings from a 12-month proof-of-concept (PoC) trial revealed that the ProACT platform was engaging and useful [21, 22]. Qualitative findings also revealed that the platform facilitated perceived improvements in participants' health and wellbeing, self-management, and support [21, 23]. Such a platform may facilitate self-management at home, and also facilitate greater coordination between PwMs and their care networks in relation to their healthcare; ensuring that healthcare systems become more sustainable and accessible to PwMs when necessary [24].

---

[1] https://cordis.europa.eu/project/id/689996.

Extensive feedback was collected during the ProACT H2020 project, resulting in updates and refinements being made to the platform, primarily in terms of aesthetics and navigation. While reviewing videos from usability testing sessions conducted with participants of the trial, it was observed that the majority of participants were reflecting on and making correlations across their various health and wellbeing data visualisations. For example, a participant might notice a high blood pressure reading on the blood pressure-specific section of the ProACT App, and subsequently navigate to other related data visualisations (e.g., heart rate, physical activity, blood oxygen) in an attempt to reflect on multiple data streams. To visualise the various related data, the user was required to switch to multiple new windows within the ProACT App, which added multiple additional steps, increasing the burden and complexity of their health data comparison. In response, a '*My Data Summary*' feature was considered as part of the platform redesign, which is the primary focus of this paper.

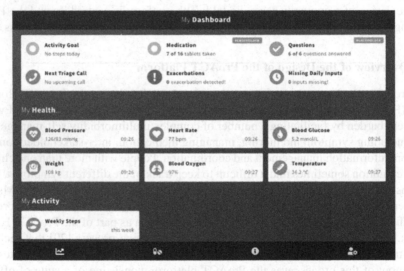

Fig. 1. Example of the ProACT App prototype.

1.2 Data Summary Feature

The '*My Data Summary*' was an additional ProACT App feature that came about through the initial design processes and a review of PoC feedback (Table 1). In essence, the concept of a data summary (DS) feature is to provide PwMs with a monthly overview of their individual health and wellbeing data. It could also support the comparison of trends across a PwMs' different health and well-being parameters and include a series of important and relevant insights to the individual about their health or disease trajectory. This type of digital health innovation aligns well with recent calls for research into data visualisation for chronic disease self-management [25]. This type of research is being highlighted due to the well-documented complexities and challenges of integrating various types and large volumes of data into health self-management technologies [25].

Table 1. Sources of information from ProACT H2020 Project underpinning the design and development of 'Data Summary' feature

Source	Extended Synopsis
Doyle et al., 2019 [20]	*Qualitative Needs Assessment* - DS as a tool for goal setting and health data communication with supporters - Consider design to support a more informed approach to goal-setting which is guided by the system e.g., contextual summary of previous and current health data - PwMs also expressed the need for support to ease the burden of managing multimorbidity. Design solutions to provide clear & concise communication of health data to supporters in seek of self-management support is critical
Doyle et al., 2021 [21]	*Proof-of-Concept Trial* - Participants spent more time reviewing their vitals than entering data or looking at their Dashboard. The 'View Readings' section (where participants could see an overview of all their health and well-being data) was one of the most frequently visited sections - Would suggest that in depth review of personal data is important to PwMs, but this appears to require a lot of over-and-back interaction with current app iteration to summarise current health status - PoC findings in line with existing literature reporting greater PwM self-efficacy due to technology-supported self-management, which enabled improved communication with health care providers. Comprehensive DS could further improve PwMs' autonomy in communicating health data to health care professionals/carers/supporters
Expert review of recorded usability testing [Unpublished]	*Review of ProACT H2020 Project Collective Outcomes* - Comprehensive view of multiple health data in one place for set time period (e.g., month) - Usability issues identified as part of the review process, that need to be addressed to provide optimal experience to future users - Important reflection was the lack of flow when PwMs are reviewing their own data. Particularly important for multi-morbidity cohort who must review multiple health measures to ascertain health status - Lack of integration/summarization of data may add to usability barriers

As the DS concept was further explored, several design questions were raised such as: what is the best timeframe for a DS (e.g., a weekly or monthly summary)?; how would it be visualised (e.g., through infographics or charts)?; and how would it be shared with care network members if desired (e.g., automatically shared monthly through ProACT App, PwM-initiated sharing via ProACT App, or an additional mechanism to download summary)? As the DS was an entirely new concept for the ProACT App, an extensive co-design process was planned to explore the construction and implementation of this feature.

Given the lack of research on designing a DS for multimorbidity self-management, a first step in this process was to engage a group of affiliated clinical triage nurses who had significant experience in using the ProACT platform to support the care of PwMs during the ProACT H2020 PoC trial, and who themselves regularly visualised multiple streams of data to fulfill their role [23].

The concept of the DS feature was presented to them during some informal group meetings and, in liaison with the study team, a number of important design considerations were developed from these discussions (Fig. 2). These discussions formed the basis for the co-design process described in this study, which was used to further explore how these DS requirements might be visualised within the ProACT App, and to further explore DS design considerations from the perspective of the PwM. Lor et al. [26] suggest that user-centered participatory approaches should be prioritised for the development of data visualisation features, with a focus on which visualisation elements work best for the desired population (PwMs) and in which contexts.

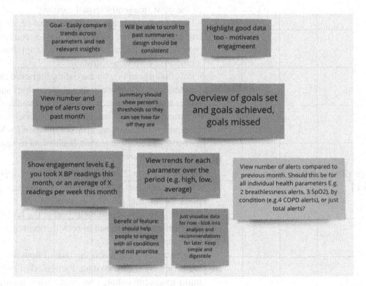

Fig. 2. Design considerations for DS feature following discussions with triage nursing teams.

1.3 Paper Objective

This paper describes the rigorous co-design process that was conducted to develop a DS feature to support PwM self-management. It outlines the proactive activity-based workshop methods used and describes the resulting design considerations for DS incorporation within future iterations of the ProACT App, and greater ProACT platform.

2 Methods

As the ProACT redesign progressed throughout 2022, co-design workshops were held with a panel of PwMs to guide the process. The five workshops were carried out on a monthly basis to allow for an ongoing process of analysis and iterative platform development (May to October 2022). The overarching goal of two of the five workshops was to explore the design of a new DS feature, that had been identified during the review process as being beneficial for inclusion within the optimised ProACT App. A working iteration of the ProACT App (which had been updated since the ProACT project trial) was used as a tangible workshop resource that could be critiqued by participants during workshop activities (Fig. 1) - which included placeholders for entirely new developments, such as the DS feature.

2.1 Participants

The workshop participant panel consisted of 7 participants, who between them participated in 5 workshops over a 5-month period. Inclusion criteria for this study were that PwMs were aged 65 or older; were community dwelling; had sufficient cognitive capacity to provide written informed consent; and had at least two of the following conditions: diabetes, chronic respiratory disease (e.g., chronic obstructive pulmonary disease (COPD), asthma), chronic heart failure, chronic heart disease. Sources of recruitment included a *Living Lab* panel, as well as participants from the previous ProACT H2020 trial who had consented to take part in additional research. PwMs were also invited to ask their informal carers if they would like to take part in the study, one of whom attended workshops.

2.2 Data Collection

Activity-based workshops were facilitated in small groups, consistent with recommendations that approximately four to six participants per session is optimum for this type of interactive research [27–29]. Two DkIT researchers facilitated the workshops. Workshops were up to 3 h in length to allow organic conversations to unfold, which is a well-regarded qualitative research technique [30]. Participants engaged in hands-on activities to stimulate discussion and inspire design ideas (Fig. 3) [31]. Techniques used in the activities were derived from multiple interrelated disciplines that have been widely used in digital health platform development, such as participatory design research and user experience design [32, 33].

The first activity was centred around discussions of participants' experiences of communicating data with their healthcare professionals. Participants worked in pairs with a fictional PwM profile that had easily identifiable similarities to their own current health situation. Questions were posed to guide the activity using techniques such as memory elicitation (Think about the last time you went to visit a doctor/nurse for one of your own conditions. Do you remember any emotions or physical sensations that were part of this experience? What types of aids do you use in your own visits that help you to communicate with your healthcare professional?) and story completion (Think about the types of goals and self-management tasks this person has to complete on a

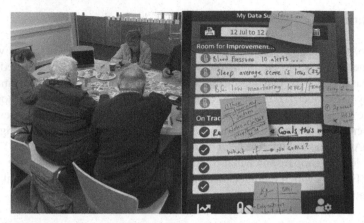

Fig. 3. Participants engaging in hands-on activities in co-design workshop.

day-to-day basis? Who are their guiding healthcare professionals? Think about what this person would like to achieve during one of their appointments? What would they need to bring with them? Are there any aids that you use in your own visits that might help you to better communicate with your healthcare professional?). The activity led to broader discussions that provided key information on time interval suggestions for a DS (e.g., weekly, fortnightly, monthly), identifying key information to be presented within the summary and how this might differ between various chronic conditions (i.e., disease-specific, healthcare professional-specific, goal-specific, individual health measures), and how a DS may be used during healthcare professional appointments (e.g., to ameliorate time barriers, improve short/long term recall, improve health literacy on medications and goals/plan).

Activity 2 explored participants' understanding and interpretation of some existing data summary styles (Fig. 4), followed by a deconstruction and reimagination of these graphical representations to co-create an appropriate DS feature for the ProACT App (Table 2).

The activity was developed with the understanding that participants' comprehension may be impacted by their own health literacy and personal health experiences. It posed questions to the PwM that related more specifically to their own lived experiences, rather than focusing on the complexity of a DS feature construction (e.g., 'Let's go back to thinking about your healthcare visits and the aids that you use to improve your communication', 'A weekly or monthly summary could potentially help you to communicate and could also help you to personally keep track of your own goals and health plan for the future', 'Take a look at these examples of summaries - at a first glance, do any of these summaries stand out to you? What do you like or dislike about it? What would you change about it? What types of information might you want to see here?').

Each of these examples are thorough in the data and details they present, but co-designing a contemporary DS feature based on reflections from PwMs' own lived experiences is an integral part of the research process. The following types of rhetoric were used to introduce this next stage of the task: "People in your position have been called 'experts of their experiences' [34] and your input can ensure ProACT caters to your

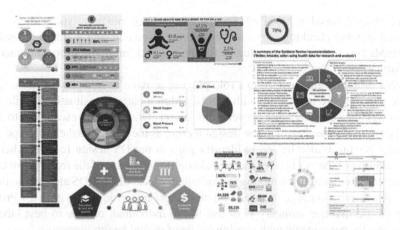

Fig. 4. Sample data summaries from various disciplines to inspire co-creation

Table 2. Sample questions to direct co-design of paper-based DS prototypes during activity.

	Timepoint
i	Use the cards on the table (or create your own) to create a bank of health information that would describe your health over the past month
ii	For each of the data points, how would you know if your progress was good/bad/average?
iii	Are there any colours or symbols that would alert you to a positive, negative, or no change in your data?
iv	Do any of the data points relate to each other? How would you describe this relationship?
V	Take a look at the different ways that the data can be laid out on the summary board e.g., charts, lines, boxes, calendars, icons and images. Using the creative tools on the table add colours, connecting lines, borders and any other details to your summary board
vi	Think about how you would explain your DS board to your GP in 5 min?
vii	Now consider if there is any information missing from your summary that may have helped you to communicate it more effectively or to review the information more comprehensively at a glance

priorities and the priorities of people like you. So, let's leverage your knowledge, experiences, and insights to design a DS tool. It can be as simplistic or as complicated as you like. There is no right or wrong way to summarise the information that is important to you."

Activities 3 and 4 were conducted as part of the second DS workshop, acting as a type of member checking session and to ensure all design recommendations had been taken into consideration. The session started with a group reflection on drafted prototypes of the DS Feature based on the previous workshop (Data Summary I). PwMs were presented with a static DS prototype and researcher-interpreted action points related to their feedback from the first workshop were communicated. A detailed discussion was then encouraged, based on how PwM input was translated into prototype designs, which facilitated member checking of researcher interpretation and captured honest feedback from PwMs by creating an opportunity for them to ask more questions and push DS ideas further.

PwMs subsequently engaged in a role-playing activity. In role playing, participants imagine that they are interacting with others within a particular situation, while using the prototype data summary as a conversation starter. This can help researchers to gauge participants' understanding of a new design feature as they describe the prototype aloud to another person. It also helped to identify gaps in the DS design feature, where the simple addition of 'helper text' or icons could optimise the use of the feature. For example, where a participant is attempting to explain an aspect of their DS aloud, researchers can use this activity to gauge the level of data interpretation required within the ProACT App to ensure that the summary is of use to the individual, or how to best label DS components for participants with varying levels of digital health literacy.

2.3 Data Analysis

As each workshop was completed, an annotated transcription of audio recorded data was collected for analysis. Between workshops, an expert panel of two researchers and two technology developers met to collaboratively review workshop data and draw ongoing design and development conclusions in a timely manner [35].

A 'live' content analysis of qualitative workshop datasets was conducted, where workshop data were utilised to make solution-focused decisions in a short time period. The ongoing iterative process of analysis and design is typically facilitated to ensure that PwMs' needs are being met through member-checking in follow-up workshops.

A summative content analysis was used for coding and categorisation of the data from the workshops. This consists of a combined manifest and latent approach. Manifest content analysis focuses on the words themselves and offers surface-level descriptions of workshop discussions/notes- which allowed researchers to quickly highlight key areas of interest for App development and refinement. For example, the number of times the word "personalisation" (or related synonyms) appears within the text would dictate whether this was a core category that required a design action for the DS feature. Following on from this, the context in which the words presented themselves in discussion (latent analysis) were used as a guide for researchers and technology developers to further consider appropriate development solutions during collaborative meetings. A deductive or 'top down' approach was used for analysis, centred around design expectations determined following the ProACT trial such as: what the timeframe would be within the feature; how it would be visualised; and how it would be shared with care network members if desired. However, it is important to note that the analysis process is not limited by predetermined categories, as the nature of co-design data collection methods (i.e., activity-based workshops) allow for open discussions which are inductive, unexpected, and guided by the participants themselves.

2.4 Ethics

Ethical approval for this co-design process was received from the School of Health and Science at Dundalk Institute of Technology.

3 Findings and Discussion

Six PwMs and one informal carer formed the workshop participant group (71% Male, Age Range 73–79 years). This study resulted in a preliminary design of the '*My Data Summary*' feature. Design recommendations from the first dedicated workshop (Data Summary I) were included in the preliminary analysis and visual protypes were produced based on PwM feedback to facilitate the follow up workshop (Data summary II). Valuable input was provided by participants as to how the DS should look, what information it should present, and how this information might be used by an individual. The following sections present findings from the workshops and discuss some of the contextual uses offered by PwM participants for a DS feature.

3.1 Visualisation of a Data Summary

3.1.1 Supporting Interpretation

Participants were not drawn to overly complex infographics or line charts. However, they noted, where there is a necessity for multiple pieces of information or extra detail, providing 'something' concrete to help them to understand their monthly summary at a glance would be preferred. These indicators could be simple icons or short text so that the PwM knows what they are looking at immediately. For example, one participant mentioned that the words 'poor' and 'room for improvement' on a sample design "struck me immediately". Despite the negative connotations, the participant valued the interpretation. This is consistent with literature which suggests that improving PwMs' interpretive capacity of their health data may lead to improved motivation [36].

Participants also mentioned the potential benefit of including an overall monthly health score incorporating all of their health data relating to their multimorbidity. Similar to the body mass index (BMI) scale, which takes a person's height and weight into account and creates an overall score- participants questioned whether this is something that could be considered for a multimorbidity-focused DS feature. This type of numeric health data summarization is well-researched in the management of chronic conditions and risk factors amongst older people [37–39], whereby the modelling of various health data information is to produce a single 'score'. Research suggests that these scores could be utilised to improve communication and shared decision-making between PwMs and their healthcare professionals [37].

Participants did not feel that a graph-style summary was the best approach- adding that if a graph was chosen as the medium for the DS, then it should be goal-oriented and "specific to the person". This aligns with a recent systematic review of health data visualisation [26] which suggests that, with a multitude of creative digital tools and software available in the digital health space, the design and dissemination of data visualisation features should extend beyond the typical bar graphs and line graphs etc.

Too much information is hard to read and can be complicated to interpret at first ["You want it to be simple"], but clear signposting could alleviate this. For example, participants liked the use of a traffic light system and a simple icon (e.g., dot, star, checkmark) to pinpoint where they fall on the colour chart, line or grid (Fig. 5). These findings are consistent with research that describes the data interpretation support required by PwMs who are self-managing their conditions [40]. A content analysis identified interrelated skills that make-up and define a person's health literacy level, including the filtering, interpretation and evaluation of health information, and subsequent engagement in informed health-related decision making [40]. People living with chronic conditions, who have lower health literacy, could achieve better levels of informed self-care if supportive technology functionalities, such as the ProACT DS feature, were made available to them for self-evaluation [40, 42].

Participants also mentioned that the colour red could signify danger to those who are managing life-threatening conditions. For one participant, red is "a bit triggering, a very worrying colour… y'know, red is danger", asking his co-participant who was admiring the traffic light system "but what about if it was red?!". To which she reacted negatively and agreed with him. Further group discussions led to the potential for a two-colour traffic light system (Fig. 5) that could incorporate amber (room for improvement) and green (good) on a scale.

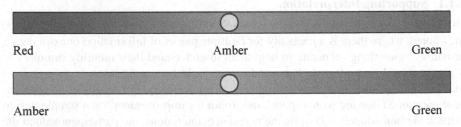

Fig. 5. Variations of potential 'traffic light system' use in DS feature

3.1.2 Personalisation and Motivation

One participant explained that personalisation using individual goals and personal thresholds are vital for a DS to work (e.g., 10,000 steps is a global recommendation, but 5,000 steps is my own personal goal). The participant added that "there's no point in telling me that I am obese. I am obese and if you give me an [impersonalised] chart I'm always going to be obese… but if you give me something that recorded my current weight and gave me a target of 10% to lose then I could be very positive moving from [from one data summary to another] by 5–10%. Instead of hitting me with the 'Boom'… the negative". In a simpler form, using an icon or colour to indicate where the PwM is at in terms of their own monthly health data or personal goal was perceived as helpful- especially if there is some indication of what "you're aiming for" (e.g., inclusion of personal goal or optimal reading).

There was an overall feeling from participants and researchers alike, that a certain "balance" is required, whereby a true summary of monthly data is provided to a PwM but with a level of appropriateness that does not alarm the reader. If a PwM's monthly DS is showing health data that is less than optimal for them as an individual, participants agree that this needs to be communicated via the ProACT App. On the other hand, there is an undercurrent of "anxiety" or "danger" that must be acknowledged in the presentation of less-than-optimal readings within a summary. A DS feature can be both informative and "stress-inducing" for the PwM and their care network. Participants emphasized that information presented within a monthly summary should act as "encouragement". Even if data is not ideal, the data should be "descriptive" rather than disheartening for a PwM: "You need 'encouragement'"; "[PwMs] want to improve themselves". Similarly, when presenting a month of multiple health data points, participants highlighted the importance of keeping successes in mind, to keep them focused and motivated. If multiple data points have been below thresholds or expectations over a month, this could affect a PwM's subsequent performance and stress levels: "The only trouble with all this, is if you are going downhill, it highlights it for you too, doesn't it?"; "It does, but you don't want to know"; "You want to think you're going to be feeling better next month"; "Yes, Yes!" Participants shared the potential negative impact that looking at a summary of multiple bad health data may have, "I'm talking about if everything is going downhill and no matter what I do y'know... I've now got my weight right, and my exercise is good, but the blood pressure is still going sky high. Certainly, I want to know in the current situation anything that's wrong".

Furthermore, having explored a range of structures (e.g., pie charts, imagery, info-graphics, line graphs), a list format that provides a monthly overview of a PwM's health and wellbeing information at a glance was preferred. Participants felt that the DS design should include a type of hierarchal structure that draws the eye to important self-management behaviours that need attention or improvement. This is consistent with existing research reporting that PwMs will prioritise their health problems which are of immediate concern, uncontrolled, or at risk of restricting their usual activities [43].

3.1.3 Supporting Self-Management

Through variations in colour (e.g., amber, green), icons (e.g., tick, exclamation mark) and basic data interpretation (e.g., comparisons with previous month over national averages), participants felt that the data summary feature could trigger important questions (e.g., 'What am I already achieving and what do I need to improve on next?') to further improve self-reflection and personal goal setting (discussed further in Sect. 3.2). For example, should a PwM's blood pressure be maintained well over the course of a month (within normal threshold ranges, with measure taken regularly), their DS would place this information further down the list (i.e., little to no attention needed). However, if this individual's blood glucose levels were regularly outside of recommended thresholds, or readings were taken sporadically throughout the month, this health measure would be placed further up the DS list to highlight it as needing more attention.

By identifying important relationships and trends within their DS (e.g., higher self-reported anxiety throughout the month could relate to lower levels of physical activity, which may affect blood pressure or weight trends), a PwM can begin to better understand their own health and wellbeing profile, which could lead to optimised goal setting and better self-management of their symptoms (Fig. 6).

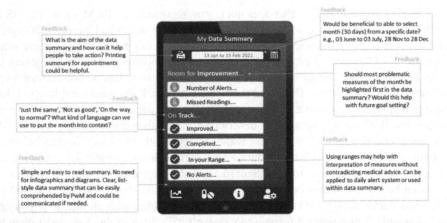

Fig. 6. Static DS prototype presented back to participants for discussion during follow-up DS workshop. Subject of discussion during activities 3 and 4 (see Sect. 2.2 for detail).

3.2 Contextualising the Use of a Data Summary

PwMs presented a multitude of uses for a DS feature within the ProACT App, three of which are presented below. Contexts for utilising a DS were both personal and as a communicative tool during interactions with healthcare professionals. A DS would provide a true representation of the individual PwM's health data and honest reflection of their disease or health trajectory. It could also act as a helpful preparatory tool for healthcare appointments, focusing topics for discussion in a time-sensitive scenario and providing a visible resource to prompt conversation. Furthermore, a primary objective of the ProACT platform, designed with the complexities of multimorbidity in mind, is optimised PwM self-management at home. A DS was highlighted by participants as a fundamental feature that could contribute to improved self-management behaviours and informed goal setting practices.

3.2.1 'Me in a Month' – the DS as a Holistic Representation

Participants valued the idea of a monthly DS for personal use, with selectable dates to coincide with healthcare appointments. They suggested that a DS representing a "running month", would be more helpful than a representation of a "month start to end". One participant provided context to this thinking, stating that: "If I have an appointment with the diabetes doctor tomorrow, I don't want to be writing up the last 13 days of data". Participants also provided important evidence to support the use of a monthly DS, as opposed to a short-term weekly or two-weekly summaries. They felt that the existing ProACT App provided useful daily representations of their individual data that would alert them to major health changes; however, it is the appearing patterns and trajectories that they felt were the primary focus of the DS: "The data summary would give a more precise reading of how the blood pressure has been. If you do it over [time] there's a pattern appearing". Another method used by healthcare professionals to capture health data patterns is ambulatory blood pressure monitoring, where the PwM would wear an

automatic cuff for a 24- or 48-h period. However, research indicates that participants
are more accepting of and prefer home-based monitoring in comparison to ambulatory
blood pressure monitoring [44]. Therefore, the use of a DS feature that permits PwMs
to display longitudinal patterns of various health data using home-based technology
devices could be a superior approach.

As mentioned previously (Sect. 3.1) participants were discussing the use of the colour
red as stress-inducing. This also prompted a discussion about the contextual use of the
feature, as one participant remarked that the use of red within daily summaries would
hypothetically mean that you may be in "danger" one day, but this can be alleviated the
next day. It was important to participants to note that the monthly DS would give them a
better overview of "where you are" with regards to your self-management: "I ended up
in hospital because I didn't manage [my data] for a month. The readings were a bit high,
and I thought 'Ah I'll leave that for a month, and I'll come back to it' and I ended up in
hospital". More simply put, participants valued the comprehensive and broad nature of
the DS, describing it as "This is me in a month!".

Through the participants' labelling of the DS feature as "me in a month", it also
emerged that there was a level of transparency that could be provided by presenting this
summary to a healthcare professional. As opposed to depending on a single reading or
an inaccurate recollection of progress, a month in review via the DS could improve
the transparency of PwMs' actual progress and increase their accountability. When
the researcher asked participants to consider a hypothetical situation where they had
taken 2–3 blood pressure readings during the week that were 'high', participants unanimously agreed that they would not communicate this to the healthcare professional
during a subsequent appointment and simply rely on the reading taken by the healthcare
professional. However, participants jovially acknowledged that this was not the best
use of their home-based self-management efforts, referring to the barriers associated
with 'white coat syndrome' and its effect on health measure accuracy during healthcare
appointments. One participant suggested that one high reading taken by a healthcare professional at an appointment could be elevated and "not represent the everyday" readings-
potentially skewing treatment decisions and there could be "some alarm bells" set off
unnecessarily. They compared this to the benefits of using the DS feature, which would
represent a months' worth of integrated health readings, giving a truer representation of
the individual and their health trajectory.

3.2.2 The DS as a Tool to Aid Collaborative Care

Participants also valued the DS feature as a comprehensive tool that could be used to
prepare for healthcare appointments. The month in review could assist PwMs to navigate the complex skill of communicating key health concerns to healthcare professionals
or people in their care network- which could optimise PwMs' use of time constrained
healthcare appointments and also improve their self-advocacy skills. When talking about
current self-management behaviours, a participant shared that he "would have brought
my [blood glucose] readings for the last few months with me. She [diabetes special-
ist] does look at them". However, he also added that this written documentation can be
cumbersome, can be missing data, and is also not easily accessible to the healthcare
professional during appointments as there are no summaries drawn on the plethora of

individual readings. Another participant agreed with this sentiment of preparing information before appointments, sharing that "the last time I went in I had just one or two
issues, but in case I forgot them, I wrote them down… for recall". However, this participant also shared her existing concerns of attending appointments without something
"concrete" to present to the healthcare professional, referring to the potential benefits of
having an easily accessible monthly DS that can be shared with others. She also emphasized the pressure felt to have her personal health data ready at a minute's notice for
unexpected appointments- stressing that she cannot always prepare her data in advance
for a visit: "I'd only go [to the healthcare professional] literally when I have to… I have
been both regularly and irregularly [attending healthcare professionals] depending on
how my [health] was. If I was going through a bad time, a very important point for me
is, I have to be seen [immediately]".

Furthermore, participants highlighted the time and resource barriers that limit the
type of care they receive during healthcare appointments. In particular, lack of communication between healthcare professionals of different specialties: "If you went in
to have your nose looked after, they look after your nose, but that's all."; "They don't
communicate. Even going back years ago you had a general consultant come in and
they dealt with everything. Where now, they're only dealing with a specific area of your
[health]". Participants felt that the integration of wide-ranging health information within
a DS feature, and the representation of them as a holistic PwM, could help to overcome
some of these barriers. Their experience is that healthcare professionals who ask about
other symptoms or are interested in reviewing general health data presented to them by
the PwM (not specific to one condition only) are of significant help to the individual,
directing them to other consultant types or educating them on what to look out for which
improves home-based self-management: "He might say to me, you've a few things going
on. They're aware of it"; "My [healthcare professional] will pick up on it [health data
that is slightly off] and send me… somewhere different".

3.2.3   The DS as a Tool to Prioritise Self-Management Activities

Participants emphasized that an accessible DS feature that helps PwMs to visualise "priority" health data could guide their self-management behaviours and subsequently assist
them with personal goal setting. Existing literature echoes this sentiment-recognising the
competing demands of each condition for a PwM and how they are tasked with priori-
tising their most significant health concerns so as to inform self-management decisions
[45]. Participants noted the potential of using a personalised DS feature to help them
to better focus their self-management practices in the coming weeks, as it would assist
them with making informed correlations across their various health and wellbeing data.
They felt that a truly comprehensive DS should certainly highlight the areas that need
work for the PwM.

Participants shared the importance of goal setting and using all resources available
to them to remain active in their self-management behaviours despite the endless distractions that life brings. They discussed "life getting in the way" and how this can lead
to certain health behaviours being abandoned: "It's not just that someone is bad at taking
their [health] readings, it's that you can get [life] interruptions… trying to manage this
and this and this, so rather than doing it all 'badly' you just abandon one and do one well,

quite well". When thinking about monthly planning, participants argued for a DS feature that could be used to guide their focus towards the health measure(s) that are not being well managed, based on a summary of data from the previous month. These findings are consistent with the concept that decision-making amongst PwMs is grounded in the personal and social context of an individual's life [45], and that PwMs will take variable levels of control of their morbidities in order to live as normally as possible [45, 46].

4 Conclusion

This paper reports on the design of the '*My Data Summary*', as part of a larger digital integrated care platform providing self-management support for those living with multiple chronic conditions. This rigorous co-design process led to a clear and concise design brief for such a feature, led by 7 individuals who shared their lived experiences of navigating these particular health challenges. This paper presents the creative methods used to actively engage PwMs and informal carers in the process. It also discusses contextual considerations around proposed design choices and collaborative decision-making throughout the process.

Acknowledgements. This work was carried out as part of the SEURO (Scaling EUROpean citizen driven transferable and transformative digital health) project which received funding from the European Union's Horizon 2020 research and innovation programme under grant agreement no. 945449. We would like to extend our gratitude to the 7 participants who dedicated an extensive amount of their valuable time to the redesign and further development of the ProACT App.

References

1. Marengoni, A., Angleman, S., Melis, R., Mangialasche, F., Karp, A., Garmen, A., et al.: Aging with multimorbidity: a systematic review of the literature. Ageing Res. Rev. **10**(4), 430–439 (2011)
2. Melchiorre, M.G., Papa, R., Rijken, M., van Ginneken, E., Hujala, A., Barbabella, F.: EHealth in integrated care programs for people with multimorbidity in Europe: insights from the ICARE4EU project. Health Policy **122**(1), 53–63 (2018)
3. Rijken, M., Struckmann, V., Dyakova, M., Gabriella, M., Rissanen, S., van Ginneken, E.: ICARE4EU: improving care for people with multiple chronic conditions in Europe. Eurohealth **19**(3), 29–31 (2013)
4. Valderas, J.M., Starfield, B., Sibbald, B., Salisbury, C., Roland, M.: Defining comorbidity: implications for understanding health and health services. Ann. Fam. Med. **7**(4), 357–363 (2009)
5. Eckerblad, J., Theander, K., Ekdahl, A., Jaarsma, T., Hellstrom, I.: To adjust and endure: a qualitative study of symptom burden in older people with multimorbidity. Appl. Nurs. Res. **28**(4), 322–327 (2015)
6. Liddy, C., Blazkho, V., Mill, K.: Challenges of self-management when living with multiple chronic conditions: systematic review of the qualitative literature. Can. Fam. Physician **60**(12), 1123–2113 (2014)

7. Ploeg, J., Matthew-Maich, N., Fraser, K., Dufour, S., McAiney, C., Kaasalainen, S., et al.: Managing multiple chronic conditions in the community: a Canadian qualitative study of the experiences of older adults, family caregivers and healthcare providers. BMC Geriatr. 17(40), 1–15 (2017)
8. Banjeree, S.: Multimorbidity - older adults need health care that can count past one. The Lancet 385(9968), 587–589 (2014)
9. Neubeck, L., Freedman, S.B., Clark, A.M., Briffa, T., Bauman, A., Redfern, J.: Participating in cardiac rehabilitation: a systematic review and meta-synthesis of qualitative data. Eur. J. Prev. Cardiol. 19(3), 494–503 (2012)
10. Clark, R.A., Conway, A., Poulsen, V., Keech, W., Tirimacco, R., Tideman, P.: Alternative models of cardiac rehabilitation: a systematic review. Eur. J. Prev. Cardiol. 22(1), 35–74 (2015)
11. Pal, K., Dack, C., Ross, J., Michie, S., May, C., Stevenson, F., et al.: Digital health interventions for adults with type 2 diabetes: qualitative study of patient perspectives on diabetes self-management education and support. J. Med. Internet Res. 20(2), e40 (2018)
12. Lahham, A., McDonald, C.F., Mahal, A., Lee, A.L., Hill, C.J., Burge, A.T., et al.: Home-based pulmonary rehabilitation for people with COPD: a qualitative study reporting the patient perspective. Chron. Respir. Dis. 15(2), 123–130 (2018)
13. Holland, A.E., Mahal, A., Hill, C.J., Lee, A.L., Burge, A.T., Cox, N.S., et al.: Home-based rehabilitation for COPD using minimal resources: a randomised, controlled equivalence trial. Thorax 72(1), 57–65 (2017)
14. Anderson, L., Sharp, G.A., Norton, R.J., Dalal, H., Dean, S.G., Jolly, K., et al.: Home-based versus centre-based cardiac rehabilitation. Cochrane Datab. Syst. Rev. 30(6), 1–151 (2017)
15. Rawstorn, J.C., Gant, N., Direito, A., Beckmann, C., Maddison, R.: Telehealth exercise-based cardiac rehabilitation: a systematic review and meta-analysis. Heart 102(15), 1183–1192 (2016)
16. Siek, K.A., Ross, S.E., Khan, D.U., Haverhals, L.M., Cali, S.R., Meyers, J.: Colorado care tablet: the design of an interoperable personal health application to help older adults with multimorbidity manage their medications. J. Biomed. Inform. 43(5), S22–S26 (2010)
17. Ongwere, T., Cantor, G., Ramirez, M.S., Shih, P., Clawson, J., Connolly, K.: Design hotspots for care of discordant chronic comorbidities: patients' perspectives. In: 10th Nordic Conference on Human Computer Interaction, pp. 571–583. Norway (2018)
18. Caldeira, C., Gui, X., Reynolds, T.L., Bietz, M., Chen, Y.: Managing healthcare conflicts when living with multiple chronic conditions. Int. J. Hum. Comput. Stud. 145, 102494 (2021)
19. Lim, C.Y., Berry, A.B.L., Hirsch, T., Hartzler, A.L., Wagner, E.H., Ludman, E.J., et al.: Understanding what is most important to individuals with multiple chronic conditions: a qualitative study of patients' perspectives. J. Gen. Intern. Med. 32(12), 1278–1284 (2017)
20. Doyle, J., et al.: Managing multimorbidity: identifying design requirements for a digital self-management tool to support older adults with multiple chronic conditions. In: Proceedings of the 2019 CHI Conference on Human Factors in Computing Systems, pp. 1–14 (2019)
21. Doyle, J., Murphy, E., Gavin, S., Pascale, A., Deparis, S., Tommasi, P., et al.: A digital platform to support self-management of multiple chronic conditions (ProACT): findings in relation to engagement during a one-year proof-of-concept trial. J. Med. Internet Res. 23(12), e22672 (2021)
22. Sheng, Y., Doyle, J., Bond, R., Jaiswal, R., Gavin, S., Dinsmore, J.: Home-based digital health technologies for older adults to self-manage multiple chronic conditions: a data-informed analysis of user engagement from a longitudinal trial. Digital Health 8, 205520762211259 (2022)
23. Doyle, J., McAleer, P., van Leeuwen, C., Smith, S., Murphy, M., Sillevis Smitt, M., et al.: The role of phone-based triage nurses in supporting older adults with multimorbidity to

digitally self-manage – findings from the ProACT proof-of-concept study. Digital Health **8**, 205520762211311 (2022)

24. Baxter, S., Johnson, M., Chambers, D., Sutton, A., Goyder, E., Booth, A.: The effects of integrated care: a systematic review of UK and international evidence. BMC Health Serv. Res. **18**(1), 1–13 (2018)

25. Lor, M., Backonja, U.: Visualizations integrated into consumer health technologies support self-management of chronic diseases: a systematic review. CIN: Comput. Inf. Nurs. **38**(3), 120–130 (2020)

26. Lor, M., Koleck, T.A., Bakken, S.: Information visualizations of symptom information for patients and providers: a systematic review. J. Am. Med. Inform. Assoc. **26**(2), 162–171 (2019)

27. Teal, G., French, T.: Spaces for participatory design innovation. In: Proceedings of the 16th Participatory Design Conference 2020, pp. 64–74. Columbia (2020)

28. Visser, F.S., Stappers, P.J., Van der Lugt, R., Sanders, E.B.: Context mapping: experiences from practice. CoDesign **1**(2), 119–149 (2005)

29. Neilsen, J.: Heuristic evaluation. In: Nielsen, J., Mack, R.L. (eds.) Usability Inspection Methods, pp. 25–64. Wiley (1994)

30. Patton, M.: Facilitating Evaluation: Principles in Practice. SAGE Publications Inc. (2018)

31. Sanders, E.B.N., Brandt, E., Binder, T.: A framework for organizing the tools and techniques of participatory design. In: Proceedings of the 11th Biennial Participatory Design Conference, pp. 195–198. Australia (2010)

32. Yardley, L., Morrison, L., Bradbury, K., Muller, I.: The person-based approach to intervention development: application to digital health-related behavior change interventions. J. Med. Internet Res. **17**(1), e4055 (2015)

33. Lupton, D.: Digital health now and in the future: findings from a participatory design stakeholder workshop. Digital Health **3**, 1–17 (2017)

34. Sanders, E.B., Stappers, P.J.: Co-creation and the new landscapes of design. Co-design **4**(1), 5–18 (2008)

35. Bengtsson, M.: How to plan and perform a qualitative study using content analysis. Nurs. Plus Open **2**, 8–14 (2016)

36. Coventry, P.A., Fisher, L., Kenning, C., Bee, P., Bower, P.: Capacity, responsibility, and motivation: a critical qualitative evaluation of patient and practitioner views about barriers to self-management in people with multimorbidity. BMC Health Serv. Res. **14**(536), 1–12 (2014)

37. SCORE2-OP Working Group. ESC Cardiovascular risk collaboration: SCORE2-OP risk prediction algorithms: estimating incident cardiovascular event risk in older persons in four geographical risk regions. Eur. Heart J. **42**(25), 2455–2467 (2021)

38. Wilson, P.W., D'Agostino, R.B., Levy, D., Belanger, A.M., Silbershatz, H., Kannel, W.B.: Prediction of coronary heart disease using risk factor categories. Circulation **97**(18), 1837–1847 (1998)

39. Stiell, I.G., et al.: Clinical characteristics associated with adverse events in patients with exacerbation of chronic obstructive pulmonary disease: a prospective cohort study. CMAJ **186**(6), E193-204 (2014)

40. Paasche-Orlow, M.K., Wolf, M.S.: The causal pathways linking health literacy to health outcomes. Am. J. Health Behav. **31**(1), S19–S26 (2007)

41. Sørensen, K., et al.: Health literacy and public health: a systematic review and integration of definitions and models. BMC Public Health **12**(1), 1–13 (2012)

42. Kim, H., Xie, B.: Health literacy in the eHealth era: a systematic review of the literature. Patient Educ. Couns. **100**(6), 1073–1082 (2017)

43. Junius-Walker, U., Schleef, T., Vogelsang, U., Dierks, M.L.: How older patients prioritise their multiple health problems: a qualitative study. BMC Geriatr. **19**(1), 1–8 (2019)

44. Nasothimiou, E.G., Karpettas, N., Dafni, M.G., Stergiou, G.S.: Patients' preference for ambulatory versus home blood pressure monitoring. J. Hum. Hypertens. **28**(4), 224–229 (2014)
45. Bratzke, L.C., Muehrer, R.J., Kehl, K.A., Lee, K.S., Ward, E.C., Kwekkeboom, K.L.: Self-management priority setting and decision-making in adults with multimorbidity: a narrative review of literature. Int. J. Nurs. Stud. **52**(3), 744–755 (2015)
46. Thorne, S., Paterson, B., Russell, C.: The structure of everyday self-care decision making in chronic illness. Qual. Health Res. **13**(10), 1337–1352 (2003)

Human Activity Recognition Using Wi-Fi CSI

Egberto Caballero$^{(\boxtimes)}$, Iandra Galdino , Julio C. H. Soto ,
Taiane C. Ramos , Raphael Guerra , Débora Muchaluat-Saade ,
and Célio Albuquerque

MidiaCom Lab, Institute of Computing - UFF, Niterói, Brazil
`{egbertocr,igaldino,jsoto,taiane,debora,celio}@midiacom.uff.br`,
`rguerra@ic.uff.br`

Abstract. Wi-Fi signals were originally developed with a focus on communication. However, beyond communication applications, Wi-Fi signals have been recently studied as a possible powerful tool for human sensing applications. In this sense, we present in this paper an original approach for obtaining human activity recognition (HAR) through the use of commercial Wi-Fi devices. Using our proposal, it is possible to infer the position of a monitored person in an indoor environment (room). To achieve this, we clean and process the amplitude of the channel state information (CSI) data collected from the Wi-Fi channel. We selected and evaluated five different classification algorithms to infer the subjects position and compare their performance. The proposed method was evaluated on a dataset of Wi-Fi CSI data collected from 125 participants. The proposed system is trained with the data collected while a person performs a variety of activities in a room. For the scenario and dataset considered in this study, the results showed that the Random Forest algorithm had the best performance for all tests, reaching an accuracy of 93.03% on average.

Keywords: Channel state information · CSI · Wi-Fi · human activity recognition · HAR

1 Introduction

It is a consensus that the worldwide population is aging, making the demand for healthcare monitoring more urgent. Therefore, monitoring elder or physically

---

This work was supported in part by Coordenação de Aperfeiçoamento de Pessoal de Nível Superior-Brazil (CAPES) under Finance Code 001, CAPES Institutional Program for Internationalization (CAPES PrInt), Brazilian National Council for Scientific and Technological Development (CNPq), Carlos Chagas Filho Foundation for Research Support in the State of Rio de Janeiro (FAPERJ), São Paulo Research Foundation (FAPESP) and National Institute of Science and Technology on Medicine Assisted by Scientific Computing (INCT-MACC).

D. Salvi et al. (Eds.): PH 2023, LNICST 572, pp. 309–321, 2024.
https://doi.org/10.1007/978-3-031-59717-6_21

impaired people during basic activities at home such as sleeping and sitting has gained a great interest mostly when discussing ambient intelligence technologies.

One of the most prominent topics regarding smart home technologies is human sensing. There is a huge amount of applications that can use human sensing to monitor people's conditions like fall detection, vital sign monitoring, identity detection, and human activity recognition (HAR) for example. HAR systems typically may use computer-vision-based technologies [1,9], wearable sensor-based technologies [19,21], or radio frequency (RF) [7,20].

Computer-vision-based systems have a limited operating area and require a direct line-of-sight (LoS) view of the environment, not to mention that users usually dislike them due to privacy concerns. Their performance is also subject to change under different lighting conditions. Wearable sensor-based HAR technologies are less user-friendly since they require users to carry or wear sensors, which may be uncomfortable or unpleasant for elderly and physically disabled people [12].

Recently, many studies have shown that Wi-Fi signals can sense human behaviors due to the interference of the human body on signal propagation [18]. The Channel State Information (CSI) of Wi-Fi communication [13], which represents how wireless signals propagate from the transmitter to the receiver at certain carrier frequencies along multiple paths, is a promising technology for human sensing and an alternative to video surveillance and sensor-based technologies. Wi-Fi CSI-based HAR systems take advantage of the widespread deployment of commercial Wi-Fi devices and ubiquity of Wi-Fi signals.

In this paper, we propose a Wi-Fi CSI-based system capable of identifying when an individual is performing each of 6 different activities: standing, sitting, lying, walking, running and sweeping in a room. We have used a CSI dataset collected from 125 participants from the eHealth CSI data set [5] available for the scientific community. The results obtained attest the effectiveness of the proposed method.

The main contributions of this work can be summarized as:

- Proposing a simplified CSI-based-HAR system.
- Performing an analysis over a huge amount of collected data compared to related work found in the literature.
- Comparison of five machine learning (ML) classification algorithms to evaluate the performance of the proposed system on human activity recognition.

The remainder of the paper is structured as follows. Section 2 gives an overview of Wi-Fi CSI systems. Section 3 gives a review of relevant related work. The data collection, processing steps, and proposed methodology are described in Sect. 4. In Sect. 5, we compare the obtained performance results of different ML algorithms. Finally, Sect. 6 brings the concluding remarks and future work directions.

2   CSI Overview

The basic properties of a Wi-Fi communication link between transmitter and receiver can be represented by the channel state information (CSI). It describes how a signal is modified while it propagates from the transmitter to the receiver. These modifications represent the combined effect of, for example, scattering due to multipath, fading, power decay with distance, etc.

The physical layer of Wi-Fi systems follows the IEEE 802.11g/n/ac specification [8], and uses the orthogonal frequency division multiplexing (OFDM) technique for both 2.4GHz and 5GHz frequency bands. OFDM is a modulation technique that divides the available bandwidth into several orthogonal subbands [23]. By doing this, the information can be independently transmitted over different OFDM symbols. The OFDM features make it a good solution for multipath channels and also for Multiple-Input Multiple-Output (MIMO) systems [10]. Besides, since the transmission over each subcarrier is orthogonal and independent, each subcarrier can be viewed as a sensor capable of collecting CSI data.

To measure CSI, the Wi-Fi transmitter sends Long Training Fields (LTFs), which contain predefined information in each subcarrier, in the frame preamble. The Wi-Fi receiver estimates the CSI using the received signal and the predefined LTFs. The amount of collected data depends on the channel bandwidth, which determines the number of subcarriers, and on the number of antennas used.

Considering a MIMO Wi-Fi system operating under IEEE 802.11n specification, and with P transmitting antennas and Q receiving antennas, the signal that contains the estimated CSI of each data stream can be mathematically expressed as:

$$h_{p,q} = |h|e^{j\theta}, \tag{1}$$

where $h_{p,q}$ represents the CSI between the p-th transmission antenna and the q-th receiving antenna.

We can also have a multipath channel, in this case, the representation of the received signal will become a vector. Let c be the number of paths, thus the state information of the channel established between a pair of antennas (p, q) can be mathematically represented by a vector with c elements. Thus we have

$$\boldsymbol{h}_{p,q} = [h_1, h_2, \ldots, h_c]^{\mathrm{T}}. \tag{2}$$

CSI data can be used to provide information about the environment and estimate changes and phenomena that occur over time, such as human presence detection, movements, and even vital signs.

3   Related Work

Wi-Fi CSI-based Human Activity Recognition (HAR) has gained high interest in recent years, as this technology takes advantage of the widespread deployment of commercial Wi-Fi devices and ubiquity of Wi-Fi signals to offer a cheap and convenient HAR system. As a consequence, we can find many studies in this area. In this section, we review the most recent works we found in the literature regarding Wi-Fi CSI-based HAR systems.

Wang et al. [22] developed a system called Wi-Fall mainly to detect falls using Wi-Fi CSI data. They analyzed different activities carried out at three different locations: a chamber, a laboratory, and a dormitory. The data was collected using three transmitting and three receiving antennas. As the first three eigenvalues of the single value decomposition (SVD) matrix describe most of the characteristics of the whole matrix, they were used for the classification. Two different classification algorithms were used, and a one-class support vector machine (SVM) was utilized to detect falls. Besides, to detect other activities in addition to falls, the random forest classifier was used.

Ding et al. [3] suggested using Deep Recurrent Neural Network (DRNN) to identify human positions. The idea was to extract features for Recurrent Neural Network (RNN) training and recognize the activity. Two features were extracted, namely channel power variation in the time domain and time-frequency analysis in the frequency domain. Then an LSTM (Long Short Term Memory) that is trained with extracted features is used to recognize an activity.

Another Wi-Fi CSI-based human activity recognition system, namely Wi-Motion, was proposed in [11], which can sensitively recognize 5 predefined different human activities. They jointly used the amplitude and phase information from the CSI sequence collected with Wi-Fi devices with three antennas. The SVM algorithm was also used to build two classifiers according to amplitude and phase information. When an unknown activity sample enters, consulting the prediction results of both classifiers, Wi-Motion performs a merge method based on the posterior probability to produce the final recognition.

Recently, Convolutional Neural Networks (CNNs) have also been applied together with bidirectional LSTM (Bi-LSTM) for the classification of human activities, including fall detection [17].

Furthermore, activity recognition using a Raspberry Pi and Nexmon firmware has also been used to extract the CSI data [4]. The only preprocessing step that was performed in that work was a low-pass filter. Additionally, a DeepConvL-STM classification model was implemented in Python using a deep learning API called Keras.

Another work focused on extracting the CSI information for different positions in the indoor LoS scenarios using Nexmon CSI tool on Raspberry Pi hardware with NIC Broadcom and Asus routers is published in [16]. Activities were classified by applying ML algorithms, SVM, and LSTM. Outliers were removed by using the Hampel filter, then a DWT (Discrete Wavelet Transform) was applied to denoise the signal and PCA to reduce the dimension of the information. Features were extracted from the preprocessed data to use in SVM and LSTM to classify the activities.

Bocus et al. [2] analyzed human position recognition using Ultra-Wideband (UWB) technology. Thy presented the techniques and addressed the feasibility of using UWB signals. They have extracted high-resolution Channel Impulse Responses (CIRs) from UWB modules and use them as features in ML algorithms for classifying different human activities. They also compared the activity classification performance using fine-grained Wi-Fi CSI in the same physical layout.

Yang et al. [24] explored three issues for recognizing human activity: (i) Based on the sensitivity of different antennas to actions, an active antenna selection approach was proposed to reduce the amount of data required for analysis; (ii) Two signal enhancement approaches were presented to strengthen the interval of active signals and weaken the impact of inactive signals; and finally, (iii) an activity segmentation algorithm was provided to detect the start and end times of an activity, which can get rid of inactive signals and retain the active signal interval.

Muaaz et al. [15] used a CNN to recognize human activities from environment-independent time-variant micro-Doppler fingerprints extracted from Wi-Fi CSI data. They also used both amplitude and phase information of the CSI data. First, they processed the CSI data to remove the noise and fixed objects present in the environment. The CSI data were then used to compute the spectogram corresponding to different human activities. The spectograms were stored as portable network graphics (PNG) images and used to train a deep CNN. The CNN used was capable of automatically extracting discriminative features from PNG images and classifying human activities.

A recent approach was proposed based on the Doppler effect [14]. First, an original phase cleaning was performed to extract micro-Doppler traces from the CSI data. The Doppler shift reveals the velocities of the scattering points during the transmission events and is not affected by static objects, allowing the gauging of the dynamic human position features. The micro-Doppler traces were used as input for a neural network architecture that was trained to recognize the activities of interest. It is important to note that this work focused on the recognition of dynamic activities. Identification of static activities, such as sitting and lying down, was outside of the scope of their work.

These works found in the literature demonstrate the sensitivity of SCI data to small body movements, allowing the identification of activities carried out by people using the collected SCI data. However, these work present proposals in controlled environments and with a limited number of people. As a difference, our work considers the recognition of human activity using a dataset with data collected from 125 people forming a very heterogeneous group, with different ages, sex, and different physical characteristics.

Based on the existing work, we proposed a simplified approach to identify the human position and/or movement based on CSI information. Furthermore, we have tested the proposed methodology on a huge amount of collected data available in the eHealth dataset [5], which corroborate its applicability. In [5] can be found more details about the data collection process and eHealth dataset construction.

4   Proposal and Experimental Methodology

Before the human activity recognition itself, it is necessary to treat the collected CSI signal to allow it to be used in Machine Learning (ML) algorithms. In this section, we describe step by step the proposed methodology. We divided our proposed system into three stages: Data collection, Signal processing, and Data treatment, as presented in Fig. 1.

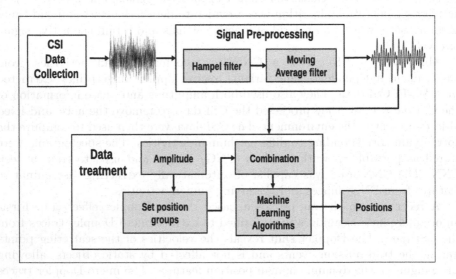

Fig. 1. Block diagram of the proposed methodology.

In the following, we describe each stage of the proposed methodology.

4.1   CSI Data Collection

For data acquisition, we have used the NEXMON firmware [6]. This firmware works on top of a Raspberry Pi 4B. NEXMON modifies the firmware of the Raspberry wireless board and allows the capture of CSI data in a wireless transmission between two devices on a Wi-Fi network. Data collection was carried out in an ordinary room with no electromagnetic isolation. We used a traditional Wi-Fi network in order to recreate an environment as close as possible to a real scenario. Figure 2 steep 1 shows the data collection scenario. The Wi-Fi network was configured in the 5 GHz frequency band, using a channel with a bandwidth of 80 MHz. For data acquisition, CSI makes use of OFDM technology, so with the configuration used, we obtain 234 subcarriers in each collection, after discarding the pilot and null subcarriers. The duration of each collection in each position was 60 seconds per participant's position, obtaining 500 samples with 234 subcarriers in each collection. More information on the functionality of NEXMON and other firmware is found in [18].

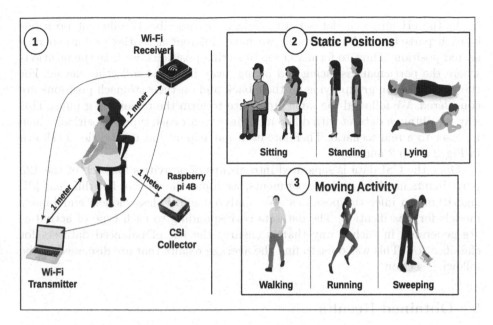

Fig. 2. (1) CSI data collection room, (2) statict positions and its different variations, (3) moving activity.

4.2 Signal Pre-processing

In the CSI data pre-processing stage, we use techniques to clean the signal from external factors. These factors perturb the signal making it harder to interpret. After collecting the data, it goes through a first filter called Hampel, which removes noise from the signal. The Hampel filter uses a sliding window of 30 and 3 standard deviations. The data then passes through another filter called Moving Average, eliminating outliers and smoothing the signal. The Moving Average filter uses a sliding window of size 10. With these two procedures, we ensure the cleaning of the signals collected by each subcarrier and that it is ready for data treatment.

4.3 Data Treatment

In the present study, we used the eHealth CSI dataset [5] created by our research group. The dataset contains the sitting, standing, and lying static positions and moving activities, such as walking and running, of 125 people, of different ages, gender, weight, and height.

In the Data treatment stage, we use as input the cleaned CSI data from the pre-processing stage. First, we use the amplitude of the signal from each subcarrier. Then we perform a data segmentation, dividing our data into four groups: sitting, standing, lying, and moving positions (walking and running).

In the eHealth CSI dataset, the collections describe 17 different positions of each participant. Among those, we have different activities performed in a seated position. Thus, to form a group of sitting positions, we take the positions where the participant is facing and facing away from the collecting device. For the lying position group, lying on their back and on their stomach positions are considered. We followed the same procedure to form the remaining groups. This way, we obtain a dataset with different variations for each type of position, which is closer to a real scenario. Therefore each participant has 6 activities as shown in Fig. 2 steep 2 and 3.

Once the CSI data is separated into groups of activities for each of the 125 participants involved in the experiments, we input the data to five different ML algorithms to infer the positions. We analyzed multi-class models and binary models for classification. The datasets corresponding to each type of activities are generated in such a way that it ensures the use of balanced datasets for classification. This was done to find the average results that are discussed in the following section.

5   Obtained Results

In our analysis, we considered the scenario of a person who requires supervision, such as an elder. In this scenario, our system could help by identifying whether the supervised person changed their position, as in a fall situation, for example.

We analyzed the classification for standing, sitting, and lying positions; walking, running, and sweeping activities. Also, the static vs. moving activities classification was analyzed. Each participant has a fully balanced dataset with a total of 1000 CSI samples for each position and 234 features representing the number of subcarriers.

The following ML algorithms were analyzed: Random Forest (RF), Support Vector Machine (SVM), Decision Tree J48 (DT-J48), MultiLayer Perceptron (MLP), and Gaussian Naïve Bayes (GNB), since they showed better performance for binary classification. For the proposed analysis, 70% of the data was used for training and 30% for testing. Metrics such as accuracy, precision, recall, and F1 measure were calculated to verify the performance of each ML model.

Initially, we performed a multi-class classification for 6 human activities: standing, sitting, lying, walking, running, and sweeping activities. As can be seen in Table 1, the Random Forest algorithm presented the best classification, reaching an accuracy of 86.65% and a precision between 85.68% and 88.35% for each class. Classification of running and sweeping classes had the best performance with a precision of 87.45% and 88.35% respectively. These results show that for activities in which people perform more body movements, the Random Forest Model achieves the best precision. This is consistent with the fact that body movement exerts greater influence over the wireless channel conditions and as a consequence, the CSI data is more affected.

Based on previous results and with the aim of improving classification results, a binary classification was performed, this time considering static positions and

Table 1. Metrics for multi-class classification (%).

Algorithm	Accuracy	Precision/ Sitting	Precision/ Standing	Precision/ Lying	Precision/ Walking	Precision/ Running	Precision/ Sweeping
RF	**86.65**	**85.68**	**86.29**	**86.67**	**86.63**	**87.45**	**88.35**
SVM	50.78	51,95	48.01	59.95	46.27	42.62	51.39
MLP	63.54	66.43	63.40	69.37	60.44	60.34	61.34
J48	41.44	45.72	42.38	49.42	37.36	38.05	38.46
GNB	30.87	34.80	30.60	39.91	26.48	26.77	27.83

moving activity. For this scenario, the moving activities group was formed by collections of each person walking and running and the static positions group contains a mixture of sitting and lying positions. Figure 3 shows the results achieved for this scenario. The best performance is achieved by Random Forest, reaching an accuracy of 91.72%. For this scenario, it is possible to identify whether a person is moving or in a static position with a precision of 93.19%.

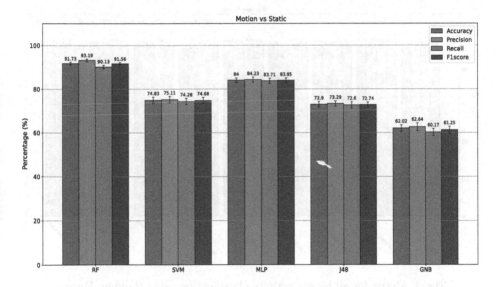

Fig. 3. Metric for motion vs static classification.

To assess the reliability of the obtained results, the classification was performed 30 times for each person, and in each round different training and test sets were randomly chosen. The same procedure was then performed for a group of 125 people. In this way, a model was generated for each person and the average of the 125 generated models was obtained with a 95% confidence interval computed through a bootstrap procedure. In Fig. 3 the average of the accuracy, precision, recall, and F1 metrics with their respective confidence intervals are presented. As shown in the figure, the results consolidate the Random Forest algorithm as the best classifier for this scenario, obtaining the highest average and the lowest confidence interval.

We also observed that when movement is detected, the RF model increases more than 5% in accuracy, and precision increases between 5% and 7.5% depending on the type of activity. In this sense, it is interesting to identify first when a person is moving and then identify what type of activity they are performing in case of movement, and in what position they are in the static case.

Further analyses were performed considering all possible combinations of static positions and movement activities, as well as the state of movement in combination with static positions. For each case, the performance of RF, SVM, MLP, DT-J48, and GNB algorithms was also analyzed based on accuracy, precision, recall, and F1 metrics.

In all cases, Random Forest presented the best performance. Figure 4 shows the values of the metrics for all classifications performed using the Random Forest algorithm, which was the best classifier. It can be seen that in all cases the metrics reach values greater than 90%.

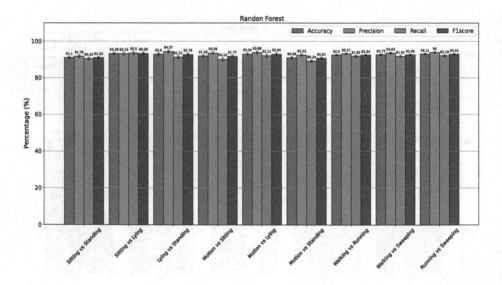

Fig. 4. Metric for all binary activity classification using Random Forest.

For static positions, analyzing sitting vs standing the classification has 91.09% accuracy and 91.79% precision. In turn, the sitting vs lying classification achieved the highest accuracy with 93.28% and 93.15% precision. For lying down vs standing the classification has 92.89% accuracy and 94.36% precision.

For moving activity, walking vs running classification achieved 92.60% accuracy and 93.27% precision. Walking vs Sweeping classification reached 92.73% accuracy and 93.62% precision. And for Running vs Sweeping the classification has 93.10% accuracy and 94% precision.

Comparing moving activity versus a specific static position also achieved values greater than 90% in the evaluation metrics. For example, for moving vs sitting, the classification has 91.95% accuracy and 93.50% precision. When classifying moving vs lying the accuracy was 93.03% and the precision was 93.87%. And for moving vs standing the classification accuracy was 90.98% and the precision was 92.51% precision.

The best results are achieved when comparing lying with any other activity. In particular, in the comparison between sitting and lying the accuracy was 93.28%, and between moving and lying it was 93.03%. This is due to the greater difference in body horizontal and vertical positions, which influences the propagation of radio waves in the environment and consequently reflects in the collected CSI data.

6   Conclusions

This work proposed a methodology based on CSI data analysis and machine learning models to recognize positions and activities of a single person in a room. This is a particularly relevant application in scenarios where a person in isolation must be monitored remotely. We evaluated our proposal using the eHealth CSI dataset with data from 125 people, of different ages, gender, weight, and height. The results consolidate the Random Forest algorithm as the best classifier for this application, obtaining the highest average and the lowest confidence interval with accuracy results between 92% and 94%.

These results for multi-class classification show that for activities in which people perform more body movements, Random Forest achieves the best precision with 87.45% for running and 88.35% for sweeping.

Also, results showed that the horizontal or vertical disposition of the body influences the propagation of radio waves in a different way and, as a result, this is reflected in the collected CSI data, allowing better classification results in the cases of sitting vs lying, standing vs lying and moving vs lying.

The proposal presented in this work achieves a increases of more than 5% in accuracy and precision increases between 5% and 7.5% depending on the type of activity, when compared with the multi-class classification. And for all scenarios analyzed, the performance metrics show values greater than 90%.

As future work, it is interesting to consider new features extracted from the CSI signal that can improve ML model performance for activity recognition. In addition, we intent to consider other more complex activities, as well as the transition between activities; Also, family environments where more than one person coexists are interesting questions to consider in future work.

References

1. Beddiar, D.R., Nini, B., Sabokrou, M., Hadid, A.: Vision-based human activity recognition: a survey. Multim. Tools Appl. **79**(41–42), 30509–30555 (2020)

2. Bocus, M., Piechocki, R., Chetty, K.: A comparison of UWB CIR and WiFi CSI for human activity recognition. In: Proceedings of the IEEE Radar Conference (RadarCon) (2021)
3. Ding, J., Wang, Y.: WiFi CSI-based human activity recognition using deep recurrent neural network. IEEE Access **7**, 174257–174269 (2019)
4. Forbes, G., Massie, S., Craw, S.: Wifi-based human activity recognition using Raspberry Pi. In: 2020 IEEE 32nd International Conference on Tools with Artificial Intelligence (ICTAI), pp. 722–730. IEEE (2020)
5. Galdino, I., et al.: eHealth CSI: a Wi-Fi CSI dataset of human activities. IEEE Access **11**, 71003–71012 (2023)
6. Gringoli, F., Schulz, M., Link, J., Hollick, M.: Free your CSI: a channel state information extraction platform for modern wi-fi chipsets. In: Proceedings of the 13th International Workshop on Wireless Network Testbeds, Experimental Evaluation and Characterization (WiNTECH 2019), pp. 21–28. Association for Computing Machinery, New York (2019). https://doi.org/10.1145/3349623.3355477
7. Hsieh, C.F., Chen, Y.C., Hsieh, C.Y., Ku, M.L.: Device-free indoor human activity recognition using wi-fi RSSI: machine learning approaches. In: 2020 IEEE International Conference on Consumer Electronics-Taiwan (ICCE-Taiwan), pp. 1–2. IEEE (2020)
8. IEEE 802.11 Working Group. IEEE 802.11ac-2013 - IEEE standard for information technology. Tech. rep., IEEE (2013). https://standards.ieee.org/standard/80211ac-2013.html
9. Kim, K., Jalal, A., Mahmood, M.: Vision-based human activity recognition system using depth silhouettes: a smart home system for monitoring the residents. J. Electric. Eng. Technol. **14**, 2567–2573 (2019)
10. Lee, S., Park, Y.D., Suh, Y.J., Jeon, S.: Design and implementation of monitoring system for breathing and heart rate pattern using WiFi signals. In: IEEE Annual Consumer Communications and Networking Conference, pp. 1–7 (2018). https://doi.org/10.1109/CCNC.2018.8319181
11. Li, H., He, X., Chen, X., Fang, Y., Fang, Q.: Wi-motion: a robust human activity recognition using WiFi signals. IEEE Access **7**, 153287–153299 (2019)
12. Loncar-Turukalo, T., Zdravevski, E., da Silva, J.M., Chouvarda, I., Trajkovik, V., et al.: Literature on wearable technology for connected health: scoping review of research trends, advances, and barriers. J. Med. Internet Res. **21**(9), e14017 (2019)
13. Ma, Y., Zhou, G., Wang, S.: Wifi sensing with channel state information: a survey. ACM Comput. Surv. **52**(3), 1–36 (2019)
14. Meneghello, F., Garlisi, D., Fabbro, N.D., Tinnirello, I., Rossi, M.: SHARP: environment and person independent activity recognition with commodity IEEE 802.11 access points. IEEE Trans. Mobile Comput. **22**(10), 6160–6175 (2023). https://doi.org/10.1109/TMC.2022.3185681
15. Muaaz, M., Chelli, A., Gerdes, M.W., Pätzold, M.: Wi-sense: a passive human activity recognition system using Wi-Fi and convolutional neural network and its integration in health information systems. Ann. Telecommun. **77**(3–4), 163–175 (2022)
16. Schäfer, J., Barrsiwal, B.R., Kokhkharova, M., Adil, H., Liebehenschel, J.: Human activity recognition using CSI information with nexmon. Appl. Sci. **11**(19), 8860 (2021)
17. Sheng, B., Xiao, F., Sha, L., Sun, L.: Deep spatial-temporal model based cross-scene action recognition using commodity WiFi. IEEE Internet Things J. **7**(4), 3592–3601 (2020)

18. Soto, J.C., Galdino, I., Caballero, E., Ferreira, V., Muchaluat-Saade, D., Albu-
    querque, C.: A survey on vital signs monitoring based on wi-fi csi data. Comput.
    Commun. **195**, 99–110 (2022). https://doi.org/10.1016/j.comcom.2022.08.004
19. Uddin, M.Z., Hassan, M.M., Alsanad, A., Savaglio, C.: A body sensor data fusion
    and deep recurrent neural network-based behavior recognition approach for robust
    healthcare. Inf. Fusion **55**, 105–115 (2020)
20. Wang, W., Liu, A.X., Shahzad, M., Ling, K., Lu, S.: Device-free human activity
    recognition using commercial wifi devices. IEEE J. Sel. Areas Commun. **35**(5),
    1118–1131 (2017)
21. Wang, Y., Cang, S., Yu, H.: A survey on wearable sensor modality centred human
    activity recognition in health care. Expert Syst. Appl. **137**, 167–190 (2019)
22. Wang, Y., Wu, K., Ni, L.M.: Wifall: device-free fall detection by wireless networks.
    IEEE Trans. Mob. Comput. **16**(2), 581–594 (2016)
23. Weinstein, S., Ebert, P.: Data transmission by frequency-division multiplexing
    using the discrete Fourier transform. IEEE Trans. Commun. Technol. **19**(5), 628–
    634 (1971)
24. Yang, J., Liu, Y., Liu, Z., Wu, Y., Li, T., Yang, Y.: A framework for human activity
    recognition based on WiFi CSI signal enhancement. Int. J. Antennas Propagat.
    2021, 1–18 (2021)

Personalized Sleep Monitoring Using Smartphones and Semi-supervised Learning

Priyanka Mary Mammen[1]($\boxtimes$) , Camellia Zakaria[2] , and Prashant Shenoy[1]

[1] University of Massachusetts Amherst, Amherst, USA
{pmammen,shenoy}@cs.umass.edu
[2] University of Toronto, Toronto, Canada
camellia.zakaria@utoronto.ca

Abstract. Sleep is a critical aspect of an individual's physical and mental well-being. Hence a large body of sleep monitoring solutions has been gaining popularity, including data-driven AI techniques with mHealth adaptations of wearable, smartphone, and contactless-sensing modalities. Regardless, proposed solutions by prior works, by and large, require gathering sufficient ground truth data to develop personalize and highly accurate sleep prediction models. This requirement inherently presents a challenge of such models underperforming when inferring sleep on new users without labeled data. However, unlabeled data is often more abundantly available in a real-world application than gathering labeled data. In this paper, we propose *SleepLess*, which uses semi-supervised learning over unlabeled data sensed from the user's smartphone network activity to develop personalized models and detect their sleep duration for the night. Specifically, it uses a pre-trained model on an existing set of users to produce pseudo labels for unlabeled data of a new user and achieves personalization by fine-tuning over selectively picking the pseudo labels. Our IRB-approved user study among 23 users found *SleepLess* model yielding around 96% accuracy, between 12–27 min of sleep time error and 18–25 min of wake time error. Comparison against other approaches that sought to predict with fewer labeled data found *SleepLess*, similarly yielding best performance. Our study demonstrates the feasibility of achieving personalization in sleep prediction models by utilizing unlabeled data extracted from network activity of users' smartphones, through the application of a semi-supervised transfer learning approach.

Keywords: Semi-supervised Learning · Time Series data · Sleep · Passive Sensing

1 Introduction

Sleep is an essential daily human activity that significantly affects a person's health and well-being. Despite its importance, sleep disorder is common among

D. Salvi et al. (Eds.): PH 2023, LNICST 572, pp. 322–338, 2024.
https://doi.org/10.1007/978-3-031-59717-6_22

adults, with prior studies reporting 20–40% adults suffering from a form of sleep disorder [5]. Sleep deprivation is a widespread problem, with a third of the population getting less sleep than the recommended 8 h of regular sleep [1]. Since poor sleep hygiene can influence various health problems, sleep monitoring has become a critical technology enabler for researchers and clinicians to understand daily sleep habits better and identify poor sleep health.

Wearable sleep trackers such as FitBit [10] and Oura ring [39] have become popular for users to keep track of their daily sleep in recent years. Although they are simple to use, these contact-based methods may be less favorable among users who prefer not to wear a device during their sleep time [2]. To overcome this challenge, researchers have responded by developing several contactless solutions. For example, radar-based approaches [2], use radio frequency signals that bounce off users to monitor their breathing and sleep. This technology, in particular, is adopted by smart speakers such as Google Nest [6] and Amazon Alexa [7] for contactless sleep tracking using a built-in radar [35]. While wearable and smart speakers can monitor sleep duration and quality, smartphones are more ubiquitous. Researchers have attempted to leverage the ubiquity of smartphones as an inexpensive means of tracking users' sleep. The primary approach of such solutions is based on indirect sensing, where passive observations of smartphone activities are used to infer a user's sleep duration. An early work [3], which utilizes smartphone screen activity as a proxy of their awake states, correspondingly estimating sleep based on users' inactivity. More recent work has successfully generalized this notion to utilizing network activity generated by smartphones and smart devices where long periods of inactivity were used to detect sleep periods [46],?. A general drawback of these solutions is the fundamental need to collect labeled ground truth data from users for training prediction models that will accurately infer their sleep. Due to a myriad of user-related issues, such as inaccurate data logging, missing data, and eventually, user attrition, conducting long-term user studies to specifically collect large amounts of ground truth data is challenging [8]. Consequently, many research efforts to study sleep have been limited to a small sample population of tens of users.

Designing models that generalize to a larger population using a small sample size and a small amount of labeled ground truth data is challenging—especially since sleep patterns can vary from one user to another. In contrast to labeled data that is difficult to collect via user studies, unlabeled data of a phone's network or screen activity is significantly easier to collect via automated apps; neither of these data sources require user involvement during data collection. Similarly, WiFi networks routinely logs client activities which can be used to infer a phone's network activity over time [9]. *The convenient availability of unlabeled data together coupled with the challenges gathering labeled data motivates the need to develop semi-supervised learning (SSL) methods* that can monitor a user's sleep using passive observations of the phone's network activity. Further, such SSL methods should enable personalization of the learnt model in order to handle each user's sleep patterns.

In this paper, we present *SleepLess*, a system that uses semi-supervised learning over unlabeled phone data to develop personalized models for detecting a user's daily sleep patterns. In designing and evaluating *SleepLess*, we make the following contributions:

1. We propose a semi-supervised training pipeline to enable personalized sleep duration estimation in users from the network activity of their mobile-phones. We use a teacher-student framework to utilize a pre-trained sleep prediction model and a few weeks of unlabeled data from the end-user.
2. We implement a complete prototype of a semi-supervised learning pipeline to demonstrate the efficacy of our approach. We conduct a user study on a campus consisting of 20 users. Further, we present a case study to demonstrate the generalizability of the approach in residential settings.
3. The model validations show that our approach achieves around 96% accuracy, between 12–27 min of sleep time error and 18–25 min of wake time error.

2   Background

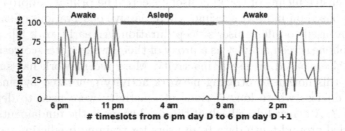

Fig. 1. Time-series data of network activity of mobile phones representing sleep and wake-up periods.

The main premise behind inferring a user's sleep through their smartphone activity is that users utilize their smartphone throughout the day, generating screen or network activity as soon as they are awake. Conversely, the lack of phone-generated activities are more likely to occur when users are asleep. This preliminary insight was leveraged by many prior work to demonstrate the feasibility of inferring sleep periods from approximating user activity through the smartphone alone [3,46]. The same concept can be applied to a phone's network activity as shown in Fig. 1. The figure shows a phone's WiFi event rate every 15 min over a day and clearly shows a low activity period during the night corresponding to the user's nocturnal sleep period.

3   Related Work

Polysomnography is the gold standard for sleep monitoring [36]. However, conducting sleep studies outside clinical settings would require less obtrusive monitoring techniques for long-term sleep monitoring. As an alternative, researchers explored using heart rate sensors and motion sensors, found in commercially available sleep trackers such as Fitbit and Apple watch [40], for detecting human activity [41]. Although such wearables are very convenient to use, there are cases where users may not always wear them to bed. Instead, contactless solutions such as doppler radar or RF signals are deployed as standalone devices to monitor breathing patterns [42,43] and predict sleep [44,45]. Other sensing techniques look into smartphone based sensing techniques for sleep tracking. These efforts utilize an array of phone sensors such as accelerometer [13,22], light sensor [13,22], microphone [13,22–24], proximity sensor [22], and WiFi network activity rates [46]. These works above have proven rich (unlabeled) data we can use to predict sleep. However, collecting labeled ground truth of users continue to be a big challenge [4]. Most of the prior sleep prediction techniques [13,22] work are based on supervised learning approaches, whereby models require large amounts of training data to build accurate prediction models . Several works developed separate models for each user in the study which require at least 2 weeks of labelled data with sleep/wake-up estimation errors less than 40 min [46]. On the other hand, unsupervised methods have been explored specifically to do away with requiring training data. For example, Cuttone et al. develop a Bayesian approach to infer bed time and wake-up time from smart-phone screen events. Although convenient, these works have reported bed time and wake-time errors in the range of 1–2 h and they don't offer any form of personalization. These results collectively informed our decision to explore semi-supervised learning (SSL) approaches, where we can leverage unlabeled data to improve the accuracy of the prediction models.

Our investigation on semi-supervised learning approaches began via Self Training, followed by other standard techniques such as Co-Training, Auto Encoder, Data Generative, and Adversarial Training. These approaches have been adopted by prior work to solve sleep stage classification [15,17,50,51]. In understanding self-training, Zhang et al. reported error accumulation as a potential problem [52]. In contrast, other works have reported lesser error accumulation with co-training [53,54], including successful detection of everyday human behavior such as walking, running, and climbing stairs [55]. In fact, much work in human activity recognition has utilized adversarial learning [56] and autoencoder [29,57] to develop a generalizable and robust classification model for everyday human behavior.

Similar to these works, we aim to predict a person's sleep duration every night as an everyday human activity. However, these works rely on fine-grained time-series data sources such as EEG and actigraphy data, which are more likely to offer data completeness. In contrast, our work aims to develop a prediction model that can leverage unlabeled data, which is also suitable for coarse-grained data.

4 *SleepLess* Design

This section presents the design of our system, *SleepLess*, beginning with its problem formulation.

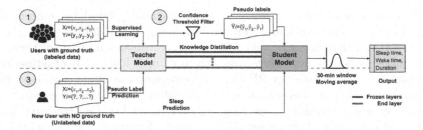

Fig. 2. *SleepLess*'s approach is a three-step process of training a Teacher model, generating high-quality pseudo labels from unlabeled data, and personalizing a Student model for a new user.

4.1 Problem Statement

The goal of our work is to develop personalized sleep detection models for each user based on unlabeled activity data from their smartphones. Our work assumes that a small amount of labeled data is available from a small group of users, which can be used for initial training. Additionally, we assume that only unlabeled data of new users is available, but their model needs to be personalized. We seek to design a semi-supervised learning approach to personalize an existing model, pre-trained on other sets of users, solely using unlabeled smartphone data for the new user. For the purpose of this paper, we consider utilizing coarse-grained WiFi activity data generated by users' smartphones as a measure of their phone activity[1]. Formally, we model this problem as a multivariate time series classification problem:

Users with Labeled Data: Consider $X^i = \{x_1, x_2....x_T\}$, which represents the multivariate time series of phone activity features for user, i, where $x_j = \{f_1, f_2....f_n\}$ is a vector of phone activity features at time, j. The features, $f_1, f_2....f_n$, in our case, are WiFi network activity features generated by user i's smartphone; for example, the number of observed WiFi events, number of WiFi access points connected by the phone. Collectively, these features represent the level of a phone's network activity. We assume time is discretized into fixed length intervals (i.e., 15-min) and these activity features are computed for each interval.

We assume a small group of users whose ground truth sleep information is available. This information includes the user's sleep duration, sleep time, T_{sleep}, and wake time T_{wake}. The ground truth yields a labeled time series for each user, i, where $Y^i = \{y_1, y_2....y_T\}$ and the label for each interval j is $y_j \in \{0, 1\}$. A label of 1 denotes the user as asleep, conversely, 0 denotes the user as being awake. All intervals between T_{sleep} and T_{wake} gets a label of 1.

---

[1] Our approach can be applied to other types of phone activity data such as screen activity. Here, phone activity data is represented by network activity rate.

New Users with Unlabeled Data: We assume a much larger group of users, whose phone activity data X^i is available but no labeled ground truth Y^i is known. In this case, the time series X^i simply represents unlabeled activity data for the user.

Henceforth, the problem is to train an (initially) supervised model on users with labeled data and personalize this model for each new user with only using their unlabeled data.

4.2   *SleepLess* Approach

Our approach to addressing the above problem involves three key steps, depicted in Fig. 2.

Step 1: Train a Teacher Model. *SleepLess* first users the set of users with ground truth data to train an initial CNN-based deep learning model. We refer to this initial model as the teacher model, $Model_{Teacher}$. $Model_{Teacher}$, discussed further in Sect. 5.3, uses a cross-entropy loss function defined as:

$$H_p(q) = -\frac{1}{N} \sum_{i=1}^{N} y_i.log(p(y_i)) + (1 - y_i).log(1 - p(y_i)) \tag{1}$$

where y is the sleep or awake label.

In solving for a binary classification problem, prior work has reported sigmoid value as a confidence metric reliable despite overconfident predictions arising from unseen classes [60]. However, due to the imbalanced nature of the dataset where there are more awake labels than sleep, the model may be biased towards predicting more prevalent label (i.e., awake). To address this issue, we calibrate our models by leveraging a validation set to improve the accuracy of our prediction probabilities.

Note that $Model_{Teacher}$ is trained to perform a binary classification task by taking the phones activity features X_j and predict whether the user is awake or asleep. The longest sequence of sleep labels over the course of each 24-h represent the sleep period for that day.

Step 2: Obtain Pseudo Labels from the Teacher Model. Given the teacher model, $Model_{Teacher}$, *SleepLess* then considers a new user, k, whose phone activity data is not accompanied with their sleep ground truth. It uses the time series of phone activity features, $X^k = \{x_1, x_2....x_T\}$, where x_T represents each time step, into $Model_{Teacher}$ to predict whether user k is asleep or awake. The output generated by $Model_{Teacher}$ constitute *pseudo labels* for the user.

It is possible that $Model_{Teacher}$ does not generalize well to the new user, likely due to low-quality pseudo labels. We use Dropout in the prediction network to improve the reliability of pseudo labels by reducing the effects of overfitting and improving the robustness of the model's predictions. Dropout works by randomly dropping out some neurons in the network during each training iteration. We also calibrate our models using a validation set. *SleepLess* performs label selection to only retain output predictions of high confidence, discarding all others. We use a confidence threshold, Δ, retaining predictions above this value as pseudo labels for the next phase. The Confidence score is chosen based on the average softmax scores of all predicted outcomes in a given 24-h period as follows:

$$C^i_{avg} = \frac{\sum c^i_t}{T} \tag{2}$$

Thus, for each new user, we obtain pseudo labels $\hat{Y} = \{\hat{y}_1, \hat{y}_2....\hat{y}_T\}$. Not all time slots will have such labels but since it is easy to collect unlabeled data, this process can continue until adequate pseudo labels are generated.

Step 3: Personalize a Student Model Using Fine-Tuning. The pseudo label data for user k can then be used to train a personalized model. Specifically, *SleepLess* performs transfer learning of the original teacher model, $Model_{Teacher}$, by freezing the initial layers of the CNN. The pseudo labels are then used to further train and fine-tune the subsequent layers, thus generating a student model, $Model_{Student}$, now personalized to the new user. This transfer learning approach helps the model re-use the learnt features in earlier layers and tailor the latter layers to specific sleep patterns of the new user.

5   *SleepLess* Implementation

We implemented *SleepLess* prototype as a cloud-based service using Python [27] and Keras libraries [28]. In what follows, we elaborate on the steps we took to build the deep learning component of the system.

5.1   Data Pre-processing

Network Activity Data. In essence, our technique utilizes users' phone activities generated from smartphone devices to predict their sleep. These activities can be represented by various measures including but not limited to the screen activity, application logs, accelerometer, and WiFi network activity logs [13].

Our work builds on utilizing WiFi network activity data for several operational reasons. As discussed in Sect. 6.1, our study sought to minimize user burdens and maximize privacy by avoiding dedicated app installations on their smartphone and, thus, directly sensing from their device. As such, we use a passive sensing technique where we acquired WiFi network activity data to collect *syslog* data directly from the WiFi APs, bypassing any connection to the user's device. In acquiring these logs, we filter out entries relevant only to our participants, specifically their primary smartphone device. The coarse granularity of WiFi data presents inherent technical errors in the measurement instrument. The coarse granularity of WiFi data presents inherent technical errors in the measurement instrument. To maintain the quality of our analysis, we cleaned these logs to reduce inaccurate and noisy data.

5.2 Feature Extraction

SleepLess processes logs of WiFi network activity rates generated from a user's phone. These logs are in the following format:

```
<date> <hh:mm:ss> <controller> <event\_ID> <severity>

<AP, MAC and IP addresses> <message text with BSSID and SSID>
```

Timestamp is given by date and time, while WiFi access point(AP) and users' device MAC addresses. Note that our collection of WiFi logs ensures user privacy by hashing users' device MAC addresses. together allow us to approximate the user's location. Event ID particularly describes three events of interest. They are i) association, when a device connects to an access point , ii) dissociation, when a device disconnects from the access point, and iii) authentication of the device, thus allowing us to approximate user activity and movement from one place to another. The result of using a *timestamp*, *event_ID*, *WiFi AP address*, and user device (hashed) *MAC address* is four input features to predict the user's sleep.

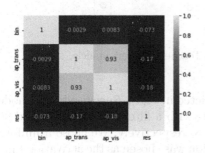

Fig. 3. Feature correlation

Table 1. Features used

Weight	Feature
0.647	Time
0.107	#WiFi AP Connections
0.132	#WiFi AP transitions
0.098	Dorm or not

- The *time of day* is marked in bins of every 15 min. Since we are interested in the nocturnal sleeping period, we consider a 24-h time span that starts from 6 pm of Day_1 and ends at 5:45 pm the next day. 6 pm of Day_1 corresponds to bin 0, while 5:45 pm of Day_2 corresponds to bin 95.
- The *number of WiFi AP connections* denotes the total number of unique access points visited over every 15 min interval.

- The *number of WiFi AP transitions* denotes the total number of transitions approximated from WiFi AP switching over every 15 min interval.
- We categorize *Dorm or not* as a user in their residential or non-residential location. This assignment is based on mapping WiFi APs specific to our campus and campus housing.

Figure 3 shows the correlation map of our features. Then, we compute feature importance through the permutation importance method. That is, we recursively measure the model performance every time the values of a feature are randomly shuffled. Table 1 summarizes the values of the most important features in our model. In this case, our top two features represent the time at which the user's device generate high network activity rate.

5.3   Model Architecture

In developing the teacher model, $Model_{Teacher}$, we extract features from the time series data of a fixed set of users into bins of 15 min intervals and include label assignments of *sleep (1)* or *awake (0)* state corresponding to their supplied ground truth. Conversely, $Model_{Student}$ is accompanied by pseudo labels of sleep.

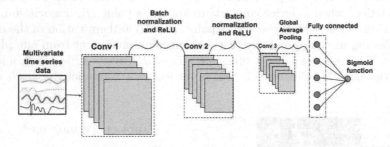

Fig. 4. CNN architecture for our Teacher-Student models.

We utilize a basic CNN architecture, depicted in Fig. 4. Specifically, the model consists of three temporal convolution layers with a filter size of 32, 64, and 96. Each layer has a kernel size of 24, 16, and 8, respectively. We chose a uniform stride of 1 for all the layers. The ReLU function was chosen as the activation function. We also chose a dropout rate of 0.1 between layers, a global 1D maximum pooling layer at the last convolutional layer. Finally, we used Adam optimizer with a learning rate of 0.0003.

6   Evaluation of *SleepLess*

In this section, we evaluate the efficacy of *SleepLess*'s semi-supervised learning model with other prediction methods employed in similar prior work. Further, we evaluate its robustness on private home users with different phone activity profiles.

Table 2. Demographic information of two different datasets.

	Student dataset (main)	Private home dataset (supplementary)
Users, N	20	3
	(18 Male, 2 Female)	(2 Male, 1 Female)
Age	18–21 years old	36–46 years old
	mean: 20, stdev.: 0.75	mean: 42, stdev.: 4.71
Study duration	4 weeks	1 week–4 weeks
Sleep summary	Bedtime: 06:00 pm–11:00 am (mean: 01:20 am), Wake time: 03:00 am–03:00 pm (mean: 10:10 am), Sleep duration: 60–660 min (mean: 420 min)	Bedtime: 11:20 pm–12:45 am (mean: 11:27 pm), Wake time: 05:30 am–08:00 am (mean: 06:16 am), Sleep duration: 300–511 min (mean: 428 min)
Sleep Tracker	Fitbit Inspire HR	Fitbit Inspire HR, Fitbit Versa 3 and manual logs
Device activity	anonymized logs of connected smartphones to campus WiFi.	unanonymized WiFi logs of connected smartphones and home devices to home WiFi

6.1   Experimental Setup

We begin by describing our user study details in acquiring two different datasets, as summarized in Table 2.

Study Protocol. We ran a month-long user study among college students living on campus upon receiving IRB approval from our institution. Our study protocol includes recruiting undergraduates and giving out Fitbit inspire HR [10] wearable to collect sleep logs automatically. The sleep logs generated from Fitbit are used as ground truth. In practice, WiFi logs generated from the campus APs only contain the timestamp and network activity rate of hashed MAC addresses per device. We specifically isolated our participants' device connection to a dedicated AP to identify our participant's smartphones, despite us dealing with only hashed records. Separately, we repeated the same protocol to a different set of private home users (non-student) over a one-week period.

Data Ethics and IRB Approval. Our user study is approved by the Institutional Review Board (IRB) and includes a Data Usage Agreement (DUA) with the campus network IT group.

6.2   Efficacy of SSL-Based Model

Our first experiment examines how *SleepLess* performs compared to a personalized supervised learning approach, which would require re-training a small amount of labeled data for a completely new user.

We utilize the student dataset in this experiment. Our results are achieved through conducting a train-test split. Specifically, models are trained on ten randomly picked student users and tested on the remaining ten users. Additionally, we set aside the first two weeks of labeled data of our test users to develop their personalized model and used the last two weeks to test the model.

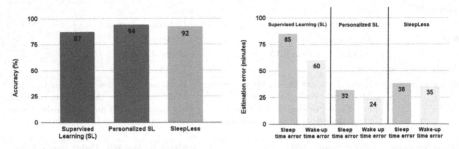

Fig. 5. Model performance comparing general and personalized supervised learning approaches with semi-supervised learning that *SleepLess* employs.

As shown in Fig. 5, the model performance for *SleepLess* is comparable to that of a personalized model. Specifically, the sleep and wake times prediction errors by *SleepLess* are approximately 10 min more than a personalized model. As expected, personalization will yield better model performance for a new user (94% accuracy, 32 min sleep time prediction error and 24 min wake-up time prediction error). In contrast, *SleepLess* achieves 92% accuracy, 38 min sleep time prediction error and 35 min wake-up time prediction error.

Table 3. Personalized supervised learning versus semi-supervised learning on home users.

Method	T_{sleep} min	T_{wake} min
Personalized SL	8 ± 5	23 ± 20
SleepLess	12 ± 4	25 ± 20

We replicated this experiment on our small group of non-student users who reside in private homes, comparing a personalized supervised learning approach with *SleepLess*. As indicated in Table 2 of our user study, the device network activity of our home participants accounted for all the personal devices connected to their home WiFi AP. Our model yielded slightly increased errors in predicted sleep and wake times. Even though *SleepLess* recorded 2% less accuracy, our results remain favorable for two reasons. First, *SleepLess*'s model decrement is insignificant ($p < .01$). Second, personalized supervised learning model will only offer practical use to new users after providing two weeks of labeled data for model retraining. In a real-world application, *SleepLess* can begin prediction for a new user without their labeled data almost instantaneously. These considerations motivate us to explore and propose *SleepLess* as a more practical approach, appealing to new users.

6.3   *SleepLess* vs. Baseline Algorithms

We follow up on the comparison of *SleepLess*'s performance with other baseline approaches proposed in prior work, including why these baselines would work less favorably for our case.

Baseline Algorithms. Given that the primary motivation of our work is to utilize fewer labeled data, we selectively picked on several methods that sought to learn with fewer labels.

The first is *semi-supervised learning using self-training*. Here, we train the teacher model using the labeled data from existing users and generate pseudo labels for the new users using their unlabeled data. The pseudo labels are picked based on the same criterion we used in *SleepLess*. The selected pseudo labels are combined with labeled data, D to train the student model. Compared to the typical self-training process, we stopped the pseudo label selection after one iteration to avoid error accumulation.

The second is *multi-head single-view co-training*. We adopt a similar structure suggested by Chen et al. [14], with several tweaks to the training pipeline. Rather than training multiple classifiers as in multi-view co-training, we will use predictions from multiple classification heads sharing a common module. First, we train the classifier using the labeled data, D, with only one classification head. Second, we generate pseudo labels for the new user using major voting by all the classification heads. Similarly, we filter the pseudo labels using the label selection criteria as per *SleepLess*. Finally, we combine the selected pseudo labels and labeled data to train the personalized model for the new user.

The third baseline employs an *encoder-decoder* approach, which exploits unlabeled data to learn the latent representation of the data [29]. The central idea of this approach is that the unlabeled data and labeled data can together help us select relevant features thus improving model robustness and generalizability. Here, we first combine unlabeled data from the new user to labeled data from existing users and train an encoder-decoder model to learn the latent representation of the new users' unlabeled data. After training the encoder-decoder model, we ingest only the labeled data, D, through the encoder decoder and obtain intermediate output from the encoder. We train the classifier using the encoded representation.

Results. Table 4 compares *SleepLess*'s model performance against the baseline models by testing on 4 weeks of data from 10 users. Specifically, *SleepLess* yields 96% accuracy, which is significantly higher than all other models ($p < .01$). Further, Fig. 6 charts the sleep and wake time errors for all methods. We observed that multi-head single-view co-training yielded the least errors among all the baseline methods; 27 min of sleep time error and 18 min of wake time error. However, this difference remains significantly higher than *SleepLess*. Co-training, which relies on the mix of new and existing user data, can be more suitable in conditions where our goal is to improve a generalized model approach.

Table 4. *SleepLess* and baseline models performance.

Method	Acc	Prec	Rec	F Scr.	p val.
SleepLess- SSL	0.96	0.98	0.87	0.93	–
Self-training	0.91	0.94	0.88	0.86	$p < .01$
Multi-head single-view Co-Training	0.92	0.87	0.88	0.88	$p < .01$
Auto encoder	0.87	0.80	0.76	0.78	$p < .05$

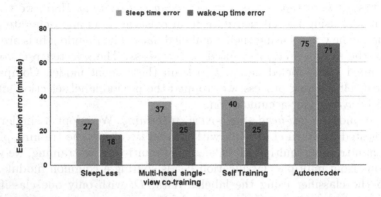

Fig. 6. Sleep and wake time errors by *SleepLess* and baselines.

Key Takeaway. Given our proposal on a semi-supervised learning approach, we compared the performance of our technique with standard SSL-based techniques such as self-training and co-training. As briefly discussed, our decision to compare these standard techniques was informed by prior work's implementation for sleep prediction, however, using fine-grained data. In this case, the consideration for a teacher-student model is primarily to address the error accumulation problem, which we hypothesized will be more prominent from using coarse-grained data such as phone network activity rate. Our results yielded significantly better performance of 96% accuracy compared to these standard techniques.

7   Conclusions

Fundamentally, the requirement of collecting a significant amount of ground truth holds for training any user behavioral models. Unlike many prior sleep detection techniques that rely on collecting and training large amounts of labeled data, *SleepLess*, w uses semi-supervised learning over unlabeled data sensed from the user's smartphone network activity to develop personalized models and detect their sleep duration for the night. By using a generalized pre-trained model on an existing set of users to produce pseudo labels for unlabeled data of a new user, it achieves personalization by fine-tuning using selected pseudo-labels for the new user without requiring any labeled data. Our user study among 23 users found *SleepLess* model yielding around 96% accuracy, between 12–27 min of sleep time error and 18–25 min of wake time error. With our prediction technique yielding the best performance, our work shows promise for sleep monitoring to be more conveniently adapted to monitor new users' sleep immediately. Where the larger goal of our work aims to improve students' health, lack of sleep is linked to many major health challenges. Our work continues investigating the efficacy of this technique in complementary domains, including sleep quality.

Acknowledgments. This work is supported in parts by NSF grants 2211302, 2211888, 2213636, 2105494, and Army grant W911NF-17-2-0196.

References

1. Krueger, P.M., Friedman, E.M.: Sleep duration in the United States: a cross-sectional population-based study. Am. J. Epidemiol. **169**(9), 1052–1063 (2009)
2. Rahman, T., et al.: Dopplesleep: a contactless unobtrusive sleep sensing system using short-range doppler radar. In: Proceedings of the 2015 ACM International Joint Conference on Pervasive and Ubiquitous Computing (2015)
3. Abdullah, S., et al.: Towards circadian computing: early to bed and early to rise makes some of us unhealthy and sleep deprived. In: Proceedings of the 2014 ACM International Joint Conference on Pervasive and Ubiquitous Computing (2014)
4. De Zambotti, M., et al.: Wearable sleep technology in clinical and research settings. Med. Sci. Sports Exercise **51**(7), 1538 (2019)
5. Ohayon, M.M.: Epidemiological overview of sleep disorders in the general population. Sleep Med. Res. **2**(1), 1–9 (2011)
6. Nest. https://support.google.com/googlenest. Accessed 27 Oct 2022
7. Amazon.   https://www.amazon.com/Paschar-LLC-Walabot-Sleep-Tracker/dp/B07C2HRYSX. Accessed 27 Oct 2022
8. Zhao, Y., et al.: Semi-supervised federated learning for activity recognition. arXiv preprint arXiv:2011.00851 (2020)
9. Trivedi, A., et al.: Wifitrace: network-based contact tracing for infectious diseases using passive wifi sensing. In: Proceedings of the ACM on Interactive, Mobile, Wearable and Ubiquitous Technologies vol. 5, no. 1, pp. 1–26 (2021)
10. Google. https://www.fitbit.com/global/be/products/-trackers/inspire. Accessed 27 Oct 2022
11. Wang, R., et al.: StudentLife: assessing mental health, academic performance and behavioral trends of college students using smartphones. In: Proceedings of the 2014 ACM International Joint Conference on Pervasive and Ubiquitous Computing (2014)
12. Hofman, J.M., Sharma, A., Watts, D.J.: Prediction and explanation in social systems. Science **355**(6324), 486–488 (2017)
13. Saeb, S., et al.: Scalable passive sleep monitoring using mobile phones: opportunities and obstacles. J. Med. Internet Res. **19**(4), e118 (2017)
14. Chen, M., et al.: Semi-supervised learning with multi-head co-training. Proc. AAAI Conf. Artif. Intell. **36**(6), 6278–6286 (2022)
15. Zhang, C., et al.: CMS2-net: semi-supervised sleep staging for diverse obstructive sleep apnea severity. IEEE J. Biomed. Health Inf. **26**(7), 3447–3457 (2022)
16. Li, Y., et al.: Adversarial learning for semi-supervised pediatric sleep staging with single-EEG channel. Methods **204**, 84–91 (2022)

17. Haoran, B., Guanze, L.: Semi-supervised end-to-end automatic sleep stage classification based on pseudo-label. In: 2021 IEEE International Conference on Power Electronics, Computer Applications (ICPECA). IEEE (2021)
18. El-Khadiri, Y., et al.: Sleep activity recognition using binary motion sensors. In: 2018 IEEE 30th International Conference on Tools with Artificial Intelligence (ICTAI). IEEE (2018)
19. Cuttone, A., et al.: Sensiblesleep: a Bayesian model for learning sleep patterns from smartphone events. PloS One 12(1), e0169901 (2017)
20. Peng, Y., et al.: Joint semi-supervised feature auto-weighting and classification model for EEG-based cross-subject sleep quality evaluation. In: ICASSP 2020-2020 IEEE International Conference on Acoustics, Speech and Signal Processing (ICASSP). IEEE (2020)
21. Heremans, E.R.M., et al.: From unsupervised to semi-supervised adversarial domain adaptation in electroencephalography-based sleep staging. J. Neural Eng. 19(3), 036044 (2022)
22. Min, J.-K., et al.: Toss'n'turn: smartphone as sleep and sleep quality detector. In: Proceedings of the SIGCHI Conference on Human Factors in Computing Systems (2014)
23. Hao, T., Xing, G., Zhou, G.: isleep: unobtrusive sleep quality monitoring using smartphones. In: Proceedings of the 11th ACM Conference on Embedded Networked Sensor Systems (2013)
24. Ren, Y., et al.: Fine-grained sleep monitoring: Hearing your breathing with smartphones. In: 2015 IEEE Conference on Computer Communications (INFOCOM). IEEE (2015)
25. Chen, Z., et al.: Unobtrusive sleep monitoring using smartphones. In: 2013 7th International Conference on Pervasive Computing Technologies for Healthcare and Workshops. IEEE (2013)
26. Gu, W., et al.: Sleep hunter: towards fine grained sleep stage tracking with smartphones. IEEE Trans. Mobile Comput. 15(6), 1514–1527 (2015)
27. Python. https://www.python.org/. Accessed 27 Oct 2022
28. keras. https://keras.io/. Accessed 27 Oct 2022
29. Bhattacharya, S., et al.: Using unlabeled data in a sparse-coding framework for human activity recognition. Pervas. Mobile Comput. 15, 242–262 (2014)
30. Munk, A.M., et al.: Semi-supervised sleep-stage scoring based on single channel EEG. In: 2018 IEEE International Conference on Acoustics, Speech and Signal Processing (ICASSP). IEEE (2018)
31. Wang, X., et al.: Smartphone sonar-based contact-free respiration rate monitoring. ACM Trans. Comput. Healthc. 2(2), 1–26 (2021)
32. Tiron, R., et al.: Screening for obstructive sleep apnea with novel hybrid acoustic smartphone app technology. J. Thoracic Dis. 12(8), 4476 (2020)
33. Kim, D.H., Kim, S.W., Hwang, S.H.: Diagnostic value of smartphone in obstructive sleep apnea syndrome: a systematic review and meta-analysis. PloS One 17(5), e0268585 (2022)
34. Goldblum, M., et al.: Dataset security for machine learning: data poisoning, backdoor attacks, and defenses. IEEE Trans. Pattern Anal. Mach. Intell. 45(2), 1563–1580 (2022)
35. Dixon, M., et al.: Sleep-wake detection with a contactless, bedside radar sleep sensing system (2021)
36. Rundo, J.V., Downey, R., III: Polysomnography. Handb. Clin. Neurol. 160, 381–392 (2019)

37. Blunck, H., et al.: On heterogeneity in mobile sensing applications aiming at representative data collection. In: Proceedings of the 2013 ACM Conference on Pervasive and Ubiquitous Computing Adjunct Publication (2013)
38. Wuzheng, X., et al.: Semi-supervised sparse representation classification for sleep EEG recognition with imbalanced sample sets. J. Mech. Med. Biol. **21**(05), 2140006 (2021)
39. ouraring. https://ouraring.com/. Accessed 27 Oct 2022
40. Apple. https://www.apple.com/watch/. Accessed 27 Oct 2022
41. Witt, D.R., et al.: Windows into human health through wearables data analytics. Curr. Opin. Biomed. Eng. **9**, 28–46 (2019)
42. Lee, Y.S., et al.: Monitoring and analysis of respiratory patterns using microwave doppler radar. IEEE J. Trans. Eng. Health Med. **2**, 1–12 (2014)
43. Gu, C., Li, C.: Assessment of human respiration patterns via noncontact sensing using doppler multi-radar system. Sensors **15**(3), 6383–6398 (2015)
44. Lin, F., et al.: SleepSense: a noncontact and cost-effective sleep monitoring system. IEEE Trans. Biomed. Circuits Syst. **11**(1), 189–202 (2016)
45. Hong, H., et al.: Microwave sensing and sleep: Noncontact sleep-monitoring technology with microwave biomedical radar. IEEE Microw. Magaz. **20**(8), 18–29 (2019)
46. Zakaria, C., et al.: SleepMore: inferring sleep duration at scale via multi-device WiFi sensing. In: Proceedings of the ACM on Interactive, Mobile, Wearable and Ubiquitous Technologies, vol. 6, no. 4, pp. 1–32 (2023)
47. Zhu, X., Goldberg, A.B.: Introduction to Semi-supervised Learning. Springer Nature (2022)
48. Zhu, X.J.: Semi-supervised learning literature survey (2005)
49. Miyato, T., et al.: Virtual adversarial training: a regularization method for supervised and semi-supervised learning. IEEE Trans. Pattern Anal. Mach. Intell. **41**(8), 1979–1993 (2018)
50. Yalniz, I.Z., et al.: Billion-scale semi-supervised learning for image classification. arXiv preprint arXiv:1905.00546 (2019)
51. Zou, Y., et al.: Unsupervised domain adaptation for semantic segmentation via class-balanced self-training. In: Proceedings of the European Conference on Computer Vision (ECCV) (2018)
52. Zhang, C., et al.: Understanding deep learning (still) requires rethinking generalization. Commun. ACM **64**(3), 107–115 (2021)
53. Zhou, Z.-H., Li, M.: Semi-supervised learning by disagreement. Knowl. Inf. Syst. **24**, 415–439 (2010)
54. Wang, W., Zhou, Z.-H.: Analyzing co-training style algorithms. In: European Conference on Machine Learning. Springer, Heidelberg (2007)
55. Guan, D., et al.: Activity recognition based on semi-supervised learning. In: 13th IEEE International Conference on Embedded and Real-Time Computing Systems and Applications (RTCSA 2007). IEEE (2007)
56. Faridee, A.Z.M., et al.: Strangan: adversarially-learnt spatial transformer for scalable human activity recognition. Smart Health **23**, 100226 (2022)
57. Gogna, A., Majumdar, A.: Semi supervised autoencoder. In: Neural Information Processing: 23rd International Conference (ICONIP 2016), Kyoto, 16–21 October 2016, Proceedings, Part II, vol. 23. Springer (2016)
58. Chakma, A., et al.: Activity recognition in wearables using adversarial multi-source domain adaptation. Smart Health **19**, 100174 (2021)
59. Pearce, T., Brintrup, A., Zhu, J.: Understanding softmax confidence and uncertainty. arXiv preprint arXiv:2106.04972 (2021)

60. Dhamija, A.R., Günther, M., Boult, T.: Reducing network agnostophobia. Adv. Neural Inf. Process. Syst. **31** (2018)
61. Japkowicz, N., Stephen, S.: The class imbalance problem: a systematic study1. Intell. Data Anal. **6**(5), 429–449 (2002). https://doi.org/10.3233/IDA-2002-6504

myAQM: Interfacing Portable Air Quality Monitor with the Apple Watch - An In-the-Wild Usability Study

Vince Nguyen[✉] [iD]

New York University Abu Dhabi, PO Box 129188, Saadiyat Island, Abu Dhabi,
United Arab Emirates
vince.nguyen@nyu.edu

Abstract. The last decade witnessed the popularization of commercial smartwatches as personal health-tracking devices. This coincided with a deeper understanding of the health effects of ambient and indoor air pollution. Consequently, there is a growing interest in interfacing data from portable sensors with commercial smartwatches, allowing users to monitor the air whenever and wherever. In the real world, it remains insufficiently investigated how and through which modalities users benefit from smartwatch interfaces. To bridge this gap, we conducted a pioneering in-the-wild usability study with myAQM (N = 9). myAQM visualizes PM2.5 and CO_2 data from a portable air quality monitor on different Apple Watch interfaces: the main application, complications (watch face's widgets), and notifications. Our qualitative analysis showed that the Apple Watch interfaces provided glanceable data, omnipresent reminders of the surrounding air, and timely alerts of changes in air quality. Through these affordances, users developed a more acute understanding of the surrounding air and reduced self-exposure to bad air quality through certain behavioral changes, if circumstances permitted. Our findings support commercial smartwatches as a convenient and readily-accessible add-on for traditional smartphone interfaces in disseminating hyperlocal air quality data.

Keywords: Personal air quality monitoring · Smartwatch · Apple Watch · Notifications · Glanceable visualization · In-the-wild usability study

1 Introduction

Air pollution is the 4th leading factor for premature death, claiming over 6 million lives worldwide in 2019 [23]. In line with growing interests in air quality monitoring, there has been growing scientific literature on personal air quality monitoring devices which provide high resolution spatio-temporal data at low cost, compared to sparsely-located reference monitoring stations [3, 26, 30, 47, 50, 51]. This data hyper-localization is important as air quality fluctuates depending on proximity to pollution sources, allowing users to monitor both ambient and household air quality more accurately [9, 27].

© ICST Institute for Computer Sciences, Social Informatics and Telecommunications Engineering 2024
Published by Springer Nature Switzerland AG 2024. All Rights Reserved
D. Salvi et al. (Eds.): PH 2023, LNICST 572, pp. 339–363, 2024.
https://doi.org/10.1007/978-3-031-59717-6_23

In the field of human-computer interaction (HCI) for health and wellness, many studies chose smartphones as the medium to display air quality data from portable sensors thanks to smartphones' ubiquitousness [9,16,18,41,47,52]. There is limited literature on interfacing hyperlocal air quality data with commercial smartwatches despite their rising popularity for health monitoring [25,29]. Furthermore, even fewer studies conducted user experiments to understand how such systems are perceived, examined, and utilized [22,56]. Thus, much remains to be investigated how the novelty of commercial smartwatch user interfaces (UIs) deliver hyperlocal air quality data and how such interfaces influence user awareness and behaviors. Deeper understanding of such concepts is key to designing better ubiquitous UIs for air quality data.

To bridge this gap, we implemented and user tested myAQM (my Air Quality Monitor), a pervasive computing system with a commercial smartwatch which visualizes air quality data obtained from a portable monitor.

myAQM's portable air quality monitor measures: particulate matter smaller than $2.5\,\mu m$ (PM2.5) and carbon dioxide (CO_2). PM2.5 is popular in the field of personal air quality monitoring [13,42] as it is one of the most hazardous ambient and household pollutants [23,33,44,54]. PM2.5 accumulates in the lung and internal organs, causing respiratory and cardiovascular diseases.

For indoor air quality, CO_2 - a by-product human respiration, was chosen as an indicator for adequate ventilation. A lack of indoor ventilation increases levels of human bioeffluents which produces stressful physiological responses and impacts cognitive performance [14,35,55,56]. Simultaneously, the COVID-19 pandemic highlights the need to monitor indoor CO_2 concentration to reduce the transmission of airborne diseases in enclosed spaces [12,45].

Air quality data is visualized on the Apple Watch interfaces. We choose the Apple Watch due to its dominance in the marketshare of commercial smartwatches (36% as of Q1 2022) [32] and frequent coverage in literature on wearables for health monitoring [25,36,56]. We evaluated myAQM in the wild with nine participants for nine days each. We conducted semi-structured interviews before and after usage. Finally, we qualitatively analyzed the interviews to answer:

- **RQ1:** How does the wrist-worn form factor of the Apple Watch and its interfaces influence how users receive air quality data in the wild?
- **RQ2:** As commercial smartwatch apps are often accompanied by similar smartphone apps, how does myAQM's Watch interfaces support its iPhone app?
- **RQ3:** How does combining a portable air quality monitor with a commercial smartwatch affect users' air quality awareness and behaviors?

We summarize the major contributions of our work below:

- **C1:** An empirical nine-day in-the-wild study of a personal air quality monitoring system whose main visualization medium is a commercial smartwatch (Apple Watch), one of the first of its kind.
- **C2:** An empirical understanding of how users interacted with air quality data on a commercial smartwatch, how it influenced their understanding of air quality, and under which circumstances they acted to reduce exposure.
- **C3:** Discussions of the implications for future work in optimizing air quality interfaces in commercial smartwatches.

2   Related Work

The last decade witnessed growing HCI literature on personal air quality monitoring systems, thanks to advances in low-cost sensor technology [3,30,50] and mounting evidence of air pollution's health effects [17,23,33]. Simultaneously, the medium for visualizing air quality data has evolved from built-in displays and dashboards [27,28,41], to smartphone apps [9,16,47] and wearable devices [22,40,56]. Table 1 summarizes relevant studies to our research.

Usability Studies of Personal Air Quality Monitoring Systems
While most studies reported the technical implementations of personal air quality monitoring systems [9,18,22,27,28,37,39,41,52,56], fewer conducted usability testing to understand how they are used and how they influence users' awareness. Early works by Kim et al. [27,28] demonstrated that their *inAir* stationary indoor air quality dashboard increased users' understanding of the environment and elicited behavioral changes to improve the air. Expanding this concept to outdoor settings, *CitiSense* by Bales et al. [9] tested a smartphone app as the visualization medium in realistic scenarios, both indoors and outdoors. Their study highlighted the importance of mobile interfaces in revealing spatio-temporal variabilities of pollutants, empowering users to reduce their exposure to bad air.

Although these early works provided evidence for the benefits of personal air quality monitoring, these systems required active engagement and environment awareness from the users to receive air quality data, such as passing by the dashboard at home (*inAir* [27,28]) or opening the smartphone application (*CitiSense* [9]). In fact, participants in *CitiSense* reported decreased user engagements over time [9].

Notifications for Personal Air Quality Monitoring Systems
Subsequent studies addressed this barrier by equipping their monitoring systems with alerts in different modalities. For instance, to notify users of air pollution spikes, Fang et al. used push notifications on their *AirSense* smartphone applications [16], while Moore et al. employed simple text messages on their *MAAV* system [41]. While both studies found that the notifications enhanced user experience by contextualizing the data and reminding users to cope with bad air quality, these findings could only be examined in the context of indoor use cases. *AirSense* employed stationary indoor sensors; MAAV employed both indoor and outdoor sensors but its outdoor sensor was installed right outside the participant's house [41], limiting its use case to when the user was nearby their home (due to outdoor air quality's spatial variation). To what extent these notification systems are usable outdoors remains unexplored.

Portable Air Quality Monitors with Commercial Smartwatches
Previous studies with stationary or smartphone interfaces hinted at unexplored research territories with commercial smartwatches as they become widely adopted for health and fitness, activities and environmental tracking, and com-

Table 1. A summarized comparison of relevant literature on different interfaces for visualizing hyperlocal air quality data from personal air quality monitors. The first column groups the studies by their main visualization medium. Our work (myAQM) is mentioned at the top.

	Literature	Portability (sensor)	Visualization Interface					Usability study		
			Description	Pollutant(s)	Notifications	Glanceability	Note	Settings	Duration	Number of Users
Commercial smartwatch	This paper myAQM (2023)	Portable	An Apple Watch app with glanceable complications and air quality change notifications, accompanied by an iPhone app	PM2.5, CO_2	Yes	Yes, with the complications		Uncontrolled, diverse real-life settings (indoors, outdoors)	nine days	9
	Zhong Hidawear (2020) [56]	Portable	A native independent Apple Watch app with 3 visualization interfaces	CO_2	Yes	-	-	Controlled, inside workplace, pre-fabricated data	At least 90 minutes	12
	Marques i4mb (2020) [40]	Stationary (Indoors)	An Apple Watch app, an iPhone app	PM10, CO_2	-	-	-	-	-	-
	Hosseini mHealth (2017) [22]	Portable	A Samsung Gear smartwatch app with child-friendly visualization, a smartphone app with detail data for caregivers	Dust density, PM2.5, spirometer data	-	-	Calculate asthma risks	Uncontrolled, in real-life (indoors, outdoors)	Several weeks	2 adult, 1 child (1 adult, 1 child)
Commercial smartphone	Bales CitiSense (2019) [9]	Portable	An Android phone app	CO, NO2, O3	-	Glanceable color scheme on phone app	-	Uncontrolled, in real-life (indoors, outdoors)	1 month	16
	Maag W-Air (2018) [37]	Wrist-worn	An Android phone app	CO_2, O3	-	-	-	-	-	-
	Fang AirSense (2016) [16]	Stationary (indoors)	An Android phone app	PM2.5, VOC	Yes	-	Identify pollution source (context-aware)	Uncontrolled, in real-life at home (indoors)	3 weeks with the phone app	5 families
	Tian MyPart (2016) [52]	Wrist-worn	An Android phone app & ambient LEDs onboard the wearable sensor	PM2.5 PM10	-	Yes, ambient LEDs		Pre-specified outdoor walking route	40-min walk	6
Dashboard	Moore MAAV (2018) [41]	Stationary (indoors, outdoors)	A tablet-based interactive visualization	PM2.5	Yes (text based)	Yes, always-on display	In-situ annotation of air quality data	Uncontrolled, in real-life (indoors at home, outdoors) and outdoors	Mean 37.7 weeks	6 families
	Kim inAir (2013) [28]	Stationary (indoors)	An iPod touch app, placed in a stationary location inside participant's home	PM count	-	Yes, always-on display		Uncontrolled, in real-life at home (indoors)	4 months	6 families

municating purposes [11,25,34]. Existing literature on commercial smartwatches as a visualization medium for air quality data is limited, with most studies only investigating the technicality of such systems, leaving the user experience inadequately understood [39,40]. Zhong et al. was one of the first to offer intriguing user experience insights with *Hilo-wear* by using an Apple Watch to display pre-fabricated CO_2 measurements in a controlled office setting (N=12) [56]. The authors leveraged the Apple Watch's form factor to deliver instant notifications regardless of the users' activities. The system was proven to facilitate user action against bad air quality (e.g. opening the windows to ventilate). That said, *Hilo-wear* was constrained within its controlled experiment setting: inside an office building, CO_2 as the only air quality marker, and a short usage duration (a few hours at most). Whether its findings would translate into real-life use cases in various types of environments (outdoors, commuting, indoors at work, indoors at home...) remained to be explored. Hosseini et al. [22] deployed in-situ their *mHealth* system, comprising a Samsung smartwatch application and a smartphone application, to an asthmatic child to assess the system in predicting and communicating asthma risk. While the author offered some glimpse into how portable the system's usability, it could not be generalized due to the extremely small sample size (N=1).

myAQM's Contributions to Current Literature
To our best knowledge, myAQM is the first study to test commercial smartwatches as UIs for hyperlocal air quality data from a portable sensor during diverse real-world usage in both indoor and outdoor environments. myAQM provides various Apple Watch interfaces for people to use from: the application itself, notifications, and complications (widgets on the watch face), catering to diverse usage patterns. By adopting the Apple Watch as one of its data visualization interfaces, our work extends *inAir*'s and *CitiSense*'s findings [9,27,28] on how pervasive air quality monitoring facilitates awareness and behavioral change, through the watch's novel form factor. myAQM also complements previous studies *Hilo-wear* [56], *MAAV* [41], and *AirSense* [16] on air quality notifications in much more diverse use cases regardless of the users' locations.

3   myAQM Portable Air Quality Monitoring System

3.1   Portable Air Quality Monitor

The portable air quality monitor is a DIY device. It employs an ESP32 microcontroller unit (MCU) that controls two air quality sensors: Sensirion SPS30 and Sensirion SCD41, see *Fig. 1(a)*. The MCU is programmed in Arduino IDE 1.8 with C++. The device measures $54 \times 70 \times 26$ mm (W × H × D), weighs 110g, and has a battery life of one full day, making it portable for daily usage. Table 2 details all components of the portable device.

Sensirion SPS30 is a light-scattering particulate matter sensor, factory-calibrated for PM2.5, and has a precision of $\pm$ [5 $\mu g/m^3$ + 5 % measured values]

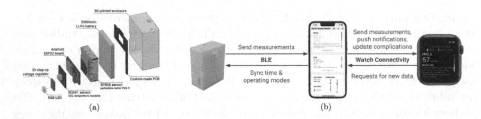

Fig. 1. An overview of the myAQM system. (a) Components of the portable air quality monitor. (b) Relationships between the 3 components of the myAQM system: air quality monitor (left), iOS app (center), and watchOS app (right).

Table 2. The components of the portable air quality monitor

	Component	Functionality
MCU	Adafruit ESP32 Feather Board	Control sensors, logics, BLE, and charging
Sensors	Sensirion SPS30	Measure PM2.5
	Sensirion SCD41	Measure CO2, temperature, humidity
Power	Li-Po Battery (3.7V, 2500mAh)	Supply power, lasting 40h in real-world testing
	Pololu 5V Voltage Regulator U1V11F5	Step-up battery's 3.7V to supply 5V for SPS30
Misc	Adafruit Diffused Piranha RGB LED	Indicate device's operating status
	LilyPad Slide Switch	Allow the device to be switched on/off
	Custom-made 1.6mm 2-layer PCB	Connect the MCU to the rest of the components
	3D-printed enclosure	Provide protection to the electronic components

(from 0 to 100 $\mu g/m^3$) and ± 10 % measured values (from 100 to 1000 $\mu g/m^3$). Meanwhile, Sensirion SCD41 is a photoacoustic NDIR CO_2 sensor, with integrated temperature and humidity sensors. The accuracy of its CO_2 measurement is $\pm(40$ PPM $+$ 5% of reading) in the concentration range 400PPM - 5,000PPM. It has automatic self-calibration which assumes that the sensor is exposed to the atmospheric concentration of 400PPM at least once a week. While the global atmospheric CO_2 concentration has surpassed 400PPM, currently around 417PPM in July 2023 [31], the relatively small difference may only have a negligible impact on the sensor's calibration, especially in indoor environments where CO_2 concentrations can be much higher [14].

3.2   iOS-watchOS myAQM Applications

The portable air quality device sends data via Bluetooth Low-Energy (BLE) to the myAQM iOS app which then relays data to the watchOS app, see Fig. 1(b). In cases when the connection is lost, the portable device saves the data onboard and sends queued-up data upon a re-connection. While a direct connection between the portable device and the Watch is possible, the Watch's low processing power would limit data update frequency. We employed this device-iOS-watchOS model to ensure data promptness and provide users with flexible use cases. In fact, most

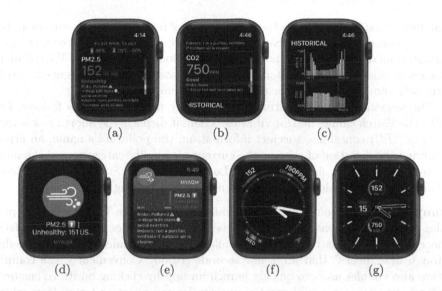

Fig. 2. myAQM's Apple Watch three interfaces: main app, notification, and complication (widget on watch face) **Main app (a), (b), (c):** (a) Connection status, portable device's battery level, temperature, humidity, and current PM2.5 air quality index (b) Current CO_2 concentration (c) Historical air quality data **Air quality change notification sequence (d), (e):** (d) Short Look, followed by (e) Long Look **Complication (widget on the watch face) (f), (g):** Two types of complications supported by myAQM, both with examples of PM2.5 and CO2 complications

watchOS apps are accompanied by corresponding iOS apps due to technical requirements and user preference [25].

We used the United States Environmental Protection Agency's Air Quality Index to categorize PM2.5 concentrations [46]. We used consensus proposed by Lowther et al. [35] to categorize CO_2 concentrations as a proxy for indoor ventilation, human bio-effluent, and other indoor air pollutants: $\leq$1,000PPM: good, 1000-1500PPM: moderate, and $\geq$1500PPM: poor. Previous studies found it challenging for some people to associate air quality thresholds with health outcomes [56] and some people were unsure how to respond to subpar air quality [27,47]. Thus, we incorporated health effects and suggestions to reduce exposure for each air quality category. While not exhaustive, they aim to encourage a remedy-oriented approach to air quality among users. An example for CO_2's Moderate category is *"Decreased cognitive performance & fatigue might be experienced → Consider: ventilate, open windows."*

3.3 watchOS Application Interfaces

Main Application: The watchOS main application shows current air quality measurements with scales, color coding schemes, health suggestions, and historical data, see *Fig. 2(a), 2(b), 2(c).*

Notifications: Notification is the major mode of interaction with smartwatches due to its promptness and convenience [11,25,53]. If either PM2.5 or CO_2 level changes from one category to another, a notification will alert users. We calculate changes in air quality with 10-minute running average measurements to avoid extremely short-burst events or random measurement errors.

The sequence of events during an air quality notification is as follows. Initially, the Watch chimes and/or vibrates. Then, it displays the Short Look screen (see *Fig. 2(d)*) containing succinct information: the pollutant's name, an arrow signifying the direction of change, the current air quality category, and the measurement. Finally, it shows the Long Look screen (see *Fig. 2(e)*), visualizing recent measurements leading to the change and suggesting what to do.

Complications: A complication is a widget on the Apple Watch's face. It provides recent data whenever the users raise their wrist to look at the watch face. The complication has been shown to allow quick dissemination of knowledge through brief"peeks" that are a few seconds [10,53]. Conveniently, the complication also enables users to quickly launch an app by clicking on it. To ensure a uniform experience, we implemented two similar complication types, from which the participants chose for their active watch face [5], see *Fig. 2(f) - Gauge text in Corner family, 2(g) - Open gauge text in Circular family*. Each complication shows the current number for the PM2.5 AQI or CO_2 concentration, accompanied by a gauge showing the color of the current air quality category.

4   Methodology - Usability Study

As we managed to build only three identical portable air quality monitors, we ran the study in batches of three participants each. Additionally, considering the strong seasonal variations in ambient PM2.5 level at the study's location (Abu Dhabi, UAE) [1,2], we must limit the total duration of the whole study to minimize differences in ambient PM2.5 level across batches. Constraints in the number of devices and in the total length of the study meant that we had to compromise between the total number of participants and the study length for each participant.

Ultimately, we recruited **nine** participants from the university mailing list and settled for a **nine-day** usage period, which totaled the whole usability study to a month to minimize the mentioned seasonal effect. Some basic demographic information of the nine participants:

- Six male, three female
- Four commuters, five on-campus residents (within walking distance to the work/study place)
- Five undergraduate students, two university professors, one researcher, and one university staff

As the study is exploratory, we did not impose selection criteria such as pre-existing medical conditions or pre-existing usage of air quality devices. We required participants to own and use: an iPhone 6 and above runnning iOS 15 and an Apple Watch 4 and above running watchOS 8. [1] Each participant was compensated AED 400 (USD 108) for their involvement in the study.

For each participant, we conducted an initial semi-structured interview with probing questions on: (1) prior understanding of air quality and air pollution, (2) prior knowledge and/or experience of using air quality monitoring devices, and (3) their Apple Watch using habits. We then used Apple's TestFlight [4] to install the iOS-watchOS applications on their personal devices. Finally, we instructed them to attach the portable device to an accessory they carried every day, such as backpacks, tote bags, and handbags, see Fig. 3.

To best approximate how people would use myAQM in real life, we advised them to interact with the system however and whenever they wanted. We opted against ecological momentary assessment (EMA) [49] to avoid reminding the participant beyond their natural usage pattern. Instead, we sent out two 20-min surveys on day 3th and 8th to help participant retroactively document their experience. After the nine-day usage period, we invited each participant for another semi-structured interview to discuss their experience, with a special emphasis on the Apple Watch's interfaces and how they worked in junction with the iPhone's counterparts.

All interviews were transcribed and open coded [48]. We went through the transcripts once to inductively uncover topics related to the RQs. We then revisited all transcripts to deductively group codes together, through axial coding, into broader categories based on similarities and possible causal relationships. Finally, we employed selective coding to construct an overarching narrative that captures the essence of how myAQM, especially its Apple Watch interfaces, affords to disseminate air quality data, impart knowledge, and induce behavioral changes.

To further support the qualitative analysis, our main method, we also measured basic app usage analytic: (1) Number of times each app (watchOS and iOS) is launched by the user, (2) Number of times the watchOS app is launched via the complications and via other methods combined (clicking on notifications and clicking on the app in the menu)[2], and (3) Screen-on time (in minutes) of each app (watchOS and iOS).

---

[1] Apple Watch 3 and below do not support myAQM's complication types [7].

[2] Due to technical limitation, we could not detect watchOS app launch via the notifications. That said, we could detect when the app is in the foreground. Thus, we report the combined number of launches via the notifications and the app menu by subtracting the number of times the complications are clicked from the total number of foreground sessions.

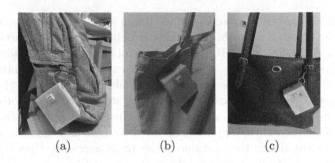

(a)   (b)   (c)

Fig. 3. Real images of how users carried the portable device throughout the day

5   Results

5.1   Prior to Using myAQM

5.1.1   Particiants' Motivations for Air Quality Tracking Prior to myAQM

To explore myAQM's influence on the participants, we examine how participants had accessed air quality data prior to using myAQM.

Air quality awareness varied among participants. Those who came from more polluted areas (P1, P3, P5, P6, P7) were familiar with air quality index and phenomena like smog and inversion. Likewise, participants who have respiratory illnesses are more acutely aware of their environment (P1, P8). However, for most, there was no regular habit of tracking air quality due to the required efforts and air quality not being an urgent health hazard. They described their non-habitual engagement with air quality data as sporadic and driven by specific events. The main sources were from publicly available platforms such as aggregate websites and search engines, live billboards on highways and in public buildings, and weather applications:

> It's not something I seek often. Occasionally, when we have dust storms, I might google to see a number. (P7)

> I was in Manila. Along the road, they put up a big sign that tells you the air quality. [...] it's just whenever I pass by, then I see it. It's useful information for me but I don't intend to check on it every day. (P9)

> When living in Paris, I would pay attention to air quality more with the weather app on my phone. Because I noticed that whenever ran outside, I would get a cough. So I started to pay attention to it. But that's really all I know. (P4)

These conversations point to convenience and urgency as important factors that can lower the entry barrier to consistently track air quality, both of which are addressed by the Watch's complications and notifications as will be discussed in Sect. 5.2.1 and Sect. 5.2.2.

5.1.2 Participants' Expectations of Using myAQM

Before using myAQM, we asked participants how they expected it would influence their understanding of air quality. Their responses varied, but two contrasting themes emerged across participants. Some participants were optimistic that it would help them identify pollution sources and take appropriate actions...

> *The air quality monitor will help me see what the current air quality is and if it's really bad, do not go outside. (P3)*

> *Concerning indoor in my home, that will trigger me to do the vent cleaning or identify items to particularly clean or remove if it's causing disturbance in the air quality. (P9)*

... while some voiced concerns over added mental burden, induced anxiety, and the inability to influence the air quality:

> *A person might forget it, or might forget to recharge or, it's just the hassle of carrying an extra device with you at all times. (P3)*

> *If I'm consistently seeing that the air quality is not good, it would make me feel a little bit paranoid. (P4)*

> *I think that sometimes having information when it's not actionable can be a stressor, particularly in situations that I can't necessarily control. If I went to a meeting and the air quality is bad, I'm not going to be like, "Everyone I have to leave, the air quality is no good." (P7)*

Even though these two themes carried opposite connotations, they were not mutually exclusive. Most participants expressed a combination of the two themes, hinting at both opportunities and hurdles of using such a system.

5.2 myAQM Provides Low-Effort Multimodal Entry Points to Monitor Air Quality

5.2.1 The Watch's Complication Is an Omnipresent Gateway to Using the Watch App

All participants reported looking at the air quality complications a few times a day. Their simple design facilitates quick glances through color differentiation:

> *Having the complications on the watch face screen makes it easy to tell how the air quality is because of the color [...] I didn't have to look at the numbers or anything to tell the air quality is good. (P2)*

The complications can also launch the user directly to the main application from the watch face. In fact, 86% of watchOS app launches were through the complications (225 out of 262) while the rest was through the app menu or by clicking on a notification. On average per participant, this translates to an average of 2.8 daily watchOS app launches via the complications (N = 225, SD = 2.5) out of 3.3 total launches (N = 262, SD = 2.5). While this finding cannot be generalized due to the limited number of participants ($N = 9$), it suggests that the complications potentially provide an important gateway to the main Apple Watch application during typical usage. Ultimately, the complications remind the users of air quality regardless if one intentionally thinks about this topic whenever looking at the Watch:

When I'm on my watch, since it's clearly shown here on the complications, I just tend to open it and then want to read more about stuff like that. (P5)

Typically I would be glancing at it [the air quality complications] when checking the time, weather or a notification, typically secondarily instead of primarily. I'd frequently click on them because I like seeing the expanded data (P7)

5.2.2 The Watch's Notifications Provide Nudges to Make the User Think About Important Air Quality Events

While the complications are passive, the Watch's notifications actively alert the users with its tactile and/or audio cues. In fact, the notification's vibration became so recognizable that many participants unanimously described it as "buzz on my wrist". Unequivocally, all participants recalled moments where the notifications helped them promptly notice air quality changes during typical daily routines, for instance:

- A marked increase in CO_2 concentration while taking a cab (P1), driving (P7), and riding the bus (P9)
- An increase in PM2.5 concentration while dining out in a restaurant where smoking was allowed (P4) and cooking at home (P1, P4, and P6)
- Changes in air quality (either PM2.5 and CO_2) while going from indoor to outdoor spaces and vice versa (all participants)

As the air quality change notifications are near instant (within 10 min of an event, as explained in Sect. 3.3), the participants were quickly able to reconcile the cause with changes in the surroundings:

[My roommate] He was making pasta and frying the garlic. I can smell that and I received a notification telling me that the PM2.5 is high, it's in the red region. It's actually working because like I've never seen the bar in red before. (P1)

I think it was my econometrics classroom, like a smallish classroom, enough space for 15 or 20 students. So when I entered it, I immediately received a notification on my watch within a couple of minutes, saying that the carbon dioxide level in this classroom is high. (P3)

These realizations were often preceded by perceived changes in the surroundings. However, it is difficult to associate these cues with changes in air quality because it requires active environmental awareness and analysis that people do not often engage during daily routines. myAQM's notifications lower this barrier, allowing users to inspect air quality events without constantly thinking about the surroundings. In fact, some participants admitted they would not have checked air quality by opening the application at all, had it not been for the notifications during these activities.

5.2.3   The Watch's Wrist-Worn Form Factor Facilitates These Micro-interactions (Complications and Notifications)

Ultimately, the Watch's wrist-worn form factor is what enables the complications and the notifications to be omnipresent and attention-grabbing entry points. *Quick, simple, convenient, provides essential info, no need to open the phone...* were how participants described the Watch application over its phone companion. Its proximity to the wearers allows for accessible data dissemination through micro-interactions, especially when smartphone use is cumbersome or unsafe:

> *I got an alert that the CO_2 was high in the car. I turned off the recirculating to pull in fresh air. I was able to see it changed from red, down to yellow, and eventually green. [...] If I was using my phone, that would have been much more dangerous. But with the watch app open, even just keeping my hands on the steering wheel, I'm able to glance at it. (P7)*

However, one drawback of the Watch's form factor is its screen size: it was awkward for P6 to hold the Watch for a long time, while P1, P7, P9 complained that the historical data was too small. With the participants' Apple Watch screen sizes ranging from 1.57 to 1.9 in. diagonally, small visual elements such as bars for historical bar chart and chart axis labels are reduced to a few millimeters.

5.3   Multimodal Entry Points Resulting in Multimodal User Experience

When designing myAQM, we were aware that watchOS apps do not exist in a vacuum: they customarily accompany and extend iOS apps [25]. Thus, we only explained to users how the pair of apps works without prescribing to them to use the apps in any certain way to avoid unrealistic use-case scenarios. This, coupled with the various low-effort multimodal entry points on the Watch, gave rise to multimodal user experiences with varying levels of synergy between the watch and the phone among participants.

On one end, P6 and P8 primarily used their watches and put their phones aside for better focus. The Watch's notifications kept P6 engaged, in his own words, *"drew me back in"*. Prior to myAQM, P6 was the only one having portable air quality monitor that sent data to his iPhone (not his watch). When being asked what he would have done if the watch had been taken away, he said:

> *I would be less likely to see the changes when active like being outside or cooking, since my phone is not in my hands then. (P6)*

In the middle, P2, P4, P5, and P7 recalled that while they heavily relied on the Watch for at-a-glance data and notifications, they would use the phone for historical data thanks to its bigger screen. The Watch was a persistent reminder nudging them to deeper examine past air quality events on the phone.

On the other end, P1, P3, and P9 preferred the iPhone application because of the bigger screen. That said, they acknowledged the minimal amount of effort when using the Watch interfaces, which complemented their primary phone use.

These findings indicate that the Watch is better suited for quick micro-interactions rather than replacing the phone application. The phone supports longer sessions than the Watch and it is the medium of choice when the user is already using the phone in that moment:

> *Strangely enough I use the iPhone app more but that's probably because I am often on my phone for checking work emails, socializing, scrolling through other apps, so my mind sometimes wanders over to check the iPhone app. (P4)*

The user statistics support this observation. *Table* 3 shows that on average, participants opened the iOS app 3 times more frequently than the watchOS app (9.5 daily launches vs 3.2 daily launches), with each session lasting almost 4 times longer (40.1 s vs. 12.4 s). Due to Apple Watch limitation, it is impossible to measure the number of glances at the complications or the notifications on the Apple Watch. Thus, this is not an absolute comparison of engagement levels between the two platforms but a relative proxy. From Fig. 4, it is worth noting that participants who spent more time on the Watch app were more likely to spend less time on the iPhone app, and vice versa. Ultimately, all participants exhibited varying degrees of mix usage across the two platforms and nobody exclusively used one or the other.

Table 3. Mean, standard deviation, and range of the number of daily app launches and the duration per foreground session across participants (N=9) between the watchOS and the iOS application.

	Number of Daily App Launches			Mean Duration per Foreground Session (s)		
	Mean	SD	Range	Mean	SD	Range
watchOS	3.2	2.3	(1.1, 8.4)	12.4	6.7	(5.7, 26.4)
iOS	9.5	4.5	(4, 14.4)	40.1	38.2	(13.1, 120.9)

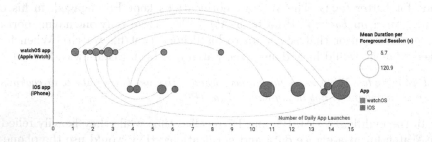

Fig. 4. Number of daily app launches of each participant (horizontal axis), grouped by either watchOS app (orange) or iOS app (blue). The size of each data point corresponds to the mean duration per foreground session in seconds. Data points of the same participant are connected by a curved line. (Color figure online)

5.4   Awareness and Behavior Impact of MyAQM

5.4.1   Positive Awareness Imparted by Constant Engagement with MyAQM

Similar to the participants' expectations outlined in Sect. 5.1.2, our finding suggests that the participants exhibited an acute increase in air quality awareness. Recurring elevated PM2.5 outdoors and elevated CO_2 in enclosed space were what prompted increased understandings of air quality among most participants. 5 out of nine participants attributed this newfound knowledge to the constant Watch notifications nudging them to be cognizant of the environment throughout the day.

Another way where myAQM helped people better understand air quality was by confirming their subjective suspicions with objective measurements:

It definitely smelled like smoke and you could tell that it wasn't well ventilated [...] In a way, the notification confirmed my suspicion, knowing that it was a smoky restaurant. I didn't realize how bad it could actually be, even if like someone was not actively smoking right next to you. (P2)

Sometimes, based on the subjective judgement of the air quality, even the act of expecting the notification to arrive was enough to prompt the users to check the air quality manually:

It was hard to breathe outside, there was a sudden [sand]storm. I was wondering if the notification will come right then or a bit later. I opened the phone up and checked: it was hazardous. I had to go back. (P8)

As the usage period progressed, feelings of curiosity was gradually replaced by feelings of anticipation and familiarity when the users receive notifications during routine activities. In some cases, reading notifications gradually became glancing at notifications as the users grew accustomed to associating certain habits and environmental settings with being alerted of air quality changes. In these cases, afforded by the Watch's wrist-worn form factor [19], its notifications habituates glancability, similar to its complications.

Especially when we were cooking, or when I'd go outside or when we were in a car, it would usually go off to tell me that the air quality was decreasing. I kind of understood what the buzzing was. And so I didn't really check it. (P2)

There's a kind of a training process that takes place with the app where you understand what a particular notification means, and you don't necessarily want to go peering down inside of it. (P6)

5.4.2   Participants Took Situational Responses to Bad Air Quality

The recurring theme across all participants in response to bad air quality events is that they would evaluate the circumstances and take actions if it was possible and/or favorable to do so.

As discussed in Sect. 5.2.2, the timely nature of the Watch's notifications empowered the participants to discover the cause of a major air quality change event. However, we also found that the lack of options to influence air quality in *certain* real-life scenarios impeded the participants from fully transforming their awareness increase to effective measures. This is in line with previous studies of personal air quality devices [9,27,47,52], implying that this remains a major issue with using portable air quality monitors regardless of the medium of the interface. From our qualitative analysis, prominent factors that influenced the participants' decision to take actions against bad air quality are: *convenience, social conformity, financial reasons, and weather/external elements*. We briefly summarize some examples pertaining to these factors below.

One of the most common actions taken among participants was wearing masks outdoors when the air quality was worse than indoor spaces. This action was made *convenient* by the mask wearing habit during the COVID-19 pandemic, as well as the low cost of masks nowadays *(financial reasons)*. Similarly, a PM2.5 spike when burning scented candles convinced P9 to opt out thanks to the ease of obtaining other inexpensive, non-polluting aroma-therapeutic treatment.

In contrast, *social conformity* contributed to P3's inaction when entering a poor-ventilated classroom:

> I don't want to get up from my seat and open all the windows, it will look super weird. If I were in a private place, then I would. (P3)

Similarly, P1's inaction against PM2.5 spikes caused by his roommate's cooking was also an example of conforming to the norm. Wearing a mask, as suggested by the Watch's notification, was perceived as *super weird*, implying that it was not socially acceptable in his situation:

> I wouldn't wear masks because people are cooking. That's just super weird. [...] But I wouldn't like stay in the kitchen for a long time. (P1)

That said, for those who could take appropriate actions when cooking, the notifications successfully prompted them to switch on the range hood (P4 and P7), replace the range hood's filter (P4), and open the door to the hallway (P7). Opening the window was also experimented by P7, however, hot and dusty weather discouraged him to rely on this method as a practical solution. The role where the *weather or other external factors* affected one's ability to act was also reflected in P1's response during a taxi ride where he could not open the window on the highway.

Overall, we found small-scale and easily-controllable changes were favored over changes that involved other people or compromises too big, similar to Bales et al.'s findings [9]. P9's response perfectly captures his sentiments of making compromises while not making air quality become the *only* wellness objective:

> It could be negative that you're limiting yourself to do more activities because you're thinking about the air quality too much. I always like to find the balance. If there's this urge for your mental health to go outside, go outside, even though the particle count is a little bit moderate. At least you're aware, compared to just making that choice and weren't aware that you're exposing yourself to certain risks [...] You can also wear proper protection. (P9)

5.4.3   Impacts of the Watch's Air Quality Notifications on Emotions

As Gilmore argued [19], smartwatches provide values in easy-to-digest modalities at the demand of the wearer's attention and labor. Given the instantaneous nature of its notifications, there were reports of anxiety and resignation among myAQM's users when they could not take an action after receiving notifications. This echoes some of their concerns before using the system. Nevertheless, this drawback was not a make-or-break factor that outright discouraged the users from further engagement with myAQM. In fact, we found evidence that suggests some participants' would rather know the bad air quality than not knowing at all:

> I think it's not so much the notifications but the fact of being in a smoky restaurant that is disturbing. The watch just confirms that it's not good. It's not the watch's fault. [...] I don't know if there's a way to like spin it positively. But I do think that when it's about your health, it should tell you bad things. (P4)

> The thing is that it has nothing to do with the app. I'm nervous for very, sometimes even small reasons. [...] But I think it's good thing, you have to know. I believe knowledge is power. I will figure out what to do with it. (P8)

Even during circumstances where immediate actions were not feasible, we found somewhat optimistic languages that implied possible future interventions should the bad air quality persist:

> I feel like it could be anxiety inducing if it's monitoring my space at work and realizing you're in a space where I don't have sort of that direct control over. Would you quit? Probably not, but maybe, reaching out to facilities and saying are there things that can be changed. (P7)

6   Discussion

6.1   Smartwatch Complication Is a Suitable Medium for Real-Time Hyperlocal Air Quality Data

Most complications on commercial smartwatches fall into either the *Health & Fitness* category or the *Weather & Planetary* category [24]. As the air quality complications belong to both categories, it will likely be increasingly used despite the limited literature focusing on understanding the user experience. By virtue of being the first study to examine the glanceable Apple Watch complications for real-time air quality data throughout real-life scenarios, our study presents insights for designing future pervasive wearable air quality interfaces.

First, our usability study supports that the complications provide a quick, easy, and omnipresent access to current air quality measurements and a direct gateway to the main smartwatch application. The complications' glanceability is specifically afforded by the wrist-worn form factor of the smartwatch, as seen in situations when the smartphone is out of reach, such as driving or working, further cementing the smartwatch as a method of getting environmental information on the go [11]. myAQM's complications were so well accepted that some users wished for more varieties that display historical measurements or combine PM2.5 and CO_2 measurements into one single complication - similar to the Apple Watch's fitness ring. This implies that smartwatch complications might be able to support more complex visualizations for more granular air quality data, something we avoided in our design. Therefore, future studies can explore a more diverse design space for glanceable air quality complications to deliver richer user experience, similar to other studies focusing on step counts [15,20] and heart rate [43].

We also found that by occupying a prominent position on the smartwatch at all times, myAQM's complications nudged the users to be aware of the surrounding air regardless of their initial intention when looking at the watch face. This is somewhat similar to *inAir*'s finding where the researchers reported that users often unintentionally glanced at the home dashboard whenever they walked by it [27]. While *inAir*'s participants could only look at the stationary indoor dashboard at home, myAQM's complications extend such glances to outdoor environments, as long as the Watch is worn, allowing the system to be truly pervasive. During the nine-day usage period, no participant recalled any decrease in engagement with the myAQM complications. This persistent engagement might be explained by the convenient position of the complications that requires little to no effort during typical usage. If anything, we hypothesize that the omnipresence of the complications will sustain user interaction with the application and portable device even after the novelty effect wears off and that commercial smartwatches' complications are the current state-of-the-art glanceable interface for real-time air quality monitoring. That said, our nine-day usability study did not allow us to gather any long-term using habit, a limitation we discuss in Sect. 6.4.

At the time of this study (May 2022), the complication is exclusive to the Apple Watch. In September 2022, Apple brought widgets to the lock screen of the iPhone [6]. This is interesting as P5 said, *"If iPhone had a complication as well, then maybe it would have been better."* We can speculate that this feature can provide at-a-glance data like the Watch's complications. That said, the Watch complications' glanceability is enabled by its proximity to the user and frequent short-bust usage [25,53]. A phone's typical placement on a desk, or inside a pocket or a bag might hinder its glanceability due to the additional steps required to look at the screen. This speculation can ascertained with a future comparative study between widgets on the iPhone and complications on the Watch.

6.2   Empowerment and Burdens of Air Quality Notifications

To summarize, we found that the Apple Watch is suitable for notifications of changes in air pollution, through which the wearers could associate activities or environmental changes that triggered the deterioration of air quality. Users gained deeper knowledge of potential pollution sources, differences in indoor and outdoor air, and the importance of indoor ventilation.

Our finding confirms and extends previous studies' findings of empowerment from air quality notifications on smartphones [16,41]. For instance, Moore et al. discovered that their text-based notifications on smartphones provided users with allow users to examine air quality spikes and subsequently enhance user engagement with their system - MAAV [41]. However, the author acknowledged people might not have their phones on hand while at home. The Apple Watch overcomes this challenge by almost always be in close proximity to the users, facilitating continuous and timely deliveries of such notifications.

Unfortunately, our study revealed that users experienced mental burden when they couldn't act on notifications, with desires ranging from adjusting notification frequency (P4) to needing a break (P2). Similarly, Moore et al. reported accounts of notification fatigue with MAAV [41]. Compared to *MAAV*'s phone text message notifications, one might reason that myAQM's Apple Watch notifications can potentially induce more fatigue because of its attention-grabbing "buzz". That said, no one reported muting or turning off myAQM's notifications. This suggests that the notifications' benefits may have outweighed their burdens in the short-term setting of our study, potentially influenced by participant compensation. The long-term effects, including the possibility of users discontinuing the use of the Apple Watch to avoid notification overload, remain uncertain. More optimized notifications to sustain long-term smartwatch user experience should be investigated in subsequent studies.

Perhaps, the users can set personal thresholds: for example, they only get urgent notifications when the air quality exceeds the "Unhealthy" category. Additionally, methods such as rate-limiting and bundling could help to lower the number of notifications [41]. Apart from addressing the quantity of notifications, we speculate that context-aware notifications [53] can minimize repetitiveness to sustain engagement for long-term usage. For instance, incorporating the type of pollution event [16] and providing less repetitive, more actionable suggestions can provide a more personal user experience, habituating users to take action in the long run even when they cannot act momentarily, as pointed out by P3:

> The notification can come with a disclaimer: It's OK if you can't do anything now. For future reference, it will be better if you avoid these environments (P3)

6.3   A Well-Designed Portable Air Quality Device is Required for a Good User Experience

While our objective was to examine the Watch interfaces, we found that the portable monitor also played a crucial role in the user experience. On the one hand, participants developed trust in its accuracy and usefulness, quoting they could often associate numerical changes in air quality measurements with changes in environmental factors and activities. On the other hand, some participants preferred the device to be half or a quarter its current size. As electronic devices are increasingly miniaturized, such as the Apple's AirTag, it is not a surprise that people have high expectations for portability. They also expressed the desire for longer battery life. To address these, future studies can re-purpose polished commercial personal monitoring devices for research. Notably, the Atmotube has been featured in previous research [21, 38] as it provides an Application Programming Interface (API) for custom-built UIs [8].

Additionally, some participants (P1, P7, P9) suggested integrating the air quality sensors physically into the Watch. In fact, there are a few studies on wrist-worn air quality sensors [18,37,52]. Even then, the authors of *MyPart* found that users preferred the sensor to be *carryable* than *wearable* because it was not small enough to be worn every day [52]. Besides, current technology does not allow air quality sensors to be integrated into existing commercial smartwatches while allowing them to be compact and offer other important functionalities such as fitness, communication, and entertainment. Thus, we believe that the most viable solution is to have a separate portable air quality monitor like our study's.

6.4   Study Limitation

6.4.1   Size and Length of the Study

Our usability study consisted of nine participants and lasted for nine days for each participant. To put our sample size in context, previous usability studies with commercial smartwatch interfaces for air quality ranged from two to twelve participants, see Table 1. As discussed in Sect. 6.3, commercial portable air quality monitoring devices could be used for future studies, which could significantly increase the number of participants. Meanwhile, to put our nine-day period in context, other studies in the fields ranged from a few hours [52], five days [22], four weeks [9,27], to a few months [28,41]. The longest study with a commercial smartwatch interface was Hosseini et al. at several weeks [22], but it was only with one child. While nine days is a moderate amount of time compared to previous literature, it does not allow us to capture long-term usage and engagement patterns compared to other longer longitudinal studies [28,41]. *Would the user find the Watch's complications useful after a year? How do they want to personalize the notifications?* These are questions to ask in a longer study that can transform our understanding of watch-based air quality interfaces from proof-of-concepts to commercialized features.

6.4.2   Lack of Comparative Study

As our study is qualitative in nature, it is not possible to isolate the influence of the Apple Watch interfaces from its iPhone counterparts'. To address this gap, we call for a future comparative study where 3 randomized groups receive either the watchOS interfaces, the iOS interfaces, or the combination of them. That said, our method allowed the participants to be more flexible and adaptive in how they used the system in their daily lives. Although our quantitative data analysis was limited, it complemented the qualitative analysis to reveal the different modalities on which the users relied, suggesting that the smartwatch complements the smartphone well in delivering air quality data and facilitating users' exploration of air quality matters with low efforts. Our work paves the way for future literature as being one of the first to test the usability of a commercial smartwatch for visualizing hyperlocal air quality data in uncontrolled settings.

7   Conclusion

We designed and user-tested myAQM which provides Apple Watch wearers with hyperlocal PM2.5 and CO_2 data from a portable monitor. Our study was the first to examine different Apple Watch interfaces (main app, notification, and complication) in realistic day-to-day scenarios. In our usability study in the wild, we discovered that the Apple Watch provided multiple entry points for receiving air quality data which generated a multimodal user experience that were quick, convenient, flexible, and in good synergy with existing smartphone interfaces.

Our findings further support the complementary role of smartwatch devices in keeping users engaged with real-time information, especially where smartphone use is restricted. The watch's value proposition is its notifications as a nudge for the users to promptly recognize sudden changes in air quality and complications as a constant reminder of the surrounding air. Together, they augment the smartphone in equipping the users with situational environmental awareness in circumstances where they might not check the measurements manually and motivating them to take actions to reduce their exposure within reason. That said, we still found instances where the watch reinforced feelings of helplessness when the users could not take actions against bad air, an observation shared by other studies with different media of visualization.

Acknowledgement. This work was supported by the NYUAD Center for Interacting Urban Networks (CITIES), funded by Tamkeen under the NYUAD Research Institute Award CG001. We sincerely thank Heather Dewey-Hagborg and Joerg Blumtritt for their kind guidance, their substantial contribution to the design iteration process, and their invaluable feedback on the design prototypes. Finally, we would like to thank Junior Garcia, Nhi Pham, Philip Rodenbough, and Yao Xu for reviewing this manuscript.

References

1. Al-Jallad, F.A., Rodrigues, C.C., Al-Thani, H.A., et al.: Ambient levels of tsp, pm10, pm2. 5 and particle number concentration in Al Samha, UAE. J. Environ. Protect. **8**(09), 1002 (2017). https://doi.org/10.4236/jep.2017.89063
2. Al-Taani, A.A., Nazzal, Y., Howari, F.M., Yousef, A.: Long-term trends in ambient fine particulate matter from 1980 to 2016 in united arab emirates. Environ. Monit. Assess. **191**, 1–19 (2019). https://doi.org/10.1007/s10661-019-7259-9
3. Alfano, B., et al.: A review of low-cost particulate matter sensors from the developers' perspectives. Sensors **20**(23), 6819 (2020). https://doi.org/10.3390/s20236819
4. Apple Developer. Beta testing made simple with testflight (2023). https://developer.apple.com/testflight/. Accessed 01 July 2023
5. Apple Developer: Complications (2023). https://developer.apple.com/design/human-interface-guidelines/components/system-experiences/complications/. Accessed 01 July 2023
6. Apple Support: How to add and edit widgets on your iphone (2022). https://support.apple.com/en-us/HT207122. Accessed 01 July 2023

7. Apple Support: Apple watch faces and their features (2023). https://support.apple.com/guide/watch/faces-and-features-apde9218b440/8.0/watchos/8.0. Accessed 01 July 2023

8. Atmotube: Bluetooth API (2023). https://atmotube.com/atmotube-support/bluetooth-api. Accessed 01 July 2023

9. Bales, E., Nikzad, N., Quick, N., Ziftci, C., Patrick, K., Griswold, W.G.: Personal pollution monitoring: mobile real-time air quality in daily life. Pers. Ubiquit. Comput. **23**(2), 309–328 (2019). https://doi.org/10.1007/s00779-019-01206-3

10. Blascheck, T., Besançon, L., Bezerianos, A., Lee, B., Isenberg, P.: Glanceable visualization: studies of data comparison performance on smartwatches. IEEE Trans. Visual Comput. Graph. **25**(1), 630–640 (2018). https://doi.org/10.1109/TVCG.2018.2865142

11. Cecchinato, M.E., Cox, A.L., Bird, J.: Always on (line)? user experience of smartwatches and their role within multi-device ecologies. In: Proceedings of the 2017 CHI Conference on Human Factors in Computing Systems, pp. 3557–3568 (2017). https://doi.org/10.1145/3025453.3025538

12. Chen, C.Y., Chen, P.H., Chen, J.K., Su, T.C.: Recommendations for ventilation of indoor spaces to reduce covid-19 transmission. J. Formos. Med. Assoc. **120**(12), 2055–2060 (2021). https://doi.org/10.1016/j.jfma.2021.08.007

13. Clements, A.L., et al.: Low-cost air quality monitoring tools: from research to practice (a workshop summary). Sensors **17**(11), 2478 (2017). https://doi.org/10.3390/s17112478

14. Du, B., Tandoc, M.C., Mack, M.L., Siegel, J.A.: Indoor co2 concentrations and cognitive function: a critical review. Indoor Air **30**(6), 1067–1082 (2020). https://doi.org/10.1111/ina.12706

15. Esakia, A., McCrickard, D.S., Harden, S., Horning, M.: Fitaware: mediating group fitness strategies with smartwatch glanceable feedback. In: Proceedings of the 12th EAI International Conference on Pervasive Computing Technologies for Healthcare, pp. 98–107 (2018). https://doi.org/10.1145/3240925.3240926

16. Fang, B., Xu, Q., Park, T., Zhang, M.: Airsense: an intelligent home-based sensing system for indoor air quality analytics. In: Proceedings of the 2016 ACM International Joint Conference on Pervasive and Ubiquitous Computing, pp. 109–119 (2016). https://doi.org/10.1145/2971648.2971720

17. Feng, S., Gao, D., Liao, F., Zhou, F., Wang, X.: The health effects of ambient pm2. 5 and potential mechanisms. Ecotoxicol. Environ. Safety **128**, 67–74 (2016). https://doi.org/10.1016/j.ecoenv.2016.01.030

18. Frampton, T.H., Tiele, A., Covington, J.A.: Development of a personalised environmental quality monitoring system (pong). IEEE Sens. J. **21**(13), 15230–15236 (2021). https://doi.org/10.1109/JSEN.2021.3073752

19. Gilmore, J.N.: From ticks and tocks to budges and nudges: the smartwatch and the haptics of informatic culture. Televis. New Media **18**(3), 189–202 (2017). https://doi.org/10.1177/1527476416658962

20. Gouveia, R., Pereira, F., Karapanos, E., Munson, S.A., Hassenzahl, M.: Exploring the design space of glanceable feedback for physical activity trackers. In: Proceedings of the 2016 ACM International Joint Conference on Pervasive and Ubiquitous Computing, pp. 144–155 (2016). https://doi.org/10.1145/2971648.2971754

21. Hart, S., Doyle, J.: Realtimeair: a real-time federated crowd sensing hyper local air quality data service. In: Proceedings of the ACM SIGCOMM Workshop on Networked Sensing Systems for a Sustainable Society, pp. 7–13 (2022). https://doi.org/10.1145/3538393.3544933

22. Hosseini, A., et al.:: Feasibility of a secure wireless sensing smartwatch application for the self-management of pediatric asthma. Sensors **17**(8), 1780 (2017). https://doi.org/10.3390/s17081780
23. Institute, H.E.: State of global air 2020 (2020). Accessed 01 July 2023
24. Islam, A., Bezerianos, A., Lee, B., Blascheck, T., Isenberg, P.: Visualizing information on watch faces: a survey with smartwatch users. In: 2020 IEEE Visualization Conference (VIS), pp. 156–160. IEEE (2020). https://doi.org/10.1109/VIS47514.2020.00038
25. Jeong, H., Kim, H., Kim, R., Lee, U., Jeong, Y.: Smartwatch wearing behavior analysis: a longitudinal study. In: Proceedings of the ACM on Interactive, Mobile, Wearable and Ubiquitous Technologies, vol. 1, no. 3, pp. 1–31 (2017). https://doi.org/10.1145/3131892
26. Kim, S., Li, M.: Awareness, understanding, and action: a conceptual framework of user experiences and expectations about indoor air quality visualizations. In: Proceedings of the 2020 CHI Conference on Human Factors in Computing Systems, pp. 1–12 (2020). https://doi.org/10.1145/3313831.3376521
27. Kim, S., Paulos, E.: Inair: sharing indoor air quality measurements and visualizations. In: Proceedings of the SIGCHI Conference on Human Factors in Computing Systems, pp. 1861–1870 (2010). https://doi.org/10.1145/1753326.1753605
28. Kim, S., Paulos, E., Mankoff, J.: inair: a longitudinal study of indoor air quality measurements and visualizations. In: Proceedings of the SIGCHI Conference on Human Factors in Computing Systems, pp. 2745–2754 (2013). https://doi.org/10.1145/2470654.2481380
29. King, C.E., Sarrafzadeh, M.: A survey of smartwatches in remote health monitoring. J. Healthc. Inform. Res. **2**, 1–24 (2018). https://doi.org/10.1007/s41666-017-0012-7
30. Kumar, P., et al.: The rise of low-cost sensing for managing air pollution in cities. Environ. Int. **75**, 199–205 (2015). https://doi.org/10.1016/j.envint.2014.11.019
31. Lan, X.T.P., Thoning, K.: Trends in globally-averaged co2 determined from NOAA global monitoring laboratory measurements, version 2023-10. NOAA Global Monitoring Laboratory (2023). https://doi.org/10.15138/9N0H-ZH07
32. Laricchia, F.: Statista - smartwatch unit shipment share worldwide 2018–2022, by vendor (2022). https://www.statista.com/statistics/910862/worldwide-smartwatch-shipment-market-share/ Accessed 01 July 2023
33. Li, D., Li, Y., Li, G., Zhang, Y., Li, J., Chen, H.: Fluorescent reconstitution on deposition of pm2. 5 in lung and extrapulmonary organs. Proc. Natl. Acad. Sci. **116**(7), 2488–2493 (2019). https://doi.org/10.1073/pnas.1818134116
34. Liu, X., et al.: Characterizing smartwatch usage in the wild. In: Proceedings of the 15th Annual International Conference on Mobile Systems, Applications, and Services, pp. 385–398 (2017). https://doi.org/10.1145/3081333.3081351
35. Lowther, S.D., et al.: Low level carbon dioxide indoors-a pollution indicator or a pollutant? a health-based perspective. Environments **8**(11), 125 (2021). https://doi.org/10.3390/environments8110125
36. Lu, X., Thomaz, E., Epstein, D.A.: Understanding people's perceptions of approaches to semi-automated dietary monitoring. In: Proceedings of the ACM on Interactive, Mobile, Wearable and Ubiquitous Technologies, vol. 6, no. 3, pp. 1–27 (2022). https://doi.org/10.1145/3550288
37. Maag, B., Zhou, Z., Thiele, L.: W-air: enabling personal air pollution monitoring on wearables. In: Proceedings of the ACM on Interactive, Mobile, Wearable and Ubiquitous Technologies, vol. 2, no. 1, pp. 1–25 (2018). https://doi.org/10.1145/3191756

362   V. Nguyen

38. Maguire, G., Chen, H., Schnall, R., Xu, W., Huang, M.C.: Smoking cessation system for preemptive smoking detection. IEEE Internet Things J. 9(5), 3204–3214 (2021). https://doi.org/10.1109/jiot.2021.3097728
39. Marques, G., Pitarma, R.: Smartwatch-based application for enhanced healthy lifestyle in indoor environments. In: Computational Intelligence in Information Systems: Proceedings of the Computational Intelligence in Information Systems Conference (CIIS 2018), LNCS, vol. 3, pp. 168–177. Springer, Cham (2019). https://doi.org/10.1007/978-3-030-03302-6_15
40. Marques, G., Pitarma, R.: Promoting health and well-being using wearable and smartphone technologies for ambient assisted living through internet of things. In: Big Data and Networks Technologies. LNCS, vol. 3, pp. 12–22. Springer, Cham (2020). https://doi.org/10.1007/978-3-030-23672-4_2
41. Moore, J., et al.: Managing in-home environments through sensing, annotating, and visualizing air quality data. In: Proceedings of the ACM on Interactive, Mobile, Wearable and Ubiquitous Technologies 2(3), 1–28 (2018). https://doi.org/10.1145/3264938
42. Morawska, L., et al.: Applications of low-cost sensing technologies for air quality monitoring and exposure assessment: how far have they gone? Environ. Int. 116, 286–299 (2018). https://doi.org/10.1016/j.envint.2018.04.018
43. Neshati, A., Leboe-Mcgowan, L., Leboe-Mcgowan, J., Serrano, M., Irani, P., et al.: G-sparks: glanceable sparklines on smartwatches. In: 45th Conference on Graphics Interface (GI 2019), pp. 1–9 (2019). https://doi.org/10.20380/GI2019.23
44. World Health Organization. WHO Global Air Quality Guidelines: Particulate Matter (PM2. 5 and PM10), Ozone, Nitrogen Dioxide, Sulfur Dioxide and Carbon Monoxide. World Health Organization (2021)
45. Peng, Z., Jimenez, J.L.: Exhaled co2 as a covid-19 infection risk proxy for different indoor environments and activities. Environ. Sci. Technol. Lett. 8(5), 392–397 (2021). https://doi.org/10.1021/acs.estlett.1c00183
46. Plaia, A., Ruggieri, M.: Air quality indices: a review. Rev. Environ. Sci. Bio/Technol. 10, 165–179 (2011). https://doi.org/10.1007/s11157-010-9227-2
47. Sakhnini, N., Yu, J.E., Jones, R.M., Chattopadhyay, D.: Personal air pollution monitoring technologies: user practices and preferences. In: Stephanidis, C., Marcus, A., Rosenzweig, E., Rau, P.L.P., Moallem, A., Rauterberg, M. (eds.) HCI International 2020 - Late Breaking Papers: User Experience Design and Case Studies, pp. 481–498. Springer, Cham (2020). https://doi.org/10.1007/978-3-030-60114-0_33
48. Saldaña, J.: The Coding Manual for Qualitative Researchers. Sage (2021)
49. Shiffman, S., Stone, A.A., Hufford, M.R.: Ecological momentary assessment. Annu. Rev. Clin. Psychol. 4, 1–32 (2008). https://doi.org/10.1146/annurev.clinpsy.3.022806.091415
50. Spinelle, L., Gerboles, M., Villani, M.G., Aleixandre, M., Bonavitacola, F.: Field calibration of a cluster of low-cost commercially available sensors for air quality monitoring. Part b: No, co and co2. Sens. Actuat. B: Chem. 238, 706–715 (2017). https://doi.org/10.1016/j.snb.2016.07.036
51. Tan, S.H., Smith, T.E.: An optimal environment for our optimal selves? an autoethnographic account of self-tracking personal exposure to air pollution. Area 53(2), 353–361 (2021). https://doi.org/10.1111/area.12671
52. Tian, R., Dierk, C., Myers, C., Paulos, E.: Mypart: personal, portable, accurate, airborne particle counting. In: Proceedings of the 2016 CHI Conference on Human Factors in Computing Systems, pp. 1338–1348 (2016). https://doi.org/10.1145/2858036.2858571

53. Visuri, A., et al.: Quantifying sources and types of smartwatch usage sessions. In: Proceedings of the 2017 CHI Conference on Human Factors in Computing Systems (CHI 2017), pp. 3569–3581. Association for Computing Machinery, New York (2017). https://doi.org/10.1145/3025453.3025817
54. Xing, Y.F., Xu, Y.H., Shi, M.H., Lian, Y.X.: The impact of pm2. 5 on the human respiratory system. J. Thoracic Dis. **8**(1), E69 (2016). https://doi.org/10.3978/j.issn.2072-1439.2016.01.19
55. Zhang, X., Wargocki, P., Lian, Z.: Physiological responses during exposure to carbon dioxide and bioeffluents at levels typically occurring indoors. Indoor Air **27**(1), 65–77 (2017). https://doi.org/10.1111/ina.12286
56. Zhong, S., Alavi, H.S., Lalanne, D.: Hilo-wear: exploring wearable interaction with indoor air quality forecast. In: Extended Abstracts of the 2020 CHI Conference on Human Factors in Computing Systems (CHI EA 2020), pp. 1–8. Association for Computing Machinery, New York (2020). https://doi.org/10.1145/3334480.3382813

Patient and User Aspects

Usability of Natural User Interfaces for People with Intellectual Disabilities

Melinda C. Braun[1,2]([✉]) and Matthias Wölfel[1,2]

[1] Institute for Intelligent Interaction and Immersive Experience, Karlsruhe
University of Applied Sciences, 76133 Karlsruhe, Germany
{melinda.braun,matthias.woelfel}@h-ka.de
[2] University of Hohenheim, 70599 Stuttgart, Germany

Abstract. In today's society, information and communication technologies are ubiquitous. They have become an essential part of people's daily lives and have the potential to improve various areas of life and daily tasks of their users. However, these technologies are usually developed for the masses rather than for specific user groups, which makes their use difficult for a large part of the population, especially for people with intellectual disabilities. A possible improvement can be achieved by adapting the user interface to the abilities of the users. This work follows up on a previous study that evaluated current interface types and their adaptability. In this study, we evaluate the usability in the daily use of different technical solutions with a questionnaire using the System Usability Scale. Our questionnaire was completed by 31 participants with varying degrees of disability for 44 solutions. The results suggest that the usability of natural user interfaces is highly dependent on factors such as age, level of customization, or the type of solution used. We found that pointing gesture interfaces are currently the most commonly used type of interfaces. These were mainly used as a standalone input modality, but usability was perceived to be higher with additional system accessibility features. Interfaces with buttons or switches required more adaptation, and interfaces with voice interaction may have potential, but currently there are too many barriers to be usable for this target group.

Keywords: usability · natural user interfaces · accessibility ·
intellectual disabilities · assistive technology · consumer technology ·
interface adaptation

1 Introduction

In today's society, information and communication technologies (ICT) are ubiquitous. They have become an important and essential part of people's daily lives [11] and have the potential to improve different areas of life and daily tasks of their users, especially those with intellectual disabilities (ID) [21]. However, these technologies tend to be developed for mainstream users and are not adapted to the needs of each user group, which makes them difficult to use for a large part of

D. Salvi et al. (Eds.): PH 2023, LNICST 572, pp. 367–385, 2024.
https://doi.org/10.1007/978-3-031-59717-6_24

the population, especially people with ID. This user group often has very individual limitations and abilities, and although design guidelines (e.g. universal design or the EU Directive 2019/882 (on accessibility requirements for products and services) [12]) exist, this range of individual characteristics and abilities can make it difficult to include everyone in the development of digital technologies and interfaces [6]. In a previous study, the current accessibility status of several natural user interfaces ("touch", "voice" and "touchless") was analyzed. This showed that there are problems when these interfaces are used by people with ID, especially in "accessing, selecting or using different types of interfaces" [7], but also a huge potential for improvement. To reduce the so-called "digital divide", which describes a gap between people with ID and mainstream users [21], and to increase the participation of those affected by this gap, different user interfaces need to be customized to the specific abilities and skills of the respective user(s) [6]. This work is an extension of a previous study that evaluated currently available interface types and their adaptability for people with ID [6]. Here we will analyze and evaluate the usability of these interface types and their adaptations when used in the daily lives of people with ID.

1.1   Continuum of Consumer and Assistive Technologies

The boundary between consumer and assistive technologies is not binary. Therefore, in [6], we introduced the *continuum of consumer and assistive technologies* (see Fig. 1). For better understanding and simplicity, it will be described again. Here, these two types of technologies represent the two extremes of the spectrum on the left and right side, respectively. In between there are hybrids with different degrees of adaptation. The categories were designated as follows [6]:

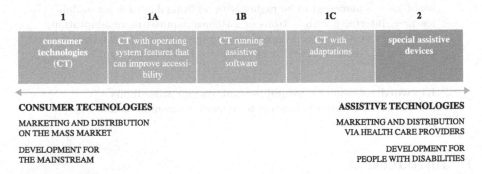

Fig. 1. Continuum of consumer and assistive technologies [6].

- **1. Consumer Technologies:** conventional consumer hardware, without specialized assistive software or hardware adaptations, e.g., an online banking-app used on a tablet or smartphone.

- **1A. Consumer Technologies with Operating System Features that can improve Accessibility:** consumer hardware with accessibility settings, e.g., usability aids, larger fonts used on a tablet or smartphone.
- **1B. Consumer Technologies running Assistive Software:** consumer hardware combined with assistive software, e.g., an app, specifically developed for people with disabilities used on a tablet or smartphone.
- **1C. Consumer Technologies with Adaptations:** adapted or customized consumer hardware, e.g., adding different sensors or buttons on a smartphone or tablet interface.
- **2. Special Assistive Devices:** assistive hardware that was specifically developed for people with disabilities e.g., speech generating devices, special interfaces.

1.2 Natural User Interfaces

The way people interact with ICT and the types of interfaces available have evolved over time and gone through different phases. Starting with the typical command line interfaces, through graphical user interfaces (GUI) to natural user interfaces (NUI). These developments allow users to interact with digital technologies in more and more diverse ways. NUIs have been developed to facilitate a more natural interaction, for example through touch interfaces, gestural interaction or voice interaction. A distinction is made between the input and output modality of an interface [35]. Since a suitable classification of the input and output modalities of current interface types did not yet exist, we introduced one that better reflects the capabilities of a given interface [6]. In this study, we focus on the input modality of each interface.

Interfaces with Buttons or Switch Elements: This describes input modalities with two states, e.g. keyboards, joysticks or buttons [6], which are not classified as NUIs. Since these input modalities are widely used in ICT today, they are also included in this study.

Interfaces with Pointing Gestures: This interface input type is controlled via a two-dimensional pointing device, such as a touchscreen, computer mouse, or pen input [6].

Interfaces with Voice Interaction: These are activated by voice or sound and are most commonly used on devices such as Amazon Echo (Alexa) or Google Home (Google Assistant), but also run on smartphones, tablets, or desktop PCs [6,7].

Interfaces with Object Interaction: Object interaction interfaces (e.g., tangible user interfaces) are operated by using real-world objects to initiate actions [29].

Interfaces with Touchless Interaction: Touchless input is controlled by 3D body or hand gestures, that allow the user to initiate actions without physically touching a device [6].

Interfaces with Multimodal Input: Interfaces with multimodal input are interfaces with more than one input modality. They can consist of two or more of the previously described input types [6]. Multimodal input types can be categorized into competing and combined input. In competing multimodal input, the user chooses one modality or the other, e.g., the user says "turn on the light by the window" or points to the light to turn it on. Here, both can be used separately. In combined multimodal input, different modalities are used together, e.g. the user points to a light by the window and says "turn on the light". In this case, both modalities must be used together.

2   Related Work

This section discusses related work in the field of people with ID and interface use. Currently, there is little research that specifically addresses people with ID and the use of NUIs or possible adaptations. It is suggested that in order to limit the digital divide and realize the full potential of a device, current digital technologies need to be made usable for people with ID through adaptation of their user interfaces or guidance from non-disabled people [4–7,20]. While simple or analogue interfaces can be easily adapted, for example by adjusting a doorknob with plasticine or replacing a button with a larger one, most NUIs rely on pattern recognition and are not easily adapted [6,7].

2.1   Interfaces with Pointing Gestures

This type of input, especially touch input, is widely used and applied in most technologies today (e.g., smartphones, tablets, desktop PCs, laptops) [18,30] and it has great potential for people with ID, e.g. for "communication, access, navigation and independence" [30]. However, there may still be usability and accessibility issues when used by people with ID. This can be caused by the often small screen or pointing area, text or button sizes, difficulties in error handling, inadequate feedback (e.g. the lack of haptic feedback) or the large number of interaction methods [32,36]. Braun et al. analyzed the accessibility of different NUIs for people with ID and found that the majority of participants faced major (29.5%) and minor (51.0%) problems when using touch interfaces, e.g., "small play button size, letting go of the button (pressing too long and using it as a physical button), keeping their whole hand on the screen and not being able to use only one finger of their hand to touch" [7]. Certain system accessibility features (category 1A, see Fig. 1), [2,17,24], applications (category 1B) [1,25], or customizations (category 1C) [27] and more intensive training can help to make this type of input more accessible to people with ID [6,30].

2.2   Interfaces with Voice Interaction

According to research, this type of input has the potential to be both accessible and inclusive for people with ID [23, 26], contributing to greater independence in everyday tasks, such as operating a smart home [10, 26] or using commands on mobile devices [4]. But especially users with speech disabilities or non-standard speech have difficulty using it. In most cases, speech recognition requires clear pronunciation [4, 26]. Differences in pronunciation, dialects, or vernaculars can have a big impact: Wenzel and Kaufman state that speech interfaces that do not take this into account can lead to not only usability problems, but also psychological problems for minorities [34]. Another difficulty for people with ID in using speech interfaces is the complexity of the commands, which require a certain level of cognitive ability. In order to use a speech interface effectively, users need to remember certain keywords or sequences of words, or to follow a particular sequence of commands [23]. Assistive applications (category 1B), such as [33], can help users with ID interact with voice interfaces [6], but customization options are still scarce. More adjustable input settings (category 1A) [4] or specific adaptation options, such as more prominent feedback, adjustable timing, or commands that include familiar words [23] are needed to make commercial voice interfaces more accessible tools for people with ID. Also, more speech data needs to be collected ethically from underrepresented groups to minimize the high error rate of speech technology [34].

2.3   Interfaces with Object Interaction

By supplementing the digital world with physical objects and materials, this type of input is intended to provide a richer sensory experience and enhance various skills, such as object manipulation or multi-sensory exploration [13, 16]. This type of interaction is meant to be natural and intuitive and can be beneficial for people with ID [22]. Gelsomini et al. highlight the potential of this type of interface for interventions with people with ID to improve performance [16]. Although this type of input is rarely used in mainstream technologies, object interaction is often used in semi-public spaces [37]. Popular examples such as [15, 31] (category 1C) demonstrate the potential for people with ID by selecting appropriate objects for the individual person. For [15], the interface and physical objects are fully customizable, but certain skills (e.g., programming, woodworking, soldering) are required, which can be a barrier for people with ID and their caregivers or families [6].

2.4   Interfaces with Touchless Interaction

Touchless input is currently mostly used in games, virtual reality, or semi-public spaces such as exhibitions or museums, and therefore few applications exist for users with ID [3, 6, 7]. This method of interaction could potentially be relevant for people with ID [6], but adaptations need to be developed as the input may be too difficult or complicated for this group of users, especially those with additional motor impairments or problems with fine motor skills [3,7]. Braun et al. tested a touchless interface using a *Leap Motion Controller* with people with ID and found that the interface and its method of interaction (touchless gestures) was often too complex for the participants with ID to understand [7]. Because this type of interface is not yet mainstream, there aren't many options for adaptation. On some devices, such as the *Leap Motion Controller*, it is already possible to train custom gestures [19].

3   Methodology

For a better understanding, this section describes the methodology of past studies, as the current study is part of a larger research project.

3.1   Target Group

People with various degrees of intellectual disabilities (ID) are included to investigate a broad audience, some with additional motor impairments. In [6] we describe three target groups:

1. *Individuals with mild ID*, who can speak and, if applicable, read and write (with motor limitations, if applicable).
2. *Persons with moderate ID*, who can understand plain language and can express themselves with limited speech (if applicable, with motor limitations).
3. *Persons with multiple disabilities* in the sense of ID with severely impaired intentionality and understanding of symbols combined with significant motor impairments.

Access to the field was gained through three institutions in the disability sector in southern Germany, where people with ID live in inpatient or outpatient facilities. Recruitment of this target group can be a time-consuming and difficult process, as some people with disabilities are not able to give consent to participate in studies themselves, and instead parents or legal representatives must give consent. In order to best represent the interests of all participants, an ethical application was approved by the German Society for Educational Science (DGfE) and the data were anonymized.

3.2   Identification of Participation Wishes and Case Selection

In an earlier study, participants with ID were asked about their most important wishes for improving their daily lives through technology. All of the following studies are based on the 150 participant wishes that were identified. The topics were mostly "independence in everyday life in various areas such as entertainment, mobility/navigation, household tasks (e.g. shopping), learning, or (digital) communication" [6]. These wishes were analyzed by the researchers according to the expected improvement of participation and technical feasibility in order to find suitable solutions for the users. In this process, inappropriate wishes were excluded.

3.3 Technology Testing and Selection

In our previous study [6], possible solutions for the previously evaluated participation wishes were tested with the participants. The goal was to find the most
suitable interface and technology, so between one and three possible solutions
were tested with each participant. This study was based on the user-centered
approach of *Scenario-Based Design* [9] and varied in execution depending on the
type of solution and the individual skills of the participants, e.g. with multiple or
written solution scenarios, testing of prototypes, wizard-of-oz testing or testing
of currently existing solutions. This process resulted in 116 possible solutions for
41 participants with varying degrees of adaptation [6].

3.4 Integration of the Solutions into Everyday Life

Once the technology was selected, each participant received a proposal with
the necessary hardware and software to purchase. A questionnaire was then
sent to each participant asking whether the proposed technology was purchased
and used, how the solutions were integrated into everyday life, and how the
participants rated the solutions. At this point, the researchers had no control
over how often or when each solution was used. Participants were not assigned
specific tasks during use. The use of the solutions was left to the participants and
their caregivers to ensure a natural interaction. Information about the frequency
and context of use, as well as the situations in which the solutions were used in
daily life, was collected later through the questionnaire.

Type and Cost of Solutions: Solutions were limited to low-cost consumer
technologies and it was always considered whether the solution could be implemented using hardware already available to the participants. Suggested hardware for the solutions included Android or iOS smartphones and tablets, PCs,
laptops, single board computers such as Raspberry Pis, smartwatches, smart
speakers such as Amazon Echo, joysticks, controllers, keyboards, or smart pens.
The software used depended on the type of solution and the level of adaptation
required (see Sect. 1.1), e.g. regular applications or software (1), system accessibility features (1A), assistive software (1B) or adapted software (1C). Special
attention was given to minimizing the cost to participants; in each case, the most
affordable options were proposed. In some cases, certain hardware was already
available, eliminating the need for new purchases. The study staff also offered
to cover the cost of some solutions with project funds and to provide them to
the individuals concerned if no other funding option was available. Ultimately,
the decision to purchase and use a solution was made by caregivers or family
members and the participants themselves.

System Usability Scale (SUS): In addition to general questions and questions about the solution, as well as duration and frequency of use, the *System
Usability Scale* (SUS) [8] with a 5-point Likert scale (strongly agree to strongly

disagree) was used to inquire about the usability of each solution. There is currently no usability evaluation questionnaire for people with intellectual disabilities, so the SUS was chosen in a slightly adapted form. It can distinguish between unusable and usable systems, and asks about issues such as complexity, need for support, training, effectiveness, and satisfaction while using a technology [8]. The 10 individual items of the SUS and the rest of the questionnaire have been translated into plain language to make it accessible to participants with ID. For scoring, the items were coded in a specific way, summed, and multiplied by 2.5. The *SUS score* goes from 0 to 100, where 100 is the best possible score, but should not be interpreted as a percentile ranking [8]. The items translated into the plain language of the SUS are as follows:

1. *Q1: I think I will continue to use the technology.*
2. *Q2: I find the technology complicated to use.*
3. *Q3: I find the technology easy to use.*
4. *Q4: I need help from another person to use the technology.*
5. *Q5: I think the functions of the technology are good.*
6. *Q6: I find the technology difficult to understand.*
7. *Q7: I think most people learn to use technology very quickly.*
8. *Q8: I find the technology very cumbersome to use.*
9. *Q9: I feel very confident using the technology.*
10. *Q10: I had to learn a lot before I could use the technology.*

Questionnaire for Observing Communicative Skills - Revision (OCS-R): In a previous study [7], we assessed certain skills that participants needed to use different types of interfaces (touch, voice, and touchless interfaces). Data on the cognitive and motor skills of participants with ID were collected using parts of the *Questionnaire for Observing Communicative Skills-Revision (OCS-R)* [28]. Then, an expert interview was conducted to analyze which important and unimportant skills are required to use each type of interface. These results should show how usable and accessible the different types of natural user interfaces are for this target group [7]. In the current study, we want to find out if there are associations between the scores on the OCS-R and the scores that participants achieve on the SUS.

4   Study

The current phase of our research began in the summer of 2022 and is still ongoing. Initially, 41 people participated in our previous study [6], where 116 solutions were proposed to them. At the moment, 40 solutions have been implemented as we proposed, 6 differ from our proposal, possibly changing the type of input. One person chose a new solution that we did not propose, which will also be evaluated. These now 47 solutions are currently in use by the participants[1]. The remaining 70 proposed solutions were not acquired or are no longer

---

[1] Supplementary material on this study can be found at: https://www.researchgate.net/profile/Melinda-Braun/research.

in use for various reasons (not accepted by the user, no further participation, no response to follow-up questions, etc.).

4.1 Participants and Questionnaire

Currently, 31 participants have completed our questionnaire for 44 of the 47 solutions. Participants range in age from 25 to 76, with an average age of 49. Of the participants, 22 identify as male and 9 as female. 14 participants belong to target group 1 (as described in Sect. 3.1), one of them with additional motor impairments and one with sensory impairments. 15 belong to target group 2, 6 of them with additional motor impairments. Two participants belong to target group 3, all of them with additional motor impairments.

The way in which the questionnaire was completed—independently, with the help of a caregiver or family member, or without the participant's involvement— depended on the individual's limitations and the caregiver's judgment. Of the 31 participants, only 1 from target group 1 completed the questionnaire independently, 15 completed it with assistance (11 from target group 1 and 4 from target group 2), and 12 had a caregiver complete it on their behalf (1 from target group 1, 9 from target group 2, and 2 from target group 3). This information is missing for 3 participants.

4.2 Solutions and Input Types

Table 1. Occurrences of the Input Modalities.

Input Modality (N)	Overall	N = 1	N = 2	N = 3
Pointing gestures	29	18	9	2
Buttons or switch elements	21	3	16	2
Object interaction	12	0	11	1
Voice interaction	7	0	6	1

Table 1 gives an overview of how often the individual input modalities occur in the different solutions. The most frequent interface type is *pointing gestures* (n = 29), 18 times as a single input modality, 9 times together with one other input modality, and two times together with two other input modalities. The second most common input type (n = 21) is interfaces with *buttons or switches*, which occur 3 times as a standalone input, 16 times alongside one other input modality, and twice alongside two other input types. Interfaces with *object interaction* occur 12 times, never as a standalone input modality, 11 times alongside another input modality, and once alongside two other input modalities, and interfaces with *voice interaction* occur a total of 7 times, 6 times alongside another input modality, and once alongside two other input modalities—also never as a standalone input modality.

Table 2. Multimodal Input (⊘ SUS Scores).

Input Modalities	Sum	Competing Input	Combined Input
Object interaction + Buttons or switch elements	10	0	10 (55.5)
Pointing gestures + Buttons or switch elements	4	0	4 (30.0)
Pointing gestures + Voice interaction	3	3 (72.5)	0
Buttons or switch elements + Voice interaction	3	3 (25.0)	0
Pointing gestures + Object interaction	1	1 (80.0)	0
Pointing gestures + Buttons or switch elements + Voice interaction	1	0	1 (50.0)
Pointing gestures + Buttons or switch elements + Object interaction	1	0	1 (50.0)
Sum	23 (49.9)	7 (53.2)	16 (48.4)

Table 3. Level of Adaptation (⊘ SUS Scores).

Input Modalities	1	1A	1B	1C	Sum
Pointing gestures	9 (68.2)	4 (83.8)	4 (52.2)	1 (70.0)	18 (68.3)
Buttons or switch elements	1 (42.5)*	0	2 (75.0)	0	3 (64.2)
Object interaction + Buttons or switch elements	1 (77.5)†	0	0	9 (53.1)	10 (55.5)
Pointing gestures + Buttons or switch elements	1 (37.5)*	0	3 (27.5)*	0	4 (30.0)
Pointing gestures + Voice interaction	0	3 (72.5)	0	0	3 (72.5)
Buttons or switch elements + Voice interaction	0	1 (25.0)	2 (25.0)	0	3 (25.0)
Pointing gestures + Object interaction	1 (80.0)	0	0	0	1 (80.0)
Pointing gestures + Buttons or switch elements + Voice interaction	0	0	1 (50.0)	0	1 (50.0)
Pointing gestures + Buttons or switch elements + Object interaction	1 (50.0)	0	0	0	1 (50.0)
Sum	14 (63.8)	8 (72.2)	12 (45.2)	10 (54.8)	44 (57.9)

Multimodal Solutions: As shown in Table 2, 23 solutions used multimodal input in different combinations. The most common combination was *object interaction and buttons or switches*—used in 10 solutions, followed by *pointing gestures and buttons or switches* (n = 4). *Voice interaction* was used with either *pointing gestures* (n = 3), *buttons or switches* (n = 3), or both (n = 1). Of the 23 multimodal solutions, 16 had to be used with all input modalities (combined multimodal input) and 7 could be used with either modality (competing multimodal input).

Level of Adaptation: Table 3 shows the level of adaptation and refers to the categorization in the *continuum of consumer and assistive technologies* as seen in Fig. 1. [6]. Most solutions belonged to category 1 (n = 14), with no adaptation, followed by category 1B (n = 12), with adaptations using assistive software, category 1C (n = 10), with hardware adaptations, and category 1A (n = 8), with operating system features that can improve accessibility.

Non-acquired Solutions: Of the 70 non-acquired solutions, 39 belonged to *pointing gestures*, 15 to *pointing gestures* combined with *voice interaction*, 5 belonged to interfaces with no input modality and 4 belonged to *pointing gestures* combined with *object interaction*. 3 belonged to interfaces with *buttons or switches* and the remaining 4 belonged to *touchless interaction, object interaction, pointing gestures* combined with *buttons or switches* and *object interaction* combined with *buttons or switches*.

5 Findings

This section will describe the findings of our work, mostly regarding usability.

5.1 Usability

SUS [8] was used to measure the usability of the different solutions and interfaces. Therefore, the *SUS scores* were evaluated. The average of all *SUS scores* is 57.9 (out of 100), with the highest individual score being 90.0 and the lowest being 25.0. Table 3 shows the average *SUS scores* for each interface input type. The input type with the highest score is *pointing gestures and object interaction* (80.0, but only used in one solution), followed by *pointing gestures and voice interaction* (72.5), and *pointing gestures* as a standalone input modality (68.3). The lowest scores were for *buttons or switches and voice interaction* (25.0) and *pointing gestures and buttons or switches"* (30.0).

Duration of Use: The questionnaire asked how long the technology had been in use (not long: 0–3 months or somewhat longer: over 3 months). 25 solutions have been in use for more than 3 months, 17 for 0–3 months. Information is missing for 2 of the solutions. The average of the *SUS scores* of the interfaces that have

M. C. Braun and M. Wölfel

been in use for 0–3 months is 54.9, the average of the solutions that have been in use for over 3 months is 60.0. No significant relationship was found between *duration of use* and *SUS score*. Long-term use and comparison of individual users between initial use and longer use need further observation.

Age: SUS Score and **Age** show a negative relationship (Spearman's Rho = -0.392, p = 0.010), this could indicate that age has an effect on the *SUS score* and the older a participant, the lower their score.

Suggested vs. Own Solution: As mentioned above, 6 solutions were not purchased or executed with the technologies or interfaces we proposed (marked with a * in Table 3. For one of these solutions, the questionnaire has not been answered yet. This was the case, when caregivers decided against a solution (mostly because of budget) and used existing hardware, e.g., an old, existing laptop instead of a new tablet or smartphone. Another solution was realized for one participant without being known to us beforehand as a participation request (marked with a †). When looking at the scores, it is noticeable that only this solution (†) has a higher score (77.5). The other solutions (*) show noticeably low scores (all between 27.5 and 42.5, with an average of 32.5), suggesting a general dissatisfaction with the execution. For solutions acquired and executed as we proposed, the average score was 60.9. *Suggested (1) vs. own solution (2)* and *SUS Score* showed a negative relationship (Spearman's Rho = −0.435, p = 0.004). Even though the sample size is small, there is an indication that more appropriate solutions can be suggested by experts. This is also supported by the statement that people with intellectual disabilities and their relatives or caregivers often do not know which technologies are available or which interfaces are usable for them [7,14].

Level of Adaptation: The level of adaptation (categories 1-1C) for each solution was determined based on the *continuum for consumer and assistive technologies* (see Fig. 1). *Level of adaptation* and *SUS score* show a negative relationship (Spearmans Rho = −0.376; p = 0.017). This shows that—in this study—the higher the level of adaptation, the lower the *SUS score*.

Competing and Combined Multimodal Input: *Competing (1) vs. combined (2)* multimodal input and *SUS score* showed a negative relationship (Spearman's Rho = −0.653, p = 0.002). This may suggest that type of multimodal input can influence usability for people with ID.

SUS and OCS-R: The *OCS-R scores* from a previous study [7] and the *SUS scores* from the present study were compared to see if there was a correlation between participants' physical, mental, and communicative abilities and their ratings of the interface they were currently using. However, since we do not have these data for all current participants, only some were evaluated (n = 18). A strong positive relationship was found between *SUS* and *OCS-R scores* of interfaces with pointing gestures (Spearman's Rho = 0.913, p =<0.001). Due to the small sample size, we could not calculate correlations for the remaining cases (n = 8). These results may indicate that *OCS-R scores* on participants' abilities and skills to use the specific interface type may predict in advance how they will later evaluate its use and whether a specific interface will be accepted. However, this comparison would need to be repeated with more data to make a clearer statement.

Table 4. Individual SUS Items.

Input	Q1	Q2	Q3	Q4	Q5	Q6	Q7	Q8	Q9	Q10
Pointing gestures	4.4	2.4	4.1	2.6	4.1	2.9	3.7	2.4	3.6	3.8
Buttons or switch elements	4.3	1.7	4.3	3.7	4.0	3.0	3.7	3.0	3.0	2.3
Object interaction + Buttons or switch elements	3.5	2.7	3.2	3.6	3.9	2.5	3.4	2.4	2.9	3.3
Pointing gestures + Buttons or switch elements	3.3	5.0	1.0	3.0	3.0	4.5	3.0	3.0	2.0	4.8
Pointing gestures + Voice interaction	5.0	1.7	3.7	3.0	5.0	2.0	3.7	1.7	2.3	2.3
Buttons or switch elements + Voice interaction	3.0	5.0	1.0	5.0	3.0	1.0	3.0	5.0	1.0	5.0
Pointing gestures + Object interaction	5.0	1.0	5.0	3.0	5.0	2.0	4.0	1.0	5.0	5.0
Pointing gestures + Buttons or switch elements + Voice interaction	1.0	4.0	2.0	5.0	4.0	2.0	4.0	2.0	3.0	1.0
Pointing gestures + Object interaction + Buttons or switch elements	3.0	3.0	3.0	3.0	3.0	4.0	2.0	2.0	3.0	2.0
Mean value	4.0	2.8	3.3	3.2	3.9	2.8	3.5	2.6	3.0	3.6

Individual Scores: It is not standard procedure, nor is it generally recommended, to report the scores for the individual items that make up the SUS. We do this to gain additional insight into how the different input modalities perform on individual items (1 = strongly disagree and 5 = strongly agree). Table 4 provides an overview of the individual results for the different input modalities.

It seems that participants tend to continue using most interfaces (Q1, mean 4.0). Regarding Q2 and Q3, which ask about the simplicity and complexity of the system, it is noticeable that there exist differences in the evaluation of simplicity and complexity between the interface types. This may be due to the input, but also to the degree of restriction of the persons. It is interesting to note that *voice interaction with pointing gestures* is generally considered low complexity and easy to use, while *voice interaction with buttons or switches* is considered rather complex and not easy to use. This may be due to the abilities of the participants: although all belong to target group 1, the participants using *voice with buttons or switches* had additional motor and communication limitations, whereas the participants using *pointing gestures and voice* did not.

Regarding Q5, in general, the functions of the solutions are sufficient (mean value = 3.9). Most of the time, the solutions are easy to understand (Q6) (mean value 2.6), but there are exceptions: *pointing gestures with buttons or switches* and *pointing gestures with object interaction, and buttons or switches* are considered difficult to understand.

Most participants did not find the solutions cumbersome to use (Q8, mean value 2.5), except with *buttons or switches and voice interaction*. Again, this probably has something to do with the abilities of the participants (with both motor and language difficulties), as it is more difficult for these cases to find a perfectly fitting solution from already existing consumer technologies.

The last question asked whether participants had to learn a lot before they could use the technology (Q10), which is more likely to be the case (mean 3.6). For some interface types, the results indicate that they had to learn a lot before using the technology. On the other hand, for other input types, participants didn't have to learn much before using the technology. It is interesting that *pointing gesture-only* interfaces are considered more complex to learn than *pointing gestures with voice interaction*, but again, the small group size must be considered.

5.2   Other Correlations

In addition to the *SUS scores*, referring to usability, the following relationships were found among the individual categories:

- **Level of Adaptation and Target Group (1–3)** show a positive relationship (Spearman's Rho = 0.519, p =< 0.001).
- **Level of Adaptation and Competing (1) or Combined (2) Input** show a positive relationship (Spearman's Rho = 0.494, p = 0.027).
- **Competing (1) or Combined (2) Input and Target Group (1–3)** show a positive relationship (Spearman's Rho = 0.527, p = 0.017).

This implies that people with more severe disabilities were more likely to use adapted technologies and more likely to use combined multimodal input. That is, the lower the person's limitation, the more often interfaces with multiple input modalities were used. Conversely, the higher the limitation, the more often interfaces were used where all input modalities were required to use the interface. These results may indicate that interfaces for people with more severe limitations need to follow a more defined pattern, with specified input modalities. Too many choices of input modalities could be too complex and lead to confusion. However, further studies would have to be conducted to investigate this in more detail.

5.3 Non-acquired Solutions

As mentioned before, 70 of the proposed solutions were not acquired or are no longer in use. This was due to various reasons (more than one reason may apply), such as:

1. *Prioritization (n = 28):* Participants had more than one participation wish and decided to implement other solutions.
2. *Not yet acquired (n = 16):* Some solutions had not yet been acquired at the time of publication of this study.
3. *No feedback (n = 12):* It is unclear why these solutions were not acquired. Since communication with people with intellectual disabilities requires multiple parties (for example, legal guardians, caregivers, parents), communication is often difficult. Often there was also no response to several queries.
4. *No acceptance (n = 7):* Solutions were acquired, but already at the beginning of usage the participant showed a rejection towards the technology.
5. *Budget (n = 6):* People with ID often have too little or no budget to purchase technology or cannot buy anything without the prior consent of a caregiver or legal representative. There were cases where the person was interested in the technology, but the caregiver or legal representative intervened, so there was no acquisition.
6. *Withdrawal from the study (n = 6):* Some participants decided themselves not to participate any longer or were obliged to do so by other circumstances (e.g., illness, death).

6 Conclusion and Outlook

In this study, different technical solutions, especially their interface types, were tested and evaluated for people with ID in everyday life. Usability was evaluated using the *System Usability Scale (SUS)* [8].

We found that the most used input type by participants with ID was *pointing gestures*, which was also the input type that could be used as a standalone interaction method a lot of the time. This makes sense, since at the moment, most consumer digital technologies use this type of input (e.g., smartphones, tablets), and some participants already owned a mobile device prior to this study. This input type was also the one that needed lesser adaptation in general and usability was perceived as acceptable (68.3), but usability was perceived higher when being used with additional system accessibility features (83.8). When used alongside other input modalities, it was mostly used with *buttons or switches*—where usability was perceived as rather low on average (30.0)—or *voice interaction*, where usability was perceived as higher (72.5).

Buttons or switch elements were the second most used type, interestingly mostly in combination with *object interaction*. Although this is an established interface type, it often required more adaptation, such as button adjustments (size, function, etc.) or finger guide grids. When used with *object interaction*, solutions had to be custom-built for participants, which can also be seen as

M. C. Braun and M. Wölfel

a barrier. This type of input was often used by participants with more severe disabilities. Despite its potential, problems were encountered when interacting with the buttons or placing the tangible objects in the right spot.

Voice interaction was never used as a standalone input modality, only alongside *pointing gestures, buttons or switches* or both. Although *voice interaction* is often seen as having great potential for this target group [23, 26], there are still major problems with its use. When this type of input was used, usability was considered relatively high, but many of the participants were not even able to try this type of interaction, so it was only used 7 times. At present, there are still too many barriers and difficulties in using voice input for people with ID, mainly due to pronunciation difficulties caused by language limitations or the complexity of the commands, and not many adaptations exist for this target group. Future developments will show whether this potential can be realized.

Interfaces with *touchless interaction* were generally too difficult for the participants to use, so the 4 initially planned solutions were not acquired. This type of input also doesn't have a lot of customization options, and in most cases other input modalities were easier to use for the participants.

Regarding the perceived usability of the solutions, the average scores were rather low (57.9), which shows that there is still a lot of room for improvement for people with ID using digital technologies. However, overcoming this is complex: we found that usability depended on many different factors, such as the age of the participants, whether the solution was suggested by experts or not, the level of adaptation used, or the type of multimodal input used—and these factors also depended on the level of disability the participants had. Solutions with no adaptation had higher scores, but were also more likely to be used by people with less severe disabilities. People with more complex and severe disabilities were more likely to use more adapted technologies and results suggest that too much choice between input modalities could possibly lead to confusion.

In the process of acquiring the individual solutions, it became clear that some solutions—even when the least expensive option was proposed by the researchers—were often quite expensive for the participants due to their limited financial resources. Successful acquisition and use of the solutions also had a lot to do with the time resources of the institution and its staff. It was noticeable that participants with a motivated carer or family member were offered more opportunities.

In conclusion, the usability of current NUIs is highly dependent on the person using them. To address this, it is important to incorporate the needs of users with ID into technology development processes, especially with regard to inclusivity and adaptability. This approach can help reduce the digital divide and increase participation in daily life. By prioritizing user-centered design and adaptability, NUIs can be developed that benefit and empower a wider range of people with ID, paving the way for a more inclusive digital future.

This study had several limitations. Not all input modalities were used equally often, so there are large differences between the group sizes. The use of an interface depended on the type of solution and the disability of the user. There are also limitations regarding the questionnaire: although we used a standardized questionnaire, it was not adapted for and tested with people with ID. The use of plain language has improved this, but it cannot be guaranteed that the questionnaire will be understood in the same way by everyone. It can never be assumed with certainty that people with ID have correctly understood or answered the questions in the questionnaire. Even though the participants with more severe disabilities always had a carer present when they completed the questionnaire, errors cannot be completely ruled out.

In the future, the long-term use of these solutions and interfaces will be further investigated. A second questionnaire will be sent out to participants who have recently started using the solution to determine possible changes in long-term use. This will allow us to determine any differences after they have become accustomed to the technology.

Acknowledgement. This study is part of a project funded by the Federal Ministry of Education and Research (BMBF) in Germany within the framework of the program "FH Sozial 2017". We would also like to thank the participating institutions for people with disabilities.

References

1. 2BIG s.r.o.: BIG Launcher (2023). https://biglauncher.com/en/. Accessed 05 May 2023
2. Apple Inc. Accessibility (2023). https://www.apple.com/accessibility/. Accessed 10 May 2023
3. Augstein, M., Kurschl, W.: Modelling touchless interaction for people with special needs. In: Koch, M., Butz, A., Schlichter, J.H. (eds.) Mensch & Computer 2014 - Workshopband. De Gruyter Oldenbourg, Berlin (2014). http://dl.gi.de/handle/20.500.12116/8164
4. Balasuriya, S.S., Sitbon, L., Bayor, A.A., Hoogstrate, M., Brereton, M.: Use of voice activated interfaces by people with intellectual disability. In: Proceedings of the 30th Australian Conference on Computer-Human Interaction, pp. 102–112. ACM, Melbourne (2018). https://doi.org/10.1145/3292147.3292161
5. Barlott, T., et al.: Connectedness and ICT: opening the door to possibilities for people with intellectual disabilities. J. Intellect. Disabil. **24**(4), 503–521 (2020). https://doi.org/10.1177/1744629519831566
6. Braun, M.C., Wölfel, M.: Demands on user interfaces for people with intellectual disabilities, their requirements, and adjustments. In: Tsanas, A., Triantafyllidis, A. (eds.) Pervasive Computing Technologies for Healthcare, pp. 540–556. Springer, Cham (2023). https://link.springer.com/10.1007/978-3-031-34586-9_36
7. Braun, M.C., Wölfel, M., Renner, G., Menschik, C.: Accessibility of different natural user interfaces for people with intellectual disabilities. In: 2020 International Conference on Cyberworlds (CW), pp. 211–218. IEEE, Caen (2020). https://doi.org/10.1109/CW49994.2020.00041
8. Brooke, J.: SUS – a quick and dirty usability scale. In: Usability Evaluation in Industry, pp. 189–194. CRC Press (1996)
9. Carroll, J.M., Rosson, M.B., Farooq, U., Xiao, L.: Beyond being aware. Inf. Organ. **19**(3), 162–185 (2009). https://doi.org/10.1016/j.infoandorg.2009.04.004

10. Domingo, M.C.: An overview of the Internet of Things for people with disabilities. J.. Netw. Comput. Appl. **35**(2), 584–596 (2012). https://doi.org/10.1016/j.jnca.2011.10.015

11. Dufva, T., Dufva, M.: Grasping the future of the digital society. Futures **107**, 17–28 (2019). https://doi.org/10.1016/j.futures.2018.11.001

12. European Parliament and Council. Directive (EU) 2019/of the European Parliament and of the Council of 17 April 2019 on the accessibility requirements for products and services. Off. J. Eur. Union 46 (2019). https://eur-lex.europa.eu/eli/dir/2019/882/oj

13. Falcao, T.P.: Action-effect mappings in tangible interaction for children with intellectual disabilities. Int. J. Learn. Technol. **12**(4), 294 (2017). https://doi.org/10.1504/IJLT.2017.089908

14. Ferreras, A., Poveda, R., Quílez, M., Poll, N.: Improving the quality of life of persons with intellectual disabilities through ICTs. Stud. Health Technol. Inf. **242**, 257–264 (2017)

15. Flor, M.: Phoniebox: the RPi-Jukebox-RFID (2023). https://github.com/MiczFlor/RPi-Jukebox-RFID. Accessed 09 Apr 2023

16. Gelsomini, M., Spitale, M., Garzotto, F.: Phygital interfaces for people with intellectual disability: an exploratory study at a social care center. Multim. Tools Appl. **80**(26–27), 34843–34874 (2021). https://doi.org/10.1007/s11042-021-11164-9

17. Google. Android Accessibility Help (2023). https://support.google.com/accessibility/android#topic=9079844. Accessed 10 Apr 2023

18. Gündogdu, R., Bejan, A., Kunze, C., Wölfel, M.: Activating people with dementia using natural user interface interaction on a surface computer. In: Proceedings of the 11th EAI International Conference on Pervasive Computing Technologies for Healthcare (PervasiveHealth 2017), pp. 386–394. ACM Press, Barcelona (2017). https://doi.org/10.1145/3154862.3154929

19. Jamaludin, N.A.N., Huey, O.: Dynamic hand gesture to text using leap motion. Int. J. Adv. Comput. Sci. Appl. **10**(11) (2019). https://doi.org/10.14569/IJACSA.2019.0101127

20. Jimenez, B.A., Alamer, K.: Using graduated guidance to teach iPad accessibility skills to high school students with severe intellectual disabilities. J. Spec. Educ. Technol. **33**(4), 237–246 (2018). https://doi.org/10.1177/0162643418766293

21. Lussier-Desrochers, D., et al.: Bridging the digital divide for people with intellectual disability. CP **11**(1) (2017). https://doi.org/10.5817/CP2017-1-1

22. Marshall, P.: Do tangible interfaces enhance learning? In: Proceedings of the 1st International conference on Tangible and embedded interaction, pp. 163–170. ACM, Baton Rouge Louisiana (2007). https://doi.org/10.1145/1226969.1227004

23. Masina, F., et al.: Investigating the accessibility of voice assistants with impaired users: mixed methods study. J. Med. Internet Res. **22**(9), e18431 (2020). https://doi.org/10.2196/18431

24. Microsoft. Windows Accessibility Features — Microsoft Accessibility (2023). https://www.microsoft.com/en-us/accessibility/windows. Accessed 08 Apr 2023

25. Pappy GmbH. Easierphone (2023). https://easierphone.com/. Accessed 05 May 2023

26. Pradhan, A., Mehta, K., Findlater, L.: Accessibility came by accident: use of voice-controlled intelligent personal assistants by people with disabilities. In: Proceedings of the 2018 CHI Conference on Human Factors in Computing Systems (CHI 2018), pp. 1–13. ACM Press, Montreal (2018). https://doi.org/10.1145/3173574.3174033

27. RehaMedia. Fingerführrraster — Lexikon & Fachbegriffe erklärt von RehaMedia (2022). https://rehamedia.de/glossar-lexikon/fingerfuehrrraster/. Accessed 10 Apr 2023

28. Scholz, M., Wagner, M., Stegkemper, J.M.: OCS-R Manual (Version 1.06). University of Education Ludwigsburg and University of Koblenz-Landau (2019)

29. Shaer, O.: Tangible user interfaces: past, present, and future directions. Found. Trends®Hum.-Comput. Interact. **3**(1–2), 1–137 (2009). https://doi.org/10.1561/1100000026

30. Skogly Kversøy, K., Kellems, R.O., Kuyini Alhassan, A.R., Bussey, H.C., Daae Kversøy, S.: The emerging promise of touchscreen devices for individuals with intellectual disabilities. Multim. Technol. Interact. **4**(4), 70 (2020). https://doi.org/10.3390/mti4040070

31. tonies GmbH. Tonies (2022). https://tonies.com/en-gb/. Accessed 09 Apr 2023

32. Saenz de Urturi Breton, Z., Jorge Hernandez, F., Mendez Zorrilla, A., Garcia Zapirain, B.: Mobile communication for intellectually challenged people: a proposed set of requirements for interface design on touch screen devices. Commun. Mob. Comput. **1**(1), 1 (2012). https://doi.org/10.1186/2192-1121-1-1

33. Voiceitt Inc. Inclusive voice AI with impact (2023). https://voiceitt.com/. Accessed 24 Oct 2023

34. Wenzel, K., Kaufman, G.: Challenges in designing racially inclusive language technologies. In: CUI@CHI: Inclusive Design of CUIs Across Modalities and Mobilities (2023). https://cui.acm.org/workshops/CHI2023/papers.html

35. Wigdor, D., Wixon, D.: Brave NUI World: Designing Natural User Interfaces for Touch and Gesture. Morgan Kaufmann, Burlington (2011)

36. Williams, P., Shekhar, S.: People with learning disabilities and smartphones: testing the usability of a touch-screen interface. Educ. Sci. **9**(4), 263 (2019). https://doi.org/10.3390/educsci9040263

37. Wölfel, M., Lintermann, B., Völzow, N.: Using tangible surfaces in opera. Re-new-IMAC (2011)

Usability of Voice Assistants in Healthcare: A Systematic Literature Review

Anh Duong[iD] and Maria Valero[✉][iD]

Kennesaw State University, Marietta, GA, USA
aduong2@students.kennesaw.edu, mvalero2@kennesaw.edu

Abstract. Over the last decades, the rapid development and applications of voice assistants (VA) have been integrated into healthcare systems worldwide. With the high acceptance rate of voice assistants, usability is the key aspect that must be examined to ensure effective and accurate performance in the critical and sensitive environment of healthcare. Based on our research, not many studies reviewed the usability of voice assistants in healthcare and thus creating a notable gap in the literature regarding the usage of VA in healthcare. This study presents a qualitative systematic review of the usability of VA in healthcare with a breakdown of five major categories where VAs serve in healthcare. A total of 18 papers contained supportive evidence for the review and summarizes the roles and usages of VA in healthcare along with existing applications in healthcare systems. Based on the reviewed studies, limitations of VA and recommendations for future research to ensure effective and reliable applications of VA in healthcare are reported.

Keywords: Voice Assistant · Healthcare · Systematic Review

1 Introduction

In today's era of rapid technological advancement and artificial intelligence, the interactive voice assistant (VA) has emerged as a critical application of AI technology [28]. Integrated into voice-controlled devices and smartphones, VA utilizes natural language processing, speech synthesis, and voice recognition to understand and execute human commands [30]. With its ability to provide prompt and purposeful responses, VA enables users to complete tasks hands-free and save valuable time [14]. Its widespread adoption is evident, with 27% of the global population using voice assistants for mobile searches [1] and approximately 41% of Americans relying on VA for multiple daily searches [4]. Acting as a bridge between human-computer interaction, VA enhances convenience, reduces multitasking, and maximizes time efficiency, making it an essential tool in our daily lives [30].

Supported by Kennesaw State University.

D. Salvi et al. (Eds.): PH 2023, LNICST 572, pp. 386–401, 2024.
https://doi.org/10.1007/978-3-031-59717-6_25

Users have enthusiastically embraced voice assistants, finding them both useful and enjoyable for their ability to engage in human-like emotional conversations, allowing users to express their social identity in the digital world [5]. Voice assistants have been adopted across various domains, serving the primary purpose of simplifying people's lives, as implied by their name. Regardless of age, ethnicity, or social class, voice assistants are utilized by a diverse group of consumers for a wide range of tasks. The most common functionality of voice assistants is conducting searches through voice commands [10]. Additionally, they perform other everyday tasks such as playing music, setting reminders, sending text messages, making calls, and controlling smart home automation systems through voice-integrated IoT devices [30].

Voice assistants go beyond being mere day-to-day assistants; they have found application in more complex settings, including education, business, and healthcare. In the education sector, teachers employ voice assistants to streamline their sessions, tracking attendance, monitoring students' performance, and providing instant and accurate answers to queries [30]. In the business realm, voice assistants serve as alternatives for customer agents, enhancing customer interactions on business websites through voice chatbot systems. These systems assist customers with support, online ordering, and product recommendations, while also enabling transactions and scheduling meetings to minimize multitasking and eliminate human error [14]. Moreover, voice assistants play a crucial role in the healthcare system, benefiting both patients and practitioners. They assist patients in their daily lives, manage mood disorders, aid in disease treatments, provide consultations, and support Covid-19 care [18]. Additionally, voice assistants help healthcare professionals optimize their workflow and efficiency within healthcare units [20]. Given the critical nature of healthcare, which involves human lives, privacy, and overall safety, the usability and efficacy of voice assistants in this context have garnered significant attention. While systematic reviews exist on topics such as voice assistants' usability [9], their applications in chronic conditions [6], and their interaction with an aging population [23], there remains a notable gap in the literature regarding the specific roles and usages of voice assistants in healthcare. This paper aims to bridge this gap by conducting a comprehensive systematic review of voice assistants in healthcare. The review seeks to summarize the diverse applications of voice assistants in healthcare settings and address research questions concerning the quality and effectiveness of voice assistants in improving healthcare outcomes.

Section 2 presents the methodology, including the research questions, search strategy, eligibility criteria, paper selection, quality assessment, data extraction and synthesis. This is followed by Sect. 3, which presents the breakdown of categories of the individual studies, descriptions of included papers, analysis, and details of each category, different usages of VA in healthcare, and the applications of VA. Section 4 presents the discussion and Sect. 5.

2 Methods

2.1 Research Questions

This systematic review aims to comprehensively examine the utilization of voice assistants in diverse healthcare settings and synthesize the available evidence on their efficacy and impact in healthcare contexts. To structure our research questions effectively, we employed the PICO (Population, Intervention, Comparison, Outcome) framework, a widely recognized criterion for formulating research questions in systematic review studies across various disciplines, including psychology, education, primary care, and software engineering [13]. The utilization of the PICO framework ensured the formulation of precise and comprehensive research questions that guided every aspect of our systematic review process, including the development of search strategies, quality assessment protocols, and data extraction procedures. By adhering to the PICO framework, we established specific criteria based on our research interests as outlined below:

- The **population** of people who work and use the healthcare system, e.g. patients, healthcare professionals, caregivers.
- The **intervention** of voice assistant.
- In **comparison** to no assistance from the voice assistant or voice-controlled devices.
- The **outcome** of changes in the targeted population and their quality of life.

We defined our research questions as the following:

- RQ1–What roles and types of voice assistants exist in healthcare?
- RQ2–How effective is voice assistant versus the absence of voice assistant for improving the quality of life of people involved in healthcare?
- RQ3–How has the use of voice assistants impacted and supported individuals in the healthcare system? What evidence exists to support these claims?

2.2 Search Strategy

In order to explore the intersection of voice assistants and healthcare, our study utilized extensive scientific databases such as Scopus and IEEE Xplore. Given the vastness of these databases and the broad scope of our research topic, which encompasses technology, health, and various aspects related to voice assistants, we employed a consistent search strategy across both databases. Our search string consisted of two keywords, 'voice assistant' and 'healthcare', connected by the operator 'AND'. This final search string, "voice assistant" AND "healthcare", was applied to titles, abstracts, and keywords of the studies.

After completing the search process, a total of 136 studies were identified, with 98 studies sourced from Scopus and 38 studies from IEEE Xplore. To facilitate further review and filtering, the data from both sources was exported and consolidated into a single Excel file.

2.3   Eligibility Criteria

In order to prevent bias and have direct evidence for the established research questions, we created the eligibility criteria–inclusion and exclusion criteria–in our protocol. We applied a set of exclusion criteria and excluded papers with at least one criterion presented to narrow down the final number of relevant papers. Papers that were qualified for further screening were the ones that matched all of the inclusion criteria. An overview of the eligibility criteria is shown in Table 1. These criteria are listed in Table 1, which include (i) duplicated papers; (ii) full-text availability; (iii) related papers to the study.

Table 1. Inclusion and Exclusion Criteria for Primary Studies

Conditions for Inclusion	Conditions for Exclusion
* The study must contain information about voice assistants and any healthcare application	* Studies focusing on other topics that do not include these keywords and are not related to healthcare
* Paper is not a duplicate existing in a different database	* Paper is already included. Copy exists in a different database
* Original research relevant to the topic in question	* Similar studies or reviews in multiple scientific databases
* Paper is written in English	* Paper is not written in English
* Peer–reviewed papers published in a conference proceeding or journal	* Non peer–reviewed papers or published in predatory venues
* Studies that are open access, i.e., have the full text available	* Studies that do not have full text available

2.4   Paper Selection

After conducting the initial search, the set of 136 studies underwent screening based on the eligibility criteria to determine the total number of papers included and excluded for further review. In the first round of screening, 13 duplicated papers were identified and removed from the set. In the second round, papers with unclear or irrelevant abstracts to the study's topic were excluded, resulting in the elimination of an additional 81 papers. The remaining 42 papers from the search process entered the third round of screening, where the eligibility criteria were applied during full-text analysis. Initially, 10 papers were removed in the first phase of this round due to the unavailability of full access to the selected databases (Scopus and IEEE Xplore) or in other libraries, despite an extensive search. Ultimately, after completing Round 3, 14 more papers were excluded, leaving 18 papers eligible for data extraction and final review. A concise overview of the paper selection process is visualized in the PRISMA flow diagram, depicted in Fig. 1.

2.5   Data Extraction and Synthesis

To address the research questions, relevant data were extracted from the 18 included papers through a meticulous data extraction process. A template

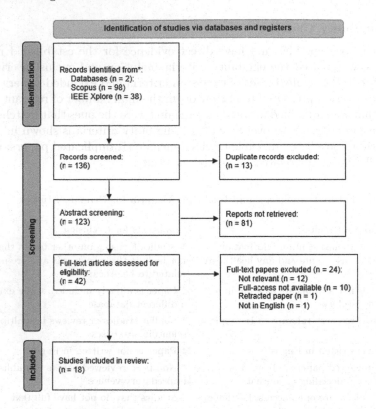

Fig. 1. PRISMA flow diagram of the selection process and final result.

(Table 2) was developed, outlining the specific items required for the review, and a spreadsheet was utilized to organize and record the extracted data. Each data item corresponded to the responses related to either the research questions or the quality assessment.

Following the data extraction phase, we employed a qualitative synthesis process, as recommended by the Cochrane Handbook for Systematic Reviews of Interventions [13]. This involved a thorough examination and analysis of the extracted data to ensure objectivity and ensure a comprehensive body of evidence for the research questions. Additionally, we investigated the connections between studies conducted in various healthcare settings and grouped similar studies into relevant categories. These categories, which will be further discussed in the Results section, are presented in Table 3, displaying the five distinct healthcare areas along with the number of papers assigned to each category.

3   Results

In this section, we provide answers to our research questions by carefully analyzing and categorizing the 18 papers that were extracted during our review process.

Table 2. Data Extraction Template

	Items	Descriptions	Category
Paper	Study Number	Keep track of papers in each category and use later in Results section. Abbreviated by Sn (for n is the number of papers)	RQ1, Study Overview
	Title	Names of the included papers	Study Overview
	Country of Study	Keep track of the origin of the papers	Study Overview
Characteristics of included studies	Aim of Study	Concisely summarize the focus of the study	Study Overview
	Roles of VA	What voice assistants serve in the study	RQ1
	Types of VA	Name of voice assistant used in the study	RQ1
	Effectiveness of VA	Data on the usability, accuracy, impact, and quality of VA	RQ2
	Evidence	Applications or innovations in the studies	RQ3
Participants	Population	Types of people use VA in each study	RQ1, RQ2, RQ3, Study Overview
	Area in Healthcare	Area where VA is integrated in	RQ1, RQ2, RQ3

Table 3. Number of paper for each category

Category	Number of papers (n)
Patient Care	7
COVID-19	2
Mood Disorder Management	3
Hospital Operation	4
Disease Management	2
Total	**18**

3.1 RQ1: What Roles and Types of Voice Assistants Exist in Healthcare?

Among the 18 papers included in our analysis, 7 papers (38.8%) exclusively utilized Amazon Alexa as their voice assistant, while 7 papers (38.8%) did not specify a particular voice assistant. Furthermore, 3 papers (16.6%) employed multiple voice assistants or included all types available, and 1 paper (5.5%) developed its own voice assistant specifically for the study.

The healthcare system comprises numerous sectors and areas, as supported by sources. Consequently, the roles of voice assistants vary depending on the specific healthcare areas. However, there are overlapping functionalities of voice assistants across multiple areas. In this study, we identified and categorized the roles of voice assistants in five distinct areas based on the findings of relevant studies. Specifically, the roles were discussed in seven studies related to Patient Care (n = 7, [7,8,11,12,22,24–26]), two studies in COVID-19 (n = 2, [15,20]), three studies in Mood Disorder Management (n = 3, [16,17,21]), four studies in Hospital Operation (n = 4, [3,18–20]), and two studies in Disease Management (n = 2, [2,29]). For detailed information on the roles of voice assistants, please refer to the respective sub-sections within each category.

Patient Care. Voice assistants play a pivotal role in assisting end-users, as supported by factual evidence. Consequently, the area of Patient Care emerged as the primary focus where voice assistants served a wide range of populations. Notably, voice assistants provided valuable support to patients, including elderly patients [7,8,11,22,24,26], caregivers of children with special healthcare needs [25], and disabled individuals [12]. An example is shown in Fig. 2.

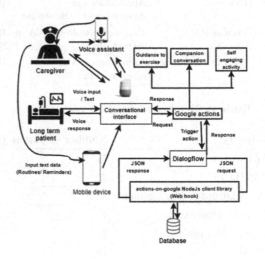

Fig. 2. System Architecture of Voice Assistant in Patient Care [11]

COVID-19. During the critical period of the global COVID-19 pandemic, healthcare professionals dedicated their time and expertise to closely support patients, prioritizing their care amidst the demanding circumstances. Technological advancements played a significant role in monitoring patients' health, with the assistance of various devices. In this context, voice assistants emerged as valuable tools, offering guidance and information specifically related to COVID-19.

Furthermore, voice assistants provided feedback to patients by analyzing essential health indicators such as body temperature, heart rate, and oxygen levels, thereby assisting in the assessment of the likelihood of a COVID-19 infection [15,20].

Mood Disorder Management. Among the 18 studies examined, three studies [16,21] shed light on the roles of voice assistants in supporting patients with mood disorders, including mild to moderate depression, anxiety, and prediagnostic depression. Notably, a study conducted in Singapore [17] highlighted the use of a voice assistant to provide information resources related to eating disorders and co-existing depression. In two distinct studies, Amazon Alexa was employed with different purposes: as a monitoring tool and pre-diagnostic depression detector [21], and as a problem-solving treatment coach [16]. In the case of a prediagnostic depression study, Alexa closely monitored patients' depressive symptoms, analyzing changes in their vocal tones [21]. This information enabled the voice assistant to provide a pre-diagnosis of depression, aiding healthcare professionals in identifying patient symptoms from their homes [21].

Hospital Operation. Within the hospital setting, voice assistants played a diverse range of roles, catering to various user groups and serving distinct purposes. In hospital triage operations, voice assistants assumed the role of front-line workers, providing assistance to patients in the emergency room. They would initially inquire about standard information, including main symptoms, body temperature, full name, and pain evaluation. Based on the collected information, the voice assistant would then assign patients a priority level [20]. Subsequently, the voice assistant would transmit the recorded data to the relevant agent and request human assistance if necessary.

Voice assistants serve various administrative purposes in healthcare settings, benefiting both patients and staff [18]. Patients can conveniently control devices, such as TVs, using voice commands directed at the voice assistant [18]. They can also rely on voice assistants to assist with tasks such as placing meal orders, calling their nurse, obtaining information, entertainment, setting reminders, and even during emergency situations [18,19]. This functionality allows nursing staff to allocate their time more efficiently towards core responsibilities [18].

Voice assistants also play a vital role in supporting hospital staff and healthcare professionals in managing electronic health records (EHRs). They can help schedule appointments, add notes, retrieve the nearest available appointments, order lab tests, and provide access to essential patient information [3]. A noteworthy example cited in [18] involved a pilot program implemented at the Boston Children's Hospital, where voice assistants were utilized to streamline pre-operative organ validation and handle administrative tasks in the intensive care unit [18,27].

Disease Management. Voice assistants were employed in studies focused on Multiple Myeloma (MM) disease and Alzheimer's disease and related dementia.

Amazon Alexa was utilized to provide medical term explanations, connect users to support groups, and offer a quiz feature specific to MM disease [2]. Additionally, Alexa extended its support to caregivers of individuals with Alzheimer's Disease and related dementia by providing explanations about food items and nutrition, suggesting meals and recipes, and offering tips for maintaining a proper diet [29].

The references cited provide valuable insights to answer the research question regarding the roles and types of voice assistants in healthcare. These studies showcase the diverse functions performed by voice assistants across different healthcare domains. They highlight how voice assistants serve as front-line workers in hospital triage operations, aid patients in obtaining information, entertainment, and emergency assistance, support administrative tasks for patients and healthcare professionals, and even offer disease-specific functionalities such as medical term explanations and connections to support groups. Furthermore, the references shed light on the types of voice assistants utilized, including Amazon Alexa, which demonstrates the variety of voice assistant technologies employed in healthcare settings.

3.2   RQ2: How Effective is Voice Assistant Versus the Absence of Voice Assistant for Improving the Quality of Life of People Involved in Healthcare?

The evaluation of voice assistants' effectiveness in healthcare involved assessing their usability, accuracy, impact, and overall quality, as reflected in the selected studies. While it is important to acknowledge the existing limitations and challenges faced by voice assistants, including algorithmic and accuracy errors [17], the overall usage of voice assistants has demonstrated a positive impact on people's lives within healthcare settings. In this review, data extraction for RQ2 was based on the discussions from 15 out of the 18 papers, highlighting the extensive exploration of the impact of voice assistants. The usage and growth of voice assistants have shown significant effects on three key aspects: the quality of patient's life, the quality of the healthcare system, and the quality of the voice assistants themselves.

Quality of the Patient's Life. A total of 6 papers [8,11,12,18,21,24] highlighted the positive impacts and benefits brought about by voice assistants for patients and their caregivers. Voice assistants were found to offer a more comfortable interactive environment compared to mobile phones or other devices when seeking assistance [21]. They enabled patients, especially the elderly, to lead a more realistic and independent life within the comfort of their own homes [11,12]. In the case of home healthcare system, voice assistants served as symptom checkers and first-aid ambulances during emergency situations, while also managing patients' health records, thereby enabling independent living [8]. Voice assistants significantly improved the quality of life for patients, including those with physical or visual impairments, by providing faster, hands-free, and user-friendly ways to meet their needs and manage daily routines [18,24].

The positive impact of voice assistants was further supported by a survey conducted in long-term patient care, where 37.5% of the respondents acknowledged that voice assistants played a role in enhancing their independence. Additionally, 26.7% referred to voice assistants as friends or companions, and among the caregivers surveyed, 83.4% out of 16% stated that voice assistants were supportive in their caregiving tasks [11].

Quality of the Healthcare System. Voice assistants have made significant contributions to the healthcare system, particularly in enhancing productivity and streamlining processes within hospital triage. They assist healthcare staff in the emergency room and also serve patients for administrative purposes, resulting in improved workflow [20]. Moreover, voice assistants have been reported to offer a more cost-efficient solution for healthcare providers compared to traditional care facilities [7]. Acting as front-line assistants and personal aides, voice assistants have proven invaluable to healthcare professionals by facilitating efficient management of electronic health records, allowing them to focus solely on their core responsibilities and increasing productivity [19].

Quality of Voice Assistant. The reviewed applications of voice assistants presented in the selected papers demonstrate a meticulous evaluation process [2] and a continuous improvement in accuracy over the years [17,22]. These advancements aim to create a patient-friendly environment and enhance users' overall experience [22]. Although voice assistants may still encounter errors and failures in fully comprehending user commands and providing the most accurate responses, studies have consistently shown the ongoing development and provision of high-quality and accurate answers. For instance, a study revealed that Amazon Alexa and Apple Siri achieved an increase of approximately 10–24% in accurately recognizing medication names within just two years [22]. Furthermore, a study from the National University of Singapore highlighted that Cortana exhibited higher quality scores and accuracy compared to the performance of Google Search [17].

The references cited in this study provide valuable insights that contribute to answering the research question concerning the effectiveness of voice assistants compared to the absence of voice assistants in improving the quality of life for individuals involved in healthcare. These references shed light on the positive impact of voice assistants on patients, caregivers, and healthcare professionals. They demonstrate how voice assistants enhance the healthcare experience, increase independence, offer personalized support, streamline processes, and improve productivity. Despite some limitations and challenges faced by voice assistants, the evidence indicates their continuous development, accuracy improvements, and commitment to providing high-quality assistance. Overall, the referenced studies suggest that voice assistants have proven effective in enhancing the quality of life for people involved in healthcare, making them valuable tools for the healthcare ecosystem.

3.3   RQ3: What Evidence is There that Voice Assistants Have Been Used to Impact and Support People's Lives in the Healthcare System?

10 papers presented the applications of voice assistants in multiple relevant categories and highlight the functionalities of voice-based devices in impacting people's lives in the healthcare system. Among the 10 applications, 5 applications belong to Patient Care (n = 5, [7,8,12,24,25]), 2 applications in Hospital Operation (n = 2, [3,20]), 1 application in Mood Disorder Management (n = 1, [16]), 1 application in COVID-19 (n = 1, [15]), and 1 application in Disease Management (n = 1, [2]). Table 4 reports the study reference, application name, type of voice assistants used, category, and description of each application.

4   Discussion

4.1   Study Limitations

In this systematic review, we conducted a thorough screening of 136 papers and identified 18 papers that presented qualitative evidence on the usability of voice assistants in healthcare. However, we acknowledge certain limitations in our approach. Firstly, our review relied on a limited number of databases to identify relevant studies, which may have constrained the breadth of our findings. To address this, we plan to expand our search to include additional databases in future studies. Secondly, we chose not to employ methods such as the snowball search or hand-searching, opting instead to focus on the database search strategy to obtain a comprehensive collection of articles spanning various aspects of healthcare. Nevertheless, we recognize that incorporating alternative search methods could provide valuable insights in future investigations. To ensure a comprehensive qualitative review of voice assistant usability, we recommend incorporating more assessments of user experience, as these technologies play an integral role in assisting individuals on a daily basis. While our review primarily focuses on the usability aspect, it provides an overview of the current state-of-the-art applications of voice assistants in healthcare and sets the stage for future research and advancements.

4.2   Challenges and Future of Voice Assistant in Healthcare

During the comprehensive process of full-text screening and data extraction, a notable observation emerged: the majority of studies investigated the challenges and limitations associated with voice assistants in healthcare, as well as the errors encountered by voice-based applications. Even though the first voice assistant was used in the early 1960s, the integration of voice assistants into people's daily life became more common within just the past decade [14]. Therefore, various errors exist in VA's algorithm design and comprehension level [17]. In the realm of EHR management, numerous studies have identified a significant

Table 4. Applications of Voice Assistants (Part I)

Study Ref.	Application Name	Type of VA	Category	Description
[15]	CovIoT	VA module developed within the application	COVID-19	An Arduino-based automatic hand sanitizer dispenser with integrated voice assistant and body monitoring feature.
[20]	Mycroft Skill for Hospital Triage	Mycroft	Hospital Operation	Using an open source voice assistant, Mycroft, to develop skills to manage hospital triage
[25]	SpeakHealth	Siri	Patient Care	A voice-enabled note-taking app for caregivers of children with special healthcare needs
[2]	Alexa Skill *Multiple Myeloma*	Alexa	Disease Management	Amazon Alexa voice assistant provides explanations for medical terms related to Multiple Myeloma disease, connections to support groups, and a quiz functionality.
[16]	Lumen	Alexa	Mood disorder management	A virtual voice-based coach and delivering 8 evidence-based and problem-solving sessions for patients with mood disorders.
[8]	Voice-enabled Healthcare System for Patients	Alexa and Google Assistant	Patient Care	A patient-focus voice application serves as a personal medical assistant and help patients with the monitoring of their body essential signs.
[7]	ACHO—Voice Assistant on Health and Care Offline	ACHO	Patient Care	A voice assistant facilitates treatment adherence among elderly adults in rural areas.
[12]	Voice Assistant and Touchscreen Operated Intelligent Wheelchair	Any commercial voice assistants	Patient Care	A voice assistant enabled wheelchair assists physically impaired people with ability to control without an active internet connection.
[3]	DocPal	Alexa	Hospital Operation	An EHR assistant in form of Amazon Alexa Skill assists health practitioners and complements the manual operation of EHR.
[24]	VoiceCare	VA module developed within the application	Patient Care	A wearable voice-interactive cognitive assistant on smartwatch for daily life healthcare

concern surrounding the storage and privacy of personal information and protected health information. These studies have shed light on the importance of addressing this issue to ensure the secure handling of sensitive data in healthcare settings [20]. At present, most commercial voice assistants have a strong possibility of not satisfying all of the requirements for the Health Insurance Portability and Accountability of 1996 (HIPAA) [19]. In addition, limitations exist in voice assistant applications based on the user's experience. Interacting with a voice assistant is not universally embraced, as some individuals may not find comfort in this mode of interaction. Furthermore, there are instances where people may actively avoid using voice assistants in public spaces due to feelings of embarrassment or shame [18].

Even though the performance of VA drastically increases over time, its AI software algorithm is still not at optimal accuracy yet. Studies on VA's comprehension level for recognizing medication names and with different accents reveal a difference in accuracy between 8–11%, which creates a gap for potential future improvements in algorithms of commercial voice assistants [22]. Furthermore, when dealing with information retrieval, VAs were reported to perform poorly in terms of source reliability and not always guarantee the accuracy of the information [17], which creates a gap for improvement in future studies. Another aspect that warrants future improvement is the speed of response exhibited by voice assistants. Notably, applications utilizing Google Assistant have reported slower response times, which may potentially impede timely and crucial responses in sensitive and urgent scenarios [12]. Addressing this issue would contribute to enhancing the overall efficiency and effectiveness of voice assistant technologies.

5   Conclusion

This systematic review critically examines the existing literature on the usability of voice assistants within the healthcare system, an area that has been relatively under-researched within the context of systematic reviews. The qualitative analysis conducted in this review reveals several significant categories where voice assistants play a crucial role in serving diverse populations in healthcare. However, it is important to acknowledge both the limitations of this review and the challenges faced by voice assistants in this domain. To comprehensively address all aspects of usability, future reviews would greatly benefit from incorporating studies that focus on the user's experience and the quality of voice assistants' algorithms specifically in healthcare settings. Given the extensive application of voice assistants in healthcare and the continuous advancement of VA technology, it is essential to place increased emphasis on training VA software to enhance its algorithmic capabilities, response speed, accuracy, voice recognition abilities, and comprehension levels. This will ensure that users in healthcare receive not only a pleasant but also a reliable and effective experience.

References

1. https://www.thinkwithgoogle.com/marketing-strategies/search/voice-search-mobile-use-statistics/
2. Baertsch, M.A., et al.: Convenient access to expert-reviewed health information via an alexa voice assistant skill for patients with multiple myeloma: development study. JMIR Cancer **8**(2), e35500 (2022). https://doi.org/10.2196/35500. https://cancer.jmir.org/2022/2/e35500
3. Bhatt, V., Li, J., Maharjan, B.: DocPal: a voice-based EHR assistant for health practitioners. In: 2020 IEEE International Conference on E-health Networking, Application & Services (HEALTHCOM), pp. 1–6 (2021). https://doi.org/10.1109/HEALTHCOM49281.2021.9399013
4. Bleu, N.: 44 latest voice search statistics for 2023, April 2023. https://bloggingwizard.com/voice-search-statistics/
5. Buteau, E., Lee, J.: Hey alexa, why do we use voice assistants? The driving factors of voice assistant technology use. Commun. Res. Rep. **38**, 1–10 (2021). https://doi.org/10.1080/08824096.2021.1980380
6. Bérubé, C., et al.: Voice-based conversational agents for the prevention and management of chronic and mental conditions: a systematic literature review. J. Med. Internet Res. **23** (2021). https://doi.org/10.2196/25933
7. David, C.C., Rivero Jiménez, B., Crespo, C., Jesús-Azabal, M., Garcia-Alonso, J., Mariano, L.: Treatment adherence in chronic conditions during ageing: uses, functionalities, and cultural adaptation of the assistant on care and health offline (ACHO) in rural areas. J. Pers. Med. **11**, 173 (2021). https://doi.org/10.3390/jpm11030173
8. Dojchinovski, D., Ilievski, A., Gusev, M.: Interactive home healthcare system with integrated voice assistant. In: 2019 42nd International Convention on Information and Communication Technology, Electronics and Microelectronics (MIPRO), pp. 284–288 (2019). https://doi.org/10.23919/MIPRO.2019.8756983
9. Faruk, L., Pal, D., Funilkul, S., Chan, J.: A systematic review of voice assistant usability: an ISO 9241-11 approach. SN Comput. Sci. **3**, 267 (2022). https://doi.org/10.1007/s42979-022-01172-3
10. Gerencer, T.: Top 10 ways to use voice assistants. https://www.hp.com/us-en/shop/tech-takes/top-10-ways-to-use-voice-assistants#:~:text=They're%20web%2Dconnected%20software,and%20even%20find%20lost%20phones
11. Gunathilaka, L.A.S.M., Weerasinghe, W.A.U.S., Wickramasinghe, I.N., Welgama, V., Weerasinghe, A.R.: The use of conversational interfaces in long term patient care. In: 2020 20th International Conference on Advances in ICT for Emerging Regions (ICTer), pp. 131–136 (2020). https://doi.org/10.1109/ICTer51097.2020.9325473
12. Sayied Haque, M.S., Tanvir Rahman, M., Tasin Khan, R., Shibli Kaysar, M.: Voice assistant and touch screen operated intelligent wheelchair for physically challenged people. In: Kaiser, M.S., Bandyopadhyay, A., Mahmud, M., Ray, K. (eds.) Proceedings of International Conference on Trends in Computational and Cognitive Engineering. AISC, vol. 1309, pp. 405–415. Springer, Singapore (2021). https://doi.org/10.1007/978-981-33-4673-4_32
13. Higgins, J.P., Thomas, J.: Cochrane Handbook for Systematic Reviews of Interventions. Wiley-Blackwell, Chichester (2020)
14. Hoy, M.: Alexa, Siri, Cortana, and more: an introduction to voice assistants. Med. Ref. Serv. Q. **37**, 81–88 (2018). https://doi.org/10.1080/02763869.2018.1404391

15. Jain, A., Prasad, J., De V. Velho, D.B.: covIoT: integrated patient monitoring and sanitization system. In: 2022 International Conference on Communication, Computing and Internet of Things (IC3IoT), pp. 1–6 (2022). https://doi.org/10.1109/IC3IOT53935.2022.9767863

16. Kannampallil, T., et al.: Design and formative evaluation of a virtual voice-based coach for problem-solving treatment: observational study. JMIR Form. Res. **6**, e38092 (2022). https://doi.org/10.2196/38092

17. Koh, M., Xie, Q., Wong, L., Yap, K.: Quality assessment of digital voice assistants on information provided in eating disorders and coexisting depression. Minerva Psychiatr. **62** (2021). https://doi.org/10.23736/S2724-6612.20.02073-7

18. Krey, M., Ramirez Garcia, R.: Voice assistants in healthcare: the patient's perception. In: 2022 8th International Conference on Information Management (ICIM), pp. 120–130 (2022). https://doi.org/10.1109/ICIM56520.2022.00029

19. Kumah-Crystal, Y., Pirtle, C., Whyte, H., Goode, E., Anders, S., Lehmann, C.: Electronic health record interactions through voice: a review, July 2018. https://doi.org/10.1055/s-0038-1666844

20. Montali, S., Lombardo, G., Mordonini, M., Tomaiuolo, M.: Voice assistants in hospital triage operations, vol. 2706, pp. 147–159 (2020). https://www.scopus.com/inward/record.uri?eid=2-s2.0-85095578981&partnerID=40&md5=c650a9270964ef04d2f759c99b7287ec, cited by: 0

21. Méndez Garduño, I., et al.: Smart homes as enablers for depression pre-diagnosis using PHQ-9 on HMI through fuzzy logic decision system. Sensors **21**, 21 (2021). https://doi.org/10.3390/s21237864

22. Palanica, A., Fossat, Y.: Medication name comprehension of intelligent virtual assistants: a comparison of Amazon Alexa, Google Assistant, and Apple Siri between 2019 and 2021. Front. Digit. Health **3** (2021). https://doi.org/10.3389/fdgth.2021.669971. https://www.frontiersin.org/articles/10.3389/fdgth.2021.669971

23. Pednekar, S., Dhirawani, P., Shah, R., Shekokar, N., Ghag, K.: Voice-based interaction for an aging population: a systematic review. In: 2023 3rd International Conference on Intelligent Communication and Computational Techniques (ICCT), pp. 1–8 (2023). https://doi.org/10.1109/ICCT56969.2023.10075801

24. Samyoun, S., Stankovic, J.: VoiceCare: a voice-interactive cognitive assistant on a smartwatch for monitoring and assisting daily healthcare activities. In: 2022 44th Annual International Conference of the IEEE Engineering in Medicine & Biology Society (EMBC), pp. 2438–2441 (2022). https://doi.org/10.1109/EMBC48229.2022.9871747

25. Sezgin, E., Oiler, B., Abbott, B., Noritz, G., Huang, Y.: "Hey Siri, help me take care of my child": a feasibility study with caregivers of children with special healthcare needs using voice interaction and automatic speech recognition in remote care management. Front. Publ. Health **10** (2022). https://doi.org/10.3389/fpubh.2022.849322. https://www.frontiersin.org/articles/10.3389/fpubh.2022.849322

26. Shade, M., Rector, K., Kupzyk, K.: Voice assistant reminders and latency of scheduled medication use in aging adults with pain: a feasibility study (preprint). JMIR Form. Res. **5** (2020). https://doi.org/10.2196/26361

27. Small, C.E., Nigrin, D., Churchwell, K., Brownstein, J.: What will health care look like once smart speakers are everywhere? October 2020. https://hbr.org/2018/03/what-will-health-care-look-like-once-smart-speakers-are-everywhere

28. Subhash, S., Srivatsa, P.N., Siddesh, S., Ullas, A., Santhosh, B.: Artificial intelligence-based voice assistant. In: 2020 Fourth World Conference on Smart

Trends in Systems, Security and Sustainability (WorldS4), pp. 593–596. IEEE (2020)

29. Tao, C., Li, J., Maharjan, B., Xie, B.: A personalized voice-based diet assistant for caregivers of Alzheimer's disease and related dementias (preprint). J. Med. Internet Res. **22** (2020). https://doi.org/10.2196/19897

30. Terzopoulos, G., Satratzemi, M.: Voice assistants and smart speakers in everyday life and in education. Inform. Educ. **19**(3), 473–490 (2020). https://doi.org/10.15388/infedu.2020.21

Gender Identity and Sexual Orientation Use in and Impact on LGBTQIA+ Healthcare

Taylor Schell Martinez(ID) and Charlotte Tang(✉)(ID)

University of Michigan-Flint, Flint, MI 48502, USA
{tschell,tcharlot}@umich.edu

Abstract. The LGBTQIA+ community has unique health experiences and needs that often go unmet by both healthcare providers and current health technologies because they are not being asked about their identity nor is their care being tailored to their unique health needs as LGBTQIA+ individuals. The purpose of this qualitative study was to improve patient care for the LGBTQIA+ community by identifying, through perceptions and experiences of LGBTQIA+ individuals, the challenges and barriers they experience when seeking health information and services. We discovered that there were several technological and societal improvements that could be made that would drastically improve their health experiences and accessibility while simultaneously alleviating the identified challenges and barriers. To improve healthcare accessibility and experiences for the LGBTQIA+ community, our study points to the need to use LGBTQIA+ gender identity in healthcare settings and technologies, training to create knowledgeable providers, a rating system to identify LGBTQIA+ competent providers and an associated national directory, a LGBTQIA+ health information repository, and improvements to social media to facilitate health information sharing.

Keywords: LGBTQIA+ · sexual orientation · gender identity · accessibility

1 Introduction

The understanding of sexual orientation and gender identity has evolved significantly over the years, with increasing recognition of diverse identities beyond the traditional binary frameworks. The LGBTQIA+ (Lesbian, Gay, Bisexual, Transgender, Queer, Intersex, and Asexual) community encompasses individuals who experience diverse sexual orientations and gender identities. The Institute of Medicine, Healthy People 2020, the Affordance Care Act, and the Joint Commission all considered the collection of sexual orientation and gender identity information in electronic health records (EMR) central to the quality assurance process [6], and highlighted the role of providers' knowledge of their patients' sexual orientation and gender identity in preventive health for improving access, quality of care, and outcomes.

Health disparities among LGBTQIA+ individuals have been well-documented. The LGBTQIA+ community constantly experiences exclusions, prejudice, and discrimination when seeking health information and services despite the gradually growing acceptance, [1, 18, 22, 26–29, 31, 35, 40]. They also experience more disparities in health than

D. Salvi et al. (Eds.): PH 2023, LNICST 572, pp. 402–419, 2024.
https://doi.org/10.1007/978-3-031-59717-6_26

the general population, such as higher rates of mental health issues, sexually transmitted infections including HIV, substance abuse, and missed reproductive cancer screenings including breast, cervical, and prostate [13, 19, 20, 23, 24, 30, 34, 38, 41], as well as lower life expectancies compared with their non-LGBTQIA+ counterparts [2, 14]. LGBTQIA+ individuals face numerous barriers when seeking healthcare, including fear of discrimination, lack of culturally competent providers, concerns about confidentiality, and delayed care. Discrimination against LGBTQIA+ individuals persists within health-care settings and is manifested in various forms such as refusal of care, verbal harassment, and differential treatment [18, 22, 27, 29, 36, 40]. The psychological and health effects of discrimination are well-documented, contributing to increased mental health issues, substance abuse, and reduced access to care [16, 31]. Despite the implementation of various legal protections and policies against LGBTQIA+ discrimination in healthcare to address these inequities, challenges persist. Delayed care due to these barriers has also contributed to adverse consequences on the health of LGBTQIA+ individuals [5, 28]. Factors contributing to the disparities in health, access to and quality of healthcare services among LGBTQIA+ individuals include providers' lack of LGBTQIA+ train-ing and knowledge, heterosexism (assumption that everyone is heterosexual), social stigma, and structural barriers such as limited or denied insurance coverage for gender-affirming treatment and differential treatment by providers [21]. As such, the Institute of Medicine (2011) emphasized the importance of addressing these disparities to ensure the well-being of LGBTQIA+ individuals. Yet, many of these health concerns have not been addressed by providers or by current health information technology.

Given the unique health needs of the LGBTQIA+ community and concerns related to their sexual orientation and gender identity which are also largely unaddressed, many LGBTQIA+ individuals constantly struggle with the abovementioned challenges in their healthcare. The collection in EMR and use of LGBTQIA+ identity information by providers could minimize the disparities and help address their unique health concerns [4, 6, 10, 11, 15, 26, 27]. Sexual orientation and gender identity information were also found to help facilitate the monitoring of risk factors and risk behaviors that contributed to negative health outcomes among this population [4]. A prior study conducted in an emergency room found that patients generally perceived the collection of sexual ori-entation and gender identity data allowed providers to better recognize their individual identity and improve therapeutic relationships [22]. Policy makers can also acquire a better understanding of the impacts of social policies and other factors on LGBTQIA+ individuals' physical and mental health with the collection of sexual orientation and gender identity data [16]. Yet, sexual orientation and gender identity are not considered part of the common clinical data set so providers are not required to collect these data [5, 7]. In fact, these data were often not collected because providers felt sexual orientation and gender identity not relevant in most clinical evaluations. Undoubtedly, this gap in perspectives could hinder patient-centered healthcare, particularly among the sexual and gender minority groups [22].

Online platforms offer a sense of anonymity, which can be beneficial for LGBTQIA+ individuals who may feel hesitant or uncomfortable discussing their health concerns in person [2]. The ability to seek information privately also allows individuals to gather knowledge, address concerns, and explore healthcare options at their own pace. Thus,

LGBTQIA+ individuals have increasingly turned to technology and the Internet as a resource for accessing health information that is relevant and sensitive to their unique needs [2, 7]. Online resources and social media platforms provide accessible and anonymous avenues for information-seeking [2, 5, 36, 38]. Moreover, LGBTQIA+ individuals often connect with others who share similar experiences or health concerns through online support networks. Other research has shown that LGBTQIA+ individuals are more likely to use HIT to address these gaps [5, 7, 24, 32, 34, 38, 42], even though there still remains huge gaps in the availability of online health information that exist for this vulnerable community and its subgroups [1, 12, 13, 16, 25, 33, 36, 40].

This paper contributes a better understanding of the challenges encountered by LGBTQIA+ in healthcare and reveals that gender identity can help shape health experiences and needs more so than sexual orientation. It also contributes several technological and societal strategies to improve health experiences for LGBTQIA+ community.

Table 1. Participant Demographics by Gender Identity Subgroups

Gender Identity (n)	Average Age	Age range	Race & Ethnicity							Marital Status			Sexual Orientation								Education						Employment						Health Insurance Coverage		Transportation Method	
			White	Black	Asian	Hispanic	Jewish	Mixed Race	Native America	Single	Married	Divorced	Heterosexual	Gay	Lesbian	Bisexual	Pansexual	Queer	Non-monosexual	Unknown	High School	Associates	Bachelors	Masters	PhD	J.D.	Full time	Part time	Self employed	Unemployed	Retired	Student	Insured	Uninsured	Owned vehicle	Public transport
Cis Men (12)	28.1	21-49	17%	58%	8%	-	-	8%	-	92%	8%	-	-	92%	-	8%	-	-	-	-	42%	-	58%	-	-	-	50%	17%	-	8%	-	25%	75%	25%	83%	17%
Cis Women (4)	33	30-37	50%	25%	-	25%	-	-	-	50%	25%	25%	-	-	75%	25%	-	-	-	-	-	-	25%	50%	25%	-	75%	25%	-	-	-	-	100%	-	75%	25%
Trans Men (3)	27.6	24-31	67%	33%	-	-	-	-	-	67%	33%	-	-	33%	33%	-	-	33%	-	-	33%	-	67%	-	-	-	33%	33%	-	33%	-	-	100%	-	67%	33%
Trans Women (6)	41.6	23-74	33%	33%	-	33%	-	-	-	67%	17%	17%	33%	-	33%	17%	-	17%	-	-	-	17%	83%	-	-	-	-	33%	50%	-	17%	-	100%	-	100%	-
Non-binary (4)	29.7	24-36	50%	-	50%	-	-	-	-	75%	25%	-	-	-	-	25%	50%	25%	-	-	-	-	50%	-	25%	25%	-	-	-	100%	-	-	100%	-	75%	25%

2 Methodology

Participants. Our participants were 29 self-identified LGBTQIA+ individuals living in the United States, and all were over the age of 18 (Table 1). They were recruited through direct emails and digital flyers posted on websites of local, regional, and national LGBTQIA+ organizations, centers, clubs, and support groups, as well as social media platforms. Our study received exempt IRB approval.

All the participants self-identified themselves into one of five commonly recognized gender identity subgroups – cisgender men, cisgender women, trans women, trans men, and non-binary people. Cisgender refers to those whose current sex matches the sex they were assigned at birth. Trans refers to those whose current sex does not match the one they were assigned at birth. Non-binary refers to those who do not identify their sex in a binary fashion and includes those who identified as non-binary, genderqueer, demigender, and those who were still figuring out their gender. Non-binary would have also included gender fluid and two spirited people had there been any in our sample.

Data Collection. In-depth semi-structured interviews were conducted with the participants to acquire a better understanding of how LGBTQIA+ individuals used technology to seek health information and services and to interact with their providers. All the interviews were conducted virtually on Zoom. Our participants were asked how they self-identified both their gender identity and sexual orientation, how they sought health information and services, about their interactions with their providers, and their healthcare experiences such as barriers and discrimination that they encountered. Each interview lasted 30 to 90 min and was recorded using the built-in recording function in Zoom with the participants' consent. The system-generated transcript was reviewed to ensure the accuracy and to anonymize the participants' identities.

Data Analysis. The qualitative data were analyzed thematically by affinity diagramming. The first author reviewed the transcripts to get familiar with the data, then examined the data to generate affinity notes which were then organized by themes that emerged. The data were initially analyzed based on three broad categories of gender identities – cisgender, trans, and non-binary. However, further examination of these three gender identity subgroups revealed the need to split the cisgender and the transgender subgroups into respective binary gender subgroups – male and female because of their unique health experiences and needs. Thus our findings are reported in accordance to five gender identity subgroups.

3   Findings

3.1   Gender Identity Impacts Healthcare Experience

Levels of 'Out' to Society Vary across Gender Identity Subgroups. For many LGBTQIA+ individuals, the decision to come 'out' to society as a member of the LGBTQIA+ community was a difficult one due to negative societal views, forcing many to hide their identity (a.k.s. staying 'in the closet'). '*Out*' or '*out of the closet*' refers to disclosing their LGBTQIA+ identity to other people.

A few participants did not feel comfortable enough to disclose their LGBTQIA+ identity to society in fear of being judged, marginalized, and discriminated against (Table 2). Some fit into multiple categories, e.g., they were out to their family and indirectly out to everyone or out to a selected few while their family was against their identity. None of the gender identity subgroups in our study were 100% fully out. Some participants were out to everyone, a few were indirectly out, some to only a small number of those they know, and others were out to no one. *Indirectly out* refers to those who had not directly announced their LGBTQIA+ identity to others but thought others assumed they were LGBTQIA+ from their behaviors. Many had conversations with their family to ascertain if they were against those who identified as LGBTQIA+, without necessarily having to disclose their own identity to their family.

The *cisgender men* we interviewed expressed a feeling of a heavy shame associated with their LGBTQIA+ identity and thus none were fully out. The other subgroups did not speak about feeling ashamed of their identities like the cisgender men did. The cisgender men only disclosed their LGBTQIA+ identity to certain people, most were out to a select trusted group of people – some were only to their friends, others to their family only, some were out to both their family and friends, only one was not out at all. P5 explained, *"the reason for not being very open to my friends and relatives and the society at large is because like fearing the stigmatization or the isolation that I could face."* Some had supportive families but for some cisgender men in our study, their family members were against their sexual orientation.

Among the **cisgender women** participants, only half considered themselves fully out, a quarter were out to family and friends while indirectly out to everyone else and the rest were not out at all. P28 discussed her being indirectly out, *"I feel like it's if I didn't have that conversation with you, it's pretty well known just through word of mouth and because of social media posts. I wear T shirts, I have the flag in my yard so like I'm not hiding or anything but it's not like, I had the conversation with every single person that I know."*

Unlike cisgender people, all trans people were out to some degree. 4/6 of the **trans women** in our study considered themselves fully out, 2/6 were out to a selected few who they trusted, one was out to their family, and another was out to their friends. Like trans women, 2/3 of the **trans men** also considered themselves out to everyone but 1/3 was out to just their family and friends.

The **trans people** we interviewed, both men and women, had the highest percentage of families who were against their trans identities – 3/9 regardless whether they identified as male or female. A trans woman explained what happened after disclosing that she was trans to her family, *"Daddy just wanted to kill me. I had to run from home just to save myself"* (P11). Some trans men said their families were also against their LGBTQIA+ identity as P21 shared, *"My father actually disowned me. She's [Mother] not okay with me being gay, but we still communicate. My family knows that but dislikes me for that."* This showed that if disclosing to one's own family could result in such an adverse response, it would certainly make trans people hesitant to disclose to other people, such as providers.

Our **non-binary** participants were out with different levels of outness for sexual orientation and gender identity. One-quarter were fully out, and another quarter were indirectly out with everyone. The other 2/4 were out in terms of sexual orientation, with half of them out to their family about their gender identity and the rest only out to a few people they carefully selected and trusted.

In summary, fear of discrimination, stigma, and marginalization continued to shape how 'out' many participants in our study were. Trans and non-binary people were more likely to disclose their LGBTQIA+ identity. This may be due to the often-visual nature of their physical transformations that occurred during gender transition and not conforming to gender norms and expectations associated with the sex they were assigned at birth. Despite being one of the most fully 'out' subgroups in our study, trans people's families were the most likely to be against their identity. None of the cisgender men was fully 'out', but it seems easier for this subgroup to hide their sexual orientation as it typically does not involve name change or physical transformations. In short, despite the growing acceptance of diversity, many participants still did not feel comfortable enough to disclose their LGBTQIA+ identity to society in fear of being judged, marginalized, and discriminated against (Table 6).

LGBTQIA+ Identities Largely Ignored in Healthcare. Many providers did not ask for LGBTQIA+ identities (Table 3), but most LGBTQIA+ participants would volunteer

Table 2. Levels of 'Out' to Society in General

	Out to everyone	Indirectly out to everyone	Family against	Out to family	Out to family & friends	Out to friends	Out to selected, trusted few	Not out
Cis Men (12)	-	8%	17%	17%	33%	58%		8%
Cis Women (4)	50%	25%	-	-	25%	-	-	25%
Trans Men (3)	67%	-	33%	-	33%	-	-	-
Trans Women (6)	67%	-	33%	17%	-	17%	33%	-
Non-binary (4)	75%	25%	-	25%	-	-	25%	-

Table 3. Disclosure and (Non)Use of LGBTQIA+ Identifiers

	Health provider asked about gender identity and sexual	Disclosed to health provider	Did not disclose to health	Did not due to fears of discrimination	Felt it was not important to	Health provider used in care	Was not used in care/acknowledged
Cis Men (12)	58%	67%	17%	17%	-	8.30%	8.30%
Cis Women (4)	25%	75%	25%	25%	25%	-	67%
Trans Men (3)	-	33%	-	33%	-	-	-
Trans Women (6)	17%	83%	17%	17%	-	80%	20%
Non-binary (4)	50%	75%	25%	25%	-	33%	33%

to give this information to their providers because they perceived it as important to their healthcare. Yet, providers often did not embrace the gender identity information in the patients' healthcare or in their interactions. This can potentially lead to patients' perception of discrimination, which could lead to negative outcomes.

When interacting with their providers, 7 *cisgender men* were asked about their sexual orientation and gender identity. Even when not asked, 8 volunteered their sexual orientation information to their provider. Yet, only 1 of those cisgender men who disclosed their sexual orientation said the information was used or acknowledged in their healthcare encounters. Fears of discrimination kept 2 of the cisgender men from disclosing their sexual orientation to their providers. Cisgender men were the second least likely to disclose their identity to their provider, second to trans men (Table 3).

Table 4. Discrimination Experienced in Health Setting

	Misgendered	Deadnamed	Discriminated due to sexual orientation	Discriminated due to gender identity	Discriminated by staff
	-	-	25%	-	-
	-	-	100%	-	-
	33%	33%	33%	-	33%
	17%	17%	17%	33%	17%
	50%	-	-	50%	25%

Table 5. LGBTQIA+ Friendly vs. Knowledgeable Primary Care Providers

	LGBTQIA+ friendly	LGBTQIA+ knowledgeable
	75%	75%
	50%	50%
	100%	67%
	67%	33%
	75%	50%

Table 6. Health Information Sources Used by LGBTQIA+

Health Professionals	Only if serious ailment	Internet	Due to privacy concerns	Social media	Enjoy social aspect
58%	14%	83%	25%	25%	17%
100%	25%	100%	-	25%	100%
67%	50%	67%	-	-	-
67%	0%	67%	17%	67%	50%
100%	50%	100%	25%	75%	67%

Of the 4 *cisgender women*, only 1 was asked about their sexual orientation and gender identity by providers, whereas the other 3 disclosed their sexual orientation to their provider either after being asked or by volunteering. Yet, 2/3 said it was never used or acknowledged in their care in any way. Such lack of use of LGBTQIA+ identifiers could have detrimental consequences like what happened to P29 in a very important moment when their spouse and the non-gestational parent were not being treated as such during the delivery of their second child. *"They didn't let [spouse's name] hold the baby, they didn't let her make decisions for the baby, she said, because she went over expecting to hold the baby and they said, oh no we give her to the mother first. So, for her it was a much different experience that second time and part of that's on us because we could have said hey this is my wife. She's the baby's other parent, you know, but I didn't know I needed to say those things until I had the experience, where they didn't know and I didn't say anything."*

Being afraid of discrimination made some of the cisgender women to not disclose their sexual orientation to their provider. P28 described her unpleasant experience after she disclosed that she was sexually active with both sexes: *"It got awkward and I don't know if that was just the nurse herself, or like the first person she's met that has answers like that or something. But suddenly it seemed like I was wrong or like I should feel ashamed and then, like all these questions followed that almost seemed like judgmental."* One cisgender woman felt disclosing gender identity to the provider was important but sexual orientation was not important for shaping health care.

Only 1 of the 6 *trans women* in our study had providers ask them about their sexual orientation and gender identity, while the others volunteered this information to their provider – more than any other subgroup. Many trans women described the medical importance of disclosing. For example, P1 explained: "[I am] *what any other 75-year-old woman would be except I have a prostate and the doctor needs to know that to properly diagnose me, to properly treat me.*" For some trans women in the study, explicitly stating their gender identity was the only way to signify their trans status to the provider because they did not physically present themselves as the gender they identified as. However, fear of discrimination has kept one trans women from disclosing their identity to providers, which could have adverse impact on the healthcare received.

Of the 5 trans women who had disclosed their LGBTQIA+ identity to their providers, 4 said it was used in their care and they felt the information was important for facilitating their health care. Their heavy use of health care services was the highest among all the subgroups. This was likely due to the medical treatments, like hormone replacement therapy and gender affirming procedures, needed by trans women to physically present themselves as and transition to female.

Providers did not ask any of our 3 *trans men* participants about their sexual orientation or gender identity which could explain why only 1 disclosed their gender identity and sexual orientation to their providers. They were the least likely of all subgroups to disclose this information. The reason that 2 did not disclose was again due to fear of discrimination. They worried that the LGBTQIA+ identity information collected by providers could be used to discriminate against them in attitude and/or care received. None of the trans men interviewed felt their provider used their LGBTQIA+ identity information to tailor the health care plans for their specific needs.

Two *non-binary* participants were asked about their sexual orientation and gender identity by their providers, the second most frequently asked of all the subgroups. Of the 2 who were not asked, 1 volunteered to disclose their LGBTQIA+ identity whereas the other withheld the information because they assumed the provider was not LGBTQIA+ friendly or knowledgeable, and feared discriminated.

Unfortunately, as we saw with the other subgroups, despite 3/4 disclosing their non-binary identity to their provider, only 1 of them said their non-binary identity was acknowledged and used in their care. P23 commented, "*It matters in a health professional yeah even if you're not talking specifically about LGBT related health issues, it's still matters that the person who's becoming very intimate with your body respects your pronouns and your identities and all of that and understands how it could affect the way that you're feeling about the language that they use with you and things like that.*"

Although many participants were not asked, they still volunteered to disclose their LGBTQIA+ identity to providers with the hopes that it would be used in their care. Unfortunately, it was largely not used to improve care or interpersonal interactions. Trans women were the subgroup that their gender identity was used the most often during their care while the other participants often felt ignored, marginalized, and discriminated against when providers assumed the patients fit in a generic binary and heteronormative classification.

Discrimination Against LGBTQIA+ Individuals Prevalent. Discrimination was widely experienced by many participants in healthcare settings and society in general. The percentage who had experienced discrimination was deeply impacted by their gender identity and sexual orientation, as shown in Table 4.

Three of the 12 *cisgender men* had experienced discrimination by a provider, which represented the lowest percentage among all the gender identity subgroups. This low number may be because only 1/12 of cisgender men's providers did not acknowledge their identity, possibly making them less likely to be discriminated. Of the cisgender men, 2/12 had not disclosed their sexual orientation to providers due to fears of discrimination.

All the *cisgender women* in our study had experienced discrimination from a provider in their life due to their sexual orientation. P29 explained: "*Like the whole you're not on birth control, how are you so certain you're not pregnant and then you can just tell that the person receiving the information is not comfortable with the information you've just shared and then the room gets awkward and you're alone in a room with this person. And it's a four-by-four room so it's more been I guess those kinds of exchanges and interactions more than outward something that's been said or done, if that makes sense?".*

Some cisgender women in our study thought it was out-and-out discrimination; others felt they were unintentional, awkward examples of the person's heteronormative biases. As P9 described, *"[It] didn't even cross their mind that could have been the reason why I wasn't using birth control, because it wasn't necessary."* Unfortunately, this was a very common experience for our cisgender women participants and one that led many to seek out LGBTQIA+ competent providers with the hope to avoid these scenarios.

One of the 3 *trans men* had been discriminated against by their providers and another one by the staff of a 'LGBTQIA friendly' provider. P15, a trans man, had been deadnamed (called by name associated with previous gender) and misgendered (identified as wrong gender) resulting in insurance coverage issues. Deadnaming and misgendering incidents have led to health care accessibility issues, lengthy battles with insurance companies, care denials, and additional costs for the patients.

Many *trans women* in our study received healthcare services for their identity. Yet, 2/6 of them was discriminated against due to their gender identity, 1/6 because of their sexual orientation, 1/6 had been misgendered, and 1/6 had been deadnamed. One trans woman (P19) was both deadnamed and misgendered by the hospital staff and anesthesiologist while undergoing gender reassignment surgery. P19 detailed her experience, *"As a trans person, it's basically like these are the things and the injustices and violations that you have to deal with in order to get the care that other people would get and it, you know, it sucks."* Such experience illustrated how the lack of inclusion and respect for these diverse identities can seriously impact their healthcare.

The gender identity information provided by *non-binary* people in our study was often disregarded or even used against them, as 2/4 had been misgendered and the other 2/4 had providers discriminate against them because of their gender identity. Even at specialized LGBTQIA+ health facilities, genders and pronouns were assumed according to the conventional binary gender identities, instead of using the ones in the medical records, thus resulting in misgendering. In fact, those who did not experience discrimination was because they had not disclosed their identity.

It is thus very unfortunate that discrimination against LGBTQIA+ individuals remains common in healthcare settings and society at large. In our study, all the cisgender women, 2/4 of the non-binary participants, 3/9 of trans people and 3/12 of cisgender men had been discriminated against. These adverse experiences LGBTQIA+ individuals encounter in society and in healthcare settings can have a significant impact on their interpersonal interactions, the quality of healthcare they receive, and their experiences in other settings such as schools, social clubs, and community at large.

LGBTQIA+ Friendly vs. LGBTQIA+ Knowledgeable. Many cisgender people in our study felt their primary care provider was both LGBTQIA+ friendly and knowledgeable. Yet trans and non-binary participants feel differently. They explained that being

LGBTQIA+ friendly did not necessarily mean the provider was LGBTQIA+ knowledgeable and knew how to interact with or provide health care to LGBTQIA+ people (Table 5).

Most cisgender men and half of cisgender women felt that their primary care providers were both LGBTQIA+ friendly and knowledgeable even though their providers did not inquire about or used proper LGBTQIA+ identifiers in the care plan. All trans men in our study felt their primary care provider was LGBTQIA+ friendly but only 2/3 perceived them being knowledgeable about their LGBTQIA+ health needs.

Four of 6 trans women felt that their primary care provider was LGBTQIA+ friendly and 3/6 thought they were knowledgeable. Unfortunately, 2/6 of the trans women interviewed felt they had to educate their health provider, as P2 commented, *"about what being trans is and where I fit within the spectrum of LGBT"* and how their trans identity related to their needed health care.

On the other hand, non-binary people thought that their primary care providers were LGBTQIA+ friendly but fell short in being knowledgeable about individual LGBTQIA+ subgroups and their respective health needs. Some discussed the struggle they faced in finding providers who were knowledgeable about the health needs of less common LGBTQIA+ identities. For example, P20 desired for providers who were *"savvy with trans folks especially who are not just trans women and trans man or like even with any kind of other sexual orientations, bisexuality, pansexuality, the asexual aromantic spectrum."*

It thus appears that providers who are LGBTQIA+ friendly are not necessarily knowledgeable about how to interact with and provide adequate care to the LGBTQIA+ community and the various, unique subgroups. This lack of knowledge may explain some of the (un)intended discrimination experienced by many of our participants as discussed in the previous subsection. This lack of knowledge also requires some to not only take an active role in advocating for their own health needs but also to educate their provider about their specific needs so that they can get the care that they need.

Gaps between Health Insurance Coverage and LGBTQIA+ Healthcare Needs. All of our participants, except 3 cisgender men, had health insurance (Table 1). Yet, many participants found it difficult to seek LGBTQIA+ knowledgeable providers who were covered by their insurance plan. As such, some participants had to pay out of their pocket to ensure they could see a LGBTQIA+ knowledgeable provider. Many also discussed the struggles of having to cover the healthcare costs, with or without insurance coverage and being employed full-time.

Cisgender men were the least insured subgroup in our study with only 9/12 insured. The lack of insurance may be due to cisgender men's lower employment rate (Table 1). In fact, 6/12 of the cisgender men found it challenging to cover healthcare cost in recent years. Hence some avoided care altogether or had family members help cover the cost.

All the *cisgender women* in the study discussed how the costs had made accessing care difficult, even with health insurance. P28 explained that cost was always a key consideration that determined whether healthcare was sought or not. *"I don't like going to the doctor in person, a lot, because I get a big fat bill. I have insurance, but it's not great and so, if it's something that I can just kind of overlook or get over, then I will I'll choose to do that."*

Half of the *trans women* subgroup considered health care cost prohibitive. The other half had to borrow money to cover copays. Trans women typically had to engage in long battles with insurance companies to have gender affirming procedures and therapies covered, and often still had to pay considerable amount out of pocket or they had to forego care altogether. P1 described her experience in appealing for insurance coverage for the medical procedures she needed, *"Fighting against the fact that Medicare would not provide gynecological procedures to me because my gender status at the time was not female. The codes existed. They had the procedures documented for women. But not for transgender individuals."* P2 was also denied voice therapy to feminize her voice because *"coverage only is if you've lost your voice completely or if your voice is damaged from surgery"*.

Some *trans* people in our study explained how insurance limited which providers were covered and sometimes those were not qualified providers for their specific LGBTQIA+ needs. For some, the only accessible surgeons on their insurance plans had higher revision rates for gender affirming surgeries, like vaginoplasty and phalloplasty, requiring the patient to have additional surgeries to repair the work that was previously done. This would undoubtedly impact how and when they were able to transition successfully. As a result, some who were desperate for their body to match their identity had to take higher risks with subpar or inexperienced surgeons, which undoubtedly increased the odds of additional revision surgeries or postponed care until they could access more qualified LGBTQIA+ healthcare professionals. Others discussed the red tape that referrals were often needed for each step of the transitioning, thus prolonging the time the process took and increasing the costs. Some in our study had insurance plans that would not cover gender transitioning. In order to receive the healthcare they needed, they had to pay out of their pocket for the gender affirming care, including masculinizing or feminizing chest surgeries, genital reconstruction surgeries, facial reconstructive surgeries, voice surgery and voice therapy, leading to substantial financial burden.

One-third of *trans men* in the study had been deadnamed and misgendered, for some it caused health care accessibility issues, lengthy battles with insurance companies, care denials, and additional costs for patients. P15 described how this complicated things for him: *"The fact that legal name and preferred name are different than the whole insurance situation gets twisted in and thrown and I'm fighting a whole big like mess with medicine and everything right now, because the clinic I was at has me listed as female and insurance doesn't want to provide testosterone."* Many trans and non-binary people also discussed how their insurance plans often did not cover the LGBTQIA+ knowledgeable providers they had found, leaving them to pay out of pocket to receive safe and quality care from a knowledgeable provider.

Non-binary participants were the second most frequently affected by cost; 3/4 cited cost as a challenge to accessing care. Some explained how they considered if the health issue was worth the financial burden it might impose on them before seeking care. *"There's always this like question where I'm like I don't know how much this is going to cost and I don't really want to like undergo this, even if it's like 10 min to only get a surprise bill for like several hundred dollars" (P20).* Some had to forgo needed care due to cost constraints despite their full-time employment, insurance coverage, and higher education level, as most were still living paycheck to paycheck and healthcare costs could have long term impacts on their economic status. Others went into debt when getting the care they needed, *"I did, for the most part, get the care that I needed it was just it just it came at a cost of having to pay back some money that I didn't have at the time (P24)."* Unexpectedly, some participants said they had been charged extra fees by their providers for asking LGBTQIA+ health information questions during routine exams, making them refrain from asking these questions during appointments in fear of being charged additional fees.

In short, most participants struggled with healthcare costs, even with insurance coverage and full-time employment. Many weighed the cost and benefits of receiving care for their health concerns prior to getting care. Thus, many had to forego the needed care while some went into debt or had to borrow money to cover the costs. Some trans participants had to resort to substandard providers for their gender affirming care they desperately needed. Some were willing to pay out of their pocket to see LGBTQIA+ friendly and knowledgeable providers even though the services were not covered by their health insurance.

3.2 LGBTQIA+ Health Information Seeking

Given their unique needs, LGBTQIA+ individuals use different resources to seek relevant health information and they encountered a variety of challenges in the course of seeking relevant health information.

Online Health Information Caused Anxiety. As with the general population, another common issue experienced was the amount of information and the alarming results returned, leaving many participants to question the trustworthiness of the results. A few cisgender men mentioned that they often struggled to decide what health information was accurate and what was not. One-third of cisgender men desired a seal of accuracy that could be used to authenticate the LGBTQIA+ health information they found online. Half the cisgender women and half the non-binary participants felt that online information often returned alarming, sometimes even fatal, health diagnoses even for mild symptoms, leaving them to question the information's credibility. As such, many had to change their search behaviors, as P27 described, *"I had to switch when I was younger. I would get myself into some anxious moments or something like that happen. I would just look up a sentence and weird stuff will come back, and I would drive myself crazy."* Only 1/3 of trans women have encountered scary or weird results while searching for health information online.

Health Literacy and Jargon Complicated Health Information Seeking. Non-binary participants were the only subgroup that mentioned how health jargon and literacy further complicated the process of finding health information. P27 explained, *"One of the big issues with online health information is probably just health literacy. People don't have the language to understand what they're reading, which is where some of the more verified sources can lose people. It's jargon."* Moreover, a few non-binary participants had trouble finding the correct terms to identify one's own identity. *"Looking back at my childhood like that makes so much sense now that I have these words to explain with what I've been feeling my whole life" (P23)*. Without proper identity language, many had no idea how to express their feelings or experiences, as P20 explained, *"I didn't* *know there was a missing puzzle piece, but then when I found it, I was like okay, a lot of things make sense."*

Fragmented LGBTQIA+ Health Information. Half of the trans women, half of the cisgender women and a few cisgender men in our study struggled with the amount of health information available online, but in different ways. P1 commented that *"one of the rare instances where more is not better"* whereas P12, a cisgender man, explained, *"compared to other health topics, before you finish typing, suggestions are already there, but for our community, it's not that easy [to find LGBTQIA+ health information]"*. Meanwhile, a few non-binary participants found health information too scattered and not centralized but unlike the other subgroups, none mentioned too much information to sort through.

Evidence-Based Subgroup-Specified Health Information Needed. Many people in the study (5/12 of cisgender men, 3/4 of cisgender women, 1/6 of trans women, and 2/4 of non-binary people) desired for a LGBTQIA+ health information repository similar to the popular WebMD and Mayo Clinic websites to improve access to credible health information. In addition, many of our participants (1/3 of cisgender men, 2/4 of cisgender women, 1/6 of trans women, 1/3 of trans men, and 4/4 of non-binary participants) would like access to evidence-based, niche health information for LGBTQIA+ individuals. Half of non-binary participants also wanted the health information to be easy to understand. P24 desired *"to have the information be displayed in a way that is easy to read and doesn't require like previous medical knowledge."* P5's statement *"each group of people have different matters"* helped explain why 2/4 of the non-binary people and 2/12 of cisgender men participants both wanted health information specific to their respective gender identity subgroups instead of having only generic LGBTQIA+ health information.

LGBTQIA+ Competent Providers in Dire Need

Directory of LGBTQIA+ Knowledgeable Provider. Our participants found it difficult to identify LGBTQIA+ competent providers. All our non-binary and 3/4 of the cisgender women participants discussed the need for a national directory of LGBTQIA+ friendly and/or knowledgeable providers. P20 had even tried to create one of their own, *"[I] wanted to work on making a more thorough queer and trans people of color health provider directory that could also include alternative or holistic medical providers because there wasn't really anything like that that exists."*

Training LGBTQIA+ Competent Providers. Half of the cisgender female participants wanted additional training for providers to improve their ability to interact with and care for the LGBTQIA+ community. One trans woman wanted providers to be trained better on how to care for and interact with trans individuals specifically. P19 explained, *"I do have a different physiology and things have happened to me and my body that would not happen to a cisgendered woman and that's important for your health care provider to know but they should be educated on how to handle that properly, and what that means, and to not treat us as if we're like some other."*

Increase Awareness of LGBTQIA+ Competency. Several cisgender women suggested the creation of a universal symbol for LGBTQIA+ inclusive health facilities and professionals to make navigating health care not only easier but also safer for the community. The iconography and medical information a health facility or professional displayed in their space, both in-person and virtual, and the organizations they were associated with has helped 2/4 of cisgender women determine how LGBTQIA+ friendly and knowledgeable the providers or facilities were. As pointed out by P28, *"If you have a sign basically that says that you are welcome and we're not going to judge you, it just feels so much better. It makes all the difference"* and *"There were rainbows on the bulletin board and workers had rainbow pins, I felt instantly welcomed."*

Overall, all sexual orientations were represented in the study. Sexual orientation played a large part in the health experience of cisgender people, while gender identity, rather than their sexual orientation, was key to shaping trans and non-binary participants' experiences.

4   Discussion

Foster Use of LGBTQIA+ Identity Information. Our research found that patients desired nuanced LGBTQIA+ identifiers to be collected and used in healthcare settings to improve patient care. Providing a more robust choice list and fill-in options for gender identity (and sexual orientation) would make the electronic health records more inclusive for LGBTQIA+ individuals. However, simply collecting gender identity information would not improve patient care. This information needs to be used by providers and institutions with their patients to shape care plans and provide holistic, inclusive care. Given the prevalent non-collection and/or non-use of the identifiers, research should be conducted with health care providers to better understand the underlying reasons and the challenges they encountered when interacting with and addressing LGBTQIA+ patients. This improved understanding can help policy makers to promote the use of LGBTQIA+ identifiers, which may facilitate access to health information and services specific to LGBTQIA+ subgroups.

Develop LGBTQIA+ Provider Competency Classification and Directory. To achieve inclusive medicine, it is important to start from the ground up by integrating LGBTQIA+ knowledge in medical education. Moreover, we believe it would be useful to design and develop a LGBTQIA+ competency classification system using inputs from LGBTQIA+ community and providers with regard to qualities a competent LGBTQIA+ provider should possess. With the proposed competency classification system, we further recommend the development of a national directory of LGBTQIA+ knowledgeable health care providers. With the growing acceptance and use of recommender systems, we further recommend a LGBTQIA+ knowledge rating system to allow patients to quickly share the perceived experience and knowledge level of their provider. Collectively, these enhancements can potentially help LGBTQIA+ individuals access providers who could provide them with the needed care and help minimize discriminatory encounters while seeking healthcare.

Create LGBTQIA+ Health Information Repository and Interactive Website. Many of our participants discussed the need for a centralized repository with credible health information for different subgroups of the LGBTQIA+ community to facilitate easy access to needed, often unique, health information. Many participants suggested that a user-friendly, trustworthy, and easily accessible LGBTQIA+ focused health website, similar to WedMD or Mayo Clinic Online designed for the general population would greatly benefit the unique LGBTQIA+ community.

Scaffolding Social Media to Facilitate Sharing and Retrieval of Health Information. Our participants frequently used social media to seek and share specific and potentially sensitive health information but the design of existing social media falls short in supporting the sharing of often personal and at times sensitive health information. We thus suggest that current social media tools should be scaffolded with enhanced features for sharing private and sensitive health information, for example, by using stronger encryption algorithms and efficient search and sorting mechanisms to facilitate data retrieval amidst the large volume of social data accumulated over time.

Limitations. This study was limited by its small sample size which became more apparent when the participants were classified into five gender identity subgroups. Moreover, the sampling method used was not truly random, thus resulting in considerable demographic differences between our sample and the US general population in terms of race, ethnicity, age, and education attainment level. Our study sample was very young, well-educated, had higher rates of insurance coverage, and represented higher rates of people of color when compared to the Unites States national averages. These demographic skews were likely due to our use of digital media for recruitment and for conducting the interviews.

5 Conclusion

Healthcare providers' and technology designers' not collecting and/or using gender identity information has huge impacts on the LGBTQIA+ subgroups' experience with health care, as revealed by our participants. Finding health information specific to individual subgroups as well as more broadly, the LGBTQIA+ community is challenging because many do not know where to find accurate LGBTQIA+ health information. Additionally, LGBTQIA+ individuals generally perceive the healthcare setting as an unwelcoming or unsafe space for their health needs and much research is needed prior to seeing a provider or facility to minimize negative experiences. Discrimination in healthcare settings is still commonly experienced by the LGBTQIA+ community, either by providers, their staff, and/or other patients. Even when asked, many LGBTQIA+ individuals choose not to disclose their LGBTQIA+ identity to providers in fear of being discriminated against. Not being able to openly discuss LGBTQIA+ health issues with their provider leaves many unanswered health questions, and likely unresolved issues as well.

The lack of use of gender identity and sexual orientation by providers normalizes and perpetuates exclusion from healthcare settings and broader mainstream culture. Thus, many LGBTQIA+ individuals feel that providers consider heterosexual and cisgender being the norm. Oftentimes, they must note their gender identity and/or sexual orientation in the margins, because of the lack of appropriate identity options on health forms. The fear of bias and discrimination as well as personal feelings of shame and worries of stigma associated with their own identity cause many to not disclose to providers even when asked, which may negatively impact their healthcare.

Finding a knowledgeable LGBTQIA+ provider is difficult, even more so to find one covered by their insurance. Our participants found many providers uneducated on LGBTQIA+ terminology other than gay, lesbian, bisexual, and trans. Many providers have trouble navigating the clinical trajectory for LGBTQIA+ patients including birth control, hormone replacement therapies, and gender affirming surgeries. Instead of reaching out to peer providers, many turn to their patients for education during appointments such as to define and explain identity terms and respective health needs. Thus, the patients are essentially providing their own care in relation to their LGBTQIA+ identity. Hence, both technology designers and health care practitioners and institutions should work together to provide LGBTQIA+ individuals better access to health information and care.

References

1. AIChE: AIChE Diversity Report Highlights Gaps in Inclusion, pp. 4–5. CEP (2019)
2. Augustaitis, L., Merrill, L., Gamarel, K.E., Haimson, O.L.: Online transgender health information seeking: facilitators, barriers, and future directors. In: Proceedings of SIGCHI Conference on Human Factors in Computing Systems (2021)
3. Banks, C.: The Cost of Homophobia: literature review on the human impact of homophobia in Canada. Gay and Lesbain Health Services (2003)
4. Bosse, J.D., Leblanc, R.G., Jackman, K., Bjarnadottir, R.I.: Benefits of implementing and improving collection of sexual orientation and gender identity data in electronic health records. Comput. Inform. Nurs. **36**(6), 267–274 (2018)
5. Cahill, S., Baker, K., Deutsch, M.B., Keatley, J., Makadon, H.J.: Inclusion of Sexual Orientation and Gender Identity in Stage 3 meaningful use guidelines: a huge step forward for LGBT health. LGBT Health **3**(2), 100–102 (2015)
6. Cahill, S., Makadon, H.: Sexual orientation and gender identity data collection in clinical settings and in electronic health records: a key to ending LGBT health disparities. LGBT Health **1**(1), 34–41 (2014)
7. CDC: Collecting Sexual Orientation and Gender Identity Information. Centers for Disease Control and Prevention. https://www.cdc.gov/hiv/clinicians/transforming-health/health-care-providers/collecting-sexual-orientation.html. Accessed 20 July 2023
8. DaHaan, S., Euper, L.E., Magee, J.C., Bigelow, L., Mustanski, B.S.: The interplay between online and offline explorations of identity, relationships, and sex: a mixed methods study with LGBT youth. J. Sex Res. **50**(5), 421–434 (2013)
9. Dahlhamer, J.M., Galinsky, A.M., Joestl, S.S., Ward, B.W.: Sexual orientation and health information technology use: a nationally representative study of U.S. adults. LGBT Health **4**(2), 121–129 (2017)
10. Dichter, M.E., Ogden, S.N.: The challenges presented around collection of patient sexual orientation and gender identity information for reduction of health disparities. Med. Care **57**(12), 945–948 (2019)
11. Donald, C., Ehrenfeld, J.M.: The opportunity for medical systems to reduce health disparities among lesbian, gay, bisexual, transgender and intersex patients. J. Med. Syst. **39**(178), 1–7 (2015)
12. Faulkner, S.L., Lannutti, P.J.: Representations of lesbian and bisexual women's sexual and relational health in online video and text-based sources. Comput. Hum. Behav. **63**, 916–921 (2016)
13. Forsberg, H., Eliason, M.J.: Healthcare providers' pregnancy prevention counseling of trans and non-binary assigned female at birth (TNB/AFAB) patients. J. Homosex. **69**, 1–28 (2020)

14. Grant, J.M., Mottet, L.A., Tanis, J.: Injustice at every turn: A report of the National Transgender Discrimination Survey. National LGBTQ Task Force (2011)
15. Grasso, C., McDowell, M.J., Goldhammer, H., Keuroghlian, A.S.: Planning and implementing sexual orientation and gender identity data collection in electronic health records. J. Am. Med. Inform. Assoc. **26**(1), 66–70 (2019)
16. Hatzenbuehler, M.L., O'Cleirigh, C., Grasso, C., Mayer, K., Safren, S., Bradford, J.: Effect of same-sex marriage laws on health care use and expenditures in sexual minority men: a quasi-natural experiment. Am. J. Public Health **102**(2), 285–291 (2012)
17. Hawkins, B.W., Morris, M., Nguyen, T., Siegel, J., Vardell, E.: Advancing the conversation: next steps for lesbian, gay, bisexual, trans, and queer (LGBTQ) health sciences librarianship. J. Med. Libr. Assoc. **105**(4), 316–327 (2017)
18. Holmes, J.J.: More anti-LGBTQ laws have been passed in the last year than any other time in American history. https://www.lgbtqnation.com/2021/05/anti-lgbtq-laws-passed-last-year-time-american-history/. Accessed 10 May 2021
19. Howard, S.D., Lee, K.L., Nathan, A.G., Wenger, H.C., Chin, M.H., Cook, S.C.: Healthcare experiences of transgender people of color. J. Gen. Intern. Med. **10**(34), 2068–2074 (2019)
20. Hsieh, N., Ruther, M.: Despite increased insurance coverage, nonwhite sexual minorities still experience disparities in access to care. Health Aff. **36**(10), 1786–1794 (2017)
21. Institute of Medicine: The Health of Lesbian, Gay, Bisexual, and Transgender People: Building a foundation for better understanding. National Academies Press (US) (2011)
22. Kodadek, L.M., et al.: Collecting sexual orientation and gender identity information in the emergency department: the divide between patient and provide perspectives. Emerg. Med. J. **36**, 136–141 (2019)
23. Laoch, A., Holmes, C.M.: Serving transgender clients in the digital age. J. LGBT Issues Couns. **12**(3), 193–208 (2018)
24. Lee, J.H., Giovenco, D., Operario, D.: Patterns of health information technology use according to sexual orientation among us adults aged 50 and older: findings from a national representative sample - national health interview survey 2013–2014. J. Health Commun. **22**, 666–671 (2017)
25. Martinez, T.S.: Designing technology to support health information and services seeking for the LGBTQIA+ community. Thesis, University of Michigan Flint (2022)
26. Martinez, T.S., Tang, C.: Design implications for health technology to support LGBTQ+ community: a literature review. In: International Conference on Pervasive Computing Technologies for Healthcare, pp. 367–370 (2020)
27. Martinez, T.S., Tang, C.: The impact of COVID-19 on LGBTQIA+ individuals' technology use to seek health information and services. In: International Conference on Pervasive Computing Technologies for Healthcare, vol. 431, pp. 53–70 (2022)
28. Mayer, K.K., Bradford, J., Makadon, H.J., Stall, R., Goldhammer, H., Landers, S.: Sexual and Gender Minority Health: what we know and what needs to be done. Am. J. Public Health **98**(6), 989–995 (2008)
29. McConnell, E.A., Clifford, A., Korpak, A.K., Phillips, G., II.: Identity, victimization, and support: Facebook experiences and mental health among LGBTQ youth. Comput. Hum. Behav. **76**, 237–244 (2017)
30. McKay, B.: Lesbian, gay, bisexual, and transgender health issues, disparities, and information resources. Med. Ref. Serv. Q. **30**(4), 393–401 (2011)
31. Meyer, I.H.: Prejudice, Social Stress, and Mental Health in Lesbian, Gay, and Bisexual Populations: conceptual issues and research evidence. Psychol. Bull. **129**(5), 674–697 (2003)
32. Mitchell, K.J., Ybarra, M.L., Korchmaros, J.D., Kosciw, J.G.: Accessing sexual health information online: use, motivations and consequences for youth with different sexual orientations. Health Educ. Res. **29**(1), 147–157 (2014)
33. Morse, B., et al.: Co-design of the transgender health information resource: web-based participatory design. J. Particip. Med. **15**, e38078 (2023)

34. Mustanski, B., Lyons, T., Garcia, S.C.: Internet use and sexual health of young men who have sex with men: a mixed-methods study. Arch. Sex. Behav. **40**(2), 289–300 (2011)
35. NCTQ: 2015 U.S. Transgender Survey: Michigan State Report. National Center for Transgender Equality, Washington, DC (2017)
36. Patterson, S.P., Hilton, S., Flowers, P., McDaid, L.M.: What are the barriers and challenges faced by adolescents when searching for sexual health information on the internet? Implications for policy and practice from a qualitative study. Sex. Transm. Infect. **95**(6), 462–467 (2019)
37. Pereira, G.C., Baranauskas, M.C.C.: Supporting people on fighting lesbian, gay, bisexual, and transgender (LGBT) prejudice: a critical codesign process. In: Proceedings of the XVI Brazilian Symposium on Human Factors in Computing Systems (IHC), Joinville Brazil (2017)
38. Perry, G.: Health information for lesbian/gay/bisexual/transgendered people on the internet. Internet Ref. Serv. Q. **6**(2), 23–34 (2001)
39. Schueller, S.M., Hunter, J.F., Figueroa, C., Aguilera, A.: Use of digital mental health for marginalized and underserved populations. Curr. Treat. Options Pscychol. **6**, 243–255 (2019)
40. Subramony, D.P.: Not in our journals - digital media technologies and the LGBTQI community. TechTrends **62**, 354–363 (2018)
41. Trinh, M.H., Agenor, M., Austin S.B., Jackson, C.L.: Health and healthcare disparities among U.S. women and men at the intersection of sexual orientation and race/ethnicity: a nationally representative cross-sectional study. BMC Publ. Health **17**(962), 1–11 (2017)
42. Ventuneac, A., John, S.A., Whitfield, T.H., Mustanski, B., Parsons, J.T.: Preferences for sexual health smartphone app features among gay and bisexual men. AIDS Behav. **22**, 3384–3394 (2018)

Motion and Rehabilitation

Exploratory Analysis of Machine Learning Methods for the Prognosis of Falls in Elderly Care Based on Accelerometer Data

Lukas Klein[1,2]([✉]) [iD], Christoph Ostrau[1] [iD], Michael Thies[2],
Wolfram Schenck[1] [iD], and Ulrich Rückert[2]

[1] Center for Health, Social Affairs and Technology (CareTech OWL),
University of Applied Sciences and Arts, Bielefeld, Germany
{lukas.klein,christoph.ostrau}@hsbi.de
[2] Center for Cognitive Interaction Technology (CITEC), Bielefeld University,
Bielefeld, Germany

Abstract. This paper investigates the feasibility of employing machine learning techniques to categorize individuals into fall-risk and non-fall-risk groups based solely on accelerometer data. The research utilizes a publicly available movement monitoring dataset, containing accelerometer data from a diverse group of individuals. The study pursues three primary objectives. First, it develops a preprocessing pipeline to prepare raw accelerometer data, which includes noise reduction, data cleaning, and identification of walking segments and the extraction of over twenty gait-related features. The second objective is to systematically explore the influence of these features on machine learning model performance. Gait stability-related parameters, known from medical literature, are of particular interest. To fulfil this objective, different machine learning algorithms are evaluated using an automated exploration framework. The third objective centres on finding a balanced combination of features and lightweight machine learning models suitable for embedded systems, which typically have limited computational resources. The emphasis here is on computational efficiency, an original aspect of this study. The results indicate that gradient boosting algorithms, such as XGBoost, LightGBM, and CatBoost, outperform other models, achieving promising performance results, including an area under the curve (AUC) score of up to 0.949.

Keywords: Machine Learning · Optimization · AutoML · Gait Analysis · Fall Risk Assessment · Feature Engineering

1 Introduction

Falls, especially among older individuals, are a serious problem in an ageing society. Elderly people are more vulnerable to falls due to various factors [21], leading to significant personal consequences such as reduced quality of life, loss

© ICST Institute for Computer Sciences, Social Informatics and Telecommunications Engineering 2024
Published by Springer Nature Switzerland AG 2024. All Rights Reserved
D. Salvi et al. (Eds.): PH 2023, LNICST 572, pp. 423–437, 2024.
https://doi.org/10.1007/978-3-031-59717-6_27

of autonomy, reduced social participation, chronic pain, and even hospitalization or mortality [22]. According to the Centers for Disease Control and Prevention (CDC), a staggering 27.5% of adults aged 65 and older in the United States experienced a fall in 2018, with around 24% of these incidents resulting in fall-related injuries [13]. Falls rank as the primary cause of injuries among adults aged 65 and older in the United States, accounting for approximately 3 million emergency department visits and 32,000 fall-related deaths annually. As the number of falls rises, so do the associated injuries and, consequently, healthcare costs [7]. To mitigate the personal, economic, and societal consequences, reducing falls among this vulnerable age group is imperative. The most effective approach to reducing falls is an early identification of individuals at risk, enabling preventive actions. However, fall risk assessments are typically conducted retrospectively through periodic medical examinations involving comprehensive questionnaires and laboratory tests [17]. To streamline ubiquitous fall risk assessment, modern sensor technology and advanced *machine learning (ML)* algorithms can be utilized (e.g. [6]). Promising approaches rely on three-dimensional motion data recorded by accelerometers, using ML techniques to predict fall risks accurately [1,24]. If these models can reliably identify fall risk, they could be integrated into cost-effective embedded systems which are continuously wearable by individuals, akin to small smartwatches. Such tools could serve as early warning systems, alerting wearers to changes in their movement patterns indicative of an increased risk of falling. This opens up the possibility of timely medical interventions to prevent impending falls and their associated consequences.

This paper assesses the applicability of ML methods for categorizing patients into two groups: those at risk of falling and those not at risk, based solely on accelerometer data from the publicly available *Long Term Movement Monitoring Database v1.0.0 (LTMM)* dataset [25]. To achieve this, we establish a comprehensive ML pipeline. The initial step is to create an effective preprocessing pipeline. This pipeline prepares raw accelerometer data by reducing noise, cleaning sensor data, and extracting walking segments. Next, we calculate features related to gait characteristics and examine their influence on ML model performance. We systematically explore various features and ML algorithms to identify an optimized combination, with a focus on lightweight models suited for resource-constrained embedded systems. In doing so, our scope does not involve implementing an embedded system, but rather evaluating the methods' feasibility and assessing optimal features in terms of computational requirements. This focus is a crucial part of our research objectives and a novel contribution to this specific application context. Furthermore, our study seeks to explore various ML techniques and to exhibit their ability to differentiate between fallers and non-fallers, based on data obtained through a single accelerometer and a constrained dataset, without extensively optimizing model architecture or preprocessing steps.

The remainder of this paper is structured as follows: In Sect. 2, the related work and research is presented. Then, the methods used to set up a preprocessing pipeline and to explore ML algorithms are explained in Sect. 3. The main findings are presented and discussed in Sect. 4 and Sect. 5 respectively. The paper is concluded in Sect. 6.

2   Related Work

Several papers have been published on the study of the LTMM dataset, as well as on predicting the risk of falling in individuals using ML algorithms with accelerometer data. The Weiss et al. research team [25], responsible for acquiring the LTMM dataset, analysed whether the acceleration data and its respective parameters display statistical correlation to the subjects' fall status in their initial publication on the dataset. They determined whether the accelerometer data of the dataset and the parameters derived from these can be used to assess the risk of falling in general. Weiss et al. calculated so-called gait-specific parameters [2] from walking segments of the raw sensor data, and performed statistical tests to compare these parameters between the class of fallers and the control group. They then used simple logistic regression to investigate the ability of the different parameters to identify the fall risk of the subjects. Weiss et al. found that there were statistically significant correlations between the sensor data and the calculated gait parameters and the subjects' fall risk status. Another paper on this dataset, published by the research team led by Ihlen et al. examined a new measure of gait stability in terms of its ability to discriminate between the fallers and the control group. The so-called'phase-dependent local dynamic stability' (λ) [10] measures how a subject's gait responds to infinitesimally small perturbations. Ihlen et al. state that this measure is very good at discriminating between fallers and non-fallers. In particular, the phase-dependent λ between 0% and 60% of the gait cycle significantly improved discrimination performance. In combination with 38 more conventional gait parameters used in the aforementioned Weiss et al. paper [25], Ihlen et al. achieved an *area under the curve (AUC)* score of 0.93 using partial least squares discriminant analysis. This is a very high value and close to a perfect result, and can be used as a reference when exploring other ML models. Van Schooten et al. [19] obtained a much larger dataset of 169 patients. They collected sensor data from an accelerometer worn on the lower back for 7 consecutive days and examined the predictive ability of features calculated from the accelerometer sensor. Using logistic regression, they obtained an area under the curve of 0.82. This result was obtained by combining data from the sensor and questionnaire data from the subjects. Other ML methods have been applied in the literature by other research groups on different data sets. Howcroft et al. [9] trained a motion dataset for fall risk prediction in older adults using multiple accelerometers at different locations on the human body. Howcroft et al. achieved an accuracy detecting people that have a higher risk of falling based on their fall history of 57%, a sensitivity of 35% and a specificity of 67%. They claimed that a fall risk screening tool should use multi-sensor data, as combining the data from all sensors improved the sensitivity of the best performing model (a neural network) to 43% and accuracy to 57%, while specificity dropped slightly to 65%. However, if one is limited to using only one sensor, they suggested attaching that sensor to the pelvic location, which is approximately the same location as the sensor worn in the LTMM data collection process. The research group of Aicha et al. [1] investigated deep learning methods to predict falls in older adults, also using accelerometer data from the lower trunk of the human body. They reached a peak performance of an AUC of 0.75 with intensive preprocessing of the data. A recent study investigated fall prediction in patients with Parkinson's disease [24], utilizing real-world data collected from foot-worn inertial sensors. Patients undertook several unsupervised 10-m walking tests daily, and data was collected over a two-week period. Patients were required to self-report any severe falls over the course of three months following the data collection period. Employing a random forest algorithm, the authors achieved a sensitivity (recall) rate of 60% and specificity rate of 88%, resulting in a balanced accuracy rate of 74%.

3 Methodology

In this chapter, we introduce the Long Term Movement Monitoring Database dataset, which comprises three-dimensional acceleration data collected from daily activities of older adults. Additionally, we provide an overview of the essential preprocessing pipeline and the process of feature engineering, setting the stage for the subsequent exploration of ML methods for fall risk prediction. Moreover, MLJAR [16], an automated ML library, is employed to delve into multiple ML algorithms and perform feature engineering.

3.1 Dataset

Traditionally, assessing the risk of falls in the elderly relied on subjective self-reports or isolated assessments, lacking objectivity. In response, the LTMM dataset [25], collected in 2016 by a consortium of researchers from various institutions, aimed to explore whether 3-dimensional acceleration data from everyday life could provide insights into the fall risk of older adults. This dataset is publicly accessible on PhysioNet [8], managed by MIT's Laboratory for Computational Physiology and supported by the National Institute of Biomedical Imaging and Bioengineering, allowing for sharing, modification, and use under the Open Data Commons Attribution Licence v1.0. The data collection process involved equipping 71 older adults, aged 65 to 87, with DynaPort Hybrid sensors from the Dutch company McRoberts. These sensors were affixed to the lower back, specifically at the fifth lumbar vertebra, for a continuous three-day monitoring period. The sensors recorded three-axis acceleration data (vertical, mediolateral, and anterior-posterior) via accelerometers and yaw, pitch, and roll velocities through triaxial gyroscopes, all sampled at a rate of 100 Hz. Based on the approaches in the literature [25] in order to make both the preprocessing pipeline and the learning algorithms least computationally intensive, only the the-axis acceleration data of the dataset was used. None of the participants had been diagnosed with balance or cognitive impairments. They were categorized as fallers or non-fallers based on self-reported fall history, with fallers having experienced two or more falls in the previous year. There were no noteworthy differences in demographic factors, such as age, gender, social status, height, weight, or body mass index, between the two groups of fallers and non-fallers. The data collection process encompassed four phases:

1. traditional laboratory-based fall risk assessments, including tests like the Dynamic Gait Index (DGI), Berg Balance Scale (BBS), Timed Up and Go test (TUG), Four Square Step Test (FSST), Mini Mental State Examination (MMSE), and Activity-specific Balance Confidence scale (ABC)
2. a laboratory gait assessment where participants walked for a minute with the same sensor belt worn during the three-day monitoring
3. three days of sensor wear in their daily routines, allowing for sensor removal during specific activities
4. a follow-up period of six months during which participants reported any falls, aiming to assess the predictive potential of accelerometer data.

While Weiss and colleagues [25] reported no significant differences in walking duration between the two participant groups, minor variations in sensor wear time, including weekdays versus weekends, can introduce variations in signal preprocessing and filtering of walking segments. These discrepancies may result in an uneven distribution of walking segments within the database, impacting the training of ML algorithms. Consequently, it is crucial to consider these potential imbalances when evaluating ML methods using diverse evaluation metrics. The data set was split into test data and training data using an 80/20 split. No explicit care was taken to perform the split according to the subjects. However, since the data was not shuffled before the split, it can be considered that the test and training data still is split according to the subjects, except for the data of the subject which may fall into the split boundary.

3.2 Preprocessing Pipeline

To employ ML methods for classifying sensor data into fallers and non-fallers, preprocessing of the raw sensor data is essential. This preprocessing, inspired by the work of Ullrich et al. [23], encompasses the three stages of signal preprocessing, movement detection, and frequency analysis. The aim of this process is to identify all data segments where the test subject is walking for a minimum of one minute. Signal preprocessing involves the removal of outliers, noise, and gravity components through high- and low-pass filters to ensure data integrity. The full preprocessing pipeline is depicted in Fig. 1. The preprocessed data undergoes segmentation using a sliding window technique with a 60-s window length and 50% overlap, enhancing temporal resolution, which is motivated by related work [18,26]. Movement detection entails determining if a data window contains movement of any kind, employing the Signal Magnitude Area threshold method as a pre-filtering step to exclude non-active sections. The *Signal Magnitude Area (SMA)* quantifies the intensity of a time-varying signal, commonly applied in physical activity analysis [12]. For a dataset with n values, it is computed as the sum of the absolute amplitudes of the signal within a specified time window. In the context of physical activity analysis, SMA is utilized to measure movement intensity and energy expenditure. For continuous time sensor data in the LTMM dataset, SMA computation is adapted as follows:

$$\text{SMA} = \frac{1}{T} \int_0^T [|X(t) - \mu_x| + |Y(t) - \mu_y| + |Z(t) - \mu_z|] \, dt \, , \tag{1}$$

428   L. Klein et al.

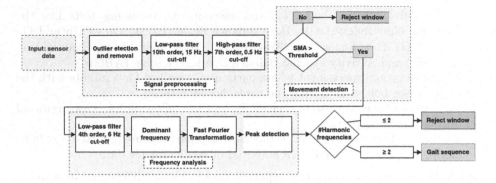

Fig. 1. Algorithm flowchart of the proposed data preprocessing and walking segment detection.

where T denotes the length of the sliding window filter, X, Y, Z represent the linear acceleration in the vertical (X), mediolateral (Y) and anterior-posterior (Z) axes. μ_i denotes the average linear acceleration of the respective axis and t represents the time step.

SMA values are evaluated against a threshold to identify movement within a given time window. Various methods are explored to establish this threshold, including visual observation, predefined thresholds from prior studies, averaging SMA values from laboratory data, and individual patient-specific thresholds. The aim is to find a threshold strategy that balances simplicity and computational efficiency while effectively detecting any activity. Subsequently, frequency analysis is performed on time windows that passed the movement detection stage. A fourth-order low-pass filter (cut-off at 6 Hz) is applied to isolate harmonic frequencies indicative of walking. The dominant frequency is computed through autocorrelation and analysed using the discrete Fourier Transform. Windows are classified as walking or non-walking based on the presence of harmonic frequencies. It is worth noting that frequency analysis is conducted solely along the vertical axis of motion, a pragmatic choice balancing accuracy and computational efficiency.

3.3   Feature Engineering

Feature engineering plays a pivotal role in ML workflows by transforming raw data into informative variables or features that enhance model performance. This process encompasses techniques such as feature extraction, selection, scaling, and transformation to represent data optimally for ML algorithms. It is iterative, relying on domain knowledge and exploration, and aims to minimize feature collinearity, maximize class separability, and reduce computational complexity. In this study, an extensive feature engineering pipeline is implemented, particularly emphasizing feature extraction. Features include gait parameters such as stride regularity, step characteristics, dominant frequencies, sensor data statistics, Signal Magnitude Area, mean swing time, time between peaks, displacement, and *Local Dynamic Stability (LDS)*. All calculated features are depicted in Table 1. These features are prepared for training with proper scaling, ensuring their effectiveness in the ML models.

To investigate the impact of the calculated feature on the performance of the ML methods, two different feature importance metrics are analysed. Firstly the permutation-based feature importance, a model inspection technique that assesses a model's reliance on specific features by measuring the reduction in its performance when individual feature values are randomly shuffled [4]. Secondly, the SHAP [11] importance scores that quantify the contribution of each feature to a model's prediction by considering all possible feature combinations and their impact on predictions based on the Shapley values [20].

Table 1. Overview of the feature that are calculated from the sensor data and used for learning with ML methods.

Feature	Abbreviation	Comment
Local Dynamic Stability	lambda_diff	Local Dynamic Stability of time window
Range of Sensor Data	acc_range_{v,ml,ap}	Range of sensor data values in each axis
Average of Sensor Data	acc_avg_{v,ml,ap}	Average of sensor data in each axis
SMA Value	SMA_value	SMA value of time window
Dominant Frequencies	{v,ml,ap}_dom_freq	Dominant frequencies of time window of each axis
Time between Peaks	time_between_peaks	Time interval between two consecutive peaks in accelerometer signal
Step Time Variation Coefficient	step_time_var_coeff	Ratio of standard deviation and mean of time between steps
Mean Step Time	mean_step_time	Average time of each step in a time window
Step Time Variation	step_tim_var_sd	Standard deviation of the step times
Number of Steps	num_steps	Number of steps in a time window
xCoM Displacement	xcom_{v,ml,ap}_displacement	Change in position of the extrapolated center of mass of the subjects
Cadence	cadence	Number of steps in a specific time period
Step Symmetry	step_symmetry	Quantifies the similarity between the movement of both feet
Mean Swing Time	mean_swing_time	Average duration of the swing phase of a step

3.4 Validation of Data Preprocessing

Validating the accuracy of identified walking segments is crucial for subsequent analyses. It ensures that the features derived from these segments are robust and contribute effectively to ML models. Validation methods include visual inspection, comparison with similar studies (limited by data availability), and an inductive approach where classical gait parameters are calculated and compared with expected values, providing confidence in the authenticity of the segments.

3.5 Exploration of ML Methods

MLJAR [16] is an *automated ML (AutoML)* library that streamlines the entire ML workflow. It is designed to facilitate intensive data analysis and comparative evaluation of various ML methods. In this study, MLJAR is leveraged to explore several ML algorithms, including Decision Trees, Random Forests, Extra

Trees, XGBoost, LightGBM, CatBoost, and simple Neural Networks consisting of fully connected layers. For training sessions, the dataset is partitioned into training and test sets using an 80/20 split. The test set is reserved for final model evaluation exclusively. In addition, a 5-fold cross-validation on the training data is conducted to assess each algorithm's performance and feature importance. MLJAR also offers preprocessing techniques like generating'Golden Features' and conducting'Feature Selection' to further enhance model performance. For the former, MLJAR generates unique feature pairs from the original input features and combines them with subtraction or division operators to obtain new features. For each (generated) feature, an importance score is calculated, the features are ranked according to their importance score, and the most important features are implanted into the training data. For Feature Selection, MLJAR inserts a random feature into the training data and trains the yet best model with this random features included. For each original feature, MLJAR calculates how many times its importance on the performance is smaller than the importance of the random feature. Every feature, that is at least on more than half the learners less important than the randomly generated feature, gets dropped from further learning.

4   Results

In this section, we delve into the outcomes of our sensor data preprocessing pipeline. Additionally, we explore feature engineering, emphasizing the significance of different features, and subsequently, we evaluate various ML models for binary classification, considering diverse evaluation metrics and the influence of feature engineering on model performance.

4.1   Walking Segment Detection

In this section, we present and analyse the results of our sensor data preprocessing pipeline, particularly focusing on the critical parameter of the Signal Magnitude Area (SMA) threshold. We experimented with various SMA thresholds, ranging from 0 to 1.0, to find the optimal value for the initial stage of preprocessing. Visual inspection of resulting movement segments was used for assessment. Using individual SMA thresholds based on each patient's 60-s laboratory walking segment data did not yield satisfactory results, as well as utilizing the mean SMA value from all participants' laboratory data, since it worsened the imbalance of the resulting dataset. The best outcome was achieved with an SMA threshold of 0.2, striking a balance between filtering stringency and dataset balance. Using this as a threshold for SMA-based movement detection, the full preprocessing pipeline resulted in an imbalanced dataset consisting of 5,951 walking segments. Of these, 68% were control group samples, whilst 32% were faller group samples. We validated the preprocessing by deriving classical gait parameters from the identified walking segments, specifically the average step duration and the dominant frequencies in the three axes of motion. The identified walking segments have an average step duration of 0.5 s, placing it in the lower range of average step duration for adults, which is between 0.49 and 0.59 s. [3,14,15]. The average dominant frequency in the vertical axis, the posterior-anterior axis and the mediolateral axis of the identified walking segments is with an average of 2.5 Hz, 2.3 Hz respectively 1.8 Hz within the 1–3 Hz which is reported as the normal range of dominant frequencies for adults [5]. The majority of values for the identified walking segments fall within the range of values found in literature, resulting in a false discovery rate of approximately 3%. However, the literature values were reported for adults of all ages, while our dataset includes solely older individuals who may have a higher risk of falling. This suggests that our preprocessing pipeline effectively extracts walking segments from sensor data.

4.2   Feature Engineering

In evaluating feature importance for predicting fall risk, we primarily examine the output of the best-performing models in MLJAR. The goal is to identify which features play a crucial role in the prediction task. Based on permutation-based importance plots, depicted in Fig. 2, the feature lambda_diff, representing the mean local dynamic stability of walking segments, consistently stands out as the most important, with weights ranging from approximately 0.16 to 0.22 across different learners. The range of vertical acceleration values follows as the second most important feature, with weights around 0.10. The average swing time feature, valued at approximately 0.10, also proves significant in both Cat-Boost and XGBoost models. Additionally, we consider SHAP importance scores, which account for feature interactions. These scores reaffirm the dominance of lambda_diff as the most critical feature, with an average weight of about 1.1 across all learners. The range of vertical acceleration values remains highly relevant. Notably, the feature cadence and the average accelerations in mediolateral and anterior-posterior directions hold very low importance in the models. This is likely because cadence is closely related to the number of steps, introducing redundancy. Ablation studies demonstrate that models lacking the three most important features (lambda_diff, vertical acceleration range, and mean swing time) perform significantly worse. This underscores the significance of these aforementioned features. Conversely, models solely trained on these top three features exhibit reduced effectiveness. While MLJAR offers automated feature generation techniques (compare Sect. 3.5), models that perform best tend to rely on manually engineered features. Nonetheless, models utilizing automatically generated features still achieve reasonable performance, suggesting their relevance. Among the generated features, those created using the Golden Features technique are the most impactful, particularly when they combine features with high importance scores. The difference between lambda_diff and time_between_peaks stands out as the most significant generated feature, reinforcing the significance of lambda_diff. In summary, lambda_diff, vertical acceleration range, and mean swing time are key features in predicting fall risk, while other features, such as

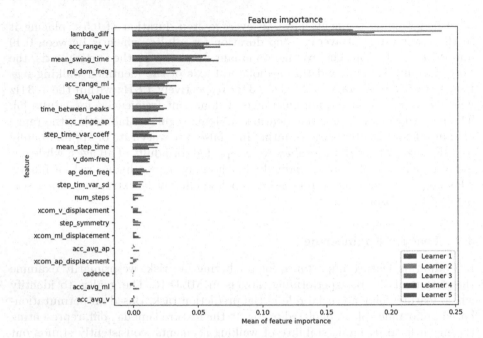

Fig. 2. Permutation based feature importance plots of best performing XGBoost model. Refer to Table 1 for an explanation of the features.

cadence, hold little importance. Automated feature generation, while less frequently used in the best models, still contributes to reasonable performance, especially when combining high-importance features. However, to achieve optimal model performance, it is advisable to utilize all manually engineered features, which is applied in the remainder of this paper.

4.3 Evaluation of ML Models

This section presents the outcomes of training runs conducted using MLJAR and identifies the most suitable ML techniques for addressing the binary classification task at hand. To determine the optimal approach for our dataset, we leveraged the insights gained from feature engineering evaluation and preprocessing. Instead of using raw sensor data, we utilized feature vectors extracted from walking segments as input data. The choice of evaluation metric significantly affects the model performance results. While log loss emerged as the top metric to optimize for to get the best results overall, we considered additional metrics like AUC, F1-score, recall, *Matthews Correlation Coefficient (MCC)* and precision due to the dataset's slight imbalance and the critical nature of the problem, where the identification of individuals at high risk of falling is crucial. To investigate the impact of using engineered features versus raw sensor data, we initially trained models solely on raw sensor data values, leading to an enormous dataset size. This approach significantly increased training times, for instance, taking more than 17 min to train a CatBoost model, compared to just 17 s when using feature vectors. Furthermore, the best results of MLJAR on the raw sensor data of walking segments also yield significantly worse results with an AUC of 0.7358, a MCC score of 0.252 and a very low recall score of 0.255 (CatBoost).

Consequently, we observed that feature engineering plays a pivotal role in model performance. The results indicated that tree-based algorithms, specifically Extra Trees and Random Forests, underperformed compared to gradient boosting methods such as LightGBM, XGBoost, and CatBoost across various evaluation metrics. Furthermore, these tree-based models exhibited longer single prediction and training times, making them less suitable for the task.

Table 2. Comparison of evaluation metrics of the best scores of CatBoost (depth: 8, random subspace method value: 0.9–1), LightGBM (number of leaves: 100–127, minimal data in leave: 10–20), XGBoost (maximal depth: 8, minimum child weights: 5) and Neural Network models (fully-connected feed-forward network, size: $22 \times 16 \times 32 \times 1$). Each cell contains the metric value.

Metric	CatBoost	LightGBM	XGBoost	Neural Network
Log Loss	**0.264**	0.290	0.291	0.415
AUC	**0.949**	0.939	0.937	0.905
F1	**0.800**	0.797	0.780	0.703
Accuracy	**0.884**	0.877	0.873	0.842
Precision	**0.858**	0.816	0.842	0.837
Recall	0.750	**0.780**	0.726	0.607
MCC	**0.723**	0.710	0.695	0.614
Predict time (s)	**0.028**	0.060	0.056	0.028
Train time (s)	81.16	28.30	31.24	**9.58**

Neural Networks, while showing reasonable performance, fell short of the best gradient boosting models in terms of metrics like log loss, F1-score, and AUC. Additionally, they incurred significantly longer prediction times, making them less efficient. The three gradient boosting techniques, LightGBM, XGBoost, and CatBoost, and a Neural Network were further examined to optimize their performance using MLJAR's 'Optuna' and 'Perform' modes. These results are displayed in Table 2. CatBoost outperformed its counterparts in log loss and AUC, achieving superior scores. LightGBM, while performing well, came in second place in these metrics. CatBoost also exhibited the highest precision, while LightGBM excelled in recall. To address class imbalance, precision-recall curves were analysed, with CatBoost demonstrating the best performance. All models displayed normal precision-recall curves without anomalies. Regarding memory consumption, CatBoost models were found to require larger file storage sizes on average, suggesting higher memory requirements compared to XGBoost and LightGBM models. In summary, gradient boosting algorithms, particularly CatBoost, LightGBM, and XGBoost, exhibited superior performance in classifying individuals at risk of falling compared to other methods. They achieved excellent results with very low prediction times, making them suitable for real-time applications. Neural Networks, while capable of achieving reasonably good results, lagged behind gradient boosting methods. Tree-based algorithms, such as Extra Trees and Random Forests, were less efficient in terms of both performance and computational speed.

5　Discussion

The data preprocessing pipeline implementation detected 5,951 walking segments, each of which were 60 s long. 68% of these segments belonged to the control group, while 32% were associated with a higher risk of falling. This preprocessing, including movement detection and feature extraction, significantly improved the accuracy of ML models for classifying individuals as fallers or controls. To enhance data quality, we applied high-pass and low-pass filters to the sensor data, reducing noise and increasing the signal-to-noise ratio. Additionally, outlier detection was employed to remove anomalous data points (e.g. caused by readout errors). However, the impact of these filtering techniques on ML model performance remains to be thoroughly investigated. These preprocessing steps allowed us to extract meaningful gait parameters from walking segments, which were crucial for fall risk assessment. We compared models trained on these engineered features with models using raw sensor data. The former consistently outperformed the latter, emphasizing the importance of feature engineering, particularly for tree-based ML algorithms. While we have diligently computed all relevant features and tested their combinations to the best of our knowledge, we must acknowledge the potential for further features that might improve ML performance. Additionally, our research focused solely on the LTMM dataset, which presents a comparatively small sample of individuals wearing the sensors. Future research could explore the impact of a more diverse dataset with a larger pool of test subjects, such as the dataset obtained by van Schooten et al., which provides data over a longer duration [19].

Another key finding is the identification of essential features for fall risk assessment, such as mean local dynamic stability, vertical acceleration range, and average swing time. Interestingly, cadence showed little significance in model performance. These results are consistent with previous studies and demonstrate the importance of stability-related features. Our analysis of various ML algorithms revealed that gradient boosting frameworks (XGBoost, CatBoost, and Light-GBM) consistently achieved the best results, with slight variations in evaluation metrics. Table 2 displays the most effective models, presenting AUC scores of up to 0.949 (CatBoost). These findings surpass the outcomes of previous studies, with Weiss et al. reaching an AUC score of up to 0.93 [25], van Schooten et al. reaching an AUC score of 0.82 [19] and Aicha et al. reaching an AUC of 0.72 [1]. Furthermore, Neural Networks consistently performed worse than gradient boosting methods, aligning with prior research [1]. In conclusion, while all three gradient boosting algorithms performed well, CatBoost stood out as a potential choice for fall risk assessment due to its strong discriminative ability. Our findings outperformed previous research and demonstrated the importance of feature engineering. Integrating these models into embedded systems seems plausible, but practical testing is necessary.

Future research will explore the ability to transfer our current findings to other sensor positions on the body. The current sensor configuration is challenging to wear and obstructs everyday use, presenting a substantial limitation to this research. Adapting the preprocessing and feature engineering strategies for accelerometers placed on alternate body locations, such as the upper back or wrist, could yield valuable insights. The next step involves implementing the findings in a real-world embedded system. In this scenario, the initial step in the preprocessing pipeline involves applying the running window SMA threshold to discard time windows with no activity. Only time windows that surpass a specific activity level will proceed for further calculations. This process is relatively straightforward and can be potentially integrated into a smart sensor, resulting in reduced power consumption. However, reducing the time resolution to ease computational loads is a topic for future research. Ultimately, this research could lead to clinical studies involving individuals wearing the embedded system for fall risk assessment based on our research.

6   Conclusion

Based on the published LTMM dataset, we have developed a pipeline that efficiently categorizes senior individuals as high-risk for falls. First, a preprocessing pipeline was designed and tested to effectively clean sensor data using frequency filter techniques and to recognize walking segments. This preprocessing substantially reduced computational overhead for feature extraction and ML model training, simultaneously enhancing model performance. From the preprocessed data, we computed over 20 distinct features, trained various ML algorithms and examined the impact of features on model outcomes. In our analysis, it became evident that features linked to gait stability held dominant importance, corroborating findings from prior studies [10]. The exploration of different ML models identified gradient boosting algorithms, namely XGBoost, LightGBM, and CatBoost, as top-performing models. Notably, these models exhibited uniform performance across various evaluation metrics, with CatBoost slightly outperforming its counterparts. Conversely, Neural Networks and tree-based methods like Extra Trees or Random Forests yielded notably inferior results. Hence, our research indicates that gradient boosting models are best suited for fall risk prediction using accelerometer data. The computational complexity of the resulting models indicates that they could be effectively integrated into embedded hardware, thereby having the potential to be used in mobile devices. In conclusion, we believe that the methods and insights from this work hold potential for the development of an embedded tool capable of accurately predicting the fall risk of elderly individuals.

Funding. This work is funded by the Ministerium für Kultur und Wissenschaft des Landes Nordrhein-Westfalen (MKW NRW).

References

1. Aicha, A.N., Englebienne, G., van Schooten, K., Pijnappels, M., Kröse, B.: Deep learning to predict falls in older adults based on daily-life trunk accelerometry. Sensors **18**(5), 1654 (2018). https://doi.org/10.3390/s18051654
2. Bobick, A.F., Johnson, A.Y.: Gait recognition using static, activity-specific parameters. In: Proceedings of the 2001 IEEE Computer Society Conference on Computer Vision and Pattern Recognition, CVPR 2001, vol. 1, p. I. IEEE (2001). https://doi.org/10.1109/CVPR.2001.990506
3. Bohannon, R.W.: Comfortable and maximum walking speed of adults aged 20–79 years: reference values and determinants. Age Ageing **26**(1), 15–19 (1997)
4. Breiman, L.: Random forests. Mach. Learn. **45**, 5–32 (2001). https://doi.org/10.1023/A:1010933404324
5. Chidean, M.I., et al.: Full band spectra analysis of gait acceleration signals for peripheral arterial disease patients. Front. Physiol. **9**, 1061 (2018)
6. Dubois, A., Bihl, T., Bresciani, J.P.: Identifying fall risk predictors by monitoring daily activities at home using a depth sensor coupled to machine learning algorithms. Sensors **21**(6) (2021). https://doi.org/10.3390/s21061957
7. Florence, C.S., Bergen, G., Atherly, A., Burns, E., Stevens, J., Drake, C.: Medical costs of fatal and nonfatal falls in older adults: medical costs of falls. J. Am. Geriatr. Soc. **66**(4), 693–698 (2018). https://doi.org/10.1111/jgs.15304
8. Goldberger, A.L., et al.: PhysioBank, PhysioToolkit, and PhysioNet. Circulation **101**(23) (2000). https://doi.org/10.1161/01.cir.101.23.e215
9. Howcroft, J., Kofman, J., Lemaire, E.D.: Prospective fall-risk prediction models for older adults based on wearable sensors. IEEE Trans. Neural Syst. Rehabil. Eng. **25**(10), 1812–1820 (2017). https://doi.org/10.1109/tnsre.2017.2687100
10. Ihlen, E.A.F., Weiss, A., Helbostad, J.L., Hausdorff, J.M.: The discriminant value of phase-dependent local dynamic stability of daily life walking in older adult community-dwelling fallers and nonfallers. Biomed. Res. Int. **2015**, 402596 (2015). https://doi.org/10.1155/2015/402596
11. Lundberg, S.M., Lee, S.I.: A unified approach to interpreting model predictions. Adv. Neural Inf. Process. Syst. **30** (2017). https://proceedings.neurips.cc/paper_files/paper/2017/file/8a20a8621978632d76c43dfd28b67767-Paper.pdf
12. Mathie, M., Coster, A., Lovell, N., Celler, B.: Detection of daily physical activities using a triaxial accelerometer. Med. Biol. Eng. Comput. **41**, 296–301 (2003). https://doi.org/10.1007/BF02348434
13. Moreland, B., Kakara, R., Henry, A.: Trends in nonfatal falls and fall-related injuries among adults aged ≥ 65 years — United States, 2012–2018. MMWR Morb. Mortal. Wkly. Rep. **69**(27), 875–881 (2020). https://doi.org/10.15585/mmwr.mm6927a5
14. Murray, M.P., Drought, A.B., Kory, R.C.: Walking patterns of normal men. JBJS **46**(2), 335–360 (1964)
15. Murray, M.P.: Walking patterns of normal woman. Arch. Phys. Med. Rehabil. **51**, 637–650 (1970)
16. Płońska, A., Płoński, P.: MLJAR: state-of-the-art automated machine learning framework for tabular data. version 0.10.3 (2021). https://github.com/mljar/mljar-supervised

17. Raîche, M., Hébert, R., Prince, F., Corriveau, H.: Screening older adults at risk of falling with the Tinetti balance scale. Lancet **356**(9234), 1001–1002 (2000). https://doi.org/10.1016/S0140-6736(00)02695-7
18. Redfield, M.T., Cagle, J.C., Hafner, B.J., Sanders, J.E.: Classifying prosthetic use via accelerometry in persons with transtibial amputations. J. Rehabil. Res. Dev. **50**(9), 1201–1212 (2013). https://doi.org/10.1682/jrrd.2012.12.0233
19. van Schooten, K.S., Pijnappels, M., Rispens, S.M., Elders, P.J.M., Lips, P., van Dieën, J.H.: Ambulatory fall-risk assessment: amount and quality of daily-life gait predict falls in older adults. J. Gerontol. A Biol. Sci. Med. Sci. **70**(5), 608–615 (2015). https://doi.org/10.1093/gerona/glu225
20. Shapley, L.S., et al.: A value for n-person games. In: Contributions to the Theory of Games, vol. 2 (1953)
21. Simpson, J.M.: Falls in older people: risk factors and strategies for prevention. Ageing Soc. **21**, 673 (2001)
22. Terroso, M., Rosa, N., Torres Marques, A., Simoes, R.: Physical consequences of falls in the elderly: a literature review from 1995 to 2010. Eur. Rev. Aging Phys. Activ. **11**, 51–59 (2014). https://doi.org/10.1007/s11556-013-0134-8
23. Ullrich, M., et al.: Detection of gait from continuous inertial sensor data using harmonic frequencies. IEEE J. Biomed. Health Inform. **24**(7), 1869–1878 (2020). https://doi.org/10.1109/JBHI.2020.2975361
24. Ullrich, M., et al.: Fall risk prediction in Parkinson's disease using real-world inertial sensor gait data. IEEE J. Biomed. Health Inform. **27**(1), 319–328 (2023). https://doi.org/10.1109/JBHI.2022.3215921
25. Weiss, A., et al.: Does the evaluation of gait quality during daily life provide insight into fall risk? A novel approach using 3-day accelerometer recordings. Neurorehabil. Neural Repair **27**(8), 742–752 (2013). https://doi.org/10.1177/1545968313491004
26. Xiao, W., Lu, Y.: Daily human physical activity recognition based on kernel discriminant analysis and extreme learning machine. Math. Probl. Eng. **2015**, 1–8 (2015). https://doi.org/10.1155/2015/790412

Unsupervised Physical Function Testing Using a Wearable Sensor System – A Cross-sectional Study with Community Dwelling Older Adults

Oonagh M. Giggins$^{(\boxtimes)}$ (iD), Grainne Vavasour(iD), and Julie Doyle(iD)

NetwellCASALA, Dundalk Institute of Technology, Dublin Road, Dundalk, Republic of Ireland
Oonagh.giggins@dkit.ie

Abstract. This study sought to investigate whether community dwelling older adults can independently undertake a Timed Up and Go (TUG) test and capture objective data related to frailty risk using a wearable sensor system. Participants were visited in their own homes and completed a sequence of TUG tests. These TUG tests were firstly supervised by the researcher. The TUG tests were then repeated by participants, unsupervised on the subsequent two days. The kinesis QTUG system was used to capture objective data during each TUG test. Fifty-one participants took part in this investigation, and 32 participants successfully obtained a frailty risk score using the QTUG system. Overall, the system usability score for the QTUG system ranged from 2.5 to 92.5 demonstrating a wide variation in participants' perception of its usability. Results of the Spearman's rank correlation coefficient (rs) indicate there was a very strong positive correlation between the supervised and the unsupervised QTUG tests for each of the two days (rs .942 and .874 day 1 and day 2 respectively $p < .001$). These results indicate that older adults can independently capture information relevant to their risk of frailty that does not depend on a clinician or researcher for analysis.

Keywords: Frailty · Older Adults · Physical Function · Wearable Sensors

1 Introduction

The global population is ageing at an unprecedented rate. Between 2015 and 2050 the proportion of the world's population over 60 years will nearly double from 12% to 22% [1]. Frailty is one of the greatest challenges facing an ageing population. It is a progressive age-related decline in physiological systems that results in decreased reserves of intrinsic capacity, which confers extreme vulnerability to stressors and increases the risk of a range of adverse health outcomes [2]. It is reflective of biological as opposed to chronological age and is influenced by physical, psychological, and social factors [2].

Frailty impacts 24% of community-dwelling adults over 65 years of age in Ireland, while the figure for pre-frailty, those at higher risk of progressing to frailty and its negative sequelae is 45% [3, 4]. Due to the heterogeneity of studies, global figures are difficult to establish, however, a systematic review of research in Europe, USA, UK, Ireland, and

D. Salvi et al. (Eds.): PH 2023, LNICST 572, pp. 438–448, 2024.
https://doi.org/10.1007/978-3-031-59717-6_28

Asia indicates that the prevalence of frailty and pre-frailty is as high as 27% and 50% respectively [5]. Frailty places older adults at increased risk for falls, disability, hospital admissions, institutionalization and mortality [6–10]. Exercise-based interventions have been shown to reverse frailty [11–13]. These interventions are particularly effective if delivered in a timely manner at the early stages of decline [14]. As a result, the early detection of frailty is critical in the development of preventive strategies against age-related conditions.

There are two major approaches to model frailty. Fried's Frailty Phenotype (FFP) model [7] identifies frailty by the presence of at least three of five physical characteristics; weight loss, exhaustion, low energy expenditure, slow walking speed and low handgrip strength. The Deficit Accumulation Index [9] identifies frailty based on the accumulation of a range of symptoms, sensory deficits, clinical signs, diseases, disabilities and abnormal laboratory test results. Other tools include the Frail Scale [15], the Tilburg Frailty Scale [16], and the Edmonton Frail Scale [17]. However, these assessment tools are time consuming and require clinical expertise within a geriatric department to complete.

Impaired physical function and declining physical activity are major precursors to frailty. Traditional assessments of physical function carried out in clinical settings are therefore frequently used to identify frailty. At present, it is common practice amongst healthcare professionals to use a combination of unstructured and structured methods to assess physical function and physical activity in older adults. Unstructured assessment methods include free observation of patient movement (e.g. walking into the room, sitting down, reaching out for an object) and questions to investigate perceived changes in the ability to complete activities of daily living. Structured assessment methods include questionnaires to investigate the impact of physical health on quality of life and physical activity, such as the CASP-19 [18], and tests to assess motor performance, such as the Berg Balance Scale [19], Elderly Mobility Scale [20], and the Timed Up and Go (TUG) test [21]. Although these methods may yield clinically relevant information and are generally easy to use, their sensitivity for quantifying small changes in physical function is limited, and therefore they may not be sensitive to identifying the early indicators of frailty. Additionally, the opportunities to undertake these assessments are limited to clinical visits, and there is the risk that the onset of frailty might go undetected or be identified too late.

Wearable sensors has become a pervasive means of measuring physical function and physical activity [22–24]. A recent systematic review has shown that wearable sensors can be used to collect objective, quantifiable parameters of mobility and physical activity that can be used to distinguish between levels of frailty [25]. The majority of studies examined were carried out in laboratory or under test conditions. While this type of assessment, in a controlled laboratory or clinical environment is important, the collection of data in the home setting is considered more valuable [26, 27]. As the onset of frailty can be more insidious, more regular or continuous assessments of physical function, in a person's naturalistic, home environment may be more useful in identifying frailty. Facilitating older adults to undertake these assessments and capture this objective data in their own homes may not only reduce the burden of testing (e.g. clinician time, traveling to a clinic for assessment) but also allow for the earlier detection of frailty and earlier intervention. However, it needs to be investigated whether these assessments of physical function can be performed by older adults independently and unsupervised in their homes. The QTUG system has been shown to be reliable in the measurement of gait and mobility [28], and is accurate in predicting falls in people with Parkinson's disease [29], and community dwelling older adults [30, 31]. In this current study, the Kinesis QTUG was used to provide an objective frailty risk score during a TUG test.

This study sought to investigate whether community-dwelling older adults can independently and safely undertake a TUG test in their own home and operate the Kinesis QTUG to capture an objective frailty risk score. This study also sought to examine the usability of the Kinesis QTUG system among older adults.

2   Methodology

2.1   Study Design

A cross-sectional study was conducted to investigate the ability of older adults to independently undertake a physical function test and capture objective data using the Kinesis QTUG sensor and software system.

2.2   Participants

Participants for this study were recruited through advertisements in local golf, bridge and church community groups. Those interested were assessed for eligibility by a member of the research team over the telephone using the study eligibility criteria; 65 years of age and over, independently mobile, physically capable of performing a series of mobility tests, had no cognitive or neurological deficits and no history in the past 6 months of lower limb orthopaedic trauma or surgery that would interfere with the ability to exercise. A sample of 52 was based on power 0.8, effect size 0.8, p value 0.05 (AI-Therapy Statistics 2018). This is justified in the literature with previous studies including similar sample sizes (Apsega et al. 2020).

2.3   Ethical Considerations

The study protocol received ethical approval from the School of Health and Science Ethics Committee in Dundalk Institute of Technology, and all participants signed a written informed consent form prior to participation.

2.4   Data Collection

Participants were visited on two occasions in their homes for data collection. Each visit was scheduled 48-h apart, and took place between September 2021 and December 2021. During the first visit, a frailty assessment was conducted with each participant based on Fried's Frailty Phenotype (FFP) [7]. Participants were also requested to perform a Timed Up and Go (TUG) test [32].

The FFP consists of five phenotypes of weight loss, exhaustion, low level of activity, weakness as measured by grip strength, and gait speed. Weight loss scored one point for unintentional weight loss >4.5 kg in the previous year or a body mass index (BMI) <18.5 kg/m^2. Exhaustion was assessed subjectively through two questions regarding perception of energy and how regularly one had rested in bed during the day over the previous four weeks – one point was scored if the answer to the first question was negative and 'every day' for the latter. Low level of activity scored one point if self-reported frequency of high *and* moderate activity was "never or hardly ever". Handgrip strength and gait speed were measured objectively and scored according to pre-determined cut-off points [7] and (www.cgakit.com 2015) respectively. One point was scored for weakness if handgrip strength was less than a pre-determined cut-off weight (in kg) for sex and BMI categories. One point was scored for slowness if time to complete the TUG test was equal to or exceeded 19 s. Individuals are considered non-frail or robust if they fulfil none of the criteria, pre-frail if they fulfil one or two and frail if they meet three or more of the five criteria.

The TUG test is a reliable and valid test of function and mobility that measures in seconds (s), the time taken by a participant to stand up from a standard chair seat height, walk a distance of 3-m (m), turn 180°, walk back to the chair and sit down [32]. Prior to performing the TUG test participants were instrumented with the Kinesis QTUG sensors. Each sensor contains a tri-axial accelerometer, tri-axial gyroscope and a magnetometer. One sensor was secured on each shin, over outer clothing using reusable straps (Fig. 1). The QTUG sensors connected via Bluetooth to the Kinesis QTUG app which uses the sensor and demographic data to produce a frailty score. Values below 50% are considered non-frail, values between 50 and 70% are considered transitionary, values above 70% are frail, while values above 90% are considered very frail.

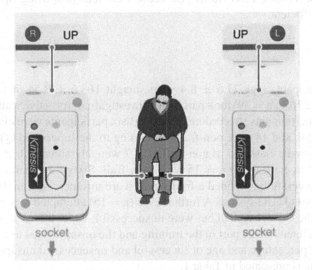

Fig. 1. Placement of the Kinesis QTUG sensors on the participant's shanks

Following the supervised TUG test, participants were requested to repeat the TUG test unsupervised, and record data using the QTUG system, once each day over the following 48-h. Participants were provided with written and verbal instructions on how to perform the test as well as a demonstration by the researcher. Participants were instructed to perform the TUG test along the same course and using the same chair as in the supervised test. Participants were provided with an illustrated information booklet and received training in the use of the QTUG. Off-site phone support was also available where required.

Participants were visited a second time 48-h after the initial visit. During this visit, participants were asked to complete the system usability score (SUS), a validated outcome measure which measures the usability of a system [33]. It consists of a 10-item questionnaire with five response options for respondents ranging from strongly disagree to strongly agree, resulting in a score between 0 and 100. The SUS for the QTUG system was calculated using standard methodology [33].

2.5 Data Analysis

Data were collated using Microsoft Office Excel (Microsoft Corp) and analyzed using SPSS software (IBM Corp). Descriptive statistics of continuous variables are presented as mean and standard deviation (SD). The frailty risk scores from the QTUG were tested for normality using the Shapiro-Wilk test. A p value of $<.05$ was considered statistically significant. The relationships between the supervised and the unsupervised QTUG frailty risk scores were analysed using Spearman's rank correlation coefficient. Correlation coefficients were interpreted as follows; very strong (0.9–1.0), strong (0.7–0.89), moderate (0.4–0.69) or weak (0.10–0.39) [34]. Because of the relatively small sample size and the non-normally distributed data, the relationships between the supervised and the unsupervised QTUG frailty risk score were analysed using Spearman's rank correlation coefficient.

3 Results

Fifty-one participants (age 77.5 $\pm$ 8.4 years, height 163.6 $\pm$ 8.54 m, weight 72.0 $\pm$ 13.5 kg, female 76%; n = 39) took part in this investigation. Assistive walking aids were used by n = 3 participants. According to the FFP, six participants were classified as frail 31 were pre-frail, and 14 were non-frail. According to the supervised QTUG data, n = 26 participants were classified as non-frail, n = 7 were classified as transitional, n = 3 were classified as frail, while n = 15 were very frail. Sixty-three percent (n = 32) of participants successfully obtained a frailty risk score unsupervised, in their own home using the Kinesis QTUG system. A further 29% (n = 15) attempted to perform the TUG test and used the QTUG system but were unsuccessful, while 8% (n = 4) (age 82.5 $\pm$ 3.19 years) declined to take part in the training and the unsupervised test. A breakdown of the number, percentage and age of successful and unsuccessful unsupervised QTUG by frailty status is presented in Table 1.

The SUS was completed by 80% of all participants (n = 41), with missing data due to participant unavailability at the second home visit. Percentile scores of the system usability score range from 2.5 to 92.5. Mean scores are presented by frailty group in Table 2.

Table 1. Number, percentage and age of successful and unsuccessful unsupervised QTUG by frailty status

	Frailty Group	n	% of each cohort	Age mean (SD)
Unsuccessful				
	Non frail	2	14	73.5 (6.4)
	Pre-frail	14	45	82.5 (5.7)
	Frail	3	50	89.7 (2.9)
	Total	**19**	**37**	**82.7 (6.6)**
Successful				
	Non frail	12	86	71.4 (7.1)
	Pre-frail	17	55	75.2 (7.8)
	Frail	3	50	81.0 (7.9)
	Total	**32**	**63**	**74.3 (7.8)**

Includes Declined; n = 4; Pre-frail n = 1; Frail n = 3; Age 82.5 (3.19)

Table 2. SUS Percentile score by Frailty Status

Frailty Status	SUS Percentile Score	
	N	Mean (SD)
Non frail	12	65.4 (17.1)
Pre-frail	26	48.1 (30.3)
Frail	3	35.0 (26.1)
Total	41	52.2 (27.8)

Results of the Spearman's rank correlation coefficient (rs) between the QTUG frailty estimate indicate there was a very strong positive correlation between the supervised QTUG and the unsupervised QTUG tests for each of the two days (rs .942 and .874 day 1 and day 2 respectively $p < .001$). There was an equally strong positive correlation between each of the two unsupervised QTUG tests (rs .938, $p < .001$). Estimates of agreement would be more appropriate for analysing the same variables however, the data violated the assumptions of normality necessary for creating and interpreting Bland Altman plots. Neither log transformation or taking the square root of variables resulted in normal distribution.

4 Discussion

Frailty is an avoidable and reversible biopsychosocial syndrome associated with ageing, resulting in adverse outcomes that are both life-changing and life-limiting, and which ultimately impacts on scarce healthcare resources. Providing older adults with a means that they can independently monitor for and identify the early signs of frailty could allow for earlier intervention and reduce the risk of developing frailty, thereby reducing the burden on the individual and society as a whole. The Kinesis QTUG is a wearable sensor system that provides an objective estimate of frailty in the form of a frailty risk score, which can be understood and used by the user without further analysis or interpretation required. This study examined the ability of older adults to independently perform a TUG test in their own home, and capture objective test data using the Kinesis QTUG system. Overall, this study found that the majority of participants were successful in undertaking the TUG tests and obtaining a frailty risk score independently using the Kinesis QTUG. Those who were successful in obtaining a frailty score unsupervised were younger (mean age 74.3 ± 7.8 years) than those who failed to undertake the TUG and use the QTUG successfully (mean age 82.7 ± 6.6 years). However, the percentage of those who were successful in the pre-frail and frail cohorts was comparable (45%–50% and 55%–50% for pre-frail and frail cohort for successful and unsuccessful respectively). The QTUG frailty estimates captured by participants unsupervised correlated strongly with the supervised QTUG frailty estimate performed by the researcher. This outcome is promising, suggesting that many older adults can independently capture information relevant to their risk of frailty that does not depend on a clinician or researcher for analysis.

Four participants who enrolled in this study declined to take part in the unsupervised TUG test, citing lack of interest or lack of confidence in their ability to perform the test independently. Twenty-nine percent of the participants who attempted to undertake the test and use the Kinesis QTUG independently were unsuccessful for reasons including system or battery failure, poor eyesight and self-reported lack of confidence to attempt the test without family support. The latter two reasons are related to biophysical restrictions and reduced confidence, both associated with ageing, and confirms the literature, which identifies these as limiting factors to the use of technology among older adults [35]. Lack of confidence in technology is referred to as digital anxiety and appears quite prevalent in the literature [36–38]. Self-confidence in digital skills is influenced by many factors including age, education and previous experience with technology, and in turn affects satisfaction, perceived usefulness and adoption or continued use of technology [39].

Training sessions that allow older adults to learn at an individual pace, with ongoing support and provision of educational literature have been shown to instill confidence and facilitate problem solving resulting in acceptance and adoption of technology among older adults [40]. It is recognised that older adults have the capacity and the interest to learn to use technology but again, the design of the training is important [41]. Participants were provided with one-to-one training and a reference manual prior to the unsupervised tests. The limited duration and once-off nature of the training provided in this study may have contributed to the participants not being equipped to manage system or battery failure. The training provided did not include the opportunity for participants to first engage with the technology and subsequently ask questions or experience success in tasks, both of which are understood to build confidence and facilitate successful adoption of technology [39].

Overall, the SUS score for the Kinesis QTUG ranged from 2.5 to 92.5 demonstrating a wide variation in participants' perception of its usability. The mean SUS score was lower with each increasing level of frailty however, the lowest score was in the pre-frail group (2.5 in the pre-frail group compared with a lowest score of 5 in the frail group) indicating that some frail participants perceived the technology more usable than their pre-frail peers. The mean score of 52 falls below the score of 68 which is considered an average and acceptable score for the system usability score [42]. However, forty-four percent of those who completed the system usability score (n = 18/41) scored ≥65 demonstrating that for many participants, the technology was deemed usable. The non-frail group came closest to the average of 68 (mean 65.4, range 45–92.5). The mean system usability score reduced in accordance with frailty status and age in keeping with previous studies [43].

While the results of this study are promising, there are some limitations which must be considered. The sampling method for recruitment of participants resulted in a lack of gender balance and a lack of diversity in frailty status. The percentage of men in the overall sample was just 25%, which is in contrast with other frailty studies where the gender balance has been more reflective of the population [44, 45]. All participants in this study were recruited from community groups, and this may have influenced the imbalance in frailty status among the participants. In addition, this study took place during the COVID-19 pandemic which may have limited the recruitment of more frail older adults. However, the 73% prevalence of frailty and pre-frailty combined in the sample is comparable with other similar studies [4, 46, 47] and reflects the population prevalence [5].

The short time frame of the study which was influenced by the COVID-19 pandemic, and the once-off training session did not facilitate self-paced learning or provide the benefit of time to explore the technology with ongoing technical support. Participants may have benefitted from a follow-up training session to address questions and provide support prior to carrying out the unsupervised QTUG test, which may have influenced the results. The Kinesis QTUG platform is designed to be administered by a clinician, and to our knowledge this is the first study to evaluate its independent use by older adults. While this system is unique, the findings of this study may be useful for deploying other smartphone apps and technologies for the independent assessment of mobility and function in older adults.

5 Conclusion

Frailty is one of the greatest challenges facing our ageing population. This study has demonstrated that older adults are capable of undertaking a TUG test and of obtaining a frailty risk score unsupervised in their own home using the Kinesis QTUG system. However, the usability of the system varied, with scores ranging from 2.5 to 92.5, indicating potential challenges in the widespread adoption of this technology among older adult. Nonetheless, these findings are important as they highlight the potential for older adults to self-monitor their mobility and physical function. Providing older adults with a means to independently identify declining physical function, may allow for the earlier detection of frailty and earlier intervention, which may mitigate some of the potential adverse sequelae.

Data Availability Statement. The data that support the findings of this study are available on request from the corresponding author, OMG.

References

1. World Health Organization. Ageing and Health.
2. World Health Organization. World Report on Ageing and Health. World Health Organization (2015)
3. O'Halloran, A., O'Shea, M.: Wellbeing and Health in Ireland's Over 50s 2009–2016. Trinity College Dublin (2018). https://doi.org/10.38018/TildaRe.2018-00
4. Roe, L., Normand, C., Wren, M.-A., Browne, J., O'Halloran, A.M.: The impact of frailty on healthcare utilisation in Ireland: evidence from the Irish longitudinal study on ageing. BMC Geriatr. **17**(1), 203 (2017). https://doi.org/10.1186/s12877-017-0579-0
5. Choi, J., Ahn, A., Kim, S., Won, C.W.: Global prevalence of physical frailty by Fried's criteria in community-dwelling elderly with national population-based surveys. J. Am. Med. Dir. Assoc. **16**(7), 548–550 (2015). https://doi.org/10.1016/j.jamda.2015.02.004
6. Chang, S.-F., Lin, H.-C., Cheng, C.-L.: The relationship of frailty and hospitalization among older people: evidence from a meta-analysis. J. Nurs. Scholarsh. **50**(4), 383–391 (2018). https://doi.org/10.1111/jnu.12397
7. Fried, L.P., et al.: Frailty in older adults: evidence for a phenotype. J. Gerontol. A Biol. Sci. Med. Sci. **56**(3), M146–M157 (2001). https://doi.org/10.1093/gerona/56.3.M146
8. Liu, H.X., et al.: Association between frailty and incident risk of disability in community-dwelling elder people: evidence from a meta-analysis. Public Health **175**, 90–100 (2019). https://doi.org/10.1016/j.puhe.2019.06.010
9. Rockwood, K.: A global clinical measure of fitness and frailty in elderly people. Can. Med. Assoc. J. **173**(5), 489–495 (2005). https://doi.org/10.1503/cmaj.050051
10. Zhang, Q., Guo, H., Gu, H., Zhao, X.: Gender-associated factors for frailty and their impact on hospitalization and mortality among community-dwelling older adults: a cross-sectional population-based study. PeerJ **6**, e4326 (2018). https://doi.org/10.7717/peerj.4326
11. Woolford, S.J., Sohan, O., Dennison, E.M., Cooper, C., Patel, H.P.: Approaches to the diagnosis and prevention of frailty. Aging Clin. Exp. Res. **32**(9), 1629–1637 (2020). https://doi.org/10.1007/s40520-020-01559-3
12. Mulasso, A., Roppolo, M., Rainoldi, A., Rabaglietti, E.: Effects of a multicomponent exercise program on prevalence and severity of the frailty syndrome in a sample of Italian community-dwelling older adults. Healthcare **10**(5), 911 (2022). https://doi.org/10.3390/healthcare10050911
13. Cesari, M., et al.: A physical activity intervention to treat the frailty syndrome in older persons-results from the LIFE-P study. J. Gerontol. A Biol. Sci. Med. Sci. **70**(2), 216–222 (2015). https://doi.org/10.1093/gerona/glu099
14. Ko, F.C.-Y.: The clinical care of frail, older adults. Clin. Geriatr. Med. **27**(1), 89–100 (2011)
15. Woo, J., Leung, J., Morley, J.E.: Comparison of frailty indicators based on clinical phenotype and the multiple deficit approach in predicting mortality and physical limitation. J. Am. Geriatr. Soc. **60**(8), 1478–1486 (2012). https://doi.org/10.1111/j.1532-5415.2012.04074.x
16. Gobbens, R.J.J., Boersma, P., Uchmanowicz, I., Santiago, L.M.: The Tilburg Frailty Indicator (TFI): New Evidence for Its Validity. Clin. Interv. Aging, 265–274 (2020)
17. Rolfson, D.B., Majumdar, S.R., Tsuyuki, R.T., Tahir, A., Rockwood, K.: Validity and reliability of the Edmonton Frail scale. Age Ageing **35**(5), 526–529 (2006). https://doi.org/10.1093/ageing/afl041

18. Hyde, M., Wiggins, R.D., Higgs, P., Blane, D.B.: A measure of quality of life in early old age: the theory, development and properties of a needs satisfaction model (CASP-19). Aging Ment. Health **7**(3), 186–194 (2003). https://doi.org/10.1080/1360786031000101157
19. Berg, K.: Measuring balance in the elderly: development and validation of an instrument (1992)
20. Prosser, L., Canby, A.: Further validation of the elderly mobility scale for measurement of mobility of hospitalized elderly people. Clin. Rehabil. **11**(4), 338–343 (1997)
21. Bohannon, R.W.: Reference values for the timed up and go test: a descriptive meta-analysis. J. Geriatr. Phys. Therapy **29**(2), 64–68 (2006)
22. Bai, Y., et al.: Comparison of consumer and research monitors under semistructured settings. Med. Sci. Sports Exerc. **48**(1), 151–158 (2016)
23. Burton, E., et al.: Reliability and validity of two fitness tracker devices in the laboratory and home environment for older community-dwelling people. BMC Geriatr. **18**(1), 1–12 (2018)
24. Hsieh, K.L., Roach, K.L., Wajda, D.A., Sosnoff, J.J.: Smartphone technology can measure postural stability and discriminate fall risk in older adults. Gait Posture **67**, 160–165 (2019)
25. Vavasour, G., Giggins, O.M., Doyle, J., Kelly, D.: How wearable sensors have been utilised to evaluate frailty in older adults: a systematic review. J. Neuroeng. Rehabil. **18**(1), 112 (2021). https://doi.org/10.1186/s12984-021-00909-0
26. Brodie, M.A., et al.: New methods to monitor stair ascents using a wearable pendant device reveal how behavior, fear, and frailty influence falls in octogenarians. IEEE Trans. Biomed. Eng. **62**(11), 2595–2601 (2015)
27. Mueller, A., et al.: Continuous digital monitoring of walking speed in frail elderly patients: noninterventional validation study and longitudinal clinical trial. JMIR Mhealth Uhealth **7**(11), e15191 (2019)
28. Smith, E., Walsh, L., Doyle, J., Greene, B., Blake, C.: The reliability of the quantitative timed up and go test (QTUG) measured over five consecutive days under single and dual-task conditions in community dwelling older adults. Gait Posture **43**, 239–244 (2016)
29. Greene, B.R., et al.: Longitudinal assessment of falls in patients with Parkinson's disease using inertial sensors and the timed up and go test. J. Rehabil. Assist. Technol. Eng. **5**, 2055668317750811 (2018)
30. Greene, B.R., Redmond, S.J., Caulfield, B.: Fall risk assessment through automatic combination of clinical fall risk factors and body-worn sensor data. IEEE J. Biomed. Health Inform. **21**(3), 725–731 (2016)
31. Greene, B.R., Doheny, E.P., Walsh, C., Cunningham, C., Crosby, L., Kenny, R.A.: Evaluation of falls risk in community-dwelling older adults using body-worn sensors. Gerontology **58**(5), 472–480 (2012)
32. Podsiadlo, D., Richardson, S.: The timed 'Up & Go': a test of basic functional mobility for Frail elderly persons. J. Am. Geriatr. Soc. **39**(2), 142–148 (1991). https://doi.org/10.1111/j.1532-5415.1991.tb01616.x
33. Brooke, J.: SUS-A quick and dirty usability scale. Usab. Eval. Indust. **189**(194), 4–7 (1996)
34. Schober, P., Boer, C., Schwarte, L.A.: Correlation coefficients: appropriate use and interpretation. Anesth. Analg. **126**(5), 1763–1768 (2018). https://doi.org/10.1213/ANE.0000000000002864
35. Wang, J., Fu, Y., Lou, V., Tan, S.Y., Chui, E.: A systematic review of factors influencing attitudes towards and intention to use the long-distance caregiving technologies for older adults. Int. J. Med. Inform. **153**, 104536 (2021)
36. Yap, Y.-Y., Tan, S.-H., Choon, S.-W.: Elderly's intention to use technologies: a systematic literature review. Heliyon **8**(1), e08765 (2022)
37. Nimrod, G.: Technophobia among older Internet users. Educ. Gerontol. **44**(2–3), 148–162 (2018)

38. Di Giacomo, D., Ranieri, J., D'Amico, M., Guerra, F., Passafiume, D.: Psychological barriers to digital living in older adults: computer anxiety as predictive mechanism for technophobia. Behav. Sci. **9**(9), 96 (2019)
39. Lee, C., Coughlin, J.F.: PERSPECTIVE: older adults' adoption of technology: an integrated approach to identifying determinants and barriers. J. Prod. Innov. Manag. **32**(5), 747–759 (2015)
40. Desai, S., McGrath, C., McNeil, H., Sveistrup, H., McMurray, J., Astell, A.: Experiential value of technologies: a qualitative study with older adults. Int. J. Environ. Res. Public Health **19**(4), 2235 (2022)
41. Schlomann, A., Even, C., Hammann, T.: How older adults learn ICT—guided and self-regulated learning in individuals with and without disabilities. Front. Comput. Sci. **3**, 140 (2022)
42. Sauro, J.: Measuring Usability with the System Usability Scale (SUS) (2011). https://measuringu.com/sus/. Accessed 12 Oct 2023
43. Bangor, A., Kortum, P., Miller, J.: Determining what individual SUS scores mean: adding an adjective rating scale. J. Usability Stud. **4**(3), 114–123 (2009)
44. Xue, Q.-L.: The frailty syndrome: definition and natural history. Clin. Geriatr. Med. **27**(1), 1–15 (2011)
45. Rodríguez-Gómez, I., et al.: Relationship between physical performance and frailty syndrome in older adults: the mediating role of physical activity, sedentary time and body composition. Int. J. Environ. Res. Publ. Health **18**(1), 203 (2021)
46. O'Halloran, A.M., Hartley, P., Moloney, D., McGarrigle, C., Kenny, R.A., Romero-Ortuno, R.: Informing patterns of health and social care utilisation in Irish older people according to the Clinical Frailty Scale. HRB Open Res. **4**, 54 (2021)
47. Pradeep Kumar, D., Wendel, C., Mohler, J., Laksari, K., Toosizadeh, N.: Between-day repeatability of sensor-based in-home gait assessment among older adults: assessing the effect of frailty. Aging Clin. Exp. Res. **33**, 1529–1537 (2021)

MARTHA - Master Therapy Assistant: Supporting the Recovery of Upper Limb Motor Function After Stroke with Digital Home Exercise Programs

Lena Rettinger(✉) [ID], Nadia Abid Aziz, Katharina Bühn, Daniela Duh,
Leon Freudenthaler, Andrea Greisberger [ID], and Carissa Klupper

FH Campus Wien, University of Applied Sciences, Vienna, Austria
lena.rettinger@fh-campuswien.ac.at

Abstract. This research aimed to develop a mobile application to support home exercise programs for persons after stroke. The study was conducted in three phases: understanding the needs, developing a prototype, and testing the application.

In the first phase, a survey with 52 physical and occupational therapists, and focus groups with 6 physical and occupational therapists were conducted to understand the needs of therapists regarding home exercise programs for persons after stroke. The second phase involved the development of the application by an interdisciplinary team following an agile software development approach. In the third phase the application's usability and feasibility was evaluated through a pilot study. The needs analysis highlighted the importance of individualized programs and adaptability in home exercise programs. 86.5% of the survey participants expressed interest in a mobile application for home exercise programs, with specific features like exercise videos, feedback mechanisms, and reminders. The usability, usefulness and satisfaction with the developed application, MARTHA, were tested in a pilot study involving 13 therapists and 18 patients and showed high scores for ease of use and learning. The study demonstrated the feasibility of using the mobile application MARTHA in supporting home exercise programs for persons after stroke. The application was found to be user-friendly and adaptable to individual needs. However, some participants raised the need for a more extensive variety of exercises, especially for patients with more severe limitations. Further development and testing are needed to address the concerns raised and to assess the long-term impact on patient outcomes.

Keywords: Home Exercise Program · Stroke · Rehabilitation · Mobile Application · mHealth · Telerehabilitation · Usability

1 Introduction

In 2019 12,2 million worldwide stroke incidents, resulting in the second-leading cause of death and 143 disability-adjusted life-years, were reported [1]. Poor health-related quality of life is, amongst others, associated with reduced upper limb function [2].

© ICST Institute for Computer Sciences, Social Informatics and Telecommunications Engineering 2024
Published by Springer Nature Switzerland AG 2024. All Rights Reserved
D. Salvi et al. (Eds.): PH 2023, LNICST 572, pp. 449–463, 2024.
https://doi.org/10.1007/978-3-031-59717-6_29

Therefore, interventions supporting the recovery of upper limb function should be a core element of rehabilitation [3] and have been studied intensively in recent years [4–6]. International stroke rehabilitation guidelines recommend repetitive task training at a high intensity and home exercise programs (HEP) to enhance learning and recovery of upper limb function [7–11]. HEP have the potential to increase frequency and intensity of upper limb training, especially when rehabilitation resources are limited [7, 12].

The beneficial effects of HEP is not questioned [12], however adherence is highly variable and sometimes unsatisfactory: between 28% and 65% of respondents actually perform a recommended HEP [12, 13]. Mahmood et al. recently developed a Delphi consensus-based framework to support home-based exercise adherence after stroke, encompassing a comprehensive list of strategies in nine domains [14]. It contains, among others, strategies targeting at methods of exercise prescription, feedback and supervision, promotion of self-efficacy, motivational strategies, and reminder strategies.

Telerehabilitative approaches could support persons after stroke in order to perform and maintain a HEP and are recommended in guidelines [15, 16]. Systematic reviews conclude that telerehabilitative interventions are equivalent to a traditional exercise setting in stroke rehabilitation [17, 18]. Users (patients, relatives, and healthcare professionals) seem to be satisfied with telemedicine services and sufficient acceptance is shown [19, 20]. To increase the acceptance of telerehabilitative approaches, it is recommended to adapt them to the needs of the users. These needs include a simple and calm interface, receiving feedback, and the ability to set a goal and evaluate it [21]. Early involvement of potential users in the development of telerehabilitative interventions is strongly recommended and ensures user-centered development [22].

1.1 Aim

Based on current views of physical therapists (PTs) and occupational therapists (OTs) on HEP for persons after stroke (PS) (Phase 1), we developed a prototype application for a mobile tablet in order to support the realization of a HEP for PS (Phase 2). The final phase involved evaluating the usage, usability and recommendations for further development of the app by applying a mixed-methods approach (Phase 3).

2 Phase 1 – Needs Assessment

2.1 Methods

This phase employed a sequential explanatory mixed methods design [23]. The process began with a quantitative online survey, which was followed by an online focus group discussion. The participants were PTs or OTs working in Vienna (Austria). They had to have experience in working with PS in an outpatient setting and to provide informed consent for participation in the study. The online survey consisted of 34 questions, primarily of a closed or semi-open type, concluding with an open-ended question. It was conducted from January 28th to February 20th, 2020, and covered topics such as demographic data, HEP prescription behavior, HEP content, patient motivation for HEP, and interest, concerns, and specifications for a video-based mobile application for HEP.

The focus group was held online via video conferencing on March 19th, 2020. The semi-structured interview guideline was based on the results of the online survey. The focus group, which lasted an hour, was audio and video recorded and aimed to give a deeper insight into the same topics as covered in the survey.

Quantitative data of the survey were analyzed using descriptive statistics. The focus group transcripts and qualitative survey data were then thoroughly analyzed using thematic qualitative content analysis based on Kuckartz [24], using the software MAXQDA. Finally, quantitative and qualitative data were combined for a comprehensive analysis.

2.2   Results

Data analysis incorporated responses from 52 participants who completed the online survey. The participants were predominantly female (92% vs. 8% male). The professional background of the participants was almost evenly split, with 48% being OTs and 52% being PTs. The focus group included six therapists, four of whom were PTs and two were OTs. The gender distribution in the focus group was five females and one male.

Prescription Behavior of HEP. Regarding the prescription behavior of HEP, participants in the online survey reported prescribing HEP PS to varying degrees (see Fig. 1).

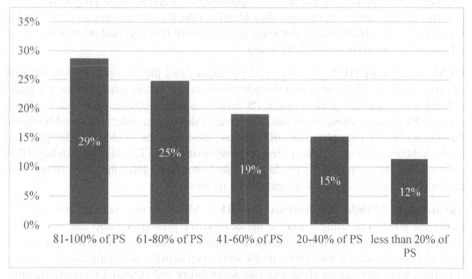

Fig. 1. Percentage of therapists (bars) prescribing HEP to different proportions of PS.

Reasons for not prescribing HEP included concerns about incorrect execution of the exercises, rejection by the PS, or a lack of time on the part of the therapists. In terms of instruction methods, 92.3% of therapists provided individual written instructions, 69.2% gave oral instructions, 17.3% used standardized paper-based instructions, and 15.4% utilized digital instructions such as videos or mobile applications. Most therapists

(72.6%) were satisfied with their chosen mode of instruction delivery, and 76.7% believed the PS were satisfied with it as well. The focus group participants reported that HEP was mostly provided in the form of individually written instructions, supplemented by hand-drawn pictures. PS involvement was facilitated by using the patients' own terminology and by having them document their exercises using their smartphones. In terms of the number of exercises prescribed, 59.6% of therapists typically prescribed three to four exercises per PS, 13% prescribed fewer, and 15.4% prescribed more. As for the frequency of the HEP, 40.4% of participants recommended once per week, 26.9% suggested several times per day, 21.2% recommended several times per week, while the rest did not specify a frequency. Frequency was individually tailored based on the PS's motivation, compliance, and physical or mental condition. The focus group participants also highlighted the importance of the timing of the HEP. This could involve a specific time of day or aligning the HEP with a specific daily activity to facilitate the integration of the HEP into the patient's routine.

Content of HEP. The content of the HEP was ranked by survey participants in terms of its importance for the rehabilitation progress. The ranking, from most to least important, was as follows: 1) Activities of daily living, 2) Tonus regulation, 3) Sensibility training, 4) Stability training, 5) Volitional motor activity in a specific plane, 6) Coordination training, 7) Strength training, 8) Improvement of passive range of motion, and 9) Endurance training. The focus group participants, however, did not specify particular exercises, emphasizing instead the importance of individualized programs and the need for adaptability. Nevertheless, they identified the following areas as most suitable for inclusion in a HEP: fine motor training, sensibility training, and integration of the affected arm into activities of daily living.

PS Motivation for HEP. The surveyed therapists rated the factors for PS motivation to carry out their HEP and found the perception of the actual rehabilitation progress, definition of a distinct goal to reach, PS involvement in exercise selection, feedback after HEP execution most important. Moreover, a digital reminder, informed relatives, monitoring by the therapist, view of progress, the relevance of the HEP for personal goals, hobbies, quality of life, a pleasant design of the HEP, a less demanding HEP, defining HEP as a part of daily productivity, and integrating HEP into daily living were mentioned to be important for increasing the motivation.

Video-Based Mobile Application for HEP. Most survey participants (86.5%) expressed interest in using a mobile application for prescribing and executing HEP, while 13.5% opposed it due to concerns about patients' tech-savviness, data privacy, or incorrect exercise execution. About 40.4% were open to using pre-made exercise videos, but others had reservations about exercise adaptability and potential misunderstanding of exercise execution.

The focus group participants suggested that exercise videos should include specific cues and should be adaptable by therapists. They also deemed it essential to have a feature for uploading individual videos. They outlined several criteria for pre-made exercise videos, including a neutral background, clearly defined initial body position, appropriate camera perspectives, detailed views, verbal instructions, and exercises for both sides of the body.

While 53.33% of surveyed therapists would use the app for communication between therapy sessions, others, including all focus group participants, declined due to concerns about maintaining professional boundaries, time constraints, lack of reimbursement, and data privacy. Those open to communication would use the app for sending HEP, text or voice messages, viewing HEP statistics, or video chatting.

Feedback for PS on HEP progress was preferred via individual text messages (40.4%), selected text modules (26.9%), or emojis (25%). The focus group suggested that feedback should be customizable, and that PS should be able to self-report feelings and to take notes. They also proposed features like checkboxes for HEP completion, a weekly HEP plan, progress statistics, goal visualization, and reminder notifications.

The design of the app should be simple, intuitive, and visually clear, with adequately sized text to enhance usability for the target group.

3   Phase 2 – Prototype

3.1 Methods

The application was developed by an interdisciplinary team comprising two PTs, one OT, and three software developers. Identified user needs (based on the survey and focus group phase 1 and literature) were articulated as user stories in the format: "As a therapist/PS, I want [...], so that [...]." Exercise videos, based on Impairment-Oriented Training [25] and results from phase 1, were created and supplemented with written instructions.

App Development. The development team followed an agile software development approach which was iterative and focused on delivering incremental improvements. The previously defined user stories were divided into smaller tasks and captured inside a product backlog. Furthermore, the development team used sprints, which are time-boxed iterations, to work on specific tasks. The sprint duration allowed the development team to focus on a specific set of user stories and deliver a working increment of the app within that timeframe. To manage their workflow, the team utilized a Kanban board, which visually represented different stages of work. Each task was represented as a card that moved across the board as it progressed through the stages.

At the beginning of each sprint, the entire team gathered to plan the sprint. They reviewed the user stories in the product backlog, selected the most important ones, and estimated the effort required for each story. Throughout the sprint, the team members collaborated and communicated regularly to ensure smooth progress. Regular stand-up meetings provided a platform for team members to discuss their work, any challenges faced, and plan for the week. To ensure code quality, the team employed code review techniques. After completing a user story or task, team members conducted code reviews, examining each other's code for potential issues, adherence to coding standards, and overall quality. At the end of each sprint, the team held a sprint review meeting to show-case the completed user stories to stakeholders, gather feedback, and ensure alignment with the product vision. Security was a paramount concern throughout the development process. The development team prioritized regular updates of core modules and libraries to ensure that the app remained up to date with the latest security patches and fixes. In addition, the team adhered to established software development principles to deliver high-quality code [26]. By implementing coding standards and guidelines, they aimed to minimize the introduction of bugs and vulnerabilities, enhancing the overall reliability of the app. To ensure data privacy, collected data is stored securely in the app's internal storage, which is only accessible by the app itself. All data reports are stored encrypted, and password protected, preventing unauthorized access or manipulation. Saving the data locally on the device rather than relying on external servers minimizes the app's attack surface, reducing the risk of potential vulnerabilities or unauthorized access.

3.2 Results

The final product is an Android tablet application named "MARTHA" (Master Therapy Assistant). MARTHA, represented as an avatar, guides the PS through the individualized HEP. The application is used collaboratively by the therapist and PS during therapy sessions, and the PS continues to use it for HEP at home between therapy sessions. The following features have been implemented.

Home Screen. The home screen features a left-sided menu, progress statistics, a reminder for performing the HEP, an overview of goals, and a button to initiate the HEP (see Fig. 2).

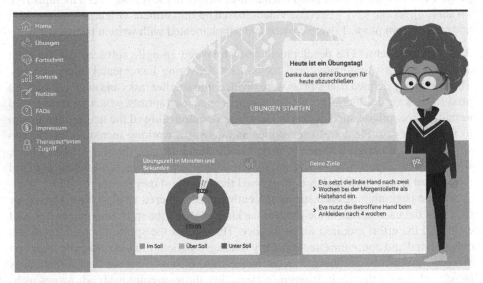

Fig. 2. Home screen of the app MARTHA.

Goal Setting and Evaluation. This section allows the PS and therapist to set one or more SMART (specific, measurable, achievable, realistic, terminated) therapy goals. The PS assesses the goal-achievement and satisfaction with this situation on a scale of 0 to 10. The therapist sets an evaluation period of two or four weeks, after which the system prompts the reassessment of the goal.

Exercise Videos. The application includes 36 videos and matching descriptions of upper limb exercises. These are categorized into grasping exercises, target-oriented exercises, object manipulation, and static/dynamic trunk exercises. Videos are available for both body sides. The therapist can select up to three relevant exercises that align with the therapy goals. Exercise frequency in terms of times per week, duration, and training cues have to be specified by the therapist as well.

Mood Assessment. The PS is prompted to assess her*his mood on a scale of 0 to 10 before and after each HEP session. Significant mood changes trigger a request which asks the PS to comment on her*his experience. These comments, which can include videos, photos, or audio recordings, can be viewed by the therapist in the next therapy session.

Progress Statistics. The home screen displays the total exercise minutes completed. In a separate statistics section of the app line graphs over time depict the goal and mood assessments. Any modifications to the exercise program are displayed as well.

Reminder and Additional Settings. Reminders for performing the HEP can be set according to the PS's needs and preferences, with or without an audio signal. Additional settings include the overall planned therapy duration and data export functions.

4 Phase 3 – Evaluation

4.1 Methods

This pilot study used a mixed-methods approach to evaluate the feasibility, usage, usability, acceptance, and satisfaction of the MARTHA application among PTs, OTs and PS.

Participants. PS inclusion criteria included being 18 years or older, having a diagnosis of ischemic or hemorrhagic stroke with resulting upper extremity impairment, undergoing occupational or physical therapy with a maximum of two sessions per week, and having the ability to use the affected upper limb for assistance. Exclusion criteria included another stroke event during the study period, hospitalization, injury of the affected upper limb, termination of occupational or physical therapy, or change of the therapist.

OTs and PTs needed to have a valid license to practice in Austria and a minimum of two years of experience in treating PS. They also needed to treat at least one PS who met the inclusion criteria and agreed to participate in the study.

The inclusion criteria were assessed by a study team member for OTs and PTs, and by the treating OT or PT for PS. Participants were recruited via professional networks and provided written informed consent.

Procedure. The study protocol was approved by the ethics committee of FH Campus Wien (EK-No. 4/2021). Before the intervention period, participating OTs and PTs received a detailed training on how to use the tablet and the MARTHA application. They were provided with the necessary hardware and software, a set of therapy material for specific exercises, and a manual with detailed instructions. Therapists were instructed to use the MARTHA application within their usual therapy routine. MARTHA was to be used over a period of minimum four weeks to a maximum of three months. During therapy sessions, PS and therapists should use goal setting, goal evaluation, selection or modification of exercises, and discussions about notes taken by the PS. Between the therapy sessions, PS were encouraged to use MARTHA at home, in order to support their individual HEP.

Demographic data and technical affinity of the participants was collected using a questionnaire at the start of the study. To gather individual information about the feasibility, acceptability, and usability of MARTHA, therapists were asked to note their experiences in a user diary after each use of the application with the PS. The usability, ease of learning, and satisfaction with MARTHA was assessed using a self-translated version of the Usefulness, Satisfaction, and Ease of use Questionnaire (USE-questionnaire) [27]. To gain insight into how and how often the application was used and which features were accessed, usage data was exported from the tablets. Finally, focus group discussions and individual interviews with therapists and PS were conducted to discuss their experience with MARTHA into more detail.

Data Analysis. Demographic data, data from app usage, and data from the USE questionnaire were analyzed using descriptive statistics. Focus group discussions and individual interviews were analyzed together with qualitative data from the usage diaries using MAXQDA. The analysis process was based on the qualitative content analysis according to Sandelowski [28], using procedures from the structural analysis according to Mayring [29] and Kuckartz [24]. Throughout the analysis process, regular team discussions were held to ensure consistency and clarity.

4.2 Results

Participants. The study involved 13 therapists (9 OTs, 4 PTs) and 18 PS. The therapists, all female, ranged in age from 25 to 66 years (median 43 years). Eight of them had prior experience with technology-assisted therapy. The duration of their participation in the study varied from one to 13 weeks (median 7 weeks).

PS (11 males; 7 females) were between 41 and 84 years (median 64 years) old. Time since stroke varied from 5 to 185 months (median 59.5 months). Out of these, 13 had experiences with HEPs and 6 had experiences with technology-assisted therapy. Seventeen PS used technology (smartphone, tablet, or laptop) in their daily life. The duration of their participation in the study ranged from 1 to 13 weeks (median 6 weeks). Two PS discontinued their participation early, after one and three weeks respectively, due to lack of enjoyment and motivation. Available data of these two drop-outs was included in the results (Table 1).

Usage Data. Therapists prescribed using the app for a duration ranging from 12 to 66 days (median 29 days), using 29 out of the 36 available videos. The app was used by PS for a period between 21 and 94 days (median 46 days). On average, two therapy goals were set per PS, with a range of 1 to 7 goals. While most PS did not make any notes in MARTHA, five PS made between 1 to 5 notes, and one PS used this function 53 times. The feature to access statistics about goal achievement was used between 0

Table 1. Technical affinity of study participants.

	PS n = 18 median (min – max)	Therapists n = 13 median (min – max)
Self-rated interest in technology (1 = no interest, 4 = high interest)	3 (2–4)	3 (2–3)
Self-rated ease of learning of new technologies (1 = very easy, 4 = very hard)	2 (1–4)	2 (1–2)
Estimation of the potential of new technologies in therapy (1 = no potential at all, 4 = very high potential)	3 (2–4)	3 (2–4)

and 109 times (median 11). The function to export training details was used by only one therapist.

Usability. The evaluation of usability based on the USE questionnaire (best possible score = 7) resulted in a median score of 6 for the subscales of usefulness (range 4–7) and satisfaction (range 3–7), and 7 for ease of use (range 5–7) and ease of learning (range 6–7) among therapists. PS gave a median score of 5 points for usefulness (range 1–7) and satisfaction (range 1–7), 6 points for ease of use (range 1–7), and 7 points for ease of learning (range 1–7) (see Fig. 3).

Focus Groups and Interviews. Three focus groups were conducted with the therapists, two in-person and one online, lasting between 1 h 7 min to 1 h 48 min. Two therapists who couldn't attend the focus groups were individually interviewed in-person. Two focus groups (duration between 50 min and 1 h and 11 min) were conducted with each three PS. Ten PS couldn't come to the focus groups, therefore individual interviews in-person took place (duration between 18 and 43 min).

Feasibility. Therapists found it easy to learn and use the app due to the manual and initial instructions from the study team. Therapists and PS noted that due to the app's simplicity prior technical experience had little influence on its usage.

"Once ... go through everything once and then again [...] I think, yes I can set that up for everybody now." (TH1, paragraph 116)

"I didn't mind exercising with the tablet. [...] that was the first time I had ever done anything like that. I never had anything to do with that." (PS 5, paragraph 71)

The structured design facilitated therapeutic routine of setting a goal and applying focused exercises.

Having such a nice package for the home exercise program. [...] these are the exercise days, we'll agree on them together, this is the exercise time, that's the goal behind it, and then we'll check again to see if you've achieved the goal. I find this a nice package that just runs smoothly. So I also have the feeling that I

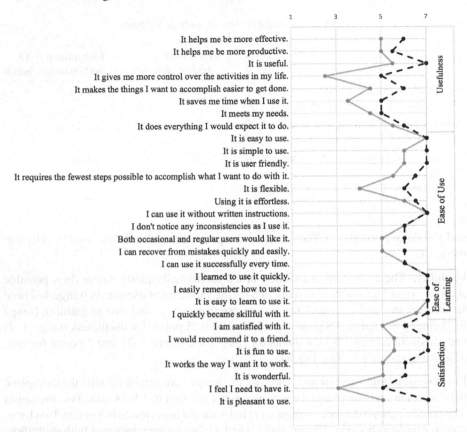

It helps me be more effective.
It helps me be more productive.
It is useful.
It gives me more control over the activities in my life.
It makes the things I want to accomplish easier to get done.
It saves me time when I use it.
It meets my needs.
It does everything I would expect it to do.
It is easy to use.
It is simple to use.
It is user friendly.
It requires the fewest steps possible to accomplish what I want to do with it.
It is flexible.
Using it is effortless.
I can use it without written instructions.
I don't notice any inconsistencies as I use it.
Both occasional and regular users would like it.
I can recover from mistakes quickly and easily.
I can use it successfully every time.
I learned to use it quickly.
I easily remember how to use it.
It is easy to learn to use it.
I quickly became skillful with it.
I am satisfied with it.
I would recommend it to a friend.
It is fun to use.
It works the way I want it to work.
It is wonderful.
I feel I need to have it.
It is pleasant to use.

Usefulness · Ease of Use · Ease of Learning · Satisfaction

Fig. 3. Usability results according to the findings from the USE questionnaire. Grey, solid line: PS; Black, dashed line: Therapists.

don't have to worry about it, it runs even when I'm not there. You're not starting from scratch every time, "And have you practiced now or not?", or "What's the situation now?", and "Where are we at the moment?". This way, it's somehow more manageable for me and gives me a good feeling when I know, ah, they're practicing when I'm not there and we can really continue next time, we don't have to start all over again. (TH2, paragraph 74)

Motivation. The motivation for therapists to participate in the study was mainly the interest in technical tools and to support therapy and HEP.

"I thought that this would motivate the patients to practice on their own. That it provides them with more structure and that they practice more regularly. And to observe this themselves." (TH1, paragraph 4)

The primary motivational aspects of PS to participate in the study and using the app were personal interest, curiosity, and the hope for improvement. The application was perceived as a useful tool for routine exercises but did not specifically alter the motivation to perform everyday HEP in all participants. PS were inconclusive if the app would support doing the HEP in the long term.

"Well, in itself, the tablet is the incentive to do the exercise." (PS 11, paragraph 85)

Acceptance of specific features of the app. Therapists appreciated the provision of exercise videos and the opportunity to add individual ones. Although this procedure was time consuming. The visualization of exercise time was also welcomed. However, the design of the pie-chart for visualizing exercise time on the home screen was criticized for complexity. Although the opportunity of taking notes was hardly used by PS, therapists liked the idea. PS found the clear structure of the app supportive. The forced answering of the "How are you?" question and compulsory video watching though were reported as annoying.

"Well, I'm not very enthusiastic about these questions, but I thought it was good that they were there. But then I had to reflect on it and I don't like thinking about how it's going [...] But yeah, wasn't bad. I think some people will need it." (PS 10, paragraph. 72)

The avatar, MARTHA, was appreciated by some, while others found it childish.

"[...]it was fun for me [...]. I was already happy when the person appeared. With 'hooray, I'm happy and so on' ... And I always said, 'yes', and 'I'm happy too'. But she didn't hear me at all." (PS 17, paragraph 47)

Similar to the therapists, PS liked the videos, and felt supported by them.

"The videos, exactly ... because somehow, the persons who showed the exercises, they had so much fun, they seemed so cheerful." (PS 10, paragraph 160)

For therapists as for PS having to define goals and evaluate these was welcomed, however this process was also perceived as complicated and sometimes too time consuming.

"For me, the goal was [...] very much in focus. Because my patients are long-term patients. And then you do lose sight of this goal. [...] where do we actually want to go specifically in the near future? This has become more present for me once again. Because these are such chronic, long-term patients, where a lot is about maintenance and so on. And to look at it again now, do we have a specific goal? And now we work towards that for a while. This has become very conscious to me with MARTHA and has been intensified." (TH 3, paragraph 32)

App integration in therapy and daily routine. Integrating the app in daily routine was substantially influenced by being part of a research project. Therapists reported that the app was incorporated into therapeutic routines at the start and end of therapy sessions. Due to the scope of the therapy it seemed to be easier for OTs to argue to use the tablet than for PTs. Expectations within occupational therapy are that PS learn how to use things in everyday life, whereas physical therapy is associated with training.

Some therapists were surprised to see the integration of the app into daily routines, as PS exercised more during the study period.

"It was really cool to observe [...] that he had much more motivation to practice on his own than usual. I've had him for about a year now, [...] and he was always like, yes, when I come, he does it for me, but on his own (laughs) he didn't really enjoy it. Even though his wife was always very supportive [...]. I called him again today and [...] you could tell, he really enjoyed it, he said so himself and he also said after the first week, that he thinks it's great and he enjoys practicing with it. And then he really made more progress than usual, because he never... did anything at home voluntarily. That was really cool." (TH1, paragraph 10)

PS also stated that the app was integrated into both therapeutic and daily routines, however, the needs of PS were quite diverse: some required the support of the therapist in every session, while others used the app autonomously once a HEP was established.

"Only the evaluation was done with the therapist [...] but everything else I did myself." (PS 13, paragraph 14)

Satisfaction with the app and related outcomes. Most therapists agreed that they would continue using the app in their daily routine, provided that the app was improved, specifically with respect to remote access. However, the selection of which PS could use it has to be done carefully and would be different based on their experience.

"We also usually address this, who do I have in front of me and what are the needs, what are the goals. And how does this patient work? How can she be motivated? What does she need to stay motivated, to stick with it? And there are those for whom I think this is really a good tool, and then there are those for whom this might be a tool, and then there are those for whom this might not be a tool at all. But I still need to have it at hand, because for many I could possibly provide a lot of support with it." (TH2, paragraph 296)

PS who have lower motivation, cognitive impairment and changing psychological status would not use the app appropriately. PS had limited expectations regarding the app's performance and outcome. The app was seen as a valuable tool, though PS were reluctant to pay for its use.

"As I said, if you look at it from the point of view: Am I motivated, do I need it at all - question mark? But if you are half-motivated, I think that's quite good and I think the program is relatively well structured. [...] So, I mean, if someone is not motivated, I don't think he will accept therapy" (PS 14, paragraph 30).

Technical Aspects. Technical issues concerning the hardware and the software hindered the usability. Especially the reminder function (for exercises and for evaluation for goal achievement) were not working reliably.

Recommendations for Further App Development. Therapists provided several recommendations, like adding audio explanations to videos, individualizing the avatar, and adding a reward system. Concerning the videos it was suggested to add videos for PS on the upper or lower edge of upper-limb functional level and for the trunk. The ability to use the app with multiple patients simultaneously and remote access for the therapists were also suggested. PS suggested including a reward system, better visual aids to enhance motivation and larger font size. They also recommended improving charts for displaying exercise data and allowing the option to disable mandatory video watching. The need for a bigger exercise variety was also highlighted, especially for patients with more severe limitations.

5 Discussion

This study aimed to develop and evaluate a tablet application for HEP execution for PS, based on a needs analysis with OTs and PTs. The results indicate that the MARTHA application is feasible and usable for both therapists and PS and was generally positively received. However, the study also identified several areas for improvement.

The development of MARTHA was based on the needs of therapists and PS, which were identified in phase 1 of the study. The results of this phase are in line with previous research, which has highlighted the importance of individualized HEPs, the involvement of PS in the selection of exercises, and the need for feedback and reminders to increase motivation for HEP [14, 21].

The evaluation of MARTHA in phase 3 of the study showed that the application was generally well accepted by both therapists and PS. The usability of the application was rated highly by both groups, which is in line with previous research showing that tablet applications can be well accepted by patients [30]. However, the study also identified several areas for improvement. For example, some therapists reported that the process of adding individual videos was time-consuming, and some PS found the mandatory video watching to be annoying. These issues could potentially be addressed by adding a bigger number and variety of exercise videos. The application could also allow for more individuality. For example, the goal and mood query could be made adjustable rather than mandatory, and there could be an option to skip certain exercise videos if PS feel confident in performing the exercises. However, this presents a challenge as it could increase the complexity of the application and it would no longer be a simple tool. Further we conclude from the feedback, that the introduction of the therapists to the application might need to be more comprehensive, as it may be necessary to explain the theory behind the mood query, goal setting, the need to watch videos, etc., in more detail.

Despite the generally positive results, the study has several limitations. First, the sample size was relatively small, and the study was conducted in a single country, which may limit the generalizability of the results. Second, the study did not include a control group, so it is not possible to determine whether the observed improvements in HEP adherence and satisfaction were due to the use of MARTHA or other factors. The integration of MARTHA into the daily routine of therapists and PS might have been influenced by being part of a research project. Finally, the study did not measure the impact of MARTHA on clinical outcomes, such as functional improvement or quality of life.

462   L. Rettinger et al.

In conclusion, this study shows that a tablet application for HEP for stroke patients, is feasible and usable, and is generally well accepted. However, further research is needed to improve the application and to evaluate its impact on clinical outcomes.

References

1. Feigin, V.L., Stark, B.A., Johnson, C.O., Roth, G.A., Bisignano, C., Abady, G.G., et al.: Global, regional, and national burden of stroke and its risk factors, 1990–2019: a systematic analysis for the Global Burden of Disease Study 2019. Lancet Neurol. **20**, 795–820 (2021). https://doi.org/10.1016/S1474-4422(21)00252-0
2. Nichols-Larsen, D.S., Clark, P.C., Zeringue, A., Greenspan, A., Blanton, S.: Factors influencing stroke survivors' quality of life during subacute recovery. Stroke **36**, 1480–1484 (2005). https://doi.org/10.1161/01.STR.0000170706.13595.4f
3. Langhorne, P., Legg, L.: Evidence behind stroke rehabilitation. J. Neurol. Neurosurg. Psychiatry. **74**(Suppl 4), iv18–iv21 (2003). https://doi.org/10.1136/jnnp.74.suppl_4.iv18
4. Gou, X., Zhang, X., Zheng, X., Zhang, Y., Ma, H.: Effect of hand intensive training on upper limb function of stroke patients with hemiplegia. Comput. Math. Methods Med. **2022**, 6844680 (2022). https://doi.org/10.1155/2022/6844680
5. Wang, L., et al.: Effects of corticospinal tract integrity on upper limb motor function recovery in stroke patients treated with repetitive transcranial magnetic stimulation. J. Integr. Neurosci. **21**, 50 (2022). https://doi.org/10.31083/j.jin2102050
6. Huang, J., et al.: Effects of physical therapy-based rehabilitation on recovery of upper limb motor function after stroke in adults: a systematic review and meta-analysis of randomized controlled trials. Ann. Palliat. Med. **11**, 521–531 (2022). https://doi.org/10.21037/apm-21-3710
7. Platz, T., Schmuck, L., Roschka, S.: S3-Leitlinie "Rehabilitative Therapie bei Armparese nach Schlaganfall" der DGNR - Langversion. [S3-Guideline "Rehabilitation therapy for arm paresis after stroke" by DGNR - long version.]. https://www.awmf.org/uploads/tx_szleitlinien/080-001l_S3_Rehabilitative_Therapie_bei_Armparese_nach_Schlaganfall_2020-07.pdf
8. Dworzynski, K., Ritchie, G., Playford, E.D.: Stroke rehabilitation: long-term rehabilitation after stroke. Clin. Med. **15**, 461–464 (2015). https://doi.org/10.7861/clinmedicine.15-5-461
9. Hebert, D., Lindsay, M.P., McIntyre, A., Kirton, A., Rumney, P.G., Bagg, S., et al.: Canadian stroke best practice recommendations: Stroke rehabilitation practice guidelines, update 2015. Int. J. Stroke **11**, 459–484 (2016). https://doi.org/10.1177/1747493016643553
10. Stroke Foundation. Clinical Guidelines for Stroke Management (2017). www.informme.org.au
11. Winstein, C.J., et al.: Guidelines for adult stroke rehabilitation and recovery: a guideline for healthcare professionals from the American Heart Association/American Stroke Association. Stroke **47** (2016). https://doi.org/10.1161/STR.0000000000000098
12. Miller, K.K., Porter, R.E., DeBaun-Sprague, E., Van Puymbroeck, M., Schmid, A.A.: Exercise after Stroke: patient adherence and beliefs after discharge from rehabilitation. Top. Stroke Rehabil. **24**, 142–148 (2017). https://doi.org/10.1080/10749357.2016.1200292
13. Mahmood, A., Solomon, J.M., English, C., Bhaskaran, U., Menon, G., Manikandan, N.: Measurement of adherence to home-based exercises among community-dwelling stroke survivors in India. Physiother. Res. Int. **25** (2020). https://doi.org/10.1002/pri.1827
14. Mahmood, A., et al.: Development of strategies to support home-based exercise adherence after stroke: a Delphi consensus. BMJ Open **12**, e055946 (2022). https://doi.org/10.1136/bmjopen-2021-055946

15. Grau-Pellicer, M., Lalanza, J., Jovell-Fernández, E., Capdevila, L.: Impact of mHealth technology on adherence to healthy PA after stroke: a randomized study. Top. Stroke Rehabil. **27**, 354–368 (2020). https://doi.org/10.1080/10749357.2019.1691816

16. Veerbeek, J.M., et al.: KNGF Clinical Practice Guideline for Physical Therapy in Patients with Stroke (2014). https://www.kngf.nl/binaries/content/assets/kennisplatform/onbeveiligd/ guidelines/stroke_practice_guidelines_2014.pdf

17. Laver, K.E., Adey-Wakeling, Z., Crotty, M., Lannin, N.A., George, S., Sherrington, C.: Telerehabilitation services for stroke. Cochrane Database Syst Rev. **1**, CD010255 (2020). https:// doi.org/10.1002/14651858.CD010255.pub3

18. Sarfo, F.S., Ulasavets, U., Opare-Sem, O.K., Ovbiagele, B.: Tele-rehabilitation after Stroke: an updated systematic review of the literature. J. Stroke Cerebrovasc. Dis. **27**, 2306–2318 (2018). https://doi.org/10.1016/j.jstrokecerebrovasdis.2018.05.013

19. Johansson, T., Wild, C.: Telerehabilitation in stroke care–a systematic review. J. Telemed. Telecare **17**, 1–6 (2011). https://doi.org/10.1258/jtt.2010.100105

20. Mahmood, A., et al.: Acceptability and attitude towards a mobile-based home exercise program among Stroke survivors and caregivers: a cross-sectional study. Int. J. Telemed. Appl. **2019**, 1–6 (2019). https://doi.org/10.1155/2019/5903106

21. Wentink, M.M., et al.: What is important in e-health interventions for Stroke rehabilitation? A survey study among patients, informal caregivers, and health professionals. Int. J, Telerehab. **10**, 15–28 (2018). https://doi.org/10.5195/IJT.2018.6247

22. Dobrics, M., Hetterle, T.: Ergebnisbericht des arbeitskreises "Erfahrungsaustausch" der AAL-Austria [Outcome report of the Working Group "Experience exchange of AAL-Austria"] (2021). https://www.aal.at/wp-content/uploads/2015/11/AK_AAL_Erfahrungsau stausch_Ergebnisbericht_20141104.pdf

23. Creswell, J.W., Creswell, J.D.: Research Design: Qualitative, Quantitative, and Mixed Methods Approaches. **388**

24. Kuckartz, U., Rädiker, S.: Analyzing Qualitative Data with MAXQDA: Text, Audio, and Video. Springer, Cham (2019). https://doi.org/10.1007/978-3-030-15671-8

25. Platz, T.: Impairment-oriented training (IOT)–scientific concept and evidence-based treatment strategies. Restor. Neurol. Neurosci. **22**, 301–315 (2004)

26. Martin, R.C. (ed.): Clean Code: A Handbook of Agile Software Craftsmanship. Prentice Hall, Upper Saddle River (2009)

27. Lund, A.M.: Measuring usability with the use questionnaire. Usab. Interface **8**, 3–6 (2001)

28. Sandelowski, M.: Whatever happened to qualitative description? Res. Nurs. Health **23**, 334–340 (2000). https://doi.org/10.1002/1098-240X(200008)23:4%3c334::AID-NUR9%3e3.0. CO;2-G

29. Mayring, P.: Qualitative Inhaltsanalyse: Grundlagen und Techniken [Qualitative content analysis. Basics and techniques.]. Beltz, Weinheim Basel (2015)

30. Mehra, S., et al.: Supporting older adults in exercising with a tablet: a usability study. JMIR Hum. Factors **6**, e11598 (2019). https://doi.org/10.2196/11598

Workshop on the Internet of Things in Health Research

The RinasciMENTE 2.0 Project: A Study Protocol for a Randomized Controlled Trial Evaluating the Efficacy of an Internet-Based Self-Help Program for Managing Psychological Distress Within the Broader Italian Population

Giada Pietrabissa[1,2]([envelope]) [iD], Gloria Marchesi[2], Michelle Semonella[3] [iD],
Gerhard Andersson[4,5] [iD], and Gianluca Castelnuovo[1,2] [iD]

[1] Clinical Psychology Research Laboratory, I.R.C.C.S. Istituto Auxologico Italiano, Milan, Italy
g.pietrabissa@auxologico.it
[2] Department of Psychology, Catholic University of Milan, Milan, Italy
[3] Department of Psychology, Bar-Ilan University, Ramat Gan, Israel
[4] Department of Behavioural Science and Learning, Linköping University, Linköping, Sweden
[5] Department of Clinical Neuroscience, Karolinska Institute, Solna, Sweden

Abstract. *Objective:* The aim of this study is to assess the feasibility and effectiveness of the RinasciMENTE 2.0 initiative, an internet-based self-help intervention grounded in the principles and techniques of Cognitive Behavioral Therapy (CBT), in assisting individuals from the general population who are dealing with mild psychological difficulties.

Methods: To accomplish this objective, a randomized controlled trial (RCT) will be carried out, with random allocation occurring at the individual level. The study intends to compare the impact of the RinasciMENTE 2.0 program with that of a waiting list control group in terms of enhancing the psychological well-being of a representative sample from the community. A minimum of 128 participants experiencing mild or subthreshold levels of psychological symptoms will be recruited. Following baseline screening, participants will be randomly assigned to the experimental group or the control condition. The program will extend over a period of two months, during which participants will engage in eight weekly modules of CBT. The effects of the RinasciMENTE 2.0 program on specific primary and secondary psychological outcomes will be evaluated post-intervention (at 2 months) and during a follow-up assessment at 12 months. *Expected Results and Conclusions*: Anticipated outcomes include an improvement in individuals' psychological functioning and the acquisition of skills and self-assurance necessary to effectively address their emotional difficulties.

Keywords: Web-based intervention · Cognitive-behavioral therapy · Self-help · Randomized controlled trial · Clinical psychology

© ICST Institute for Computer Sciences, Social Informatics and Telecommunications Engineering 2024
Published by Springer Nature Switzerland AG 2024. All Rights Reserved
D. Salvi et al. (Eds.): PH 2023, LNICST 572, pp. 467–477, 2024.
https://doi.org/10.1007/978-3-031-59717-6_30

1 Background

Recent research has highlighted a concerning decline in global mental health, as evidenced by clinical assessments and statistical data [1, 2]. This alarming trend is expected to continue, underscoring the urgent need for practical psychological interventions that can meet the specific needs of the population [3–6].

In this context, cognitive-behavioral techniques, such as cognitive bias restructuring, planning activities, and relaxation strategies, have demonstrated significant effectiveness in managing emotional problems [7, 8]. CBT is a structured form of psychotherapy designed to help individuals identify and change harmful or ineffective thought and behavior patterns, replacing them with more helpful thoughts and functional behaviors [9].

However, because traditional face-to-face therapy is not always feasible [10–14], there is a growing need for innovative methods to deliver psychological treatments, and remote therapy has emerged as a potentially viable solution.

Numerous randomized controlled trials (RCTs) and systematic reviews have shown the usefulness and effectiveness of internet-based interventions in helping individuals facing psychological issues [15–18]. CBT is particularly well-suited to remote therapy for several reasons. It is a talk-based therapy, making it relatively easy to adapt for remote delivery, and it encourages individuals to take an active role in engaging in modifications and focusing on particular assignments between sessions, which aligns seamlessly with remote therapy [19]. Furthermore, remote therapy can enhance the sense of self-efficacy [20], empowering individuals to become their therapists by equipping them with skills they can use independently to maintain their well-being after treatment.

Studies have indicated that the use of digitally administered Cognitive-Behavioral Therapy (iCBT) has proven effective in alleviating symptoms associated with a range of mental health conditions, including social anxiety disorder, generalized anxiety disorder, panic disorder, major depressive disorder, obsessive-compulsive disorder, and insomnia [21–26], whether in guided or unguided self-help programs.

Despite the increasing attention given to digital interventions, internet-based self-help programs rooted in CBT have not yet reached their full potential. To close this notable research gap, it is essential to conduct comprehensive investigations into the effects of internet-based interventions on improving personal emotional health.

2 Main Hypotheses and Objectives

This RCT aims to investigate the effectiveness of an innovative internet-based Cognitive Behavioral Therapy (CBT) self-help program designed to address mild psychological distress in both Italian residents and Italians living abroad. To evaluate its impact, we will compare the outcomes of participants in the RinasciMENTE 2.0 program with those on a waiting list (WL) using self-reported measures immediately after the 8-week intervention and at a 12-month follow-up.

The primary hypothesis we will examine is whether the program is both feasible and effective in enhancing individuals' psychological well-being.

The secondary hypothesis will assess whether individuals assigned to the experimental group experienced a reduction in levels of stress, anxiety, and depression, along with improvements in emotion regulation skills, self-efficacy, and perceived quality of life compared to those in the WL condition at the end of the treatment.

Furthermore, we anticipate that participants in the experimental group will maintain or further decrease their psychological symptoms at the 12-month follow-up after completing the treatment program.

3 Methods

3.1 Design

This project entails a randomized, open-label, and parallel-group comparative study comprising two groups: an experimental group, which will receive 8 weekly online CBT self-help sessions, and a control group placed on a waiting list (WL).

The research received approval from the Ethical Committee at the Catholic University of Milan, Italy, under the identification number 25–21. All actions conducted as part of the study will adhere to the ethical guidelines set forth by the institutional and/or national research committee, following the principles outlined in the Helsinki Declaration and its subsequent revisions or equivalent ethical norms.

3.2 Participants

Participants will be sourced from the general populace using advertisements posted on various social media platforms such as Facebook, Instagram, and Twitter, as well as through online webinars centered around the study's subject matter. The recruitment materials will contain information regarding the study's objectives, the treatment provided, and the prerequisites for participation, along with a web link to access the program.

To be eligible for participation in the study, individuals must meet the following criteria: (A) possess fluency in the Italian language, regardless of their country of origin; (B) be at least 18 years old; (C) provide informed consent online; and (D) exhibit mild or subthreshold levels of symptoms on the Web Screening Questionnaire (WSQ) [27]. This 15-item online questionnaire was designed by Cuijpers et al. [28] to quickly (about 5 min) identify the following psychiatric conditions: depressive disorder, alcohol abuse/dependence, generalized anxiety disorder (GAD), post-traumatic stress disorder (PTSD), social phobia, panic disorder, agoraphobia, specific phobia, and obsessive-compulsive disorder (OCD). Cut-off scores are set as follow: Depression: item #1 $\geq$ 5 & item #2 = 1; GAD: item #3 $\geq$ 2; Panic: item #4 $\geq$ 1; Panic with Agoraphobia: item #4 $\geq$ 1 & item #5 = 1; Agoraphobia: item #5 = 1; Specific phobia: item #6 or item #6 $\geq$ 1; Social phobia: item #8 = 1 & item #9 = 1; PTSD: item #10 = 1 or item #11 = 1; OCD: item #12 $\geq$ 1; Alcohol Abuse/Dependence: item #13 $\geq$ 2 & item #14 $\geq$ 3; Suicide: item #5 $\geq$ 3.

Exclusion from the program will apply to individuals who: (A) have visual, hearing, or cognitive impairments that hinder their ability to receive and follow the intervention; (B) suffer from severe psychiatric disorders as defined by the Diagnostic and Statistical Manual of Mental Disorders (DSM-5) [29]; (C) lack basic computer skills or access to the internet. Participants will not be eliminated even if they are currently undergoing psychopharmacological treatment or receiving psychological or psychotherapeutic assistance.

3.3 Sample Size Calculation

We determined the minimum sample size required for this study using a predefined sample size calculator (specifically, G*Power 3.1.9.2 software) designed for F tests [30–32]. Subjects were randomly assigned to the iCBT self-help group and the waiting list group. Additionally, they will be assessed at three different time points: (1) before the intervention, (2) after the intervention (two months later), and (3) 12 months after treatment completion.

Given the innovative nature of the study, realistic estimates of effect sizes were derived, with a predefined partial η2 set at 0.02, indicating a small effect size [33, 34]. This corresponds to a Cohen's f value of 0.143. Furthermore, we established a type I error rate (α) of 0.05 (two-sided), a Power ($1 - \beta$) of 0.95, and a predetermined correlation between repeated measures of 0.50, following standard guidelines [33].

The adjustment for non-sphericity was established at a factor of 1.

Results indicated that with a total of 128 participants (64 in each group), there is a 95% probability of correctly rejecting the null hypothesis, indicating a significant effect of the interaction.

3.4 Randomization Procedure

The randomization plan and allocation will be created using the Randomization.com website [35]. To maintain allocation concealment, the program will generate an anonymous code for each participant, which will correspond to the randomization sequence. However, because of the nature of the intervention, it will not be possible to conceal the treatment group allocation from the participants, the research team, or the outcome assessors. Nevertheless, the clinical psychologist conducting the sessions, as well as the participants and observers, will remain unaware of the research objectives. Subjects will be allocated to the two conditions in two days from the initial assessment (Fig. 1).

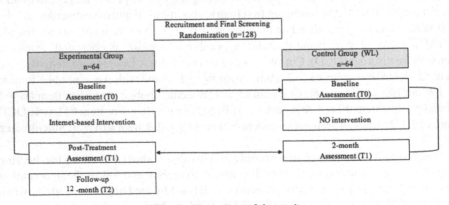

Fig. 1. Flow chart of the study

3.5 Measures

Participants will be asked to provide self-reported demographic and clinical information at the baseline assessment. This information will include age, gender, educational background, marital status, as well as their current weight, and height, which will be used to determine Body Mass Index (BMI, kg/m^2).

Furthermore, the Italian version of the following psychological measures will be administered at baseline (T0), after 2 months (T1), and at the 12-month follow-up (T2):

Primary Outcome Measure

The primary outcome will be assessed using the *Outcome Questionnaire* (OQ-45) [36], which consists of 45 items. Participants will rate these items on a 5-point Likert scale, ranging from 0 (Never) to 4 (Almost always). The OQ-45 evaluates treatment progress in three distinct domains: Symptom Distress (SD – 25 items); Interpersonal Relations (IR - 11 items), and Social Role (SR – 9 items). The total OQ-45 score is derived by summing the scores of these three subscales. The total score can range from 0 to 180. A total score equal to or greater than 63 suggests the existence of important symptoms. More specifically, a score equal to or greater than 36 in the SD subscale signifies significant symptom distress, a score equal to or greater than 15 in the IR subscale indicates dysfunctional relationships and a score equal to or greater than 12 in the SR subscale suggests an ill-defined social role.

Secondary Outcome Measure

Perceived Stress Scale (PSS) [37]: This scale consists of 10 items, and participants rate their responses on a 5-point Likert scale, ranging from 0 (Never) to 4 (Very often). It assesses the extent to which individuals perceive situations in their lives as stressful. PSS scores are calculated by reversing responses to items 4, 5, 7, and 8 and then adding up all scale items. The overall score can vary between 0 and 40.

Emotional Regulation Questionnaire (ERQ) [38]: This questionnaire consists of 10 statements that participants rate on a 7-point Likert scale, ranging from 1 (Strongly disagree) to 7 (Strongly agree). It evaluates how individuals manage their emotions in two ways: Cognitive Reappraisal and Expressive Suppression. The total score can vary between 7 and 70.

Depression Anxiety Stress Scales-Short Version (DASS-21) [39]: This scale includes 21 statements rated on a 4-point Likert scale, ranging from 0 (Did not apply to me at all) to 3 (Applied to me very much). It assesses negative emotional states, including depression, anxiety, and stress. Each scale comprises 7 items. The total scores for each subscale are obtained by summing the scores of the individual items and then doubling the result. The DASS-total score can range between 0 and 126, with each subscale score ranging between 0 and 42.

General Self-efficacy Scale (GSES) [40]: This scale comprises 10 items rated on a 4-point Likert scale, ranging from 1 (Not at all true) to 4 (Exactly true). It assesses individuals' confidence in their ability to cope with challenging or stressful events. The total score is calculated by summing all items, and it ranges from 10 to 40, with higher scores indicating greater self-efficacy.

World Health Organization Quality of Life (WHOQOL-BREF) [41]: This questionnaire includes 26 items rated on a 5-point Likert scale and assesses four domains: physical health, psychological health, social relationships, and environmental health. Scores that originally fall within the range of 25 to 130, are transformed using a conversion to fit a 0 to 100 scale.

Furthermore, adherence to the program will be assessed by examining factors like the proportion of pages visited or the frequency of access. To gauge *acceptability,* we will track participant attrition rates and, for the experimental group, by employing the *System Usability Scale* (SUS) [42]. The SUS involves responding to 10 statements using a 5-point Likert scale, with possible scores spanning from 0 to 100. A score exceeding 68 suggests there are no significant usability issues.

3.6 Procedure

Individuals interested in participating will be guided to the RinasciMENTE 2.0 website (https://www.iterapi.se/sites/rinascimente/login).

There, they will find an online consent form, and upon acceptance, each participant will receive a document outlining the study's objectives and requirements.

The initial step will involve participants completing the Web Screening Questionnaire (WSQ). Subsequently, over the following 5 days, participants will select a convenient time slot for a clinical semi-structured interview. This interview, lasting approximately 45 min, will be conducted by a certified psychotherapist who is not affiliated with the study. The purpose of this interview is to further assess each individual's eligibility for participation in the study. Additional information regarding the study and the randomization process will be provided to all respondents.

The decision regarding the inclusion of participants in the study will be made collectively by the professional conducting the interview and the research investigators. Participants will be informed of the decision via email within a week. In cases where exclusion is necessary, individuals will be provided with explanations, and if there are indications of severe psychological distress, they will be encouraged to seek professional assistance.

Eligible participants will then be randomly assigned to either the experimental group (iCBT self-help) or the control group (WL). They will receive an email containing a username and a personalized link to create a password, which will grant them access to the *iterapi* platform [43, 44]. The *iterapi* platform is a secure platform with demonstrated effectiveness in alleviating symptoms of various disorders [45–48]. In the present study, the platform content and activities will be for the first time re-design to adapt to the psychological needs of the broader Italian population.

Participants assigned to the experimental group have to log in to the platform and provide electronic informed consent. In contrast, individuals in the control group will gain access to the online treatment once the experimental group has finished its two-month intervention period. The *iterapi* platform will be the main channel for communication between mental health professionals and participants, as well as for delivering the intervention and collecting quantitative assessments. Before starting the program, participants will be required to fill out self-report questionnaires evaluating primary and secondary outcomes (T0).

The treatment itself will consist of 8 weekly modules focused on: 1) setting goals; 2) anxiety management; 3) effective communication; 4) stress management; 5) anger management; 6) taking care of yourself; 7) sleep problems; 8) plan of completion and maintenance.

Throughout the intervention, participants will receive weekly email updates notifying them of new materials available on the platform. Participants who will not access the materials or fail to complete recommended tasks and exercises will receive weekly reminders, along with brief, encouraging messages.

Upon completion of the program (after two months – T1), participants in both groups will be asked to complete the baseline questionnaires once more. Additionally, the experimental group will undergo assessments at 12-month intervals following the conclusion of the treatment (T2) (Fig. 1).

We do not anticipate any adverse or unintended effects resulting from trial participation. However, if participants experience any form of psychological discomfort, they can consult with the responsible psychologist. Moreover, participants can reach out to the study's coordinator for any doubts or information needs. Once enrolled, participants retain the freedom to withdraw from the study at any point without impacting their future treatment.

3.7 Statistical Analysis

Statistical analyses will be conducted using SPSS software version 24.0 [49].

Initially, preliminary analyses will be carried out to evaluate the assumptions related to univariate and multivariate normality. In cases where significant violations of these assumptions will be detected, robust methods or data transformations will be applied. Participants who dropped out of the study will be excluded during these preliminary analyses.

To handle missing data, a missing values analysis will be conducted to determine if the missing values were Missing Completely at Random (MCAR) or if there will be a discernible pattern among them. If no patterns are identified, then either pairwise or listwise deletion will be employed to manage missing data. However, if a pattern is identified through the missing value analysis, imputation techniques will be used.

Demographic attributes will be displayed using means and standard deviations for continuous variables, while categorical variables will be presented as frequencies and percentages.

The association between treatment groups and socio-demographic variables will be examined using the chi-square statistic, and correlation analysis will be used to explore associations among quantitative variables.

To assess treatment outcomes, an Intention-To-Treat (ITT) approach will be utilized, with a significance level set at 5%. A repeated-measures ANOVA will be employed to investigate potential differences both between and within groups in the selected outcomes from baseline to the end of treatment. Subsequently, repeated measures within-group ANOVAs will be used to assess outcome differences over time, specifically at baseline, end of treatment, and 12-month follow-up. Effect sizes, corrected for bias (Cohen's d), and their significance at a 95% confidence interval will be computed for group differences. For the overall effect, Cohen's f will be computed.

The analysis will be conducted by an independent statistician blinded to the treatment allocation.

4 Expected Results and Conclusions

The outcomes of this RCT will furnish valuable insights into the feasibility and effectiveness of the RinasciMENTE 2.0 program in enhancing the emotional health of the Italian population. Specifically, we anticipate that participants will experience reductions in stress, anxiety, and depression, along with improvements in their emotional regulation strategies and self-efficacy. Furthermore, the levels of adherence to and dropout from the program will serve as important indicators of the study's feasibility.

Still, limitations of this study might be individuals' lack of internet access and digital literacy skills, particularly among non-digital natives.

Therefore, before commencing the trial, a usability analysis was conducted to identify and address any usability challenges associated with the platform, especially for older participants [50]. The results of this study not only help identify and address usability issues but also contribute to the adaptation and refinement of self-help CBT programs.

Consistent with prior studies, it is plausible that dropout rates could be more pronounced in web-based interventions than in traditional in-person therapy, particularly when self-help programs are utilized. To address this concern, subjects will receive reminders and messages aimed at stimulating their involvement with online resources.

Emphasis will also be placed on cultivating a positive relationship between each participant and their referring therapist. While the professional remains available for support when needed, the participant is encouraged to take responsibility for their treatment as successes. This approach highlights the importance of the learning process, empowering individuals to enhance their self-management skills and to develop strategies for addressing emotional challenges.

The RinasciMENTE 2.0 program has the potential to provide individuals with a range of self-help techniques to address psychological challenges while helping to reduce the financial burden on the healthcare system.

Acknowledgment. This research is partially supported by the Fondazione Cariplo – SENIOR project [SystEm for Nudge theory-based Information and Communication Technology (ICT) applications for OlderR citizens] as part of the main SENIOR project.

References

1. Thachil, A.: A new approach to global mental health action. Int. J. Soc. Psychiatry **69**(1), 235–236 (2023)
2. Pinto da Costa, M., Dixon, L.B.: Global mental health. Psychiatr Serv. **74**(5), 559–560 (2023)
3. Pedersen, G.A., et al.: Identifying core competencies for remote delivery of psychological interventions: a rapid review. Psychiatr. Serv. **74**(3), 292–304 (2023)
4. Johnson, L.R., Drescher, C.F., Bordieri, M.J.: Intervention: Enhancing Mental Health and Well-Being Around the World. American Psychological Association (2023). **4**

5. Castelnuovo, G., et al.: Not only clinical efficacy in psychological treatments: clinical psychology must promote cost-benefit, cost-effectiveness, and cost-utility analysis. Front. Psychol. **7**, 563 (2016)
6. Bertuzzi, V., et al.: Single-session therapy by appointment for the treatment of anxiety disorders in youth and adults: a systematic review of the literature. Front. Psychol. **12**, 721382 (2021)
7. Fordham, B., et al.: The evidence for cognitive behavioural therapy in any condition, population or context: a meta-review of systematic reviews and panoramic meta-analysis. Psychol. Med. **51**(1), 21–29 (2021)
8. Pettman, D., et al.: Effectiveness of cognitive behavioural therapy-based interventions for maternal perinatal depression: a systematic review and meta-analysis. BMC Psychiatry **23**(1), 208 (2023)
9. Jackson, J.B., et al.: Brief strategic therapy and cognitive behavioral therapy for women with binge eating disorder and comorbid obesity: a randomized clinical trial one-year follow-up. J. Consult. Clin. Psychol. **86**(8), 688–701 (2018)
10. Bertuzzi, V., et al.: Psychological support interventions for healthcare providers and informal caregivers during the COVID-19 pandemic: a systematic review of the literature. Int. J. Environ. Res. Public Health **18**(13), 6939 (2021)
11. Semonella, M., et al.: Making a virtue out of necessity: COVID-19 as a catalyst for applying internet-based psychological interventions for informal caregivers. Front. Psychol. **13**, 856016 (2022)
12. Stadler, M., et al.: Remote psychotherapy during the COVID-19 pandemic: a mixed-methods study on the changes experienced by Austrian psychotherapists. Life (Basel) **13**(2), 360 (2023)
13. Stefan, R., et al.: Remote psychotherapy during the COVID-19 pandemic. experiences with the transition and the therapeutic relationship. A longitudinal mixed-methods study. Front. Psychol. **12**, 743430 (2021)
14. Humer, E., et al.: Experiences of psychotherapists with remote psychotherapy during the COVID-19 pandemic: cross-sectional web-based survey study. J. Med. Internet Res. **22**(11), e20246 (2020)
15. Beukes, E.W., et al.: Internet-based interventions for adults with hearing loss, tinnitus, and vestibular disorders: a systematic review and meta-analysis. Trends Hear **23**, 2331216519851749 (2019)
16. Bendig, E., et al.: Internet- based interventions in chronic somatic disease. Dtsch. Arztebl. Int. **115**(40), 659–665 (2018)
17. Karyotaki, E., et al.: Do guided internet-based interventions result in clinically relevant changes for patients with depression? An individual participant data meta-analysis. Clin. Psychol. Rev. **63**, 80–92 (2018)
18. Cammisuli, D.M., Pietrabissa, G., Castelnuovo, G.: Improving wellbeing of community-dwelling people with mild cognitive impairment: the SENIOR (SystEm of Nudge theory based ICT applications for OldeR citizens) project. Neural Regen. Res. **16**(5), 963–966 (2021)
19. Andersson, G.: Using the Internet to provide cognitive behaviour therapy. Behav. Res. Ther. **47**(3), 175–180 (2009)
20. Berg, M., et al.: Self-esteem in new light: a qualitative study of experiences of internet-based cognitive behaviour therapy for low self-esteem in adolescents. BMC Psychiatry **23**(1), 810 (2023)
21. Andersson, G., et al.: Internet-based psychodynamic versus cognitive behavioral guided self-help for generalized anxiety disorder: a randomized controlled trial. Psychother. Psychosom. **81**(6), 344–355 (2012)
22. Van't Hof, E., Cuijpers, P., Stein, D.J.: Self-help and Internet-guided interventions in depression and anxiety disorders: a systematic review of meta-analyses. CNS Spectr. **14**(2 Suppl 3), 34–40 (2009)

23. Ciuca, A.M., et al.: Internet-based treatment for panic disorder: a three-arm randomized controlled trial comparing guided (via real-time video sessions) with unguided self-help treatment and a waitlist control. PAXPD study results. J. Anxiety Disord. **56**, 43–55 (2018)
24. Reins, J.A., et al.: The more I got, the less I need? Efficacy of Internet-based guided self-help compared to online psychoeducation for major depressive disorder. J. Affect. Disord. **246**, 695–705 (2019)
25. Vernmark, K., et al.: Internet administered guided self-help versus individualized e-mail therapy: a randomized trial of two versions of CBT for major depression. Behav. Res. Ther. **48**(5), 368–376 (2010)
26. Andersson, E., et al.: Internet-based cognitive behaviour therapy for obsessive-compulsive disorder: a randomized controlled trial. Psychol. Med. **42**(10), 2193–2203 (2012)
27. Pietrabissa, G., et al.: Validation of the Italian version of the web screening questionnaire for common mental disorders. J. Clin. Med. **13**, 1170 (2023)
28. Donker, T., et al.: A brief Web-based screening questionnaire for common mental disorders: development and validation. J. Med. Internet Res. **11**(3), e19 (2009)
29. American Psychiatric Association: Diagnostic and Statistical Manual of Mental Disorders, 5th edn., Washington, DC (2013)
30. Faul, F., et al.: Statistical power analyses using G*Power 3.1: tests for correlation and regression analyses. Behav. Res. Methods **41**(4), 1149–1160 (2009)
31. Pietrabissa, G., et al.: Brief strategic therapy for bulimia nervosa and binge eating disorder: a clinical and research protocol. Front. Psychol. **10**, 373 (2019)
32. Cattivelli, R., et al.: ACTonHEALTH study protocol: promoting psychological flexibility with activity tracker and mHealth tools to foster healthful lifestyle for obesity and other chronic health conditions. Trials **19**(1), 659 (2018)
33. Cohen, J.: Statistical Power Analysis for the Behavioral Sciences. A. Press, London (2013)
34. Eid, M., Gollwitzer, M., Schmitt, M.: Statistik und forschungsmethoden (2017)
35. Castelnuovo, G., et al.: The STRATOB study: design of a randomized controlled clinical trial of Cognitive Behavioral Therapy and Brief Strategic Therapy with telecare in patients with obesity and binge-eating disorder referred to residential nutritional rehabilitation. Trials **12**, 114 (2011)
36. Chiappelli, M., et al.: The Outcome Questionnaire 45.2. Italian validation of an instrument for the assessment of psychological treatments. Epidemiologia e Psichiatria Sociale **17**(2), 152–161 (2008)
37. Mondo, M., Sechi, C., Cabras, C.: Psychometric evaluation of three versions of the Italian Perceived Stress Scale. Curr. Psychol. **40**, 1884–1892 (2019)
38. Balzarotti, S., John, O.P., Gross, J.J.: An Italian adaptation of the emotion regulation questionnaire. Eur. J. Psychol. Assess. **26**(1), 61–67 (2010)
39. Balzarotti, S., John, O.P., Gross, J.J.: An Italian adaptation of the emotion regulation questionnaire. Eur. J. Psychol. Assess. **26**(1), 61–67 (2010)
40. Sibilia, L., Schwarzer, R., Jerusalem, M.: Italian Adaptation of the General Self-Efficacy Scale: Self-Efficacy Generalizzata (1995). http://userpage.fu-berlin.de/~health/italian.htm
41. De Girolamo, G., et al.: Quality of life assessment: validation of the Italian version of the WHOQOL-Brief. Epidemiol. Psichiatr. Soc. **9**(1), 45–55 (2000)
42. Brooke, J.: SUS: a "quick and dirty" usability scale. In: Jordan, P.W., et al. (eds.) Usability Evaluation in Industry, pp. 189–194. Taylor & Francis, London (1996)
43. Vlaescu, G., et al.: Features and functionality of the Iterapi platform for internet-based psychological treatment. Internet Interv. **6**, 107–114 (2016)
44. Semonella, M., et al.: SOSteniamoci: an internet-based intervention to support informal caregivers. In: PSYCHOBIT (2020)
45. Thoren, E.S., et al.: A randomized controlled trial evaluating the effects of online rehabilitative intervention for adult hearing-aid users. Int. J. Audiol. **53**(7), 452–461 (2014)

46. Hesser, H., et al.: A randomized controlled trial of Internet-delivered cognitive behavior therapy and acceptance and commitment therapy in the treatment of tinnitus. J. Consult. Clin. Psychol. **80**(4), 649–661 (2012)
47. Tulbure, B.T., et al.: Internet-delivered cognitive-behavioral therapy for social anxiety disorder in Romania: a randomized controlled trial. PLoS ONE **10**(5), e0123997 (2015)
48. Johansson, R., et al.: Tailored vs. standardized internet-based cognitive behavior therapy for depression and comorbid symptoms: a randomized controlled trial. PLoS One **7**(5), e36905 (2012)
49. IBM Corp.: IBM SPSS Statistics for Windows, Version 24.0, N.I.C. Armonk, Editor. Released 2016
50. Bertuzzi, V., et al.: Internet-delivered emotional self-management program for the general population during the COVID-19 pandemic: usability testing. Front. Psychol. - Health Psychology (2023)

An IoT-Based Method for Collecting Reference Walked Distance for the 6-Minute Walk Test

Sara Caramaschi[1]($\boxtimes$) (iD), Jérémy Bezançon[2] (iD), Carl Magnus Olsson[1] (iD), and Dario Salvi[1] (iD)

[1] Internet of Things and People, Malmö University, Malmö, Sweden
`sara.caramaschi@mau.se`
[2] Université de Montpellier, Montpellier, France

Abstract. This paper addresses the need for accurate and continuous measurement of walked distance in applications such as indoor localisation, gait analysis or the 6-minute walk test (6MWT). We propose a method to continuously collect ground truth data of walked distance using an IoT-based trundle wheel. The wheel is connected via Bluetooth Low Energy to a smartphone application which allows the collection of inertial sensor data and GPS location information in addition to the reference distance. We prove the usefulness of this data collection approach in a use case where we derive walked distance from inertial data. We train a 1-dimensional CNN on inertial data collected by one researcher in 15 walking sessions of 1 km length at varying speeds. The training is facilitated by the continuous nature of the reference data. The accuracy of the algorithm is then tested on holdout data of a 6-min duration for which the error of the inferred distance is within clinically significant limits. The proposed approach is useful for the efficient collection of input and reference data for the development of algorithms used to estimate walked distance, such as for the 6MWT.

Keywords: 6MWT · odometer · walk distance · IoT · inertial sensors

1 Introduction

Measuring walked distance is of relevance to several applications, including indoor localisation [1], pedestrian dead reckoning (PDR) [2], gait analysis [3], fitness tracking and medicine [4] and, more broadly, where the main interest is to measure the distance between two points or of a path. In PDR applications, for example, step length is an important parameter used to obtain the subject's location, and a common way to estimate the step length is to divide the walked distance by the number of detected steps [5–7].

Among clinical applications, the walked distance is particularly relevant in the 6-Minute Walk Test (6MWT), a sub-maximal physical capacity exercise that patients, mostly with pulmonary and cardiac diseases, perform to monitor

© ICST Institute for Computer Sciences, Social Informatics and Telecommunications Engineering 2024
Published by Springer Nature Switzerland AG 2024. All Rights Reserved
D. Salvi et al. (Eds.): PH 2023, LNICST 572, pp. 478–489, 2024.
https://doi.org/10.1007/978-3-031-59717-6_31

the progress or deterioration of their condition [8]. The test is usually run in a clinic and is performed by measuring the distance walked in six minutes, i.e. the 6-Minute Walked Distance (6MWD). The current gold-standard 6MWD is measured either using a trundle wheel or by counting how many laps a patient walks on a 30-m long track, such as a hospital hallway. Technology advances allow the remote execution of this test, thus easing the burden and reducing costs for both clinicians and patients. Additionally, performing the test in patients' natural environments promotes more frequent monitoring [9,10]. Typically Inertial Measurements Units (IMUs) such as accelerometers and gyroscopes are used to measure the 6MWD [11] or, in outdoor environments, the Global Positioning System (GPS) is also often used [12]. However, weather conditions and privacy issues can make this type of environment inconvenient for patients.

To develop and test algorithms for the estimation of walked distance, be it for step length estimation or the 6MWT, a fundamental requirement is the collection of data from human subjects. To allow data collection in natural conditions, for example in indoor environments where positioning is not available or when the walk does not happen on a straight line [6], a simple-to-use, reliable, (semi)automatic approach is needed. Standardised methodologies and datasets do not exist yet for this type of problem [13], therefore the challenge of capturing human mobility information using sensors with unconstrained placement remains open [6].

With this paper, we propose a method to continuously collect IMU and distance data at every meter based on an Internet of Things (IoT)-based trundle wheel which is connected to a mobile phone. The work has four main contributions:

1. An IoT-based trundle wheel which measures the distance in a continuous fashion and sends the measurements over Bluetooth Low Energy (BLE).
2. A smartphone app to collect data from the BLE connected trundle wheel and the sensors embedded in the phone - including IMU (acceleration, rotation rate, orientation) and positioning (such as GPS).
3. A dataset of walking activity, including continuous reference distances, collected by one researcher at different speeds.
4. An example of a Convolutional Neural Network (CNN) model that accurately (compared with reference distance) computes the walked distance using only the inertial sensors data from the smartphone.

This paper is structured as follows: Sect. 2 introduces related work, Sect. 3 describes the methods we employed, Sect. 4 shows the results we have obtained and Sect. 5 discusses and reflects on them. Finally, Sect. 6 summarises our main conclusions based on this research and proposes future directions.

2   Related Work

In the domain of supervised algorithms for estimating walked distance, a multitude of data sources and sensor configurations have been explored, each with its unique considerations. This section explores sensor choices, methods to collect reference distance measurements and distance estimation approaches.

IMUs sensors found in smartphones and wearable devices are common for tracking human activity. Sensor's location on the body affects data patterns [10,14]. In outdoor environments, satellite positioning signals such as the GPS are usually considered [12,15,16], while in indoor environments BLE or WiFi are used to compute walked distances, e.g., in PDR applications [7]. While satellite positioning is considered accurate, smartphone users may find outdoor environments problematic, especially when physical conditions or weather do not allow outdoor activities. This paper focuses on computing the walked distance through smartphone IMU sensors, as this could be used both indoors and outdoors.

To ensure accurate walking distance estimates and compare approaches, it's crucial to consider standardised methods for reference measurements. In the 6MWT, clinical personnel typically count laps walked and measure the remaining distance of the final lap at the end of 6 min [17]. In research settings, a simple but reliable approach involves using a trundle wheel to measure walked distance [12,15]. More complex approaches have been used in other studies, such as video recording or sensorised carpets [18–20]. Providing public datasets including both sensor data and a reference walked distance is thus valuable for developing algorithms that extract the walked distance from the input sensor data. For example, Yan et al. published a dataset comprising 150 min of walking data from individuals who carried smartphones in various body locations, with ground truth positioning obtained via a Visual Inertial Odometry system [21]. However, as highlighted in the review by Diez et al. [13], there is an absence of established methodologies and datasets for step length estimation, notwithstanding the potential of inertial sensor-based algorithm to estimate walked distance [17].

Modelling of walked distance using inertial sensors has been approached with rule-based algorithms such as the one proposed by Capela et al. for the 6MWT [19] and the indoor algorithm proposed by Salvi et al. [12,22] or by means of Machine Learning (ML) models [23], where the latter approach is showing promise within gait analysis [24]. Furthermore, Juen et al. [23] proposed support vector machine models for computing walking speed and to compute 6MWD, obtaining an average 3.23% error. A more sophisticated approach is used by Klein et al. [2], who proposed a framework which outputs a regression value of change in distance or in step length. They used data coming from the public dataset RIDI [21] to train algorithms to estimate step length, either directly or through the change in distance or the Weinberg gain. Of these algorithms, the best performing was the change in distance estimator with an average error of 2.1% on six considered trajectories. The architecture considered as input was the smartphone body location and the raw inertial data which were then fed into a neural network based on a modified version of the ResNet-18 [25].

In this paper, we present both an IoT-trundle wheel for the collection of walked distances useful for supervised modelling approaches and an example of a regression model to estimate the distance from inertial sensor data. This example highlights how the trundle wheel allows the collection of distance information with finer granularity compared to current golden-standard approaches.

3   Materials and Methods

3.1   IoT Trundle Wheel

The IoT trundle wheel was developed at Malmö University using off-the-shelf electronic components. It consists of an electronic board based on the ESP32 chip, a reed switch and a magnet. The reed switch serves as a magnetic sensor: when a magnet passes by the sensor, the switch's blades come into contact with each other allowing current to flow. By attaching the magnet to one spoke of the wheel it becomes possible to detect each revolution of the wheel. The reed switch is connected between the reference voltage (3.3 V) and a GPIO port of the ESP32. The ESP32 and the reed switch are soldered onto a protoboard, which is then attached to the wheel handle using velcro in order to be easily attached and detached as needed. The firmware, running on the ESP32 and developed using the Arduino libraries, counts the number of revolutions of the wheel and transmits the measured distance, one per revolution, to the smartphone via BLE at each wheel revolution. If no wheel revolution is detected for 5 s, the overall walked distance until that time is sent. Figure 1.a provides a visual representation of the trundle wheel with the incorporated components.

3.2   Smartphone Application

The mobile application, developed using the Apache Cordova framework, enables the collection of data from the IoT trundle wheel and the embedded sensors in the phone simultaneously. The collected information is stored in a text file, including data on distance travelled, acceleration, rotation rate, orientation, steps taken, and GPS signal. Figure 1.b shows the main screen of the smartphone application. The user starts data collection by pressing the "connect" button. This scans for nearby BLE devices, connects to the ESP32 board if found, and displays the connection state on the main screen of the app. After connecting, the user can press "Start" which initiates a timer, resets the distance to zero and activates wheel rotation detection on the ESP32. Concurrently, the application writes the sensor data as well as the time at which the data is captured. When completing the walk, the user presses "End" to stop writing to the file and stops reading the IMU and GPS data. The BLE connection remains active until the smartphone Bluetooth is turned off.

3.3   Data Collection

Data used in this research paper correspond to inertial measurements of accelerometer and gyroscope sensors embedded in the smartphone from fifteen recordings made by a single researcher walking outdoors. Each recording corresponds to a walked distance of approximately one kilometre performed while

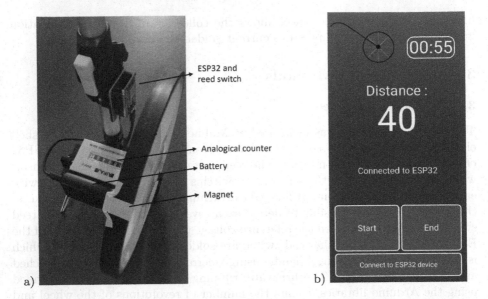

a)   b)

Fig. 1. a) IoT-based trundle wheel and its components, b) Screenshot of the smart-phone application to retrieve data.

keeping the smartphone in one hand, and the IoT trundle-wheel in the other hand. The data was recorded with different speeds and waking styles, according to the following protocol: 3 walks at normal speed, 3 walks at fast speed, 3 walks at slow speed, 3 walks at varying speed (from standing still to walking fast), and 3 walks at mixed speed. The dataset, the Arduino code, the smartphone application and the CNN model code are published with an open-source license at https://github.com/Jeremy618/TrundleWheel. An example of recorded acceleration and rotation rate in a 5-second chunk is shown in Fig. 2.

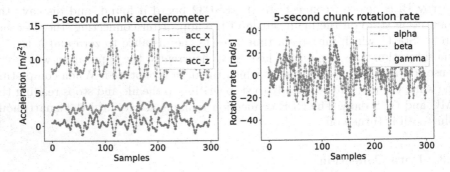

Fig. 2. Acceleration and rotation rate example in a 5-second chunk

3.4 Distance Estimation Algorithm

As an example of how this dataset can be used, we propose a CNN-based model for estimating the walked distance. This example illustrates the potential of having a high-fidelity reference dataset for walked distance estimations. The architecture of the algorithm is represented in Fig. 3 where we considered time windows of 5 s, which would allow us to capture the movement produced by at least 2 or 3 steps. The model input is a [300 × 6] matrix where the first dimension corresponds to 5 s of recording using a sampling frequency of 60 Hz and the second dimension corresponds to the six input signals of the IMU: three-axial acceleration and three-axial rotation rate. The corresponding output for each input is the distance walked within that segment, which was interpolated from the reference data collected from the IoT trundle wheel.

The model architecture develops through three 1-D convolutional layers to extract relevant features from the provided inputs [26]. These layers are interspersed with batch normalisation, max pooling and dropout layers. The convolutional layers employ a Rectifier Linear Unit (ReLU) activation function, have kernel sizes of 32, 16, and 3, and a number of filters of 64, 32, and 8 respectively. The max pooling layer uses a pooling size of three. The network ends with a flattening layer and a dense layer with a single unit which provides the desired output of dimension 1 (one distance per input). To develop the model architecture, we considered examples of CNNs fed with inertial sensors from previous work that studied activity recognition using inertial sensors [27,28]. However, since these tasks were different, we empirically selected the model's hyper-parameters as the number of filters and kernel size, epochs, batch size, and the number of considered convolutional layers.

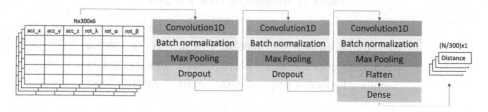

Fig. 3. CNN model architecture. Input data corresponds to three-axial accelerometer and gyroscope, while the output is the walked distance every 5 s.

To evaluate model performances throughout the training process, the Mean Square Error (MSE), the loss function and the Mean Absolute Error (MAE) are monitored. The model is trained over 150 epochs with a batch size of 32. Data were initially divided into two primary sets: one for cross-validation (54.83%) and the other for holdout testing (45.17%). The holdout test data covers the first six minutes of each recording. Nevertheless, the model is suitable to estimate distance in any time window, and can therefore be applied to other purposes (e.g., a 2-minute walk test, which is sometimes used in clinical practice). The model

S. Caramaschi et al.

is trained using a 5-fold cross-validation, which, at each iteration, separates the
data into training set (53.5%), validation set (13.2%), and test set (33.3%).
Early stopping is used to mitigate overfitting while training. Of the five obtained
models, the one which performs the best on the test data of the respective fold is
selected and is used to predict the outcomes from holdout test data and related
statistics. Holdout estimation results are finally evaluated by examining various
error statistics, including the Mean Absolute Percentage Error (MAPE) and
the Bland-Altman limits of agreement. This approach allows for a meaningful
comparison with results from the existing literature, including applications for
the 6MWT.

4   Results

Data includes 15 walks in the city of Malmö (Table 1), gathered by a healthy
researcher using a Xiaomi Redmi Note 9 Pro smartphone. Electronic and
mechanical measurements matched, verifying reliability. In Fig. 4 we observe
that the absolute errors mostly stay below three meters in a 5-s time window,
and they remain below 30 m in a 6-min duration, except for one instance reaching
34.53 m. Key evaluation metrics are presented in Table 2. Among other promising statistical results, the correlation between the estimated distance and the
ground truth distance is 0.93 for the 5-second chunks and 0.99 for the 6-min
duration. Performance variations can be attributed to factors like variations in
speed, walking style and the presence of noise and confounders, such as the way
the phone was held and how the arms were moving.

Table 1. Statistics on collected data.

	Mean	STD	Max	Min
Recordings distance [m]	1005.39	5.74	1014.98	999.99
Recordings duration [s]	796.79	133.08	1058.14	581.43
Sampling frequency [Hz]	59.92	0.04	59.96	59.83

5   Discussion

This paper proposes a method to collect walked distance reference values by
using an IoT trundle wheel and a smartphone app. The IoT-trundle wheel is
composed of a conventional trundle wheel with commercially available electronics
components mounted to it. It is possible to use the IoT-trundle wheel both
indoors and outdoors, as well as for trajectories that are not straight lines since
the distance is measured even when a user makes turns. This approach allows
users to walk in more natural conditions, with any kind of desired walk pattern

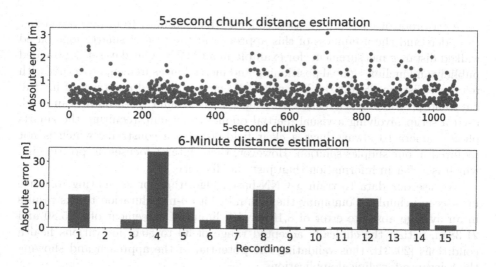

Fig. 4. Absolute error of the estimated distance for the holdout test data (first 6 min of every recording). Results are shown for the 5-second chunks and for the whole 6-minute distance.

Table 2. 5-second chunk and 6-minute statistics of the error computed as the difference between the reference value and the estimated one. All values are in meters. MAPE is not available for 5-second chunks because of the presence of zeros.

	5-second chunk	6-minute cumulative
MSE	0.33	149.73
RMSE	0.57	12.24
ABS median	0.31	3.79
ABS mean	0.41	8.15
ABS SD	0.4	9.12
ABS min	0	0.11
ABS max	3.16	34.53
CORR	0.93	0.99
MAPE	–	1.97
LoA_low	−1.15	−25.80
LoA_high	1.10	21.38

and speed. It, however, requires keeping the trundle wheel in one hand, which makes it not suitable for people who require walking support. The IoT trundle wheel produces distance information at each revolution of the wheel, thus at each meter. Considering that the average walking speed of an healthy adult is 4.5 km/h (1.25 m/s), we can estimate the trundle wheel sampling frequency as 1.25 Hz. Thus, we consider both spatial resolution (1 m) and sampling frequency (1.25 Hz) as acceptable for the purposes of measuring human walking activity.

As a proof of concept, we used collected inertial data from one researcher to understand the usefulness of this approach in the case of smartphone-based walked distance measurement, for example in a 6MWT. Our dataset is provided publicly and includes global positioning and inertial measurements together with reference distance. Similarly, Yan et al. [21] have published a dataset of inertial data and positioning references. To collect their ground truth data, Yan et al. used a setup involving a visual inertial odometry system, requiring the smartphone camera to always have a clear field-of-view, a constraint which is not required in our simpler solution. However, their dataset focuses on positioning, which is richer in information than just the distance.

We use our data to train a CNN-based algorithm for estimating distance in 5-second chunks. Combining these chunks into 6-min duration tracks results in an average absolute error of 8.15 m with limits of agreement of −25.80 and 21.38 m. within the clinically accepted range of 30 to 50 m for various health conditions [29–31], thus validating the potential of the approach and showing the relevance for clinical applications.

Compared to other studies reported in the literature, our algorithm performs similarly or better. For example, a study from Juen et al. [23] proposed a model trained on a walking lap with fixed distance and it estimates walked distance in a 6MWT with a 3.23% error. The percentage error that we obtained not only is smaller (MAPE: 1.97%) but also allows for distance estimation at any path length. Our obtained errors are also smaller than Klein et al. [2] (2.1%) who proposed a regression model predicting change in distance along six different trajectories.

Capela et al. [19] achieved a better result with an average percentage difference of 0.12%. However, they used a smartphone attached to a waist belt, which reduces noise and motion artefacts, whereas we opted for a more user-friendly approach of holding the phone in one hand, better suited for natural environments.

An inertial-based algorithm for 6MWT was proposed in [12,22]. Their indoor approach reached Bland-Altman limits of agreement of −133.35 to 162.55 m, which are significantly higher than ours. Their tests were conducted imitating a classic 6MWT, that is, walking back and forth a walkway, whereas our approach allows a more natural walking activity. It has to be noted, however, that their tests included different users and mobile phones, whereas our example only employed one user and one smartphone. They also developed an algorithm based on GPS data which could inspire future developments, i.e., mixing both positioning and inertial data for higher accuracy.

5.1   Limitations and Future Works

Our data collection method is limited to estimating walked distance, in addition, the data are restricted to one user and smartphone, limiting its generalizability. Despite these limitations, we see our approach as a promising proof of concept that highlights the data's potential applications and the need for further research in this direction.

This work provides a foundation for multiple directions to be developed in the future. For example, given the open challenge of step length estimation, heading towards its estimation is likely to be relevant. A more thorough dataset involving several users, different mobile phones and walking styles would be needed to be able to assess the extent to which supervised algorithms can estimate walked distance on a wide population. The algorithm was developed by only using a CNN architecture to obtain a proof-of-concept model on this type of data. Further exploration is necessary to improve the model by considering hyperparameter tuning and other Deep Learning (DL) approaches such as the use of recurrent layers like in Long Short-Term Memory (LSTM). Some simplifications of the model should also be considered, for example, considering the magnitude of the signals, instead of the three axial components, or using data augmentation techniques [27,32].

6   Conclusions

This article presents a novel approach to continuously measuring walking activity, using IMU sensors and positioning data while providing reference walked distance throughout the whole path. The results show that this approach performs as well or better than existing methods, particularly in the context of the 6MWT. It offers enhanced reliability and information, enabling distance measurements in diverse, natural settings, indoors and outdoors, facilitating continuous and unobtrusive health monitoring.

While this study illustrates the potential of this approach, it suffers from limitations related to a single user and smartphone. The results should be viewed as groundwork for future research in the field.

References

1. Mariakakis, A.T., et al.: SAIL: single access point-based indoor localization. In: Proceedings of the 12th Annual International Conference on Mobile Systems, Applications, and Services, pp. 315–328 (2014)
2. Klein, I., Asraf, O.: StepNet–deep learning approaches for step length estimation. IEEE Access **8**, 85706–85713 (2020)
3. Wang, J.-S., et al.: Walking pattern classification and walking distance estimation algorithms using gait phase information. IEEE Trans. Biomed. Eng. **59**(10), 2884–2892 (2012)
4. Xie, J., et al.: Evaluating the validity of current mainstream wearable devices in fitness tracking under various physical activities: comparative study. JMIR Mhealth Uhealth **6**(4), e9754 (2018)
5. Ho, N.-H., Truong, P.H., Jeong, G.-M.: Step-detection and adaptive step-length estimation for pedestrian dead-reckoning at various walking speeds using a smartphone. Sensors **16**(9), 1423 (2016)
6. Yang, Z., et al.: Mobility increases localizability: a survey on wireless indoor localization using inertial sensors. ACM Comput. Surv. **47**(3), 1–34 (2015). https://doi.org/10.1145/2676430. ISSN 0360-0300, 1557-7341

7. Kunhoth, J., et al.: Indoor positioning and wayfinding systems: a survey. Hum.-centric Comput. Inf. Sci **10**(1), 1–41 (2020)
8. Enright, P.L.: The six-minute walk test. Respir. Care **48**(8), 783–785 (2003)
9. Mak, J., et al.: Reliability and repeatability of a smartphone-based 6-min walk test as a patient-centred outcome measure **2**, 77–87 (2021). https://doi.org/10.1093/ehjdh/ztab018. ISSN 2634–3916
10. Pires, I.M., et al.: Development technologies for the monitoring of six-minute walk test: a systematic review. Sensors **22**(22), 581 (2022). https://doi.org/10.3390/s22020581. ISSN 1424-8220
11. Storm, F.A., et al.: Wearable inertial sensors to assess gait during the 6-minute walk test: a systematic review. Sensors **20**(9), 2660 (2020)
12. Salvi, D., et al.: The mobile-based 6-minute walk test: usability study and algorithm development and validation. JMIR mHealth uHealth **8**(1), e13756 (2020). https://doi.org/10.2196/13756. Company: JMIR mHealth and uHealth Distributor: JMIR mHealth and uHealth Institution: JMIR mHealth and uHealth Label: JMIR mHealth and uHealth publisher: JMIR Publications Inc., Toronto, Canada
13. Díez, L.E., et al.: Step length estimation methods based on inertial sensors: a review. IEEE Sens. J. **18**(17), 6908–6926 (2018)
14. Kunze, K., Lukowicz, P.: Sensor placement variations in wearable activity recognition. IEEE Pervasive Comput. **13**(4), 32–41 (2014). https://doi.org/10.1109/MPRV.2014.73
15. Ziegl, A., et al.: mHealth 6-minute walk test – accuracy for detecting clinically relevant differences in heart failure patients. In: 2021 43rd Annual International Conference of the IEEE Engineering in Medicine & Biology Society (EMBC), pp. 7095–7098, November 2021. https://doi.org/10.1109/EMBC46164.2021.9630118
16. Gray, A.J., et al.: Validity and reliability of GPS for measuring distance travelled in field-based team sports. J. Sports Sci. **28**(12), 1319–1325 (2010)
17. Shah, V.V., et al.: Inertial sensor algorithm to estimate walk distance. Sensors **22**(33), 1077 (2022). ISSN 1424–8220. https://doi.org/10.3390/s22031077
18. Li, S.-H., et al.: Design of wearable and wireless multi-parameter monitoring system for evaluating cardiopulmonary function. Med. Eng. Phys. **47**, 144–150 (2017)
19. Capela, N.A., Lemaire, E.D., Baddour, N.: Novel algorithm for a smartphone-based 6-minute walk test application: algorithm, application development, and evaluation. J. NeuroEng. Rehabil. **12**(1), 19 (2015). https://doi.org/10.1186/s12984-015-0013-9. ISSN 1743–0003
20. A smartphone approach for the 2 and 6-minute walk test. In: Chicago, IL, August 2014, pp. 958–961 (2014). https://doi.org/10.1109/EMBC.2014.6943751. http://ieeexplore.ieee.org/document/6943751/. ISBN 978-1-4244-7929-0
21. Yan, H., Shan, Q., Furukawa, Y.: RIDI: robust IMU double integration. In: Ferrari, V., Hebert, M., Sminchisescu, C., Weiss, Y. (eds.) ECCV 2018. LNCS, vol. 11217, pp. 641–656. Springer, Cham (2018). https://doi.org/10.1007/978-3-030-01261-8_38
22. Salvi, D., et al.: App-based versus standard six-minute walk test in pulmonary hypertension: mixed methods study. JMIR Mhealth Uhealth **9**(6), e22748 (2021)
23. Juen, J., Cheng, Q., Schatz, B.: A natural walking monitor for pulmonary patients using mobile phones. IEEE J. Biomed. Health Inform. **19**(4), 1399–1405 (2015)
24. Caldas, R., et al.: A systematic review of gait analysis methods based on inertial sensors and adaptive algorithms. Gait Posture **57**, 204–210 (2017)
25. He, K., et al.: Deep residual learning for image recognition. In: Proceedings of the IEEE Conference on Computer Vision and Pattern Recognition, pp. 770–778 (2016)

26. Zhao, B., et al.: Convolutional neural networks for time series classification. J. Syst. Eng. Electron. **28**(1), 162–169 (2017)
27. Caramaschi, S., Papini, G.B., Caiani, E.G.: Device orientation independent human activity recognition model for patient monitoring based on triaxial acceleration. Appl. Sci. **13**(7), 4175 (2023)
28. Fridriksdottir, E., Bonomi, A.G.: Accelerometer-based human activity recognition for patient monitoring using a deep neural network. Sensors **20**(22), 6424 (2020)
29. Ries, J.D., et al.: Test-retest reliability and minimal detectable change scores for the timed "up & go" test, the six-minute walk test, and gait speed in people with Alzheimer disease. Phys. Ther. **89**(6), 569–579 (2009)
30. Macchia, A., et al.: A meta-analysis of trials of pulmonary hypertension: a clinical condition looking for drugs and research methodology. Am. Heart J. **153**(6), 1037–1047 (2007)
31. Chan, W.L.S., Pin, T.W.: Reliability, validity and minimal detectable change of 2-minute walk test, 6-minute walk test and 10-meter walk test in frail older adults with dementia. Exp. Gerontol. **115**, 9–18 (2019)
32. Ohashi, H., et al.: Augmenting wearable sensor data with physical constraint for DNN-based human-action recognition. In: ICML 2017 Times Series Workshop, pp. 6–11 (2017)

Dozzz: Exploring Voice-Based Sleep Experience Sampling for Children

Shanshan Chen(✉) [iD], Panos Markopoulos [iD], and Jun Hu [iD]

Department of Industrial Design, Eindhoven University of Technology, 5612 Eindhoven, AZ, The Netherlands
{s.chen1,p.markopoulos,j.hu}@tue.nl

Abstract. Text-based digital diaries are an essential tool for sleep clinicians to assess how their patients experience sleep. However, text-entry can be challenging for children. Voice entry represents a plausible and yet unexplored alternative for supporting children's self-report in sleep diaries. We introduce Dozzz, a voice-based digital sleep diary that empowers children to record their sleep experiences using a smartphone. We present the result of usability evaluation involving ten children aged six to twelve. This evaluation confirmed that children were able to understand and interact with Dozzz effectively. Our study demonstrates the feasibility of voice-user interfaces (VUIs) to support sleep diaries for children. Future work needs to assess the use of diaries in real-life settings and evaluate the quality of responses children provide when using the system independently at home.

Keywords: voice-user interfaces · experience sampling method · children-computer interaction · sleep diary · self-tracking

1 Introduction

Sleep problems can have a significant impact on children's mental and physical health and development; they are very common and often chronic, with a prevalence estimated between 25–40% [4]. Sleep problems may refer to difficulties in falling asleep, interrupted sleep, drowsiness during the day, etc. To assess and subsequently treat sleep problems health care specialists like pediatricians, psychiatrists and psychologists, need to identify sleep-related patterns and behaviours such as bedtimes, routines related to going to sleep and waking up, co-sleeping, habits relating to watching television or using digital media, nocturnal behaviours such as snoring and nightmares, and daytime behaviours affected by sleep [1].

There are various ways for health care specialists to collect information about sleep, which include discussing with children and their parents and technical means such as actigraphy and polysomnography. Next to these, diaries can be useful for tracking daily sleep behaviour and experiences, allowing the assessment of night-to-night variability and other patterns over time. Diaries can be filled by the parents, but also there are sleep

D. Salvi et al. (Eds.): PH 2023, LNICST 572, pp. 490–500, 2024.
https://doi.org/10.1007/978-3-031-59717-6_32

diaries specially developed for children to report their sleep experience independently [16, 17]. Children's reports in a sleep diary have been argued to be more valid as children are actively engaged in their experiences throughout the entire time, compared with a sleep diary for parents [8, 18]. Additionally, previous research has found low correlations between parent and child reports regarding a child's behaviors and emotions [19]. Hence, it is necessary to develop sleep diaries that enable children to self-report their sleep experiences accurately and reliably, which may be particularly difficult for children.

Traditional paper-based diaries are not always completed within the instructed time-frame, potentially leading to inaccurate responses [7]. For this reason, digital media, such as websites and mobile applications, are increasingly used for self-tracking purposes. These digital systems can help in recording and managing personal data, eliminating the inconvenience of editing, recording, and analyzing data with pen and paper [6, 10], especially with the widespread use of digital devices such as mobile phones [22], laptops [23], and wearables [24]. On the other hand, most digital sleep diaries and sleep questionnaires, like the Consensus Sleep Diary [20] and Graphical diaries [12], have primarily targeted adults and have not been tailored for use by children. Snoozy [11] is a chatbot-based sleep diary that assists children in recording their sleep experiences. In a week-long evaluation with children (N = 5) having sleep disorders, Snoozy was deemed feasible and enjoyable for children, offering clinical practitioners and sleep scientists a direct source of sleep quality data from children instead of relying on parents. Participants, however, indicated their preference for a voice-based version of the chatbot as it would be more fun to have a vocal conversation.

This paper introduces Dozzz, a voice-based sleep diary designed for children, using Google recognizer technology on the Android platform. It employs voice-user interfaces (VUIs) to facilitate children's self-reporting of sleep related behaviours and experiences. The evaluation involved ten children aged six to twelve, combining quantitative and qualitative methods, including a user test and a semi-structured interview to assess the system's usability and opinions of users regarding its potential for long-term usage.

This study revealed that the children were able to successfully complete the sleep survey entirely by independent voice input. Through data analysis, we found that children were willing to use voice entry for sleep diary self-reporting. Dozzz provides an alternative for researchers to explore voice-based sleep diaries for children in a conversational context, which paves the way for future work to facilitate more natural conversation on portable devices and in more complex contexts, while maintaining the sustained engagement of children.

2 Materials and Methods

2.1 Materials

Software Dozzz, our chatbot-based self-reporting method with voice-based response, was developed in Java, based on the children's sleep diary [11]. Dozzz implements voice input/output using the Google recognizer. It utilizes the voice recognizer APIs for backend infrastructure and capabilities such as voice recognition and transcription. SQLite is used to store user's answers on client devices. (see in Fig. 1).

To enhance the chatbot's conversational naturalness with human-like sound, the system utilizes a matching regulation approach, which seeks to offer responses that are relatable to children. Rather than utilizing complex machine learning algorithms, we employ preset search rules based on keyword classification using Regular Expressions (Regex), as depicted in Fig. 1.

Dozzz has been meticulously designed to accommodate the following scenarios:

(1) Clarification of Questions: Dozzz responds by kindly rephrasing the last question to ensure children's comprehension when they express confusion.
(2) Empathetic Responses: In response to children's answers, Dozzz maintains a warm and empathetic tone, fostering a kind and understanding interaction.
(3) Personalization: Dozzz enhances the conversational experience by remembering children's names and addressing them by name when asking follow-up questions, creating a more personal connection.

For added transparency and flexibility, the configuration files are publicly accessible through the project's GitHub examples repository [30].

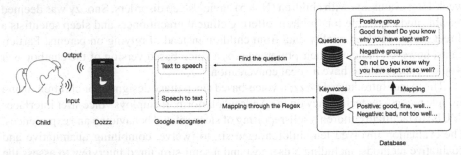

Fig. 1. Overview of the data processing approach involves mapping emotional responses based on children's answers by utilizing keyword searches with predefined regex regulations.

2.2 Methods

User Study A structured user test was carried out in a field setting, where we asked children to interact with Dozzz and respond to its questions about their sleep. Our aim was to examine whether children understood Dozzz and could carry their end of the conversation and to gauge their attitudes towards it.

Recruitment. We recruited ten children by making announcements on social media platforms and sharing them widely in parent-social groups, and child centers in public libraries. The recruitment process aimed to reach a diverse group of children.

Experiment Duration. Each session with a participant lasted 20 to 30 min and was conducted one-on-one with a researcher. To ensure the child's comfort, sessions were held in locations like the public library or their home.

Number of Participants. Due to recruitment constraints and privacy concerns, we received consent from ten children's parents, concluding the evaluation with children aged six to twelve (M = 8.5 years, SD = 1.65), including four boys and six girls.

User Test. Each child completed the chatbot survey independently, with their behavior recorded by a camera during the 20 to 30 min.

Semi-structure Interview. We conducted a semi-structured interview with the children, covering their chatbot experience, technology usage at home (including voice technology), and daily routine, with parental consent for audio recording.

Data Collection. In the current system, participant responses lack timestamps in SQLite database. To address this, video recordings are employed to monitor response duration and wait time.

Ethical Considerations We received ethics approval from the Ethical Review Board of our university. Data will be deleted after the study, with consent obtained from ten participants and their parents.

Data Analysis

Transcription Accuracy. We assessed transcription accuracy using methods like Google Cloud Speech and real-time transcription, comparing them to a gold-standard reference corpus. The word error rate (WER) was the primary metric for evaluating speech recognition precision [31]. We also introduced Carly's calculation method for accuracy evaluation [3]. See Eq. 1.

$$WER_w = \sum_{i=1}^{n} WER_{u_i} \frac{L_{u_i}}{L_T} \tag{1}$$

WER_{u_i} is each utterances' individual word error rate, where $i \in 1, \ldots, n$, n is the number of utterances. L_{u_i} is the number of words in the utterance. L_T is the total number of words (TNW) in the transcription. WER_{u_i} is calculated by summing the number of insertions, substitutions, and deletions, and then divided by the TNW through comparing the transcript and real recordings.

Turn-Taking Analysis. We introduce "pause" in turn-taking, a mechanism for analyzing discourse through phrasing, intonation, and pausing. These pauses, also known as "wait time," are essential for interpreting interactional behaviors and emotions [32], potentially signaling lower confidence. We aim to define wait time for different types of Turn Constructional Units (TCU) [26] (see Fig. 2).

Affinity Diagramming and Thematic Analysis. Affinity diagramming and thematic analysis [27, 28], involving spatially clustering related insights or ideas to analyze qualitive data obtained from observational studies and user interviews [25, 26], was used to group and cluster insights derived from the semi-structured interviews with children in this study and then generate themes from the clustered data. In this study, we use thematic analysis to identify patterns, themes, or categories within the data and using those themes as codes to organize and analyze the children's interview data. Figure 3 shows the resulting clustering of children's statements.

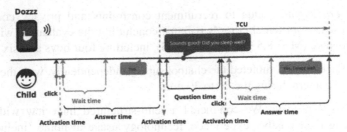

Fig. 2. The conversation with Dozzz starts when the user activates the system by clicking a button.

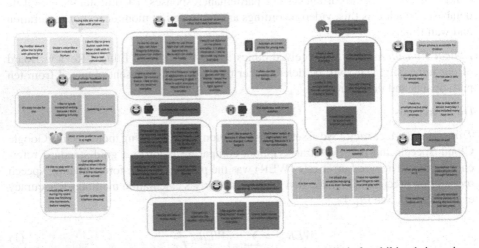

Fig. 3. The visualization of affinity diagramming and thematic analysis for children's interviews with experience of voice interaction and daily activities with voice-based devices

3   Results

The analysis of the video recordings provides insights into the participants' activities with Dozzz, an overview of temporal aspects is shown in Table 1. The average answer duration was found to be 2.49s (SD = 1.73). The average wait time was 2.02s (SD = 1.53). Notably, when children answered yes-no questions, the average wait time was just 1.54s (SD = 0.37). However, when participants were asked wh-questions like "Where do you need to go today?", they took more time to think, resulting in an average wait time of 4.04s (SD = 1.15).

Table 1. Indices on ten children's answers

Answer duration	Wait time	Wait time for yes-no unit	Wait time for wh- unit	WER
2.49s (1.73)	2.02s (1.53)	1.54s (0.37)	4.04s (1.15)	14.9%(0.061)

3.1 Transcription Accuracy

Based on Eq. 1, we calculated a Word Error Rate (WER) of 0.149 (SD = 0.061) (see Table 1), indicating acceptable transcription accuracy [2]. The left of Fig. 4 displays WER distribution for the 'wh-unit' and 'yes-no-unit' groups. Although no significant difference was observed, it is notable that the primary cause of recognition errors differs between the groups. In the 'wh-unit' group, word substitution is the primary issue, while in the 'yes-no-unit' group, word deletion prevails. Importantly, many 'yes-no-unit' recognition errors occurred when the child pressed the button before the system fully activated (as shown in Fig. 2), suggesting a readiness issue with voice recognition.

3.2 Turn-Taking Analysis

In the right of Fig. 4, we observe a notable difference in wait times between the 'wh-unit' and the 'yes-no-unit' group. Upon reviewing video recordings, it became evident that when children were presented with questions pertaining to future plans or preferences that had not yet occurred, such as "What do you plan to do today?" or "Where do you want to go today?", they frequently responded with phrases like "I don't know" or "I have no idea" after contemplating for a few seconds. These responses suggest that children often felt uncertain or lacked specific intentions or preferences in those situations. This also suggests younger children may face challenges in comprehending and responding to certain questions due to factors like memory limitations, restricted vocabulary, and social factors. Designing voice-based interfaces for children should consider these challenges to enhance the user experience [21, 29].

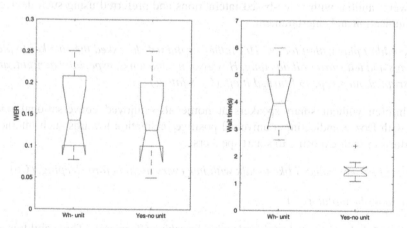

Fig. 4. Box plots show WER and wait time for ten children in 'wh-unit' and 'yes-no-unit' groups. In the 'wh-unit' group, WER is slightly higher, while wait time are significantly higher compared to the 'yes-no-unit' group.

3.3 Qualitative Feedback

All the children had previous experience with VUIs on different terminal devices such as smart speakers, phones, and watches. Among the participants, five children (50%) had speakers at home, four children (40%) owned smartwatches, and three children (30%) had tablet computers. Additionally, all the children had the opportunity to interact with smartphones in their daily lives.

The youngest participant favored smart speakers over smartphones. Listening to music and stories was popular among all children, averaging 30 min daily. Asking questions through speakers was also popular, averaging ten minutes daily. They used smartwatches to stay in touch with friends and for location tracking. Of the three tablet owners, gaming and online courses were common activities. Preferences for the moments, devices, and activities of engagement varied among different age groups.

Out of the ten participants, 90% expressed willingness to continue self-reporting with their sleep diary. Among these, 66.6% preferred reporting at night, while 33.4% reported whenever they remembered. Additionally, 30% of children aged nine or older had prior experience with similar diary apps using templates instead of typing.

Summary of Themes

The analysis of the data revealed two main themes: enablers and barriers in conversations, and enablers and barriers in digital sleep-diaries. These themes provide insights into children's needs, preferences, and communication activities.

Theme 1: Enablers and Barriers in Conversations

Subtheme 1.1: Voice input/output (Enablers). Children found Dozzz easy to use and enjoyable. They also found it funny, enhancing their positive experience. Children who owned smart speakers at home were particularly enthusiastic users of Dozzz, as they were familiar with voice-based interactions and preferred using such devices for communication and entertainment.

> 'I couldn't play with it today.' Her father explained she asked the speaker to play songs and tell stories all day long. However, it's too noisy, especially at night, and disrupted our sleep, so I turned it off. (C2's father)

Children without smart speakers at home also enjoyed conversational interactions with Dozzz, indicating a universal positive inclination towards such interactions regardless of their exposure to smart speakers.

> Dozzz likes my friend. I like to talk with her every night before sleeping. (C6)

> She looks beautiful. (C7)

Subtheme 1.2: Redundant Activities During Speaking (Barriers). Three children above 9 years old preferred Dozzz's hands-free voice interaction over the button-based voice recording method. This highlights the importance of user-friendly interfaces for children of different ages.

> I don't like to click each time. It feels a bit inconvenient. (C9)

Theme 2: Enablers and barriers in sustained engagement with digital sleep diaries

Subtheme 1: Gamification as the Continuous Trigger for Children (Enablers). About half of the children suggested adding gamification elements like point-based rankings and progress tracking to boost motivation and encourage regular app use. This indicates that gamification features and progress tracking can enhance engagement, promote commitment to the self-reporting process, and provide a sense of achievement for consistent sleep diary reporting.

I like 'Jumping Every Day'. Because I enjoy earning points every day. (C3)

I use the learning app primarily to keep a record. I clock in everyday. (C5)

One child highlighted the significance of social features in sustaining app usage. This indicates that incorporating features like progress sharing and friend interactions can boost children's motivation and engagement in self-reporting, fostering a sense of community and encouraging ongoing app use.

I love playing Pokémon Go on my phone almost every day because I can team up with friends. (C8)

Subtheme 2: Parent's Role in Promoting Sustained Engagement (Enablers). Parent's habits, like exercise and eating, can shape children's long-term behavior, emphasizing the role of parental modeling and the family environment. Including family-related questions and promoting healthy behaviors in the self-reporting method can reinforce positive habits and offer a holistic view of children's well-being and sleep patterns.

My mother and I use 'Balance' for meditation every morning and night. It helps me sleep better, and I enjoy the music. (C10)

Subtheme 3: Limitations in Younger Ages (Barriers). Children above 8 years old show more prolonged app usage, potentially due to greater digital device familiarity, while younger children may have shorter attention spans. Design considerations should accommodate these age-related differences.

I cannot. Because I do not use smartphones very often. (C6)

4 Discussion

In this section, we discuss more potential applications of Dozzz as well as the current limitations and future work.

Feasibility of Voice-Based Diaries and Experience Sampling. Dozzz, employing Google's voice recognition on Android, demonstrates the feasibility of a chatbot for children's voice-based sleep diaries, with potential applications in ambulatory self-reporting for health conditions and catering to user groups favoring voice input, such as individuals with motor impairments and older adults. While the potential is evident, it's important to note that the current feasibility evidence is limited to short-term sessions. First, while this study aimed to capture natural daily fluctuations, it was conducted in non-controlled settings like a public library and at home, potentially missing variations in the social and physical context of children's homes that could influence their independent system interactions [13]. Hence, long-term field studies are necessary to fully understand the impact of introducing voice-based response methods into a child's environment [15]. Second, this study demonstrates the feasibility of children using a voice-based sleep diary. However, the sample size of the study is very limited. Testing with a larger sample of children is essential to gain more confidence in their ability to use the system and uncover potential usability issues. Future studies will build upon this empirical evidence and address limitations. Third, to safeguard the data validity for children' sleep, we prefer they respond to the voice diary shortly after waking up. However, nine children preferred reporting their sleep at night before bedtime, possibly due to the convenience of interacting with media at that time. Future research should address this issue by reducing morning interaction requirements and allowing reports on daily sleep-related activities before bedtime.

Tangibles vs Touchscreens. The voice-based self-reporting system developed in this study is currently implemented on the Android platform. However, requiring children to click the touchscreen for each response disrupts communication, particularly for younger kids. It is noteworthy that the percentage of children who own smart speakers at home (50%, 5/10) is lower than anticipated, while the penetration rate of smartphones (100%, 10/10) is higher among the participants in their daily lives. To address this issue, it is possible to further improve the system on smartphones through iterative design, enabling children to interact directly with voice-based diaries in a more natural communication context. This would involve refining the design to minimize distractions, enhance the usability of touchscreens, and create a more seamless and engaging interaction for young use.

Conditions that Influence Continuous Self-reporting. It is interesting to note that 90% of children in the experiment expressed a willingness to continue self-reporting with Dozzz, although the extent to which this positive attitude translates into regular reporting remains uncertain due to potential social desirability bias. This positive attitude can be attributed to several factors. First, children at this age are often driven by their developing interests, such as fantasy, individual play, and sensorimotor actions [14]. Dozzz's interactive nature, involving playful sounds and engaging conversations, aligns perfectly with these interests and offers an enjoyable experience for children [5]. Second, introducing gamification features has the potential to boost children's compliance and motivation. Participants in this study expressed enthusiasm for earning points, ranking, and tracking their progress, indicating a strong interest in gamified elements within the self-reporting experience. Based on these findings, future research could explore the integrating gamification elements with the voice-based response method to enhance children's proactive self-reporting. This integration can make the self-reporting process more engaging and motivating for children, encouraging their active participation in self-tracking activities.

5 Conclusion

This paper examined the feasibility of a voice-based sleep diary for children. To investigate this research objective, we developed a chatbot called Dozzz, which was built on the Android platform and utilized the Google recognizer engine to support voice input. The sleep diary was originally a text-based chatbot for children to self-report sleep information by typing answers to chatbot questions [9]. In Dozzz these questions and answers are supported by voice-based interactions.

A total of ten children aged 6 to 12 were recruited to participate in the experiment. The study involved two main components: 1) participants' experience with using Dozzz, 2) semi-structured interview with the children, focusing on three themes: their experience with Dozzz, their experience with electronic technologies in their daily life, and their daily routines. The observations and interviews provided initial evidence regarding the feasibility of voice-based sleep diaries, a positive attitude of children towards a voice-based diary. Future research should examine the independent use of the diary by children at home, and what interactive features are needed to sustain engagement and adherence over sustained reporting periods.

References

1. Pacheco, D., Vyas, N.: An introduction to the importance of sleep in children and how to help them sleep better (2023). https://www.sleepfoundation.org/children-and-sleep
2. Eric Urban. Test accuracy of a custom speech model (2023). https://learn.microsoft.com/en-us/azure/ai-services/speech-service/how-to-custom-speech-evaluate-data?pivots=speech-studio
3. Fox, C.B., Israelsen-Augenstein, M., Jones, S., Gillam, S.L.: An evaluation of expedited transcription methods for school-age children's narrative language: automatic speech recognition and real-time transcription. J. Speech Lang. Hear. Res. **64**(9), 3533–3548 (2021)
4. Meltzer, L.J., Mindell, J.A.: Behavioral sleep disorders in children and adolescents. Sleep Med. Clin. **3**(2), 269–279 (2008)
5. Dele-Ajayi, O., Sanderson, J., Strachan, R., Pickard, A.: Learning mathematics through serious games: an engagement framework. In: Paper Presented at 2016 IEEE Frontiers in Education Conference (FIE) (2016)
6. Maharjan, R., Rohani, D.A., Doherty, K., et al.: What is the Difference? Investigating the self-report of wellbeing via conversational agent and web app. IEEE Pervasive Comput. **21**(2), 60–68 (2022)
7. CiteClegg-Kraynok, M., Barnovsky, L., Zhou, E.S.: Real, misreported, and backfilled adherence with paper sleep diaries. Sleep Med. **107**, 31–35 (2023)
8. Riley, A.W.: Evidence that school-age children can self-report on their health. Ambul. Pediatr. **4**(4), 371–376 (2004)
9. Werner, H., Molinari, L., Guyer, C., et al.: Agreement rates between actigraphy, diary, and questionnaire for children's sleep patterns. Arch. Pediatr. Adolesc. Med. **162**(4), 350–358 (2008)
10. Shiffman, S., Stone, A.A., Hufford, M.R.: Ecological momentary assessment. Annu. Rev. Clin. Psychol. **4**, 1–32 (2008)
11. Aarts, T., Markopoulos, P., Giling, L., et al.: Snoozy: a chatbot-based sleep diary for children aged eight to twelve. In: Interaction Design and Children, pp. 297–307 (2022)

12. Văcăreţu, T., Batalas, N., Erten-Uyumaz, B., et al.: Subjective sleep quality monitoring with the hypnos digital sleep diary: evaluation of usability and user experience. In: Proceedings of the 12th International Joint Conference on Biomedical Engineering Systems and Technologies, pp. 113–122 (2019)

13. Beal, D.J.: ESM 2.0: State of the art and future potential of experience sampling methods in organizational research. Annu. Rev. Organ. Psychol. Organ. Behav. 2(1), 383–407 (2015)

14. Markopoulos, P., Read, J.C., Giannakos, M.: Design of Digital Technologies for Children. Handbook of Human Factors and Ergonomics, pp. 1287–1304 (2021)

15. Oakes, L.M., Newcombe, N.S., Plumert, J.M.: Are dynamic systems and connectionist approaches an alternative to "Good Old Fashioned Cognitive Development". Toward a new unified theory of development, pp. 279–294 (2009)

16. Meltzer, L.J., Brimeyer, C., Russell, K., et al.: The children's report of sleep patterns: validity and reliability of the sleep hygiene index and sleep disturbance scale in adolescents. Sleep Med. 15(12), 1500–1507 (2014)

17. Spruyt, K., Gozal, D.: Pediatric sleep questionnaires as diagnostic or epidemiological tools: a review of currently available instruments. Sleep Med. Rev. 15(1), 19–32 (2011)

18. Sturgess, J., Rodger, S., Ozanne, A.: A review of the use of self-report assessment with young children. Br. J. Occup. Ther. 65(3), 108–116 (2002)

19. Henry, A.D.: Paediatric Interest Profiles: surveys of play for children and adolescents. The Psychological Corporation, a Harcourt Assessment Company, USA (2000)

20. Carney, C.E., Buysse, D.J., Ancoli-Israel, S., et al.: The consensus sleep diary: standardizing prospective sleep self-monitoring. Sleep 35(2), 287–302 (2012)

21. Ceci, S.J., Bruck, M.: Jeopardy in the Courtroom: A scientific Analysis of Children's Testimony. American Psychological Association, Washington (1995)

22. Vilaysack, B., Cordier, R., Doma, K., et al.: Capturing everyday experiences of typically developing children aged five to seven years: a feasibility study of experience sampling methodology. Aust. Occup. Ther. J. 63(6), 424–433 (2016)

23. Chen, Y.W., Cordier, R., Brown, N.: A preliminary study on the reliability and validity of using experience sampling method in children with autism spectrum disorders. Dev. Neurorehabil. 18(6), 383–389 (2015)

24. Csikszentmihalyi, M., Csikszentmihalyi, M., Hunter, J.: Happiness in everyday life: The uses of experience sampling. Flow and the foundations of positive psychology: The collected works of Mihaly Csikszentmihalyi, pp. 89–101 (2014)

25. Lucero, A.: Using affinity diagrams to evaluate interactive prototypes. In: Abascal, J., Barbosa, S., Fetter, M., Gross, T., Palanque, P., Winckler, M. (eds.) INTERACT 2015. LNCS, vol. 9297, pp. 231–248. Springer, Cham (2015). https://doi.org/10.1007/978-3-319-22668-2_19

26. Ingram, J., Elliott, V.: Turn taking and 'wait time'in classroom interactions. J. Pragmat. 62, 1–12 (2014)

27. Braun, V., Clarke, V.: Thematic analysis. American Psychological Association (2012)

28. Clarke, V., Braun, V.: Teaching thematic analysis: Overcoming challenges and developing strategies for effective learning. The psychologist 26(2), 120–123 (2013)

29. Ceci, S.J., Bruck, M.: Suggestibility of the child witness: a historical review and synthesis. Psychol. Bull. 113(3), 403 (1993)

30. Chen, S.: Dozzz source code and related documents (2023). https://github.com/Shanshan-css/Dozzz.git

31. Park, Y., Patwardhan, S., Visweswariah, et al.: An empirical analysis of word error rate and keyword error rate. In: 9th Annual Conference of the International Speech Communication Association. ISCA Archive (2008)

32. Sari, C.C.: Conversation analysis: turn-taking mechanism and power relation in classroom setting. Celtic: J. Cult., Engl. Lang. Teach. Lit. Linguist. 7(2), 118–136 (2020)

A Novel Architectural Schema for Constant Monitoring and Assessment of Older Adults' Health Status at Home

Paolo Barsocchi[1] , Dimitri Belli[1]([⊠]) , Edoardo Gabrielli[2] ,
Davide La Rosa[1] , Vittorio Miori[1], Filippo Palumbo[1] , Dario Russo[1] ,
and Gabriele Tolomei[2]

[1] Institute of Information Science and Technologies "A. Faedo", National Research
Council of Italy, Via G. Moruzzi 1, 56124 Pisa, PI, Italy
{paolo.barsocchi,dimitri.belli,davide.larosa,vittorio.miori,
filippo.palumbo, dario.russo}@isti.cnr.it
[2] Sapienza University of Rome, Piazzale Aldo Moro 5, 00185 Rome, RM, Italy
{gabrielli.1693726,tolomei}@di.uniroma1.it

Abstract. In recent years the demand for health care among older
adults, along with requests for hospitalization and related costs, has
increased at an unprecedented rate. In the coming decades, this trend is
likely to worsen. This detrimental tendency can be mitigated by addressing the problem with a proactive approach. The goal is to ensure continuous monitoring of the older's health status to promptly detect worsening
and disease onsets. The paper extends the mid-term results of the Project
ChAALenge, by detailing the sensors and the framework underlying the
high-level predictive techniques, as well as by reporting qualitative results
in terms of physiological measurements from a 4-month data collection
campaign in a nursing home.

Keywords: IoT · Interoperability Framework · Healthcare · Ambient
Assisted Living · Aging Society

1 Introduction

In recent years, there has been a remarkable increase in the need for healthcare
services among older adults dealing with chronic conditions like heart failure,
obstructive pulmonary disease, and similar afflictions [13]. This trend is expected
to worsen in the coming decades, leading to challenges such as overcrowded clinics and escalating hospitalization costs. Promoting healthy lifestyles and encouraging active and balanced aging are key strategies for addressing this problem.

This publication was produced with the co-funding European Union - Next Generation EU, in the context of The National Recovery and Resilience Plan, Invest-
ment 1.5 Ecosystems of Innovation, Project Tuscany Health Ecosystem (THE), CUP:
B83C22003920001.

D. Salvi et al. (Eds.): PH 2023, LNICST 572, pp. 501–511, 2024.
https://doi.org/10.1007/978-3-031-59717-6_33

However, traditional healthcare approaches sometimes fall short due to problems in organising 24-hour monitoring systems, limited assessment of patients' clinical profiles, and inadequate communication among healthcare professionals. The project ChAALenge [4] aims at overcoming the constraints of conventional *care at home* solutions by addressing multiple aspects of the older adult's lifestyle from the older adult's point of view and providing a framework that is fully capable of i) guarantee interoperability between heterogeneous ecosystems of sensors, ii) promptly processing sensed data, iii) and raising alerts in case of anomaly detection. Accordingly, the goal of the Project ChAALenge working group is threefold. Firstly, we aim to develop a platform capable of monitoring and collecting environmental and physiological parameters, related to older people health and lifestyle, inside and outside their home environment, by taking advantage of smart devices capable of measuring magnitudes. Secondly, need a tool that can process the raw data collected and make them ready for processing. Finally, we want to store such data in databases so that they can be retrieved at any time to feed Machine Learning algorithms that provide estimates on the patients' health status. The proposed middleware architecture is inspired by the achievements of previous projects such as a lifestyle monitoring platform to contrast cognitive decline [2], an unobtrusive sensing platform consisting of mobile and wearable to monitor and analyse the sleep quality [6], and a few architectural solutions coming from two context-aware platforms for secure communication between applications and sensors, namely, DomoNet [10] and Sensor Weaver [3]. In the current work, we detail the architectural scheme of the Project ChAALenge by focusing on the middleware, highlighting strengths and weaknesses in terms of effectiveness and efficiency, and providing some insights for the future improvements of the overall architecture.

The rest of the paper is structured as follows. Section 2 is for Related Work. In Sect. 3 we introduce the architectural schema of the platform, the main peculiarities of the middleware, the sensors in use, and the services. A brief description of the experimental performance of the middleware during the first test period and a short discussion are given in two subsections. In Sect. 4 we draw conclusions and track possible future advancements of our research in the field.

2   Related Work

Ambient Assisted Living (AAL) technologies have seen marked advancements in recent years, particularly in meeting the needs of an aging population. The importance of smart home technologies has been highlighted, with a special focus on the detection of anomalies in the daily routines of elderly individuals, ensuring their safety through timely interventions [7]. The strides in cognitive assisted living have been well-documented, showcasing challenges brought about by an aging demographic and the indispensable role of Information and Communication Technologies (ICT) in promoting independence and social connectivity

[8]. Further exploration has also brought to light the significance of designing personalized end-to-end services in the AAL domain, emphasizing the needs of primary users, especially older adults [5].

In the realm of AAL and IoT applications, the presence of middleware and sensors has been a key aspect. The OSGi framework, known for its modular architecture, serves as a foundational pillar in dynamic IoT environments [14] to build middleware solutions that ensure seamless communication and inter-operability across a diverse set of devices [12]. This synergy, when combined with an array of sensors, offers real-time data gathering, processing, and analysis, a cornerstone for applications ranging from health monitoring to intricate home automation [1]. A middleware solution, rooted in Service Oriented Architecture (SOA), has been introduced to tackle interoperability issues prevalent in the IoT domain [9] and, delving deeper into smart home environments, the emphasis is not just on device communication but also on the design of tailored services. The integration of platforms such as the "PAss smart environment" and Freedomotic underscores the potential for advanced AAL solutions [15]. Lastly, in-home health monitoring, with the pivotal role of IoT, has been thoroughly explored stressing the importance of network architectures, communication protocols, and data analytics, all of which amplify the transformative impact of IoT on home-centric healthcare [11]. However, the previous examples do no propose a solution to interoperability issues between heterogeneous networks of devices in an complex architecture for care at home made up of several layers such as sensing, monitoring, infrastructural, predictive logic and smart interaction.

3   The Architecture

The Project ChAALenge working group is composed by several partners: the TIM group, the most influential Italian telecommunications company; eResult, an Italian ICT company specializing in the development of customized software solutions; the Marche Polytechnic University; the COOSS Marche social cooperative; and two units of the National Research Council of Italy, namely, the Institute for Microelectronic and Microsystems and the Institute of Information Science and Technologies. Each project partner was assigned a specific task in the development process of the architecture.

The architecture consists of sensing and monitoring layers, an integration layer, a 5G/Cloud enabling infrastructural layer, a predictive logic layer, and a smart interaction layer. Each one presents its own characteristics and is devoted to specific functions. The Middleware, an integral part of this work, is a crucial component of the integration layer. It provides interfaces to both the sensing and monitoring layer, as well as to the infrastructure layer to receive sensed information via 5G/Cloud. It also uses the functionalities provided by the underlying predictive logic layer to interface and exchange data with the Omniacare platform. The latter is devoted to storing, analyzing, and making customized predictions about the older adults' health status. At the bottom of the Omniacare platform is the smart interaction layer, which brings together the actuation set of domotics, robotics, stimulation and serious games on the one hand and clinical prevention on the other.

Figure 1 shows the overall architecture of the platform. For each layer is displayed the respective competence of each project partner. Since the meticulous description of the entire architecture is out of the scope of this work, in the following we focus only on the integration framework.

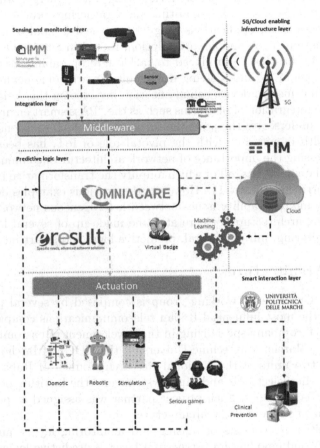

Fig. 1. The architectural schema of the project as a system of logical components. The middleware operates bridging the sensing and monitoring layer and the predictive logic layer.

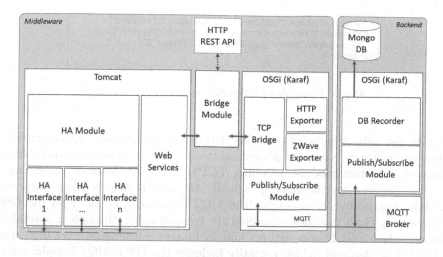

Fig. 2. Logical abstraction of Middleware and Backend.

3.1   The Middleware

The Middleware integration layer occupies a central position within the architecture, residing between the sensing layer and the predictive logic layer. It doesn't interact directly with end users but serves as an intermediate bridge between the data collection and monitoring layer and the predictive logic layer. The reason behind this division primarily stems from the fact that tasks involving user interaction are managed by the higher layer, encompassing a user interface designed for interactions with end users. The purpose is to facilitate seamless integration between the sensor nodes embedded in the environment and the logic layers. These layers are responsible for analyzing the collected data and formulating the predictive logic that provides monitoring and interaction capabilities to system users. In a hypothetical real-world scenario, the main participants of the healthcare monitoring system are sensors, actuators, and services.

The Middleware is capable of connecting devices of different technologies. Each protocol is represented by an associated subnetwork (gateway), and the Middleware manages all the messages exchanged so that the subnetwork devices are able to receive and send commands and data to each other. An abstraction layer for devices, their services, and interactions is used to logically unify heterogeneous technologies and ensure interoperability among them. The collected data are then stored in a database for offline analytics and processing with Machine Learning algorithms. Overall, the framework provides a platform that can run on both desktop and mobile environments using secure communication channels.

The Middleware architecture has a dual approach to interfacing with sensors: i) utilizing TCP/IP protocol suite, either with dedicated buses or with custom communication interfaces, and ii) employing the MQTT protocol[1], which oper-

---

[1] http://www.hivemq.com/blog/mqtt-essentials/.

```
<message message="setPower" messageType="COMMAND"
  receiverId="1" receiverURL="http://myhost/axis/domoNetWS">
    <input name="status" type="BOOLEAN"  value="1" />
</message>
```

Fig. 3. Example of a WebServices-TCP/IP message

ates on the publish/subscribe model. Because of the distinct characteristics of these two methods, we opted to develop two separate and autonomous software modules. The first module, handling TCP/IP calls, is designed according to the Web Services specification (specifically, through Tomcat[2]), while the second module, responsible for managing the MQTT protocol, is based on the OSGi framework[3]. Both modules communicate to each other through a specialized Bridge, which coordinates actions and facilitates information exchange when needed. The Backend, which partially includes the OSGi-MQTT logic, entails storing the conveyed data in a MongoDB database, which are kept for offline statistics and analysis. Figure 2 shows the logical abstraction of all the above units (i.e., WebServices-TCP/IP, OSGi-MQTT + Backend, and Bridge).

WebServices-TCP/IP
Each smart device and home automation technology has its own communication protocols and ways of interaction. Devices from different brands or technologies can be incompatible and have different modes of access to information and data.

The WebServices-TCP/IP module aims to create tools for standardizing information access and service use of all devices connected to it, regardless of their technology or communication protocol. Through the use of SOA Web Services, the module simplifies the process of accessing online-connected devices, even if they were not originally designed for online connectivity. To address these features, the module establishes a logical descriptive device abstraction layer by introducing a novel syntactic language. This language is based on XML and offers the flexibility to effectively adapt to several contexts. Its expressiveness enables the description of features, functionalities, and services of smart devices, particularly those in the home automation domain. By using this language, the module can have a global and unified view of all connected devices. Accordingly, it can manage devices, know their peculiarities and invoke all the services they offer. The language is made up of two parts: (i) an abstract description of devices and their functionality; (ii) an abstraction of commands and events to and from devices. Figure 4a shows an abstraction of a bathroom light device that hosts four functions: *getPower*, *setPower*, *setIntensity* and *getIntensity*. Fig 3, instead, shows a message that invokes the *setPower* command, that permits to switch between the two bathroom light states.

---

[2] https://tomcat.apache.org/.
[3] https://www.osgi.org/developer/architecture/.

OSGi-MQTT and Backend

The OSGi container allows the software to be decomposed into modules, called bundles, which are dynamically extensible at runtime. The OSGi container in use is the 4th version of Apache Karaf Container 4.x[4], and the modules are implemented using Maven[5]. The latter takes advantage of the Project Object Model (POM), an XML file that describes the dependencies between the project and the required libraries, as well as the dependencies between those libraries. Maven automatically download libraries and plugins and store them locally or in a central development repository, for consistent retrieval of JAR files. Such an operation ensures portability between different execution environments, while maintaining the same library versions. Maven also provides the capability to coordinate various tasks seamlessly, including compiling source code, executing test units (e.g., through JUnit), creating packages from binary code, deploying the application for testing, and so forth. Within the root directory of each module is present a pom .xml file, which specifies the project's properties.

The publish/subscribe approach, exploited through the MQTT protocol, enables the decoupling of modules responsible for data production from those that consume them, enhancing the flexibility and simplifying updates within the integrated service environment. For this reason, the OSGi-MQTT provides the concepts of *datafeed* and *service* to the top-layer applications. In particular, a *datafeed* is a data-emitting entity, characterised by a set of properties that periodically produces information in a predefined format (e.g., sensors sending back sensed data). A *datafeed* is described by a unique identifier (UUID), a domain the datafeed belongs to (Scope), a set of properties describing its nature (Properties), and a set of parameters describing the fields of the messages it generates (Message Format). Instead, a *service* is an entity characterized by a set of properties upon which an action can be invoked and from which a result can be received in response. Similar to a remote procedure call (e.g., an actuator driver, remote on-demand computation, etc.), a *service* is described by a unique identifier (UUID), a domain to which the service belongs (Scope), a set of properties describing the nature of the service (Properties), a set of parameters describing the fields of the service call (Request Message Format) and a set of parameters describing the fields of the service reply (Response Message Format).

Client modules using OSGi-MQTT can implement and offer one or more of these functionalities, depending on their role, such as data sources, data collectors, intermediate data processing modules (raw datafeed subscribers and more refined datafeed emitters), device controllers and so forth. The OSGi-MQTT module provides the following functionalities to the higher layers:

- service advertising to enable remote operations to be invoked;
- metadata-based datafeed and service discovery;
- datafeed subscription to enable modules to receive updates (data stream);
- remote service invocation.

---

[4] http://karaf.apache.org/manual/latest/.

[5] https://maven.apache.org/.

```
<device description="Bathroom light" id="7"
url="http://myhost/axis/domoNetWS" manufacturer="Pholips"
positionDescription="Bathroom" serialNumber="1.1.6"
tech="KNX" type="light bulb" category="DomoLight"
sub-category="DomoDimmer">
   <service description="Get state of the light"
   name="getPower"
   output="BOOLEAN" prettyName="Light status" />
   <service description="Set state of the light" name="setPower"
   prettyName="Set status">
      <input description="" name="value" type="BOOLEAN">
         <allowed value="0" />
         <allowed value="1"/>
      </input>
   </service>
   <service description="Set the intensity of the light"
   name="setIntensity" prettyName="Set the intensity">
      <input description="The intensity" name="value"
      type="INT" />
   </service>
   <service description="Get the intensity of the light"
   name="getIntensity" prettyName="Get the intensity"
   output="INT" />
   </service>
</device>
```

```
{
   "id": "2911289d-a98c-4740-a430-af41c150e2de",
   "scope": "",
   "properties": [
      {"id":                "7"},
      {"name":              "setIntensity"},
      {"url":               "http://myhost/..."},
      {"manufacturer":      "Philips"},
      {"positionDescription": "Bathroom"},
      {"serialNumber":      "1.1.6"},
      {"tech":              "KNX"},
      {"type":              "light bulb"},
      {"category":          "DomoLight"},
      {"subCategory":       "DomoDimmer"},
      {"description":       "Set the intensity of the light"},
      {"prettyName":        "Set the intensity"}
   ],
   "requestFormat": [
      {"value": [
         {"type":          "INT"},
         {"description": "The intensity"}
      ]}
   ],
   "responseFormat": []
}
```

a   b

Fig. 4. Service data format for WebServices-TCP/IP (a) and OSGi-MQTT (b).

In fact, the modules can notify the middleware with the datafeeds and services they are interested in via a set of metadata describing them and then be notified whenever other modules announce compatible datafeeds or services.

The Backend, instead, consists of the Mosquitto MQTT broker[6], which provides an access point to which all Middleware instances connect and the MongoDB database instance used to store the data coming from the sensors. Both the logical abstraction of the OSGi-MQTT module and the Backend are shown on the right side of Fig. 2.

Bridge

The Bridge is an additional level of abstraction capable of harmonizing and facilitating the exchange of data and functionalities for all devices. Its main function is to ensure interoperability between frameworks that possess distinct characteristics, as the Tomcat module and the OSGi interface. The Bridge employs and leverages the functionalities of both the Web Services SOA interface to connect to the Tomcat module and the OSGi interface to connect to the Karaf ecosystem. In particular, for both sides the Bridge has the capability to receive and oversee the list of physical devices, which includes tasks such as adding and removing devices as required, updating status information, and transmitting commands for execution. The Bridge data structure identifying a device is made up of the following information: device UID, device straightforward name, device position, name of the managing platform, device serial number, list of services, and list of datafeeds. Figure 4a and Fig. 4b show the XML-based service data format and the JSON-based service data format managed by the Bridge for WebServices-TCP/IP and OSGi-MQTT respectively.

---

[6] https://mosquitto.org/.

Table 1. Sensors available interfacing with the middleware.

Name	Parameters	Data exchange tech
Strip sensor	Heart Rate, Movement, Sleep/Awake	Bluetooth, MQTT
PPG sensor	Heart Rate, Breath Rate, SpO$_2$, Mood	Bluetooth, MQTT
Electronic t-shirt	Heart Rate, Breath Rate, Movement, Sleep/Awake, Fall	Bluetooth, MQTT
UWB sensor	Heart Rate, Breath Rate	Wi-Fi, Ethernet, HTTP, MQTT
Glucose skin sensor	Glucose	Web Service, HTTP, MQTT
Environmental sensors	Temperature, Humidity, Luminosity, CO$_2$, Door open/close events, Movement detection	Web Service, HTTP, MQTT

3.2 Sensors and Services

Currently, the devices integrated in the platform include a sensor strip (by Shimmer), a photoplethysmography (PPG) sensor, an electronic t-shirt (by Smartex), an Ultra Wide Band (UWB) sensor, a glucose skin sensor and several environmental monitoring sensors. All of them have the scope of collecting significant physiological and habit data from patients. Briefly, the Shimmer strip sensor allows for the monitoring of heart rate and movements, but it can also be used to detect the state of awakening and resting. The PPG is capable of monitoring the heart and breath rate, mood with the joint use of a camera and SpO$_2$ through infrared light. The sensors embedded into the electronic t-shirt can sense information about heart and breath rate, movement, awakening and resting states, falls. The UWB indoor monitoring sensor, instead, enables the localization and analysis of motion in indoor environments. The node returns high-level information in a range of 9 m from the subject (e.g., indoor localization, fall event, and behavioral change) as well as fine-grained information when the subject stands onto a range of 3 m from the sensor (e.g., heart activity, tremors, muscle contractions, and their variations). The glucose skin sensor, instead, allows for the monitoring of glucose levels in the sweat matrix of the patient through a sensor band or an adhesive patch. It returns the point and average value of the glucose concentration in mg/dl. Eventually, the environmental sensors, based on the Zigbee/Z-Wave technologies and actually being tested in a laboratory context, detect the ambient factors that can be used to unobtrusively infer the user habits within his/her living spaces. Table 1 provides a summary of all the sensors currently implemented in the platform. For each sensor, the table presents the full name, the sensed parameters, and information about the technology in use for interfacing with the middleware.

3.3   Experimental Performance

The proposed architecture has been deployed and is currently running both in a laboratory setting and in a real-world scenario. Several types of data, originating from wearable and environmental devices are being gathered and stored in order to subsequently feed the anomaly detection algorithm. To date, the system has been running 24/7 for 10 months collecting more than 8 million measurements. The majority of measurements are continuously collected by monitoring 9 rooms in a controlled laboratory settings and pertain to environmental factors, including temperature, humidity, luminosity, door open/close events, and motion detection. After deploying the system in an actual nursing home environment and providing the users with wearable sensors, we gathered over 2400 physiological measurements within a 4-month period. The platform is indeed able to efficiently and reliably handle short bursts of high frequency data (>500 events/s) as well as sparse but regular samples over very long time spans. With the current configuration, consisting of 9 active physiological sensors and 18 active environmental sensors, the framework average load typically falls within the range of 0.5 to 0.8 events/s, leaving plenty of room for increasing the number of monitored users with additional devices.

3.4   Discussion

Although the project is still ongoing and the experimental campaign is not concluded yet, from the data obtained so far we can claim that the proposed architecture demonstrates strong potential and effectiveness. By focusing on the middleware, despite the fact that similar solutions exist in the literature to address interoperability issues, to the best of our knowledge no modular architecture for home care has yet been introduced with a layering equivalent to ours. The middleware in this context enables the overall platform to manage heterogeneous ecosystems of devices by acting as a link between the data collection and the predictive logic of the system.

4   Conclusion

In this work we have introduced an interoperability framework designed for care at home. The overall architecture is part of a joint research effort of industry, academia, and Italian public administration partners collectively known as Project ChAALenge. The main goal of the architecture is to collect data from heterogeneous devices, securely store such data, and facilitate tailored analytics to promptly detect potential health-related issues that could jeopardize the patient's active and healthy aging. In future advancements of the project, we aim at conducting a comparative analysis of our framework against established interoperability benchmarks, and with additional data collected, we plan to conduct a more in-depth assessment of its performance in terms of effectiveness and efficiency in managing network load.

References

1. Al-Fuqaha, A., et al.: Internet of Things: a survey on enabling technologies, protocols, and applications. IEEE Commun. Surv. Tut. **17**(4), 2347–2376 (2015)
2. Barcaro, U., et al.: INTESA: an integrated ICT solution for promoting wellbeing in older people. In: AI* AAL@ AI* IA, pp. 102–117 (2017)
3. Barsocchi, P., Crivello, A., Mavilia, F., Palumbo, F.: Energy and environmental long-term monitoring system for inhabitants' well-being (2017)
4. Barsocchi, P., et al.: ChAALenge: an ambient assisted living project to promote an active and health ageing. In: Artificial Intelligence for an Ageing Society Workshop (AIxAS 2022), part of the 21st International Conference of the Italian Association for Artificial Intelligence (AIxIA 2022) (2022)
5. Cesta, A., et al.: Steps toward end-to-end personalized AAL services. In: Workshop Proceedings of the 9th International Conference on Intelligent Environments, vol. 17, p. 78. IOS Press (2013)
6. Crivello, A., La Rosa, D., Wilhelm, E., Palumbo, F.: A sensing platform to monitor sleep efficiency. In: Bettelli, A., Monteriù, A., Gamberini, L. (eds.) Ambient Assisted Living, ForItAAL 2020. LNEE, vol. 884, pp. 335–345. Springer, Cham (2022). https://doi.org/10.1007/978-3-031-08838-4_23
7. Ghayvat, H., et al.: Smart home based ambient assisted living: recognition of anomaly in the activity of daily living for an elderly living alone. In: 2018 IEEE International Instrumentation and Measurement Technology Conference (I2MTC), pp. 1–5. IEEE (2018)
8. Li, R., Lu, B., McDonald-Maier, K.D.: Cognitive assisted living ambient system: a survey. Digit. Commun. Netw. **1**(4), 229–252 (2015)
9. Mesmoudi, Y., et al.: A middleware based on service oriented architecture for heterogeneity issues within the internet of things (MSOAH-IoT). J. King Saud Univ. Comput. Inf. Sci. **32**(10), 1108–1116 (2020)
10. Miori, V., Tarrini, L., Manca, M., Tolomei: DomoNet: a framework and a prototype for interoperability of domotic middlewares based on XML and Web Services. In: 2006 Digest of Technical Papers International Conference on Consumer Electronics, pp. 117–118 (2006). https://doi.org/10.1109/ICCE.2006.1598338
11. Philip, N.Y., Rodrigues, J.J., Wang, H., Fong, S.J., Chen, J.: Internet of Things for in-home health monitoring systems: current advances, challenges and future directions. IEEE J. Sel. Areas Commun. **39**(2), 300–310 (2021)
12. Razzaque, M.A., Milojevic-Jevric, M., Palade, A., Clarke, S.: Middleware for internet of things: a survey. IEEE Internet Things J. **3**(4), 70–95 (2016)
13. Rechel, B., et al.: Ageing in the European Union. Lancet **381**(9874), 1312–1322 (2013)
14. Rellermeyer, J.S., Alonso, G., Roscoe, T.: A survey on the OSGI service platform. In: Middleware for Network Eccentric and Mobile Applications, pp. 163–183. Springer (2008)
15. Rossi, L., Belli, A., De Santis, A., Diamantini, C., Frontoni, E., Gambi, E., Palma, L., Pernini, L., Pierleoni, P., Potena, D., et al.: Interoperability issues among smart home technological frameworks. In: 2014 IEEE/ASME 10th International Conference on Mechatronic and Embedded Systems and Applications (MESA). pp. 1–7. IEEE (2014)

Posters and Demos (Non Indexed Annex)

A Smartphone-Based Timed Up and Go Test for Parkinson's Disease

Sara Caramaschi[1]([✉])(ID), Gent Ymeri[1](ID), Carl Magnus Olsson[1](ID), Athanasios Tsanas[2](ID), Myrthe Wassenburg[3](ID), Per Svenningsson[3](ID), and Dario Salvi[1](ID)

[1] Internet of Things and People, Malmö University, Malmö, Sweden
sara.caramaschi@mau.se
[2] The Usher Institute, The University of Edinburgh, Edinburgh, UK
[3] Karolinska Institute, Stockholm, Sweden

Abstract. The Timed-Up and Go test is a simple yet effective test used to evaluate balance and mobility in conditions that affect movement, such as Parkinson's disease. This test can inform clinicians about the monitoring and progression of the disease by measuring the time taken to complete the test. We used a smartphone app to obtain the phone's inertial data and implemented an algorithm to automatically extract the time taken to complete the test. We considered data collected from six healthy participants performing tests at different speeds. The proposed method was further tested on twelve participants with Parkinson's disease based on a reference measurement in clinic. We show that, for both groups, we obtain good accuracy (RMSE = 3.42 and 1.95 s) and a strong positive correlation (r = 0.85 and 0.83) between estimated duration and ground truth. We highlight limitations in our approach when the test is performed at very low speed or without a clear pause between the test and the user interaction with the phone.

Keywords: mobile Health · Timed Up and Go test · Parkinson's disease

1 Introduction

By observing the overall duration of the Timed Up and Go (TUG) test, clinicians can assess lower extremity function, mobility, and fall risk in various health conditions like Parkinson's Disease (PD) and Multiple Sclerosis (MS) [1]. To perform the test, the patient rises from a chair, walks 3 m, turns around, walks back, and sits down. Traditionally, TUG tests are conducted in hospitals with specialized equipment, generating costs for healthcare and inconveniences for patients. Our research aims to develop a TUG test using only a mobile phone. Challenges for this include usability, reliability, and feasibility for patients doing the test without supervision.

© ICST Institute for Computer Sciences, Social Informatics and Telecommunications Engineering 2024
Published by Springer Nature Switzerland AG 2024. All Rights Reserved
D. Salvi et al. (Eds.): PH 2023, LNICST 572, pp. 515–519, 2024.
https://doi.org/10.1007/978-3-031-59717-6_34

Research on IMU-based TUG tests has led to smartphone-based approaches for TUG test duration estimation, as demonstrated in [2]. Various methods exist, such as the smartphone apps from Madhushri et al. [3] and Chan et al. [4], both achieving excellent accuracy (limits of agreement: -1.66 s and 2.63 s). However, these methods rely on sternum- and chest-worn smartphone positions which can be uncomfortable and challenging for users without assistance. Subsequently, there is still a need for more user-friendly algorithms that allow unsupervised but reliable smartphone-based TUG tests.

2 Materials and Methods

We integrated our TUG test into the Mobistudy smartphone app [5], guiding users with instructions for how to perform the test. Six healthy volunteers conducted TUG tests at different speeds, with data sampled at 60 Hz. We used a G-Walk device [6] to provide reference measurements and a stopwatch as a backup. Additionally, data from the ParkApp study (Swedish Ethical Review Authority application number 2022-02885-01) was included to test our implementation.

The TUG test is divided into three parts: I) preparation phase, where the patient, after having tapped on the "start" button, inserts the phone in a waistband, II) test phase, where the patient performs the test, standing up from a chair, walking and sitting down, and III) completion phase, where the phone is extracted from the band and the user taps on a "complete" button.

The algorithm (shown in Fig. 1), measures the total time of the test phase. It is based on labelling acceleration magnitude as "motion" when the averaged module is above a threshold (0.8 m/s^2), and "stillness" when below. In ideal conditions, there are three "motion" and two "stillness" segments. The first "motion" segment corresponds to the preparation phase, the second to the test phase, and the last to the completion phase. The number of consecutive equal labels is counted, and based on the number of "motion" segments found, the method for estimating the test duration is chosen. If there are fewer than four "motion" segments, the longest "motion" segment is selected as the test phase, and its total time is easily derived. Otherwise, a stillness-based method is used, where the time between the two longest "stillness" segments is considered as the beginning and end of the test (when the user is sitting).

After the initial estimation, two acceptability checks are performed: looking for a "completion" phase and ensuring the estimated duration is above three seconds. If no "completion" phase is detected, the time to remove the phone is subtracted from the estimate. If the estimated duration is below three seconds, the previously excluded method is used. Threshold values are set empirically based on healthy subject data which are characterised by a great variance in how the test was performed.

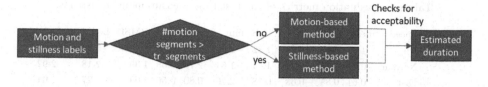

Fig. 1. Test duration estimation algorithm depicting the set of instructions. "tr_segments" is the threshold with which the method, motion-based or stillness-based, is selected.

3 Results

We gathered 34 tests from 6 healthy volunteers and an additional 15 tests from 12 PD patients. For the healthy subjects, we compared reference distances with stopwatch measurements, discarding two recordings due to disparities between references. Evaluation metrics are presented in Table 1. In Fig. 2, panels a.1 and a.2 depict the Bland Altman plot, while panels b.1 and b.2 display the correlation between estimated and reference values.

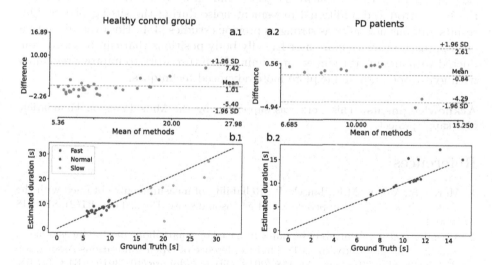

Fig. 2. Plots a.1 and a.2 show the Bland-Altman analysis while plots b.1 and b.2 show the estimated and the reference values match. The Pearson's correlation is 0.85 for the healthy control group and 0.83 for PD patients.

Table 1. Evaluation metrics of the test time measurement in seconds.

	Speed	mean	SD	median	IQR	min	max	corr	RMSE	LoA_low	LoA_high
6 Healthy	All	1.01	3.27	0.33	1.32	−2.26	16.89	0.85	3.42	−5.40	7.42
	Normal	0.37	1.30	0.31	1.54	−1.84	2.72	0.58	1.35	−2.18	2.92
	Fast	−0.61	0.85	−0.63	0.78	−2.26	0.80	0.56	1.04	−2.27	1.04
	Slow	3.08	4.59	0.81	3.35	−0.14	16.89	0.59	5.53	−5.91	12.07
12 PD	All	−0.84	1.76	−0.12	0.74	−4.94	0.56	0.83	1.95	−4.29	2.61

4   Discussion and Conclusion

This study shows how smartphones hand-held can be used to implement a TUG test. Our algorithm was developed on data collected from healthy participants and later validated with data from PD patients. Our TUG duration estimation performs well overall but may result in outliers, especially at extremely slow speeds. The TUG test's Minimal Detectable Change for Parkinson's disease is typically below 3.5 s [7] which is smaller than our limits of agreements.

Errors in the detection of the time are introduced especially in tests at very slow speed from three healthy subjects, and three tests from patients where the user introduced additional movement noise during the sitting phases. Our results are thus not quite as strong as previous studies [3, 4]. However, given that our approach provides more user-friendly body positions that can be easily conducted without supervision, we are aiming for future work to improve reliability with gyroscope data and explore more advanced techniques.

Acknowledgments. This work was supported by the Mats Paulsson Foundation, "Parkapp" project.

References

1. Morris, S., Morris, M.E., Iansek, R.: Reliability of measurements obtained with the timed "Up & Go" test in people with Parkinson disease. Phys. Ther. **81**(2), 810–818 (2001)
2. Meigal, A., et al.: Analysis of human gait based on smartphone inertial measurement unit: a feasibility study. In: 2018 22nd Conference of Open Innovations Association (FRUCT), May 2018, pp. 151–158 (2018). https://doi.org/10.23919/FRUCT.2018.8468264.
3. Madhushri, P., et al.: A smartphone application suite for assessing mobility. In: 2016 38th Annual International Conference of the IEEE Engineering in Medicine and Biology Society (EMBC), August 2016, pp. 3117–3120 (2016). https://doi.org/10.1109/EMBC.2016.7591389.
4. Chan, M.H.M., et al.: A validation study of a smartphone application for functional mobility assessment of the elderly. Hong Kong Physiother. J. **35**, 1–4 (2016). ISSN 1013-7025. https://doi.org/10.1016/j.hkpj.2015.11.001
5. Salvi, D., et al.: Mobistudy: mobile-based, platform-independent, multidimensional data collection for clinical studies. In: Proceedings of the 11th International Conference on the Internet of Things, pp. 219–222 (2021)

6. BTS Engineering: G-Walk. https://www.btsbioengineering.com/products/g-walk/. Accessed July 2023
7. Huang, S.-L., et al.: Minimal detectable change of the timed "up & go" test and the dynamic gait index in people with Parkinson disease. Phys. Ther. **91**(1), 114–121 (2011)

Developmental Evaluation of an e-Counselling and Learning Application for Parents of Children with Attention Deficit Hyperactivity Disorder

Andrea Kerschbaumer[1]([✉])[iD], Lisa-Sophie Gstöttner[1][iD], Erna Schönthaler[2][iD],
Károly Szabó[3][iD], Peter Putz[4][iD], Carina Hauser[1][iD], and Franz Werner[1][iD]

[1] Health Assisting Engineering, University of Applied Sciences Campus Vienna, 1100 Vienna,
Austria
andrea.kerschbaumer@fh-campuswien.ac.at
[2] Occupational Therapy, University of Applied Sciences Campus Vienna, 1100 Vienna, Austria
[3] Computer Science and Digital Communications, University of Applied Sciences Campus
Vienna, 1100 Vienna, Austria
[4] Competence Center Indication, University of Applied Sciences Campus Vienna, 1100 Vienna,
Austria

Abstract. Attention deficit hyperactivity disorder (ADHD) is a common mental disorder among children and adolescents. In Austria, approximately 5% of children and adolescents have ADHD, which includes 89,000 children. This paper describes our approach of developmental evaluation of a smartphone app designed to support parents of children with ADHD. We conducted usability tests and interviews involving eleven parents and four children iteratively. Although the general feedback was positive, the high number of identified optimizations highlights the importance of user testing.

Keywords: Developmental Evaluation · Application · ADHD

1 Introduction

1.1 Attention Deficit Hyperactivity Disorder

Attention deficit hyperactivity disorder (ADHD) is one of the most common mental disorders among children and adolescents [1]. With a prevalence of approximately 5% [2], approximately 89,000 children in Austria meet the diagnostic criteria for ADHD. The main symptoms are attention deficits, hyperactivity and impulsivity [3], which result in increased daily stress and dysfunction in family life [4].

Occupational therapy can make an important contribution to improving symptoms in daily life, independent of medication [5]. However, there is a lack of occupational therapy and support in the home environment in Austria. Apps could provide effective,

D. Salvi et al. (Eds.): PH 2023, LNICST 572, pp. 520–523, 2024.
https://doi.org/10.1007/978-3-031-59717-6_35

low-threshold access to professional guidance. Yet, the existing apps for ADHD are mainly aimed at assessing or treating symptoms [6].

Thus, the aim of the project is the development of an app with evidence-based occupational content and tips to support parents with ADHD-diagnosed children in everyday life.

1.2 Description of the Initial ELSA Prototype

Navigation through the interface is facilitated by a home screen, a burger menu in the right-hand corner and a bottom navigation bar. The home screen displays graphical icons for three sections: Home, School, and Leisure. When starting the application, users assess twenty everyday situations with a Likert scale (never - very often). According to the answers, an individual selection of recommendations is provided. Each tip consists of an instructional text and a video, which shows the situation and application of the tip. A lexicon gives background information. Printable templates (e.g. checklists), a list with contacts (e.g. hospitals) and an online forum for exchange are embedded. The burger menu provides sub-categories such as "profile", "statistics" "settings" and "legal notice". Users are accompanied by an avatar, which goes through five stages of evolution.

2   Methods

This developmental evaluation was conducted iteratively throughout the development of the application. Parents of children with ADHD and their children participated in the research. Ethical approval was obtained.

Parents evaluated the app on a smartphone provided under the observation of a researcher. As part of the usability tests, the participants used the think-aloud method [7].

Subsequently, they were asked questions in a semi-structured interview. In this iterative process, the findings from interviews were fed back to the development team, who adapted the app. The systematic data analysis was conducted according to the content structuring qualitative content analysis by Kuckartz [8].

3   Results

A total of eleven parents of children with ADHD and four children diagnosed with ADHD participated in the study. The results of the user feedback and the changes to the first prototype version are as follows:

Two of the initial questions required revision to make them self-explanatory. The slider to answer the questions was not recognized as such, which resulted in the addition of a short demo animation. A further problem occurred when reinstalling the app after removal from the home screen. This issue was rectified by saving the answers and taking the user directly to the home screen.

Since not all participants could clearly comprehend which tips had been selected for them, colors were introduced to mark the selected tips and headings such as "especially interesting for you" and "also interesting for you" were added. Some participants stated that the texts should stand alone. Therefore, the texts were adapted to stand-alone texts that complement the videos.

To establish comprehensible connections between the various parts of the app, terms that appear elsewhere in the app were connected via hyperlink to the lexicon. The templates were made more attractive and appealing. The prototype version merely allowed downloading all templates at the same time, which was adapted to enable the selection of templates. The contact addresses appeared as a list, which did not clearly indicate the option of selection. This was solved by using a different, more intuitive design. The options "structure of the app" and "about us" were added in the burger menu including general app information.

All participants liked the design of the avatar except for one child who preferred a more realistic avatar. Two other children wished for more than five evolution stages of the avatar and one child would enjoy a game to play within the app.

4 Discussion

The feedback during the iterative development process shows the importance of involving the target group in this ongoing process. When including users in this process their needs can be met better [7].

As expected, a few technical problems that occurred within the app had to be overcome. Some feedback showed that not all functions were obvious or self-explaining. Feedback concerning the wording stressed the importance of precise wording that is understandable to non-specialists.

In the future, the app should be accessible and meet the needs of a wide variety of users. It should be intuitive, clearly structured and easy to use. Recent literature stresses that the likelihood of siblings or parents of a child with ADHD also having ADHD in the range from 10 to 35% [9]. Therefore, the app was adapted to offer even more structure, shorter text passages and ready-made templates.

We encourage parents to adapt the tips to their needs and family life. The app is not intended to replace therapy. It shall provide low-threshold assistance for families while waiting for occupational therapy treatment or in addition to it.

5 Conclusion

This study highlights the importance of target group involvement in the development and evaluation, as this allows requirements, performance and usability issues to be captured.

Results show that every person has individual needs and ideas on how the app should look. The next step in this project is testing the final version of the app.

Acknowledgements. This work was funded by the Municipal Department of Vienna 23 for economy, labor and statistics (MA23, call number: 30-33). We would like to thank Anna Höchsmann for her assistance with data collection.

References

1. Dilling, H., Mombour, W., Schmidt, M.H., Schulte-Markwort, E.: Internationale Klassifikation psychischer Störungen: ICD-10 Kapitel V (F) Klinisch-diagnostische Leitlinien. Hogrefe, Göttingen (2018)
2. Falkai, P., et al.: Diagnostisches und statistisches Manual psychischer Störungen. Hogrefe, Göttingen (2015)
3. Paulzen, M., Habel, U., Schneider, F.: Aufmerksamkeitsdefizit-/ Hyperaktivitätsstörung (ADHS) (F90) im Erwachsenenalter. In: Schneider, F. (ed.) Klinikmanual Psychiatrie, Psychosomatik und Psychotherapie, pp. 539–551. Springer, Heidelberg (2016). https://doi.org/10.1007/978-3-642-54571-9_23
4. Kendall, J., Shelton, K.: A typology of management styles in families with children with ADHD. J. Fam. Nurs. **9**(3), 257–280 (2003)
5. Popow, C., Ohmann, S.: ADHS im Kindes- und Jugendalter. Pädiatrie Pädologie **55**, 1–22 (2020)
6. Păsărelu, C.R., Andersson, G., Dobrean, A.: Attention-deficit/hyperactivity disorder mobile apps: a systematic review. Int. J. Med. Inform. **138**, 104133 (2020)
7. Task-centered user interface design. A practical introduction. https://www.hcibib.org/tcuid/. Accessed 27 Jun 2023
8. Kuckartz, U.: Qualitative Inhaltsanalyse. Methoden, Praxis, Computerunterstützung, 4th edn. Beltz Juventa, Weinheim, Basel (2018)
9. Long version of the interdisciplinary evidence- and consensus-based (S3) guideline "Attention-Deficit/Hyperactivity Disorder (ADHD) in children, adolescents and adults" AWMF Registration No. 028-045. https://register.awmf.org/de/leitlinien/detail/028-045. Accessed 4 Jul 2023

Author Index

Printed in the United States
by Baker & Taylor Publisher Services

Printed in the United States
by Baker & Taylor Publisher Services